P9-CMV-396

3 1271 00

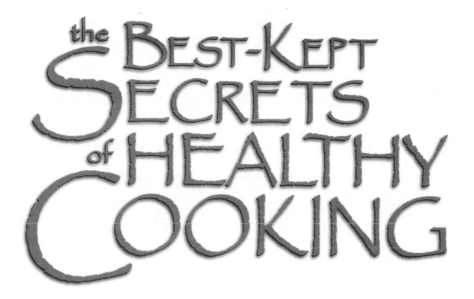

the BEST-KEPT SECRETS of HEALTHY COOKING

SANDRA WOODRUFF, RD

AVERY

a member of Penguin Putnam Inc.   *New York*

Most Avery books are available at special quantity discounts for bulk purchase for sales promotions, premiums, fund-raising, and educational needs. Special books or book excerpts also can be created to fit specific needs. For details, write Putnam Special Markets, 375 Hudson Street, New York, NY 10014.

Avery
A member of Penguin Putnam Inc.
375 Hudson Street
New York, NY 10014
www.penguinputnam.com

Library of Congress Cataloging-in-Publication
Woodruff, Sandra L.
    The best-kept secrets of healthy cooking: more than 600 kitchen-tested,
  easy-to-make, light and healthy recipes / Sandra Woodruff.
        p. cm.
    Includes index.
    ISBN 0-89529-880-5
        1. Low-fat diet—Recipes. 2. Low-calorie diet—Recipes.
    3. Nutrition. I. Title: Best-kept secrets of healthy cooking. II. Title.

RM237.7 W657 2000   99-048011
641.5′63—dc21

Printed in the United States of America

10 9 8 7 6 5 4

Front cover photograph: PhotoDisc
Back cover photograph: Victor Giordano
Cover design: Phaedra Mastrocola
Interior photographs: PhotoDisc
Typesetting: Gary A. Rosenberg
In-house editor: Joanne Abrams

Contents

*This book is dedicated to
my favorite taste testers,
Wiley, C.D., and Belle.*

Acknowledgments

I am most grateful to have had the opportunity to do work that I love, and to work with great people while doing it. It has truly been a pleasure to produce another book with the talented and dedicated professionals at Avery Publishing Group, who lend their support and creativity at every stage of production. Special thanks go to Rudy Shur and Ken Rajman for providing the opportunity to publish this book, and to my editor, Joanne Abrams, whose hard work, diligent attention to detail, and endless patience are appreciated more than I can say! I would also like to express my heartfelt gratitude to Evan Schwartz and Beth Croteau, who have been instrumental in making my books a huge success.

Thanks also go to my husband, Tom, and to my dear friends and family members for their long-term support and encouragement. And last but not least, I would like to thank all of the clients and coworkers whose many questions, ideas, and suggestions keep me learning and experimenting with new things.

Preface

As a nutritionist who has helped people improve their eating habits for well over a decade, I have witnessed first-hand the profound changes that occur when people start choosing healthier foods. I have been delighted to see a wide range of people enjoy greater success in losing and maintaining weight, dramatic drops in blood cholesterol and triglycerides, reduced blood pressure, and greatly enhanced energy levels and feelings of well-being—all as a result of improved diets.

I also know that a good cookbook can be instrumental in helping people make the dietary changes that can maximize health. Over the past six years, it has been my pleasure to write a number of cookbooks for healthy living. From the very start, my primary goal was to prove that eating healthfully can be both easy and enjoyable. Using suggestions and feedback from clients, students, friends, and family, I sought to create tantalizing user-friendly recipes that would appeal to the entire family. In each of my books, I provided detailed information on choosing and using healthful new ingredients as they entered the marketplace. And I presented guidelines that would allow readers to give their own favorite recipes a healthy makeover so that they needn't sacrifice their favorite foods in the name of nutrition.

I am now delighted to select the best recipes from each of my previous books and present them in *The Best-Kept Secrets of Healthy Cooking*, a collection of over 600 recipes designed to help you maximize taste and nutrition while controlling fat and calories. As I selected recipes from my earlier books—such as *Secrets of Fat-Free Cooking, Secrets of Fat-Free Italian Cooking, Brand Name Fat-Fighter's Cookbook, Secrets of Cooking for Long Life, Secrets of Fat-Free Baking,* and *Secrets of Fat-Free Desserts*—I updated and improved them to reflect the availability of new products or to accommodate changes in existing products. Whenever possible, I also streamlined or simplified recipes using newer and better techniques that I learned over the past few years. Recipes from my book *Fat-Free Holiday Recipes* were scaled down to serve four to six people, making them easier to enjoy all year round. In addition, like the books from which this collection was derived, *Best-Kept Secrets* includes a wealth of information on new products and healthful ingredients, as well as the most up-to-date guidelines for transforming your own favorite recipes into light and healthy classics.

Over the past several years, the science of nutrition has evolved, and while the fundamentals of good nutrition remain the same, some new thoughts have emerged on what constitutes a healthy diet. *Best-Kept Secrets* reflects these changes. The emphasis is on getting a healthy balance of fats by limiting ingredients that are high in saturated and trans fats, and instead using small amounts of healthful fats like olive oil and canola oil, as well as moderate amounts of nuts and seeds. Lean meats and low-fat dairy products are featured in many recipes, and vegetables, fruits, and whole grains are used in generous amounts. Most of the recipes in this book are compatible with a diet that gets 20 to 25 percent of its calories from fat, and is rich in fiber, vitamins, minerals, and health-promoting phytochemicals and antioxidants. In addition, sugar and salt have been kept at low to moderate levels.

I am pleased to have seen an increased focus on the health effects of dietary carbohydrates over the past few years. It is long overdue. Numerous research studies have demonstrated the tremendous health benefits that can be derived simply by choosing more *unrefined* carbohydrates and more foods with a low glycemic index, or a low potential to raise blood sugar and insulin levels. It has become abundantly clear that choosing the right carbohydrates is every bit as important in the pursuit of optimal health as is controlling fat and calories. How does *Best-Kept Secrets* fit

into this picture? Exceptionally well. Unlike the vast majority of mainstream "healthy" cookbooks that have been produced over the years, the *Secrets* series has embraced a healthy carbohydrate philosophy since its inception. For instance, entrées, soups, salads, and side dishes have always featured wholesome whole grains like brown rice, barley, bulgur wheat, and whole wheat couscous. Quick breads, muffins, pancakes, waffles, and other baked goods have always been made with ingredients like whole wheat flour, wheat bran, wheat germ, oat bran, and rolled oats. And, of course, it has always been a primary goal to reduce the amount of sugar needed in baked goods and desserts. Furthermore, many of the ingredients that are staples throughout this book—ingredients such as legumes, pasta, oats, vegetables, fruits, lean meats, and low-fat dairy products—naturally have a gentle effect on blood sugar, and fit very well into a low-glycemic index eating plan.

I am pleased to present my best, most complete collection of healthy recipes to date. It is my hope that you will find *The Best-Kept Secrets of Healthy Cooking* both a source of inspiration and a useful reference book that will enable you to create a variety of healthy and delicious meals for years to come.

Introduction

Many people believe that healthy eating means limited choices, deprivation, and extra hours spent shopping and cooking. If you have ever held this view, *The Best-Kept Secrets of Healthy Cooking* will change your mind once and for all. Here are over 600 kitchen-tested recipes for low-fat, low-calorie, high-nutrient dishes. And from Skillet Stroganoff and Greek Grilled Chicken Salad to Crispy Onion Rings and Classic Berry-Topped Cheesecake, every dish is as easy to prepare as it is absolutely delicious.

Secrets begins by presenting the simple guidelines for healthy eating upon which the recipes in this book are based. You will learn how much fat is allowable in a healthy diet, and what kinds of fat are the best choices. You will also learn the role that calories play in planning a healthful diet, and you will discover how choosing a diet rich in vegetables, fruits, legumes, and whole grains can help you obtain both an appropriate body weight and excellent health. Next, you will learn about the many healthful, readily available ingredients that will allow you to reduce fat and calories and maximize nutrition without sacrificing taste, and you will learn about the nutritional analysis that accompanies each and every recipe in this book.

Following this important information, each chapter focuses on a specific meal of the day or a specific type of dish. Looking for breakfast foods that are not only tempting enough to lure family members out of bed, but also nutritious enough to give them the energy they'll need until lunch time? Chapter 2, "Breakfast and Brunch Favorites," presents a wide selection of dishes, from Country Morning Omelette and Sausage and Potato Strata to Cinnamon-Vanilla French Toast. Or perhaps you want to serve fresh-baked breads, rolls, muffins, and biscuits that will add that special touch to family meals without wreaking havoc on your healthy lifestyle. "The Healthy Bread Basket" will lead the way with a sumptuous selection of low- and no-fat homemade goodies that are as easy to prepare as they are satisfying. Still other chapters will show you how to make palate-pleasing hot and cold finger foods like Flaky Spinach Pies, hearty sandwiches like Skinny Sloppy Joes, warming soups and stews like Golden Chicken and Dumpling Soup, refreshing salads like Tuscan Tuna and Pasta Salad, wholesome side dishes like Southwestern Roasted Sweet Potatoes, comforting pasta dishes like Fabulous Fettuccine Alfredo, hearty home-style entrées like Honey Crunch Chicken, and meatless main dishes like Spicy Lentils and Rice. And because for some of us, the meal isn't complete until we've enjoyed a taste of something sweet, the final chapter presents a tempting selection of cakes, cobblers, crisps, pies, puddings, and many other treats that will satisfy your sweet tooth without blowing your fat or sugar budgets.

Besides offering 600-plus tantalizing recipes, *Secrets* features a wealth of tips designed to guide you in creating more healthful versions of your own favorite creations. You will discover how to use smart ingredient substitutions and creative cooking techniques to trim fat and calories, and how to boost flavor with herbs, spices, and other seasonings. Perhaps the best part of this book, however, is the simplicity of the recipes. Each recipe is pre-sented in a straightforward, easy-to-follow format, and every effort has been made to keep the number of ingredients, pots, pans, and utensils to a minimum. This will save you time and make cleanup a breeze—important considerations for most people today.

It is my hope that *The Best-Kept Secrets of Healthy Cooking* will prove to you, your family, and your friends that any dish imaginable can be luscious and satisfying without being rich and fattening. So eat well and enjoy! As you will see it is possible to do both—at every meal, and on every day of the year.

1. Mastering Healthy Cooking

Who says you can't have your cake and eat it, too? If you know the secrets of healthy cooking, you can have just about anything you want—crispy Cajun chicken, creamy capellini carbonara, old-fashioned pot roast, hearty Western omelettes, sour cream apple pie, and much, much more.

For too many years, eating healthfully has meant limited choices, deprivation, and extra hours spent shopping and cooking. "If it tastes good, it must be bad for you," was the attitude that emerged. Fortunately, this is far from true. *The Best-Kept Secrets of Healthy Cooking* introduces you to a variety of innovative cooking techniques, and shows you how to use the latest fat- and calorie-saving products, as well as many traditional ingredients. The result? Healthy home-style favorites that are never bland or boring, that are simple to prepare, and that your whole family will love.

In these pages, you will find recipes for a wide variety of deliciously light dishes that are perfect for any day of the week. You will be delighted by slimmed-down versions of old favorites, as well as tempting new creations that will let you eat the foods you love without guilt. Perhaps just as important, this book will show you that, contrary to popular belief, changing to a light and healthy lifestyle does not have to be an ordeal. As you will see, the recipes in this book will save you not just fat and calories, but time and effort, too. Most of these recipes are very simple to prepare, even for beginners, and are designed to create as little mess as possible, saving you cleanup time.

This chapter will explain the basics of light and healthy eating, and will guide you in budgeting your daily fat and calorie intakes. In addition, you will learn about the best ingredients to use in your light and healthy dishes, and you will discover how to use these foods to create great-tasting surefire family favorites that will be requested again and again.

SIMPLE STEPS TO A HEALTHIER DIET

In recent years, volumes of research have proven that we have enormous power to prevent disease, slow the rate of aging, increase our energy level, and promote natural weight control simply by making smart food choices. The old saying "You are what you eat" has proven truer than anyone could have guessed. And despite headlines that are often contradictory and confusing, eating healthfully is a lot easier than most people think.

Following are some simple strategies that can help bring your diet into balance. In fact, these strategies are so simple that people often dismiss them. But don't let their simplicity fool you—they are very powerful. By implementing the following guidelines, you will automatically get more of the antioxidants, phytochemicals, vitamins, minerals, fiber, and other nutrients that your body needs, and less of the harmful fats, sugar, salt, and calories that you don't need.

❏ Eat Two to Three Servings of Protein-Rich Foods Every Day

An adequate protein intake is critical for maintaining lean body mass and muscular strength, and for keeping your immune system going strong. But many people who follow low-fat diets do not eat enough protein. The reason? In an effort to reduce fat and cholesterol, people often choose to eat less meat, or even to give it up entirely. And while it is not necessary to eat meat to get enough protein, you must substitute a protein-rich alternative like dried beans, soy foods, or eggs. Unfortunately, many people do not do this. If you are watching your weight, you should know that it is especially important to include two to three ounces of protein in each meal. Why? Protein-rich foods are the most filling of all foods, so they help stave off hunger and keep you feeling satisfied until your next meal.

Fat-fighters will be happy to know that a wide selection of ultra-lean red meats, pork, poultry, and even lunchmeats and sausages are now available. This means that you can have your protein without a counterproductive dose of saturated fat. Where does seafood fit in? Fish range from practically fat-free to moderately fatty. However, the oil in fish provides an essential kind of fat, known as omega-3 fat, that most people do not eat in sufficient quantities. Therefore, all kinds of fish—and especially the more oily ones like salmon and mackerel—are considered health-

ful, and are excellent alternatives to meat and poultry. In fact, fish should be substituted for meat at least twice a week.

Prefer not to eat meat? Plenty of protein-rich plant-based alternatives are available. And even if you are a meat-eater, these vegetarian alternatives should constitute at least half of your protein choices. Why? Plant foods are naturally low in fat and contain no cholesterol. In addition, plant foods supply the dietary fiber and health-promoting phytochemicals that meats, poultry, and seafood do not.

Some of the best and most widely available alternatives to meat are legumes—dried beans, peas, and lentils. Besides being rich in protein and nutrients, legumes are loaded with soluble fibers that both lower cholesterol and help stabilize blood sugar levels. One type of legume that is gaining popularity in this country is the soybean. Once relegated only to health food stores, a wide variety of soy products, including tofu, burgers, and ground meat alternatives, are now available at your local grocery store. The last part of this chapter provides more information on selecting these healthful meat alternatives.

❏ Eat Two to Three Servings of Calcium-Rich Foods Every Day

Everyone knows that calcium is essential for building strong bones. But calcium also helps maintain normal blood pressure, may help prevent colon cancer, and performs many other vital functions in the body. Yet most people's diets fall short of the recommended 1,000 to 1,200 milligrams per day. Why do so many people lack calcium? Many avoid calcium-rich dairy products, believing them to be high in fat and calories. While this used to be true, these days, a multitude of no- and low-fat reduced-calorie dairy products are widely available. The last part of this chapter will introduce you to these products, which can beautifully replace full-fat cheeses, sour cream, and other popular foods.

Prefer not to eat dairy products? No problem. But you must substitute other calcium-rich foods such as calcium-fortified soymilk, cheese, and yogurt. As a bonus, soy products also contain phytochemicals and nutrients that help protect against osteoporosis, cancer, and heart disease. Many green leafy vegetables—including broccoli greens, kale, and bok choy—are also loaded with calcium. And legumes and tofu can add significant amounts of calcium to the diet.

❏ Eat at Least Five Servings of Fruits and Vegetables Every Day

Fruits and vegetables offer a bounty of nutrients, fiber, and phytochemicals—all powerful preventive medicines against cancer, heart disease, and many other health problems. Since not all of the protective substances present in these foods have been identified, and some of them probably never will be, it is impossible to get all the benefits of fruits and vegetables from pills or supplements. Currently, fruits and vegetables are placed on the second tier of the USDA Food Guide Pyramid, while grains form the larger foundation. Some health professionals believe that this order should be reversed, making fruits and vegetables the core of the diet, and giving grains the secondary role.

Watching your weight? You just might benefit from including generous portions of produce in your meals. People who skip the vegetables and fruits at a mere 25 to 50 calories per cup, and pile on extra rice or pasta at 200 calories per cup—or who have an extra slice of bread at 80 to 100 calories—will probably find weight loss slower than they expect-

ed. Realize that starchy vegetables like potatoes, corn, and peas contain about the same amount of calories as rice or pasta, so be careful not to overdo portions of these veggies.

Sadly, the average American does not consume even the minimum recommended amount of vegetables and fruits. Even worse, much of the time, these foods are laden with butter, margarine, cheese sauce, or other fats. But, as the remaining chapters in this book will show, getting your five-a-day is not as hard as you may think. A medium-sized piece of fruit, a half cup of cooked or raw fruits or vegetables, a cup of leafy salad greens, a quarter cup of dried fruit, or three-fourths of a cup of fruit or vegetable juice each constitute a serving. So if you include at least one cup of fruit or vegetables at each meal, and replace snacks like pretzels, crackers, chips, and cookies with fruits and vegetables, you will easily meet or exceed the five-a-day recommendation. Finally, remember that five servings are the *minimum* recommended amount. To maximize your health, aim for eight to ten servings.

❏ Choose Whole Grains Over Refined Grains

Grain products like bread, cereal, rice, and pasta form the base of the USDA Food Guide Pyramid, with six to eleven servings recommended daily. But you should know that not all grains are created equal. To get the most from this food group, it is crucial to choose whole grain products—products such as 100-percent whole grain breads and cereals, oats, barley, brown rice, and bulgur wheat. Why? In recent years, whole grains have emerged as one of the foremost health-protective foods. In fact, several major studies have shown that people who eat whole grains are about 30 percent less likely to develop heart disease and diabetes than people who eat mostly refined grain products like white bread, white flour, white rice, and refined breakfast cereals. This should come as no surprise. Many of the nutrients that are present in whole grains—magnesium, copper, chromium, selenium, folate, vitamin E, and fiber, for instance—are essential for the protection of the cardiovascular system and the metabolism of carbohydrates. In addition, whole grains contain health-promoting phytochemicals, the benefits of which are just being recognized.

Unfortunately, most people are not reaping the benefits of whole grains. In fact, a whopping 83 percent of all grains eaten by Americans are refined! Refining strips grains of most of their fiber, vitamins, and minerals, and causes a 200- to 300-fold loss of phytochemicals. Therefore, a diet based on refined products can actually hasten the development of certain health problems. Need another reason to switch to whole grains? Fiber-rich whole grains are more filling and satisfying than their refined counterparts, and so can help prevent overeating. In contrast, a diet of low-fiber refined foods will leave you feeling constantly hungry.

When made properly, breads, muffins, casseroles, side dishes, soups, and even desserts can include wholesome whole grains. The last part of this chapter will introduce you to a variety of versatile whole grain products, and the recipes in this book will show you how to use these and other foods to create hearty and wholesome dishes in your own kitchen.

❏ Limit Your Use of Table and Cooking Fats

One of the most effective ways to trim fat and calories from your diet is to cut down on butter, oil, and other fats used in cooking and baking, as well as table fats found in products such as margarine, mayonnaise, and salad dressings. In their full-fat versions, just one tablespoon of any of these products will add about 10 grams of fat and 100 calories to your meal, so it is well worth finding ways to cut back on these products. In addition, a diet that is low in fat leaves more room for healthful foods like vegetables, fruits, and whole grains. But can you cut back on fat and still have flavor? Absolutely! For each of these foods there is now a lighter alternative that can substitute beautifully in your favorite dishes. The last part of this chapter will introduce you to many of these exciting new products, and will help you select the vegetable oils with the most healthful nutritional profiles.

❏ Eat Sugar Only in Moderation

Too much sugar has long been a problem in many people's diets. And the mind-boggling array of low-fat cookies, brownies, pastries, candies, and other goodies produced in recent years has only added to the problem. You should realize that while these products may contain little or no fat, they usually contain just as much sugar as their high-fat counterparts—and sometimes more! What health threats are posed by sugar? First and foremost, sugar contains no nutrients, and, when eaten in excess, can actually deplete your body's stores of chromium, the B vitamins, and other vitamins and minerals. Second, sugary foods are typically eaten in place of nutritious foods. Third, by overwhelming the taste buds and increasing the taste threshold for sweet flavors, diets rich in sugary foods can cause you to lose your taste for the more subtle flavors of wholesome, natural foods. Last but not least, sugary foods are usually loaded with calories, making them a real menace if you're watching your weight.

The good news is that, in moderation, sugar can be enjoyed without harm to your health. What's a moderate amount? A person who needs 2,200 calories per day to maintain his or her weight should aim for an upper limit of 48 grams of sugar per day, or about 12 teaspoons. If you need only 1,600 calories per day, your upper limit should be 24 grams, or about 6 teaspoons—the amount present in 8 ounces of sugar-sweetened soda. Unfortunately, consumption of sodas, ice cream, pastries, cookies, and other sweets has risen dramatically in the past decade. Currently, the average American diet—which includes over 30 teaspoons of sugar per day—can hardly be considered moderate.

❏ Limit Your Sodium Intake to 2,400 Milligrams Per Day

A limited sodium intake has many benefits, ranging from better-controlled blood pressure to stronger bones. But of all the guidelines for good eating, this one can be the most difficult to follow, since many lower-fat foods contain extra salt. Fortunately, with a just a little effort, even this dietary goal can be met. The most effective sodium-control strategy is to cut back on the salt used for cooking and at the table. Believe it or not, just one teaspoon of salt contains 2,300 milligrams of sodium—almost your entire daily allowance—so it pays to put the salt shaker away. You can also cut back on sodium by switching to a "light" salt, which is half sodium chloride and half potassium chloride. (Note that people with certain medical conditions should not use light salt due to its high potassium content.)

Another effective strategy is to limit your intake of high-sodium processed foods. Read labels, and choose the lower-sodium frozen meals, canned goods, broths, cheeses, and other products. Also, whenever you make a recipe that contains high-sodium cheeses, processed meats, or other salty ingredients, avoid adding any extra salt. The recipes in this book will show you how to balance high-sodium products with low-sodium ingredients, herbs, and spices to make dishes that are lower in sodium but high in flavor.

These guidelines aren't glamorous and they don't make headlines, but, as many people have discovered, they do produce results. The fact is that it is the simple things you do day in and day out that have the biggest impact on your health. You'll find that the tips provided throughout this book make it surprisingly easy to follow these steps and to build a healthful, enjoyable eating plan.

WINNING THE BATTLE OF THE BULGE

What's the number-one reason people seek to make dietary changes? Better weight control. And with over half of all Americans now fitting into the overweight category, this problem is getting a lot of attention. Unfortunately, this is also an area that is fraught with misinformation, fad diets, and quick fixes. But if you look at the primary causes of obesity today, it's easy to see why quick fix diets don't offer permanent success.

Over the past few decades, our environment has changed dramatically. We now have labor-saving devices that do much of the work we used to do ourselves. Many people also have sedentary jobs, and then go home at night and sit in front of a television or a computer. To make matters worse, the vast majority of Americans do not engage in regular exercise. The bottom line is that people just don't burn as many calories as they used to.

At the same time, portion sizes have grown dramatically—just compare the size of the average muffin or bagel today with that of two decades ago!—and we are constantly being bombarded with advertisements that encourage us to eat. The fact is that, on average, people eat 200 to 300 calories more per day than they did twenty years ago. And when you eat more calories than you burn, the excess gets stored as fat.

How can you bring your lifestyle back into balance? First, be aware of portion sizes. The simple consumption of too much food may well be the number-one dietary problem in America. Watching your fat intake is another important strategy for controlling calories, since fat contains more than twice the calories of carbohydrate or protein. And, of course, increasing your daily activity level is a must for permanent weight control.

Following the Simple Steps to a Healthier Diet listed above will go a long way toward helping you maintain calorie control, because an eating plan based on these strategies is low in fat and sugar and high in foods that are filling and satisfying. For many people, these guidelines alone will promote natural weight control because they will get full before they overeat. However, everyone should have a sense of how many calories they need to maintain a healthy weight, and how much fat is reasonable in a healthy eating plan. The following table presents daily calorie budgets based on a variety of body weights. (If you are overweight, go by the weight you would like to be.) These budgets are based on the fact that most people need about 13 to 15 calories per pound to maintain their weight. Of course, some people will need more or less calories than the table states, depending on their activity level and metabolic rate.

The following table also shows two recommended daily fat-gram budgets to go along with each range of calorie intakes. Most health experts recommend that fat constitute

no more than 30 percent of your daily calorie intake. In fact, 20 to 25 percent would be better in most cases. Realize, though, that you do need some fat for good health, so it is neither necessary nor healthy to eliminate all of the fat from your diet. The inset "Getting a Smart Balance of Fats," found on page 10, will help you spend your fat budget wisely so that you can get the essential fats you need, while avoiding the harmful fats that you don't need.

Keep in mind that although you shouldn't become obsessed with counting calories or fat grams, this "budget" can help you make wise decisions when purchasing and preparing foods. And realize that small changes, practiced consistently, can make a big difference. For instance, simply trimming 100 calories from your daily diet can produce a ten-pound weight loss over the course of a year. If you are unable to get your weight under control on your own, seek the help of a health professional such as a registered or licensed dietitian who specializes in weight control. She or he can help you set some realistic weight-management goals, fine-tune a healthful eating plan, and recommend exercise and behavior strategies that will meet your individual needs.

ABOUT THE INGREDIENTS

Never before has it been so easy to eat healthfully. Light and healthy alternatives are available for just about any ingredient you can think of. This makes it possible to create a dazzling array of healthful and delicious foods, including dramatically slimmed-down versions of many of your favorite dishes. In the pages that follow, we'll take a look at the low-fat dairy products, spreads and dressings, eggs and egg substitutes, ultra-lean meats, and many other ingredients that will insure success in all your healthy cooking adventures.

RECOMMENDED DAILY CALORIE AND FAT INTAKES

Weight (pounds)	Recommended Daily Calorie Intake (13–15 calories per pound)	Daily Fat Gram Intake (20% of calorie intake)	Daily Fat Gram Intake (25% of calorie intake)
100	1,300–1,500	29–33	36–42
110	1,430–1,650	32–37	40–46
120	1,560–1,800	34–40	43–50
130	1,690–1,950	38–43	47–54
140	1,820–2,100	40–46	51–58
150	1,950–2,250	43–50	54–62
160	2,080–2,400	46–53	58–67
170	2,210–2,550	49–57	61–71
180	2,340–2,700	52–60	65–75
190	2,470–2,850	55–63	69–79
200	2,600–3,000	58–66	72–83

Low-Fat and Nonfat Cheeses

Cheese is an excellent source of calcium and high-quality protein. Unfortunately, these nutrients often come packaged with a large dose of artery-clogging saturated fat. But take heart, as an amazing array of low-fat and nonfat products are now also available, making it possible to have your cheese and eat it, too. Let's learn about some of the cheeses that you'll be using in your light and healthy recipes.

Cottage Cheese. Although often thought of as a "diet food," full-fat cottage cheese has 5 grams of fat per 4-ounce serving, making it far from diet fare. Instead, choose nonfat or low-fat cottage cheese. When puréed until smooth, these versatile products make a great base for dips, spreads, and salad dressings. Cottage cheese also adds richness and body to casseroles, quiches, cheesecakes, and many other recipes. Select brands with 1 percent or less milk fat, such as Breakstone's Free and Light n' Lively. Most brands of cottage cheese are quite high in sodium, with about 400 milligrams per half cup, so it is best to avoid adding salt whenever this cheese is a recipe ingredient. As an alternative, use unsalted cottage cheese, which is available in some stores.

Another option when buying cottage cheese is dry curd cottage cheese. This nonfat version is made without the "dressing" or creaming mixture. Minus the dressing, cottage cheese has a drier consistency; hence its name, dry curd. Unlike most cottage cheese, dry curd is low in sodium. Dry curd cottage cheese can be substituted cup-for-cup for nonfat or low-fat cottage cheese in your favorite recipes. (In some cases, you might need to add a tablespoon or two of milk to the recipe to compensate for the drier consistency.) Look for brands like Breakstone's Dry Curd.

Getting a Smart Balance of Fats

While limiting your fat intake is an important strategy for better weight control, the type of fat you eat is equally important to your pursuit of optimal health. Why? Certain kinds of fats are harmful and should be avoided, while others are actually necessary for life. Here are the basics of what you should know about choosing fats.

Saturated Fat

Best known for its role in promoting heart disease, saturated fat raises blood cholesterol levels, thus contributing to clogged arteries. The vast majority of saturated fat in most people's diets comes from high-fat meat and dairy products, so simply switching to low- and no-fat alternatives can go a long way towards reducing your intake of this harmful substance. Coconuts and tropical oils such as palm kernel oil also contain saturated fats, and should be limited as well.

A similar kind of fat that you should be aware of is hydrogenated fat. This is a chemically altered fat that is produced by adding hydrogen to liquid vegetable oils. This process, called hydrogenation, transforms the liquid vegetable oils into solid margarines and shortenings. While hydrogenation improves the cooking and baking qualities of oils, and extends their shelf life as well, it also makes the oils more saturated and creates undesirable by-products known as trans-fatty acids, or trans fats. And trans fats act much like saturated fats to raise levels of LDL, or "bad" cholesterol, and at the same time lower levels of HDL, or "good" cholesterol. The best way to trim your intake of trans fats is to avoid hard margarines as well as baked goods, snack foods, and other products that contain hydrogenated vegetable oils.

Monounsaturated Fat

Monounsaturated fats—found in olive oil, canola oil, avocados, and some nuts—are the fats of choice these days. Unlike saturated and hydrogenated fats, monounsaturated fats do not promote heart disease. In fact, in Mediterranean countries where olive oil is used liberally, the incidence of heart disease is much lower than it is in countries like the United States. Keep in mind, though, that olive oil is just one component of the Mediterranean diet. This style of eating also includes generous amounts of fish, fruits, vegetables, legumes, and garlic, and contains less sugar, red meat, and processed foods than Western diets. It is

Cream Cheese. This product adds creamy richness to dips, spreads, sauces, fillings, frostings, and many other dishes, but with 10 grams of fat per ounce, this popular spread can blow your fat budget in a hurry. Just one block of full-fat cream cheese contains 80 grams of fat—the equivalent of a stick of butter! But don't fear, as there are many lower-fat alternatives. Neufchâtel cheese, with 6 grams of fat per ounce, was once the only lower-fat alternative available. However, these days, a variety of light brands with 3 to 5 grams of fat per ounce are also widely sold in grocery stores. Better still are the many brands of non-fat cream cheese that can also be found in the dairy case. Look for brands like Philadelphia Free, and be sure to use the block-style cheese for best results in all your recipes.

Feta Cheese. With 6 grams of fat per ounce,

the total Mediterranean diet—not just the olive oil—that is responsible for protection against heart disease. Realize, too, that like all fats, monounsaturated fats are a concentrated source of calories.

Polyunsaturated Fat

Some of the most exciting research in recent years centers on polyunsaturated fats—especially on two classes of essential fatty acids known as omega-6 and omega-3 fats. Why are these fats attracting so much attention? Omega-6 and omega-3 fats have very powerful—and very different—effects in the body. For instance, omega-6 fat promotes blood clotting, while omega-3 fat inhibits clot formation. Omega-6 fat acts to raise blood pressure, while omega-3 fat helps to lower blood pressure. Because of their powerful and opposing effects, the balance of these essential fats in your diet can greatly affect your susceptibility to a variety of disorders.

Researchers believe that humans evolved on a diet that provided about equal amounts of these two fats. But over time—and especially during the twentieth century—our diets changed dramatically. First, technology made it possible to mass-produce vegetable oils, and our food supply became inundated with polyunsaturated vegetable oils that are concentrated sources of omega-6 fat, and practically devoid of omega-3 fat. Then, farmers began feeding livestock grains, which made the animals fatter as well as higher in saturated and omega-6 fats. To make matters worse, manufacturers began using omega-6-rich oils as the main ingredient in foods like mayonnaise, margarine, and salad dressings. As a result, the ratio of omega-6 to omega-3 fat in the diet rose from about 1 to 1 to as high as 20 to 1, creating an imbalance that alters body chemistry to favor the development of heart disease, cancer, inflammatory and autoimmune disorders, and many other health problems.

Fortunately, it is a simple matter to bring your intake of these two fats into balance. How? Eat fish at least twice a week, since fish is a rich source of especially potent omega-3 fatty acids. Also include generous amounts of green plant foods in your diet, as they, too, supply omega-3 fats. For most of your cooking needs, choose oils like canola, olive, walnut, and soybean, which have a healthier balance of omega-6 to omega-3 fats than do oils like safflower, sunflower, and corn. When purchasing products like mayonnaise and salad dressings, choose lower-fat versions, and read the label to see which oils they contain. Finally, try using omega-3-rich flaxseeds (page 23) in baking, or sprinkle some over your cereal. These simple strategies will help you consume both a healthy amount and a healthy balance of fats.

this semi-soft cheese has about a third less fat than most other kinds of cheese, and is considered moderately high in fat. However, a little bit goes a long way, so used moderately in recipes that contain little or no other fats, this product can be enjoyed without blowing your fat budget. An even better choice, though, is a reduced-fat brand like Athenos reduced-fat feta cheese. With 4 grams of fat per ounce, this product is now widely available in grocery stores. Nonfat feta is also available in some grocery stores.

Firm and Hard Cheeses. Both low-fat and nonfat cheeses of many types—including Cheddar, Monterey jack, mozzarella, provolone, and Swiss—are widely available in grocery stores. Reduced-fat cheeses generally have 3 to 6 grams of fat and 60 to 80 calories per ounce, while nonfat cheeses contain about

40 calories per ounce and no fat at all. Compare this with whole milk varieties, which contain 9 to 10 grams of fat and 100 to 110 calories per ounce, and you'll realize your savings. Look for brands like Alpine Lace, Borden Low-Fat, Cabot Light, Cracker Barrel Reduced-Fat, Healthy Choice, Jarlsberg Lite Swiss, Kraft Reduced-Fat and Kraft Free, Lifetime, Sargento Light, Sorrento Low-Fat, Polly-O Light, Smart Beat, and Weight Watchers.

Parmesan Cheese. Parmesan typically contains 8 grams of fat and 400 milligrams of sodium per ounce. As with most cheeses, reduced-fat and nonfat versions—brands such as Kraft Free and Weight Watchers—are available. A little bit of this flavorful cheese goes a long way, so used moderately in recipes that call for few or no other high-fat ingredients, even the "real thing" will not blow your fat budget. Some of the recipes in this book specifically call for nonfat Parmesan, some call for regular Parmesan, and still others give you a choice. Why? Nonfat Parmesan works beautifully in sauces and creamy soups, where it adds thickness and body. It also works well in casseroles and recipes like lasagna. However, it is too dry to be used as a topping for casseroles and other dishes. In these instances, a few tablespoons of regular Parmesan will produce the best results.

If you are following a white sauce or cream soup recipe that calls for nonfat Parmesan cheese, and all you have on hand is the regular product, simply add $1/2$ teaspoon of cornstarch for each tablespoon of Parmesan being used. Stir the cornstarch into the Parmesan before adding it to the recipe, and your sauce or soup will both be flavorful and have body.

Process Cheese. Typically sold in one- or two-pound blocks, as well as in preshredded and sliced forms, this cheese is designed to melt smoothly, and so is a good choice for use in macaroni and cheese, cheese sauces, and similar dishes. Most grocery stores sell brands like Velveeta Light. Process cheeses tend to be quite high in sodium and artificial ingredients, but you can avoid a sodium overload when using these cheeses by leaving out the salt and avoiding the use of other high-sodium ingredients in your recipe. As for artificial ingredients, you can avoid these by choosing a brand like Lifetime, which contains none.

Ricotta Cheese. Ricotta is a mild, slightly sweet, creamy cheese that may be used in dips, spreads, and traditional Italian dishes like lasagna. As the name implies, nonfat ricotta contains no fat at all. Low-fat and light ricottas, on the other hand, have 1 to 3 grams of fat per ounce, while whole milk ricotta has 4 grams of fat per ounce. Look for brands like Frigo Fat-Free, Polly-O Free, Maggio Nonfat, and Sorrento Fat-Free. Many stores and regional dairies offer their own nonfat and low-fat brands, as well.

Soft Curd Farmer Cheese. Blended until smooth, this soft, slightly crumbly white cheese makes a good low-fat substitute for cream cheese. Brands made with skim milk have about 3 grams of fat per ounce compared with cream cheese's 10 grams. Nonfat brands are also available in some grocery stores and specialty shops. Soft curd farmer cheese may be used in dips, spreads, fillings, frostings, and many other recipes. Some brands are made with whole milk, so read the label before you buy. Look for a brand like Friendship farmer cheese.

Yogurt Cheese. A good substitute for cream cheese in dips, spreads, and cheesecakes, yogurt cheese can be made at home with any brand of plain or flavored yogurt that does not contain gelatin or vegetable thickeners such as carrageenan or guar gum. Simply place the yogurt in a funnel lined with cheesecloth or a coffee filter, and let it drain into a jar in the refrigerator for eight hours or overnight. When the yogurt is reduced by half, it is ready to use. The whey that collects in the jar may be used in place of the liquid in breads and other baked goods.

Nondairy Cheese Alternatives. If you choose to avoid dairy products because of a lactose intolerance or for another reason, you'll be glad to know that low-fat cheeses made from soymilk, almond milk, and Brazil nut milk are now available in a variety of flavors. Look for brands like Almondrella, Veganrella, Tofurella, Soy Kaas, and Nu Tofu. Be aware that some nondairy cheeses do contain casein, a milk protein that you may want to avoid.

Other Low-Fat and Nonfat Dairy Products

Of course, cheese isn't the only dairy product you use in your everyday cooking. How about the sour cream in dips, casseroles, and sauces, and the buttermilk in your favorite cornbread? Fortunately, there are low-fat and nonfat versions of these and other dairy products as well.

Buttermilk. An essential ingredient in the low-fat kitchen, buttermilk adds a rich flavor and texture to all kinds of breads and baked goods, and lends a "cheesy" taste to sauces, dressings, frozen desserts, and many other recipes. But isn't buttermilk high in fat? Contrary to what its name implies, most buttermilk is quite low in fat. Originally a by-product of butter making, buttermilk should perhaps be called "butterless" milk. Low-fat brands of buttermilk are widely available in grocery stores, and many stores offer nonfat brands, as well. Choose these for your low-fat cooking needs.

The flavor and texture of real buttermilk works best in the recipes in this book, but if you do not have buttermilk on hand, you can make a substitute by mixing equal parts of plain nonfat yogurt and skim or low-fat milk. Alternatively, place a tablespoon of vinegar or lemon juice in a one-cup measure, and fill to the one-cup mark with skim or low-fat milk. Let the mixture sit for five minutes before using.

Evaporated Skim Milk. This ingredient can be substituted for cream in sauces, gravies, quiches, puddings, and many other dishes. Not only do you save 620 calories and 88 grams of fat for each cup of evaporated skim milk you substitute for cream, but you add extra calcium, protein, potassium, and other nutrients to your recipe. If you don't have any evaporated skim milk on hand, you can make a substitute by mixing $1/3$ cup of instant nonfat dry milk powder with $7/8$ cup of skim or low-fat milk. This will yield one cup.

Milk. One gallon of whole milk contains 130 grams of fat—the equivalent of about $1^1/_2$ sticks of butter! And while you may not drink a gallon at one sitting, the fat you consume from milk can really add up over time. What are the best milk choices? Choose nonfat (skim) milk for the very least fat. Next in line is 1% low-fat milk with about 2.5 grams ($1/_2$ teaspoon) of fat per cup. What about 2-percent milk? By legal definition, a low-fat product can have no more than 3 grams of fat per serving. With 5 grams of fat per cup, 2-percent milk is not low-fat. People who cannot tolerate milk sugar (lactose) will be glad to know that most supermarkets stock Lactaid milk in a nonfat version. Nonfat Lactaid milk may be used in place of milk in any recipe.

Nonfat Dry Milk. Like evaporated skim milk, this product adds creamy richness, as well as important nutrients, to quiches, cream soups, sauces, custards, puddings, and many other dishes. Try adding 1 to 2 tablespoons of nonfat dry milk powder to each cup of skim or low-fat milk used for drinking or cooking. To replace one cup of cream in a favorite recipe, try mixing $1/3$ cup of nonfat dry milk powder with $7/8$ cup of skim or low-fat milk. Or add a few tablespoons of this ingredient to low-fat baked goods to enhance flavor and promote browning. For best results, always use instant nonfat dry milk powder, as this product will not clump.

Sour Cream. As calorie- and fat-conscious people know, full-fat sour cream contains 48 grams of fat and almost 500 calories per cup! Use nonfat sour cream, though, and you'll eliminate at least half of the calories and all of the fat. Light sour cream, with half the fat of regular sour cream, is another good option. Made from cultured nonfat or low-fat milk thickened with vegetable gums, these products beautifully replace their fatty counterpart in dips, spreads, sauces, and many other dishes. Look for brands like Breakstone's Free, Friendship Light, Land O Lakes nonfat and light, and Naturally Yours fat-free.

Yogurt. Yogurt adds creamy richness and flavor to sauces, baked goods, and casseroles. And, of course, it is a perfect base for many dips and dressings. Be aware, though, that yogurt will curdle if added to hot sauces or gravies. To prevent this, first let the yogurt warm to room temperature. Then stir 1 tablespoon of cornstarch or 2 tablespoons of unbleached flour into the yogurt for every cup of yogurt being used. You will then be able to add this tasty ingredient to your dish without fear of separation. In your low-fat cooking,

select brands of yogurt with 1 percent or less milkfat.

Fat-Free and Low-Fat Spreads and Dressings

Like dairy products, spreads and dressings have long been a major source of fat and calories in many people's diets. Happily, many lighter alternatives to our high-fat favorites are now available. Let's learn a little more about these fat-saving products.

Butter and Margarine. Which is better, butter or margarine? Neither should have a prominent place in your diet. Butter is a concentrated source of artery-clogging saturated fat, while margarine usually contains harmful trans fats. In addition, both are pure fat and loaded with calories. If you are used to spreading foods with butter or margarine, you can easily reduce your dietary fat by switching to a nonfat or reduced-fat spread, and using it sparingly. Every tablespoon of nonfat margarine that you substitute for regular margarine or butter will save you 11 grams of fat and 85 to 95 calories. Replacing regular butter or margarine with a reduced-fat version will save about 4 to 7 grams of fat and 40 to 70 calories per tablespoon.

Although you cannot sauté with nonfat or low-fat spreads, you can use these products for many of your other cooking needs. For instance, most brands melt well enough to toss with steamed vegetables or rice dishes when you want added moisture and flavor. In many cases, you can also bake with light butter and reduced-fat margarine. Simply replace the desired amount of full-fat butter or margarine with three-fourths as much of a light brand. For baking, select a light spread that contains 5 to 6 grams of fat per tablespoon, as brands with less fat generally do not perform

Cooking With Nonfat and Low-Fat Firm and Hard Cheeses

If you have been cooking with nonfat cheeses for a while, you may have noticed that some brands do not melt as well as their full-fat counterparts. So what do you do when you want to prepare a cheese sauce, a cheese soup, or another smooth and creamy dish? One option is to use a finely shredded brand of nonfat cheese. Often referred to on the package label as "fancy" shredded cheese, these products melt better than coarsely shredded brands—although they still may not melt completely. Or use a process nonfat cheese. Process cheeses are specially made to melt, so they will work in any sauce recipe. What about reduced-fat cheeses? Most brands melt nicely and can be substituted for full-fat brands in any sauce recipe, with very little difference in taste or texture.

What's your best choice for casseroles, lasagna, and pizza? Both nonfat and low-fat brands can be used, although low-fat and reduced-fat brands have more "stretch" as a pizza topping. As for topping salads, tacos, or a bowl of chili or black bean soup, any of the nonfat or low-fat shredded brands work nicely. Only your waistline will know the difference.

well for this use. Finally, to help insure that your diet provides a healthy balance of essential fatty acids, choose spreads that list liquid canola or liquid soybean oil as the first ingredient. (See the inset "Getting a Smart Balance of Fats" on page 10 for information on essential fatty acids.)

Butter-Flavored Sprinkles. Made mostly of cornstarch with natural butter flavor, these products add buttery flavor—but no fat—to foods. Look for brands like Butter Buds and Molly McButter, which are packaged in handy shaker containers for sprinkling onto moist foods like baked potatoes and steamed vegetables. The Butter Buds product that comes in packets can be mixed with water to make a pourable butter substitute.

Mayonnaise. Nonfat and reduced-fat mayonnaise is highly recommended over regular mayonnaise, which provides about 11 grams of fat and 100 calories per tablespoon. How can mayonnaise be made without all that oil? Manufacturers use more water and vegetable

thickeners to create creamy spreads that can replace the full-fat versions in all of your favorite recipes. Look for brands like Hellmann's Low-Fat, Kraft Free, Miracle Whip Free, Smart Beat, and Weight Watchers.

Salad Dressings. Available in a wide variety of flavors, from creamy ranch and honey Dijon to balsamic and raspberry vinaigrettes, fat-free dressings contain either no oil or so little oil that they have less than 0.5 gram of fat per 2-tablespoon serving. Low-fat dressings contain no more than 3 grams of fat per serving, while light dressings contain half the fat of the traditional product. Compare these lighter dressings with their full-fat counterparts, which provide 12 to 18 grams of fat per 2-tablespoon serving, and your savings are clear.

Use these lighter products to dress your favorite salads or as a delicious basting sauce for grilled foods. Beware, though—many light dressings are quite high in sodium, so compare brands and flavors, and choose those that are on the lower end of the sodium range.

Another option is to dress your salads with flavored vinegars. Try raspberry, rice, balsamic, herb, and red wine vinegars. And keep in mind that most vinegars are salt-free as well as fat-free.

Oils

Like butter and margarine, oils used in cooking, baking, and salad dressings can blow your fat budget in a hurry. Many people are confused about oils because liquid vegetable oils have long been promoted as being "heart healthy." The reason? These oils are low in artery-clogging saturated fat, and contain no cholesterol. Unfortunately, many people also assume that these products are low in total fat and calories, and therefore may be used liberally. Not so. The fact is that *all* oils are pure fat. Just one tablespoon of any oil has 13.6 grams of fat and 120 calories. However, for those times when you do need a little oil for cooking, be aware that some oils are more useful than others in light and healthy cooking. Here are a few products that you should know about.

Canola Oil. Low in saturated fats and rich in monounsaturated fats, canola oil also contains alpha-linolenic acid, an essential omega-3 fat that is deficient in most people's diets. For these reasons, canola oil should be one of your primary cooking oils. Canola oil has a very mild, bland taste, so it is a good all-purpose oil for cooking and baking when you want no interfering flavors.

Extra Virgin Olive Oil. Along with canola oil, olive oil should be one of your primary cooking oils. Rich in monounsaturated fat, olive oil also contains phytochemicals that may help lower blood cholesterol levels and protect against cancer. Unlike most vegetable oils, which are very bland, olive oil adds its own

delicious flavor to foods. Extra virgin olive oil is the least processed and most flavorful type of olive oil. And a little bit goes a long way, making this product a good choice for use in low-fat recipes. What about "light" olive oil? In this case, light refers to flavor, which is mild and bland compared with that of other olive oils. This means that you have to use more oil for the same amount of flavor—not a good bargain.

Macadamia Nut Oil. This oil has a delicious, light macadamia nut flavor, making it especially complementary to fish, chicken, vegetables, baked goods, and salads. Its high smoking point also makes macadamia nut oil ideal for stir-frying and sautéing. Like olive oil, macadamia nut oil is highly monounsaturated. Look for macadamia nut oil in health food and specialty stores.

Sesame Oil. Sesame oil has a rich, nutty flavor that enhances the flavors of many foods. And when used in small amounts, this ingredient will add a distinctive taste to recipes without blowing your fat budget. Use toasted (dark) sesame oil for the most flavor.

Soybean Oil. Most cooking oils that are simply labelled "vegetable oil" are made from soybean oil. Soybean oil is also used as an ingredient in many brands of margarine, mayonnaise, and salad dressing. This oil supplies a fair amount of omega-3 fat, though not as much as canola and walnut oils do. Like canola oil, soybean oil has a bland flavor that works well when you want to avoid adding any interfering flavors to your dish.

Walnut Oil. With a delicate nutty flavor, walnut oil is an excellent choice for baking, cooking, and salad making. Most grocery stores sell as least one brand of walnut oil such as Lorvia California Walnut Oil. Like canola oil, walnut oil contains a substantial amount of omega-3 fats. Most brands of walnut oil have been only minimally processed and can turn rancid quickly, so once opened, they should be refrigerated.

Nonstick Vegetable Oil Cooking Spray. Available unflavored and in butter, olive oil, and garlic flavors, these products are pure fat. The advantage to using them is that the amount that comes out during a one-second spray is so small that it adds an insignificant amount of fat to a recipe. Nonstick cooking sprays are very useful to the low-fat cook, as they promote the browning of foods and prevent foods from sticking to pots and pans.

Eggs and Egg Substitutes

From hearty breakfast omelettes to quiches, casseroles, and puddings, eggs are star ingredients in many foods. Most people know that eggs are also loaded with cholesterol. In fact, just one large egg uses up two-thirds of your daily cholesterol budget. One egg also contains about 5 grams of fat. This may not seem like all that much until you consider that a three-egg omelette contains 15 grams of fat—and that's *without* the cheese filling or the butter used in the skillet! The good news is that it is a simple matter to make dishes with more whites—which are fat- and cholesterol-free—and fewer yolks. Or you can use a fat-free egg substitute, and enjoy your favorite egg dishes with absolutely no fat or cholesterol at all.

Just what are egg substitutes? Contrary to what the term "substitute" implies, these products are 99 percent pure egg whites. The remaining 1 percent consists of vegetable thickeners, vitamins and minerals, and yellow coloring—usually beta-carotene or the plant-based coloring agents anatto or turmeric. You will find egg substitutes in both the refrigerat-ed foods section and the freezer case of your grocery store. When selecting an egg substitute, look for fat-free brands like Egg Beaters, Better'n Eggs, and Scramblers. Many stores also have their own brand of fat-free egg substitute. Beware, though, as some brands contain vegetable oil, and so have almost as much fat as the eggs you are replacing.

You may wonder why some of the recipes in this book call for egg whites or a combination of whole eggs and egg whites, while others call for egg substitute. In some cases, one ingredient does, in fact, work better than the other. For instance, because they have been pasteurized (heat treated), egg substitutes are safe to use uncooked in eggnogs and salad dressings. On the other hand, when recipes require whipped egg whites, egg substitutes do not work. And because egg substitute looks just like whole eggs when cooked, you may prefer to use egg substitute or a combination of whole eggs and egg whites when making omelettes, frittatas, quiches, and custards.

In most recipes, egg whites and egg substitutes can be used interchangeably. When replacing egg whites with egg substitutes, or whole eggs with egg whites or egg substitutes, use the following guidelines:

1 large egg = 1½ large egg whites
1 large egg = 3 tablespoons egg substitute
1 large egg white = 2 tablespoons egg substitute

Realize, too, that most people can eat four egg yolks a week and still stay within the bounds of a healthy diet. So if you want to occasionally eat whole eggs or use them in recipes, feel free to do so within the context of these guidelines. Some manufacturers are now feeding hens a diet that is enriched with vitamin E and ingredients like flaxseeds, marine algae, and fish meal. This produces eggs that are nutritionally superior to regular eggs because the yolks are higher in vitamin E and omega-3 fatty acids. Look for brands like Gold Circle Farms, Pilgrims Pride Eggs Plus, and Eggland's Best in health food and grocery stores.

Ultra-Lean Poultry, Meat, and Vegetarian Alternatives

Because of the high fat and cholesterol contents of meats, many people have sharply reduced their consumption of meat, have limited themselves to white meat chicken or turkey, or have totally eliminated meat and poultry from their diets. Happily, whether you are a sworn meat eater, someone who only occasionally eats meat dishes, or a confirmed vegetarian, plenty of lean meats, lean poultry, and excellent meat substitutes are now available. Here are some suggestions for choosing the leanest possible poultry and meat.

Turkey

Once relegated only to Thanksgiving dinner, turkey is now a big seller all year round. Of course, skinless turkey breast is the leanest cut available, with just 119 calories and 1 gram of fat per 3-ounce serving. Below, you will learn about the turkey breast cuts that you're likely to find at your local supermarket.

Turkey Cutlets. Turkey cutlets, which are slices of fresh turkey breast, are usually about $1/4$ inch thick and weigh about 2 to 3 ounces each. These cutlets may be used as a delicious ultra-lean alternative to boneless chicken breast, pork tenderloin slices, or veal.

Turkey Medallions. Sliced from turkey tenderloins, medallions are about 1 inch thick and weigh about 2 to 3 ounces each. Turkey medallions can be substituted for pork or veal medallions.

Turkey Steaks. Cut from the turkey breast, these steaks are about $1/2$ to 1 inch in thickness. Turkey steaks may be baked, broiled, grilled, cut into stir-fry pieces or kabobs, or ground for burgers.

Turkey Tenderloins. Large sections of fresh turkey breast, tenderloins usually weigh about 8 ounces each. Tenderloins may be sliced into cutlets or medallions, cut into stir-fry or kabob pieces, ground for burgers, or grilled or roasted as is.

Whole Turkey Breasts. Perfect for people who love roast turkey but want only the breast meat, turkey breasts weigh 4 to 8 pounds each. These breasts may be roasted with or without stuffing.

Ground Turkey. Ground turkey is an excellent ingredient for use in meatballs, chili, burgers—in any dish that uses ground meat. When shopping for ground turkey, you'll find that different products have different percentages of fat. Some are simply labelled "ground turkey," and bear no Nutrition Facts label. These products are often made with added skin and fat, and are usually about 15 percent fat by weight—which is more than twice the amount of fat found in some kinds of lean ground beef. At the other end of the spectrum is ground turkey breast, which is only 1 percent fat by weight, and is the leanest ground meat you can buy. However, many people find this product too dry and tough for their taste. A good compromise is a mixture that is labelled somewhere between 93- and 96-percent lean. Or look for a product that is labelled "ground turkey meat," as this should contain no added skin.

Chicken

Although not as low in fat as turkey, chicken is still lower in fat than most cuts of beef and pork, and therefore is a valuable ingredient in light and healthy cooking. Beware, though. If eaten with the skin on, many cuts of chicken contain more fat than some cuts of beef and pork. For the least amount of fat, choose the chicken breast, and always remove the skin—preferably, before cooking.

Where does ground chicken fit in? Like ground turkey, ground chicken often contains skin and fat. In fact, most brands contain at least 15 percent fat by weight, so read the labels before you buy.

Beef and Pork

Although not as lean as turkey, beef and pork are both considerably leaner today than in decades past. Spurred by competition from the poultry industry, beef and pork producers have changed breeding and feeding practices to reduce the fat content of these products. In addition, butchers are now trimming away more of the fat from retail cuts of meat. The result? On average, grocery store cuts of beef are 27 percent leaner today than they were in the early 1980s, and retail cuts of pork are 43 percent leaner.

Of course, some cuts of beef and pork are leaner than others. Which are the smartest choices? The following table will guide you in selecting those cuts that are lowest in fat. Also be aware that some manufacturers, such as Maverick Ranch NaturaLite beef and Smithfield Lean Generation pork, are now offering cuts of meat that are even leaner than the ones listed in this table. Look for these in your local grocery store.

While identifying the lowest-fat cuts of meat is an important first step in healthy

THE LEANEST BEEF AND PORK CUTS

Cut (3-ounce cooked portion)	Calories	Fat
Beef		
Eye of Round	143	4.2 g
Top Round	153	4.2 g
Round Tip	157	5.9 g
Top Sirloin	165	6.1 g
Pork		
Tenderloin	139	4.1 g
Ham (95% lean)	112	4.3 g
Boneless Sirloin Chops	164	5.7 g
Boneless Loin Roast	165	6.1 g
Boneless Loin Chops	173	6.6 g

cooking, be aware that even lean cuts have varying amounts of fat because of differences in grades. In general, the higher and more expensive grades of meat, like USDA Prime and Choice, have more fat due to a higher degree of marbling—internal fat that cannot be trimmed away. USDA Select meats have the least amount of marbling, and therefore the lowest amount of fat. How important are these differences? A USDA Choice piece of meat may have 15 to 20 percent more fat than a USDA Select cut, and USDA Prime may have even more fat. Clearly, the difference is significant. So when choosing beef and pork for your table, by all means check the package for grade. Then look for the least amount of marbling in the cut you have chosen, and let appearance be your final guide.

Ground Beef. If you are not fond of ground turkey as a hamburger substitute, you will be happy to learn that lean mixtures of ground beef are now widely available, giving you another choice. Always check the label before you buy ground beef, because—like ground turkey—this product varies greatly in its fat and calorie content. At its worst, ground beef is almost one-third pure fat. But grocery stores also commonly sell ground beef that is 93- to 96-percent lean. As an alternative to ready-made ground beef, you can select a piece of top round, and ask the butcher to trim off the fat and grind the remaining meat. The resulting product will be about 95-percent lean.

How different is the leaner ground beef from the more commonly sold product? Beef that is 95-percent lean contains 4.9 grams of fat and 132 calories per 3-ounce cooked serving. Compare this with regular ground beef, which is 73-percent lean and has 17.9 grams of fat and 248 calories per serving, and your savings are clear.

Lean Processed Meats

Because of our new health-consciousness, low-fat bacon, ham, and sausages are now available, with just a fraction of the fat of regular processed meats. Some of these low-fat products are used in the recipes in this book. Here are some examples of what you are likely to find in your local grocery store.

Bacon. Turkey bacon, made with strips of light and dark turkey meat, looks and tastes much like pork bacon. But with 20 to 30 calories and 0.5 to 2 grams of fat per strip, turkey bacon has at least 50 percent less fat than crisp-cooked pork bacon, and shrinks much less during cooking. Besides being a leaner alternative to regular breakfast bacon, turkey bacon may be substituted for pork bacon in vegetables, casseroles, salads, and other dishes.

For the best results when cooking turkey bacon, prepare it in a microwave oven. This will produce a crisp texture instead of the chewy texture that results when turkey bacon is cooked in a skillet. Place the bacon slices on a microwave-safe plate, and cover with a paper towel. Then cook on high power for about one minute per slice, or until browned and crisp. Or follow the manufacturer's directions for making crisp bacon.

Canadian bacon, which has always been about 95-percent lean, is another useful ingredient to the low-fat cook. Use this flavorful product in breakfast casseroles and soups, and as a topping for pizzas.

Ham. Low-fat hams are made from either pork or turkey. These products contain as little as 0.5 gram of fat per ounce. Of course, all cured hams, including the leaner brands, are very high in sodium. However, used in moderation—to flavor bean soups or breakfast casseroles, for instance—these products can be incorporated into a healthy diet. Just avoid adding further salt to your recipes.

Sausage. A variety of low-fat smoked sausages and kielbasa made from turkey, or a combination of turkey, beef, and pork, are now available. These products contain a mere 30 to 40 calories and from less than 0.5 gram to 3 grams of fat per ounce. Compare this with an ounce of full-fat pork sausage, which contains over 100 calories and almost 9 grams of fat, and you'll see what a boon these new healthier mixtures are. Beware, though: While labeled "light," some brands of sausage contain as much as 10 grams of fat per 2.5-ounce serving. This is half the amount of fat found in the same-size serving of regular pork sausage, but is still a hefty dose of fat for such a small portion of food.

When a recipe calls for smoked sausage or kielbasa, try a brand like Butterball, Healthy

Choice, Hillshire Farm 97% Fat-Free, Jennie-O, Louis Rich, or Mr. Turkey—all of which contain significantly less fat than traditional brands. When buying bulk ground turkey breakfast sausage, try a brand like Louis Rich, which contains 75 percent less fat than most ground pork sausage. Many stores also make their own fresh turkey sausage, including turkey Italian sausage. When buying fresh sausage, always check the package labels and choose the leanest mixture available.

Vegetarian Alternatives

Soy foods have been in the spotlight in recent years, as researchers have discovered that the isoflavones in soy foods may help prevent heart disease and cancer, and can help ease the symptoms of menopause. As a result, a variety of soy foods have become mainstream, and people everywhere are discovering the "joy of soy."

Following are descriptions of some of the soy products that are now widely available. Several of these products—tofu hamburger, for instance—make great ground meat substitutes in dishes like chili, and can replace up to a third of the ground meat in burgers, meat loaves, and meatballs. Plain tofu is so versatile that it can be used to fill a number of culinary roles. And soy nuts can be used as a lower-fat alternative to regular nuts.

Meatless Recipe Crumbles. Made from soy and other vegetable proteins, these products—which include Green Giant's Harvest Burger for recipes—can be found in the freezer case of most grocery stores. Two cups of crumbles is the equivalent of one pound of cooked ground beef.

Soy Nuts. Made from soaked soybeans that are roasted until brown and crisp, these crunchy treats look like roasted peanuts, and have a similar texture and a nutty flavor. Sprinkle them over salads or add to casseroles, stir-fries, and veggie burgers as you would any other nut. With about 100 calories and 5 grams of fat per 1/4-cup serving, soy nuts have half the calories and 75 percent less fat than most nuts.

Texturized Vegetable Protein (TVP). This product has long been a staple in health food stores, and can now be found in some grocery stores, as well. TVP is made from defatted soy flour and comes packaged as small nuggets that you rehydrate with water. To rehydrate TVP, simply place 1 cup of the nuggets in a bowl, pour 7/8 cup of boiling water or broth over the nuggets, and let the mixture sit for five minutes. The rehydrated product is equivalent to one pound of cooked ground beef.

Tofu. Made from soybeans in a process similar to cheese-making, tofu has long been a staple in Oriental diets. Tofu's naturally bland flavor and unique texture make it a versatile product that can take on a wide variety of flavors. From spicy stir-fries, savory burgers, tacos, and chili, to smooth and creamy dips, cheesecakes, and puddings, tofu can star in just about any dish, and can replace many common cooking ingredients.

Tofu Hamburger. Located in the produce section alongside the regular tofu, these mildly seasoned bits of tofu look like cooked ground beef. One 10-ounce package—about 2 cups—is the equivalent of one pound of cooked ground beef. Look for brands like Tofu Crumbles and Ready Ground Tofu.

Fish and Other Seafood

Of the many kinds of fish and other seafood now available, some types are almost fat-free, while some are moderately fatty. However, the oil in fish provides an essential kind of fat—known as omega-3 fatty acids—that most people do not eat in sufficient quantities. These healthful fats can reduce your risk of cardiovascular disease, cancer, and inflammatory and autoimmune diseases, and may even help improve memory and fight depression. This means that all kinds of fish, especially the more oily ones, are considered healthful.

What about the cholesterol content of shellfish? It may not be as high as you think it is. With the exception of shrimp and oysters, a 3-ounce serving of most shellfish contains about 60 milligrams of cholesterol—well under the daily upper limit of 300 milligrams. The same-size serving of shrimp has about 166 milligrams of cholesterol, which is just over half the recommended daily limit. Oysters have about 90 milligrams of cholesterol. However, all seafood, including shellfish, is very low in saturated fat, which has a greater cholesterol-raising effect than does cholesterol.

Fish is highly perishable, so it is important to know how to select a high-quality product. First, make sure that the fish is firm and springy to the touch. Second, buy fish only if it has a clean seaweed odor, rather than a "fishy" smell. Third, when purchasing whole fish, choose those fish whose gills are bright red in color, and whose eyes are clear and bulging, not sunken or cloudy. Finally, refrigerate fish as soon as you get it home, and be sure to cook it within forty-eight hours of purchase.

Grains and Flours

One of the best-kept secrets of healthy eating is the benefits that can be derived simply by switching from refined grains and refined flours to whole grain products. While refined grains are practically devoid of fiber, nutrients, and phytochemicals, whole grains are loaded with these health-promoting substances. In fact, a number of studies have shown that whole grains offer protection against cardiovascular disease, cancer, and diabetes. And because they are more filling and satisfying than refined grains, making the switch can help you control your weight, as well.

Unfortunately, people who grew up eating refined grains often find whole grains too heavy for their taste. But once accustomed to the heartier taste and texture of whole grain products, most people prefer them over refined grains, which are bland and tasteless in comparison. In addition, making the switch to whole grains opens up a whole new world of flavors, textures, and meal-planning possibilities.

If you have never used whole grain flours before, a word should be said about storing these products. Since whole grain flours naturally contain a small amount of oil, they can become rancid more quickly than their refined counterparts. For this reason, be sure to purchase them in a store that has a high turnover rate, and to keep them in the refrigerator or freezer after you take them home. Following are descriptions of some of the grain products that you will find in your local grocery store or health food store.

Barley. This grain has a light nutty flavor, making it a great substitute for rice in casseroles, soups, pilafs, and other dishes. Hulled or pearled barley cooks in about 50 minutes. Quick-cooking barley is also widely available. With all the fiber of hulled barley, this product—which is available from both Mother's and Quaker—cooks in about 12 minutes. **Barley flour** is also available in health food stores and some grocery stores. This mildly sweet flour is perfect for cakes, muffins, and other baked goods, and can replace up to half of the wheat flour in these products.

Brown Rice. Brown rice is whole kernel rice, meaning that all nutrients are intact. With a slightly chewy texture and a pleasant nutty flavor, brown rice can replace white rice in any of your favorite recipes. For a real treat, try **basmati brown rice,** which has a richer, nuttier flavor than regular brown rice. Most grocery stores sell basmati brown rice alongside regular brown rice. Brown rice does take 45 to 50 minutes to cook, so when you are in a hurry, try one of the many brands of quick-cooking brown rice that are now available. These products cook in just 10 to 12 minutes. **Brown rice flour,** which is available in many grocery stores, makes a nutritious addition to baked goods, where it adds a pleasant corn-meal-like texture.

Buckwheat. Buckwheat is technically not a grain, but the edible fruit seed of a plant that is closely related to rhubarb. Roasted buck-wheat kernels, commonly known as **kasha,** are delicious in pilafs and hot breakfast cereals. **Buckwheat flour,** made from finely ground whole buckwheat kernels, is delicious in pancakes, waffles, breads, and muffins.

Cornmeal. This grain adds a sweet flavor, a lovely golden color, and a crunchy texture to baked goods. Select whole grain (unbolted) cornmeal for the most nutrition. Your next best choice is bolted cornmeal, which is nearly whole grain. By contrast, degermed cornmeal is refined. If you find all this confusing, just look at the Nutrition Facts label and choose a brand that contains at least 2 grams of fiber per 3-tablespoon serving. Cornmeal may be fine, medium, or coarsely ground, and is available in white, yellow, and even blue colors. Unlike the color of bread, the color of cornmeal—white versus yellow or blue—does not indicate the product's nutritional value or the degree to which it was refined.

Couscous. This is actually a tiny pasta, and not a grain. Couscous, which cooks in less than 5 minutes, makes a great substitute for rice in pilafs and salads, and is an excellent accompaniment to stews and stir-fries. Be sure to choose whole wheat couscous for the most nutrition.

Flax Meal. This product, which resembles wheat bran, is simply ground flaxseeds. Widely available in health food stores, this is one ingredient that you should definitely add to your shopping list. Why? The richest known plant source of health-promoting omega-3 fatty acids, flax is also loaded with lignans, a type of phytoestrogen that may help prevent cancer and ease menopausal symptoms.

To add the goodness of flax to your diet, try sprinkling a spoonful of the meal over cereals and other foods, as you would wheat bran. Flax meal is also a superior baking ingredient, and has long been popular with bakers in Europe and Canada because it adds a slightly sweet, nutty flavor to baked goods. And because the meal contains fibers and gums, it actually holds in moisture and adds tenderness to your baked goods, reducing the need for fat.

It is a simple matter to substitute flax meal for 10 to 15 percent of the flour in baked goods like breads, muffins, cookies, and pancakes. Just place $1\frac{1}{2}$ to 2 tablespoons of flax meal in a measuring cup, and fill the cup with your usual flour. Used like this, in small amounts, flax will actually improve the flavor and texture of most baked goods without adding a noticeable flavor.

You can also make your own flax meal at home by purchasing the whole flaxseeds and grinding them in a coffee grinder or blender. By doing this, you can be assured of getting the freshest product possible. This is important because once ground into meal, the oils in flax will more readily turn rancid. Whether you are purchasing ready-made flax meal or making your own, be sure to store the meal in an opaque container in the refrigerator, and to use it within one week. Keep in mind that you can also use the whole seeds in a variety of ways. Try sprinkling these reddish-brown seeds over your breakfast cereal or adding them to baked goods for a nutty crunch and a nutrient boost. The whole seeds can be stored at room temperature for up to a year.

Looking for a healthy egg substitute for use in your baked goods? Flaxseeds may be the answer. When the meal is mixed with water, it develops a texture and binding capacity similar to that of eggs. Simply place 1 tablespoon of flax meal and 3 tablespoons of water in a small bowl, and stir to mix well. Let the mixture sit for about 5 minutes, or until it has the consistency of raw egg whites. Use this mixture to replace one whole egg, or use 2 tablespoons of the mixture to replace one egg white.

Kamut. This ancient variety of wheat has made a comeback in recent years. **Kamut kernels,** which are also called berries, are about three times the size of wheat berries and have a delicate, buttery flavor and a chewy texture. Kamut berries may be cooked whole and incorporated into pilafs, casseroles, and other dishes. Also available are **kamut flakes,** which can be cooked like oatmeal. In addition, many health food stores sell **kamut flour,** which can

be substituted for regular whole wheat flour in yeast breads, quick breads, and other baked goods. Kamut is closely related to durum wheat, which is used for making pasta. For this reason, kamut makes a superior whole wheat pasta with a mild flavor and smooth texture.

Oats. Loaded with cholesterol-lowering soluble fiber, oats aren't just for breakfast. Use this healthful product to add a chewy texture and sweet flavor to muffins, quick breads, pancakes, cookies, and crumb toppings, or use oats as a filler for meat loaves and meatballs.

Another fiber-rich product to look for is **oat bran.** Made of the outer part of the oat kernel, oat bran has a sweet, mild flavor and is a concentrated source of cholesterol-lowering soluble fiber. Great as a hot and hearty breakfast cereal, oat bran can also replace 25 to 50 percent of the flour in many baked goods, where its soluble fibers add tenderness and retain moisture, reducing the need for fat. In fact, oat fibers are used in a variety of commercial fat substitutes. Look for oat bran in the hot cereal section of your grocery store, alongside the rolled oats. The softer products, like Quaker and Mother's, work best in baked goods.

Still another oat product to stock up on is **oat flour.** This mildly sweet flour is perfect for cakes, muffins, and other baked goods. Like oat bran, oat flour retains moisture and adds tenderness to baked goods, reducing the need for fat. To add extra fiber and nutrients, substitute oat flour for up to half of the refined wheat flour in recipes. Look for brands like Arrowhead Mills oat flour in grocery and health food stores, or make your own oat flour by finely grinding quick-cooking rolled oats in a food processor.

Quinoa *(keen'wa).* Rich in iron, magnesium, copper, vitamin B_6, and protein, quinoa has a unique light taste and a fluffy texture. It cooks in just 15 minutes, and is delicious in pilafs and puddings, and as a hot cereal. Be sure to rinse quinoa well with cool water before cooking to remove the bitter saponins—a natural repellent to birds and insects that coats the outside of the grains.

Soy Flour. Made from ground soybeans, soy flour contains health-promoting isoflavones and is rich in protein and other nutrients. You can use this product to add the goodness of soy to many of your baked goods. Simply substitute soy flour for 10 to 15 percent of the flour in baked goods. (Place $1^1/_2$ to 2 tablespoons of soy flour in a measuring cup, and fill the cup with your usual flour.) Used in small amounts, soy flour actually adds moistness and tenderness to baked goods. When larger amounts are used, though, baked goods can brown excessively and develop an unpleasant flavor. Look for soy flour in your local health food store.

Spelt. Like kamut, spelt is an ancient variety of wheat that is gaining renewed interest. Spelt looks similar to whole grain wheat, but has a milder flavor. Whole **spelt kernels,** also called spelt berries, may be cooked and incorporated into pilafs, casseroles, and other dishes. Also available are **spelt flakes,** which can be cooked like oatmeal. In addition, many health food stores sell **spelt flour,** which can be substituted for regular whole wheat flour in yeast breads, quick breads, muffins, and other baked goods.

Toasted Garbanzo Flour. Made from ground garbanzo beans (chickpeas), this golden flour is high in protein, fiber, and minerals. Toasted garbanzo flour is an excellent thickener for soups, stews, and gravies, where it adds a rich nutty flavor. This product can also replace up to 15 percent of the wheat flour in baked goods, and can be used as a binder in veggie burgers and other recipes. Look for toasted garbanzo flour in health food stores.

Unbleached Flour. This is refined white flour that has not been subjected to a bleaching process. Unbleached white flour lacks significant amounts of nutrients compared with whole wheat flour, but does contain more vitamin E than bleached flour. Arrowhead Mills, Gold Medal, Hodgson Mill, and Pillsbury's Best all make unbleached flour.

Wheat Germ. Use this ingredient to add crunch and nutty flavor to a wide range of dishes. A supernutritious food, wheat germ is loaded with B vitamins, vitamin E, zinc, magnesium, and many other nutrients. Two kinds of wheat germ are commonly available in the cereal section of grocery stores—plain toasted and honey crunch. Try substituting toasted wheat germ for part of the flour in quick breads, muffins, and coffee cakes. It also makes a nutritious filler for meat loaves or burgers, and a crunchy coating for oven-fried foods. Honey crunch wheat germ has a nugget-like texture, and makes an excellent substitute for chopped nuts, but with 90 percent less fat. It is also delicious sprinkled over cereal, fruit, or yogurt.

White Whole Wheat Flour. This is a good whole grain flour for all your baking needs, including yeast breads. Made from hard white wheat instead of the hard red wheat used to make regular whole wheat flour, white whole wheat flour contains all the fiber and nutrients of regular whole wheat flour, but is sweeter and lighter tasting than its red wheat counterpart. King Arthur white whole wheat flour is available in many grocery stores and by mail order.

Whole Grain Wheat. Available in many forms, this grain is perhaps easiest to use in the form of bulgur wheat. Cracked wheat that is precooked and dried, bulgur wheat can be prepared in a matter of minutes and can replace rice in any recipe. Look for it in grocery and health food stores.

Whole Wheat Flour. Made of ground whole grain wheat kernels, whole wheat flour includes the grain's nutrient-rich bran and germ. A good way to learn to enjoy whole grain flour is to use part whole wheat and part unbleached flour in recipes, and gradually increase the amount of whole wheat used over time. Most grocery stores stock Gold Medal, Pillsbury's Best, Hodgson Mill, Arrowhead Mills, or Heckers whole wheat flour. If you find these brands too heavy for your taste, try either whole wheat pastry flour or white whole wheat flour.

Whole Wheat Pastry Flour. When muffin, quick bread, cake, pastry, pancake, pie crust, and cookie recipes call for whole wheat flour, whole wheat pastry flour is, by far, the best choice. The reason? Made from a finely ground, soft (low-protein) wheat, whole wheat pastry flour has a milder, sweeter flavor and produces lighter, softer-textured baked goods than regular whole wheat flour does. Look for Bob's Red Mill Whole Wheat Pastry Flour and Arrowhead Mills Whole Grain Pastry Flour in health foods stores and many grocery stores. Keep in mind, though, that whole wheat pastry flour is not suitable for most yeast breads. Regular whole wheat and white whole wheat flours, which are higher in gluten, will allow your yeast breads to rise better.

As you can see, there are a wide variety of flours available for use in baking. Experiment with various flours to see which kinds you like best. Here are some general guidelines that will allow you to substitute various flours for refined wheat flour in your own favorite recipes.

1 cup refined wheat flour equals:

❏ 1 cup unbleached flour

❏ 1 cup whole wheat pastry flour

❏ 1 cup minus 1 tablespoon white whole wheat flour

❏ 1 cup minus 2 tablespoons regular whole wheat flour

❏ 1 cup brown rice flour

❏ 1 cup barley flour

❏ 1 cup minus 3 tablespoons kamut flour

❏ 1 cup oat flour

❏ 1 cup spelt flour

Sweeteners

Refined white sugar contains no nutrients. In fact, when eaten in excess, refined sugar can actually deplete the body's stores of essential nutrients like chromium and B vitamins. Of course, a moderate amount of sugar is usually not a problem for people who eat an otherwise healthy diet. Most of the sweet bread and dessert recipes in this book contain about 25 percent less sugar than traditional recipes do. Ingredients like fruit juices, fruit purées, and dried fruits; flavorings and spices like vanilla extract, nutmeg, cinnamon, and orange rind; and mildly sweet grains such as whole wheat pastry flour, oats, and oat bran have often been used to reduce the need for sugar. In addition, glazes and lower-sugar frostings are used to top cakes instead of traditional high-sugar frostings.

The recipes in this book call for moderate amounts of white sugar, brown sugar, and different liquid sweeteners. However, a large number of sweeteners are now available, and you should feel free to substitute one sweetener for another, using your own tastes, your desire for high-nutrient ingredients, and your pocketbook as a guide. (Some of the newer less-refined sweeteners are far more expensive than traditional sweeteners.) For best results, replace granular sweeteners with other granular sweeteners, and substitute liquid sweeteners for other liquid sweeteners. You can, of course, replace a liquid with granules, or vice versa, but adjustments in other recipe ingredients will have to be made. (For each cup of liquid sweetener substituted for a granulated sweetener, reduce the liquid by $1/4$ to $1/3$ cup.) Also be aware that each sweetener has its own unique flavor and its own degree of sweetness, making some sweeteners better suited to particular recipes. Following is a description of some of the sweeteners commonly available in grocery stores, health food stores, and gourmet shops.

Brown Sugar. This granulated sweetener is simply refined white sugar that has been coated with a thin film of molasses. Light brown sugar is lighter in color than regular brown sugar, but not lower in calories, as the name might imply. Because this sweetener contains some molasses, brown sugar has more calcium, iron, and potassium than white sugar. But like most sugars, brown sugar is no nutritional powerhouse. The advantage to using this sweetener instead of white sugar is that it is more flavorful, and so often can be used in smaller quantities.

Date Sugar. Made from ground dried dates, date sugar provides copper, magnesium, iron, and B vitamins. With a distinct date flavor, this product is delicious in breads, cakes, and muffins. Because it does not dissolve as readily as white sugar does, it is best to mix date sugar with the recipe's liquid ingredients and let it sit for a few minutes before proceeding with the recipe. Date sugar is less dense than white sugar, and so is only about two-thirds as sweet. However, date sugar is more flavorful, and so can often be substituted for white sugar on a cup-for-cup basis.

Fruit Juice Concentrates. Frozen juice concentrates add sweetness and flavor to baked goods while enhancing nutritional value. Use the concentrates as you would honey or other liquid sweeteners, but beware, as too much will be overpowering. Always keep cans of frozen orange and apple juice concentrate in the freezer just for cooking and baking. Pineapple and tropical fruit blends also make good sweeteners, and white grape juice is ideal when you want a more neutral flavor.

Fruit Source. Made from white grape juice and brown rice, this sweetener has a rather neutral flavor and is about as sweet as white sugar. Fruit Source is available in both granular and liquid forms. Use the liquid as you would honey, and the granules as you would sugar. The granules do not dissolve as readily as sugar does, so mix Fruit Source with the recipe's liquid ingredients and let it sit for a few minutes before proceeding with the recipe.

Fruit Spreads, Jams, and Preserves. Available in a variety of flavors, these products make delicious sweeteners. For the best flavor and nutrition, choose a brand made from fruits and fruit juice concentrate, with little or no added sugar, and select a flavor that is compatible with the baked goods you're making. Use as you would any liquid sweetener.

Honey. Contrary to popular belief, honey is not significantly more nutritious than sugar, but it does add a nice flavor to baked goods. It also adds moistness, reducing the need for fat. The sweetest of the liquid sweeteners, honey is generally 20 to 30 percent sweeter than sugar. Be sure to consider this when making substitutions.

Maple Sugar. Made from dehydrated maple syrup, granulated maple sugar adds a distinct maple flavor to baked goods. Powdered maple sugar is also available, and can be used to replace powdered white sugar in glazes.

Maple Syrup. The boiled-down sap of sugar maple trees, maple syrup adds delicious flavor to all baked goods, and also provides some potassium and other nutrients. Use it as you would honey or molasses.

Molasses. Light, or Barbados, molasses is pure sugar cane juice boiled down into a thick syrup. Light molasses provides some calcium, potassium, and iron, and is delicious in spice cakes, muffins, breads, and cookies. Blackstrap molasses is a by-product of the sugar-refining process. Very rich in calcium, potassium, and iron, it has a slightly bitter, strong flavor, and is half as sweet as refined sugar. Because of its distinctive taste, more than a few tablespoons of blackstrap in a recipe is overwhelming.

Sucanat. Granules of evaporated sugar cane juice, Sucanat provides small amounts of potassium, chromium, calcium, iron, and vitamins A and C. Use it as you would any other granulated sugar.

Herbs, Spices, and Flavorings

Herbs, spices, and other flavorings play an essential role in light and healthy cooking. Wisely used, these ingredients enhance the flavors of your dish, allowing you to reduce or eliminate fat and salt. Most of the seasonings that are used in the recipes in this book—basil, oregano, thyme, Italian seasoning, and garlic, for instance—are probably already in your pantry. A few others, like those listed below, may be new to you.

Curry Paste. A flavorful blend of curry spices mixed with canola oil, curry paste has a deeper, richer flavor than curry powder. Brands like Patak's curry paste are widely available in the imported foods section of many grocery stores and in specialty shops, and can be found in hot, medium, or mild varieties. Although curry paste contains oil, a teaspoon or two is generally enough to flavor an entire recipe, so that this ingredient will add very little fat to your dish. Most brands of curry paste contain salt, but by limiting any other salt added to your recipe, you can keep sodium under control. If you do not have curry paste on hand, substitute an equal amount of curry powder and add a little extra salt to the recipe.

Fines Herbes. A blend of thyme, oregano, sage, rosemary, marjoram, and basil, this herb blend can be found in the dried spice section of most grocery stores. Or you can make your own fines herbes blend by mixing equal parts of each of these herbs, and storing them in an airtight container.

Szechuan Seasoning. A spicy-hot mixture of ginger, garlic, pepper, and Asian seasonings, Szechuan seasoning can be found in the spice section of most grocery stores. Or make 3 tablespoons of Szechuan seasoning by combining 1 tablespoon of ground ginger, 2$\frac{1}{4}$ teaspoons of dry mustard, 2$\frac{1}{4}$ teaspoons of lemon pepper, 1$\frac{1}{2}$ teaspoons of garlic powder, and 1 to 1$\frac{1}{2}$ teaspoons of crushed red pepper. Stir to mix well, and store in an airtight container until ready to use.

ABOUT THE NUTRITIONAL ANALYSIS

The Food Processor II (ESHA Research) computer nutrition analysis system, along with product information from manufacturers, was used to calculate the nutritional information for the recipes in this book. Nutrients are always listed per one piece, one muffin, one slice, one serving, etc.

Sometimes recipes give you options regarding ingredients. For instance, you might be able to choose between wheat germ and nuts, nonfat and reduced-fat cheese, or nonfat and reduced-fat mayonnaise. This will help you create dishes that suit your tastes. Just keep in mind that the nutritional analysis is based on the first ingredient listed.

This book is filled with creative dishes that help promote good health. But more important, these dishes are so simple to make, so satisfying, and so delicious that you will truly enjoy serving them to your family and friends. So get ready to create some new family favorites and to experience the pleasures and rewards of healthful cooking.

2. Breakfast and Brunch Favorites

When it comes to high-fat, high-calorie foods, few meals can top a traditional breakfast. For decades, whole eggs, cheese, sausage, and bacon were considered an essential part of morning fare. Of course, we now know that these foods are far from healthy. But for many of us, breakfast just isn't breakfast without a stack of golden French toast or a hearty Western omelette. What to do, what to do?

Fortunately, you need not discard your favorite breakfast fare in order to banish high-fat foods from the breakfast table. There is now a healthier fat-free or low-fat alternative to just about any breakfast food that comes to mind. Fat-free egg substitutes have been the biggest boon to breakfast lovers. With none of the fat or cholesterol of eggs, these substitutes can replace the eggs in all of your breakfast casseroles and omelettes. Fat-free and reduced-fat cheeses and ultra-lean sausage, ham, and bacon are other breakfast favorites that can now take their place in a healthful lifestyle. In fact, many of the recipes in this chapter combine these new no- and low-fat ingredients to create delicious versions of dishes that were previously taboo in many people's diets.

Can pancakes, waffles, and French toast also be part of a light and healthy breakfast menu? Happily, many of the traditional recipes for these treats have always been fairly low in fat. However, most recipes do contain unnecessary oil, egg yolks, and salt—unhealthy ingredients that can easily be trimmed away without sacrificing the flavors you love. Replace the usual refined white flour with whole grain ingredients, add some sweet yet wholesome toppings, and these dishes are more than just low in fat. They are high in many important nutrients.

When creating breakfast menus, you need not confine your choices to the selections in this chapter. Fresh juices, in-season fruits, and whole grain breads and muffins will add both diversity and balance to your menu. So heat up the griddle and get ready for high-nutrient, taste-tempting breakfast foods that will not only get you out of bed, but will keep you going all morning long!

Multigrain Pancakes

YIELD: 12 PANCAKES

1 cup plus 2 tablespoons whole wheat pastry flour
2 tablespoons yellow cornmeal
2 tablespoons oat bran
2 tablespoons toasted wheat germ or flax meal (page 23)
1 tablespoon sugar
1 teaspoon baking soda
1$^3/_4$ cups nonfat or low-fat buttermilk
2 egg whites, lightly beaten, or $^1/_4$ cup fat-free egg substitute

1. Place the flour, cornmeal, oat bran, wheat germ or flax meal, sugar, and baking soda in a large bowl, and stir to mix well. Add the buttermilk and the egg whites or egg substitute, and mix with a wire whisk to blend well.

2. Coat a griddle or large nonstick skillet with nonstick cooking spray, and preheat over medium heat until a drop of water sizzles when it hits the surface. (If using an electric griddle, preheat the griddle according to the manufacturer's directions.)

3. For each pancake, pour $^1/_4$ cup of batter onto the griddle, and spread into a 4-inch circle. Cook for about 1 minute and 30 seconds, or until the top is bubbly and the edges are dry. Turn and cook for an additional minute, or until the second side is golden brown. As the pancakes are done, transfer them to a serving plate and keep warm in a preheated oven.

4. Serve hot, topped with honey, maple syrup, Berry Fresh Fruit Sauce (page 35), or Fast and Easy Fruit Sauce (page 34).

NUTRITIONAL FACTS (PER PANCAKE)
Cal: 70   Carbs: 13.2 g   Chol: 1 mg   Fat: 0.7 g
Fiber: 1.8 g   Protein: 3.8 g   Sodium: 151 mg

VARIATION

To make Multigrain Banana Pancakes, add 1$^1/_2$ cups of sliced bananas to the batter, and proceed with recipe as directed to make 15 pancakes. Top with maple syrup or honey and a sprinkling of toasted pecans, if desired.

NUTRITIONAL FACTS (PER PANCAKE)
Cal: 70   Carbs: 14 g   Chol: 1 mg   Fat: 0.7 g
Fiber: 1.8 g   Protein: 3.2 g   Sodium: 121 mg

Banana Buttermilk Pancakes

YIELD: 15 PANCAKES

1$^1/_2$ cups whole wheat pastry flour
1 tablespoon sugar
1 teaspoon baking soda
1$^3/_4$ cups nonfat or low-fat buttermilk
$^1/_4$ cup fat-free egg substitute, or 2 egg whites, lightly beaten
1$^1/_2$ cups sliced banana (about 1$^1/_2$ medium)
$^1/_4$ cup honey crunch wheat germ or chopped toasted pecans (page 348)

1. Place the flour, sugar, and baking soda in a medium-sized bowl, and stir to mix well. Add the buttermilk and egg substitute or egg whites, and stir to mix well. Fold in the banana and wheat germ or pecans.

2. Coat a griddle or large skillet with nonstick cooking spray, and preheat over medium heat until a drop of water sizzles when it hits the heated surface. (If using an electric griddle, heat the griddle according to the manufacturer's directions.)

3. For each pancake, pour $^1/_4$ cup of batter onto the griddle, and spread into a 4-inch circle. Cook for about 1 minute and 30 seconds, or until the top is bubbly and the edges are dry. Turn and cook for an additional minute, or until the second side is golden brown. As the pancakes are done, transfer them to a serving plate and keep warm in a preheated oven.

4. Serve hot, topped with honey or maple syrup.

VARIATION

To make Banana Buckwheat Pancakes, substitute $^3/_4$ cup of buckwheat flour for $^3/_4$ cup of the whole wheat pastry flour.

NUTRITIONAL FACTS (PER PANCAKE)
Cal: 78   Carbs: 14 g   Chol: 1 mg   Fat: 0.7 g
Fiber: 1.9 g   Protein: 3.6 g   Sodium: 121 mg

Cottage-Apple Pancakes

YIELD: 20 PANCAKES

| 1⅓ cups whole wheat pastry flour |
| 1 tablespoon sugar |
| 1 tablespoon baking powder |
| 1 cup skim or low-fat milk |
| 1 cup nonfat or low-fat cottage cheese |
| ¼ cup plus 2 tablespoons fat-free egg substitute, or 3 egg whites, lightly beaten |
| 1¼ cups finely chopped peeled apple (about 2 medium) |

1. Place the flour, sugar, and baking powder in a large bowl, and stir to mix well. Add the milk, cottage cheese, and egg substitute or egg whites, and stir to mix well. Stir in the apples.

2. Coat a griddle or large nonstick skillet with nonstick cooking spray, and preheat over medium heat until a drop of water sizzles when it hits the surface. (If using an electric griddle, preheat the griddle according to the manufacturer's directions.)

3. For each pancake, pour 3 tablespoons of batter onto the griddle, and spread into a 3-inch circle. Cook for about 1 minute and 30 seconds, or until the top is bubbly and the edges are dry. Turn and cook for an additional minute, or until the second side is golden brown. As the pancakes are done, transfer them to a serving plate and keep warm in a preheated oven.

4. Serve hot, topped with honey or maple syrup.

NUTRITIONAL FACTS (PER PANCAKE)
Cal: 48   Carbs: 9 g   Chol: 1 mg   Fat: 0.2 g
Fiber: 1.3 g   Protein: 3.5 g   Sodium: 105 mg

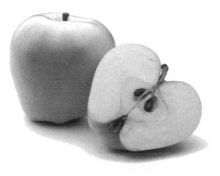

Blueberry-Cornmeal Cakes

YIELD: 15 PANCAKES

| ¾ cup whole wheat pastry flour |
| ¾ cup yellow cornmeal |
| 1 tablespoon sugar |
| 1 teaspoon baking soda |
| 1¾ cups nonfat or low-fat buttermilk |
| ¼ cup fat-free egg substitute, or 2 egg whites, lightly beaten |
| 1½ cups fresh or frozen (unthawed) blueberries |

1. Place the flour, cornmeal, sugar, and baking soda in a medium-sized bowl, and stir to mix well. Add the buttermilk and egg substitute or egg whites, and stir to mix well. Fold in the blueberries.

2. Coat a griddle or large skillet with nonstick cooking spray, and preheat over medium heat until a drop of water sizzles when it hits the surface. (If using an electric griddle, heat the griddle according to the manufacturer's directions.)

3. For each pancake, pour ¼ cup of batter onto the griddle, and spread into a 4-inch circle. Cook for 1 minute and 30 seconds, or until the top is bubbly and the edges are dry. Turn and cook for an additional minute, or until the second side is golden brown. As the pancakes are done, transfer them to a serving plate and keep warm in a preheated oven.

4. Serve hot, topped with Honey-Orange Syrup (page 34), honey, or maple syrup.

NUTRITIONAL FACTS (PER PANCAKE)
Cal: 67   Carbs: 12.6 g   Chol: 1 mg   Fat: 0.6 g
Fiber: 1.6 g   Protein: 2.8 g   Sodium: 124 mg

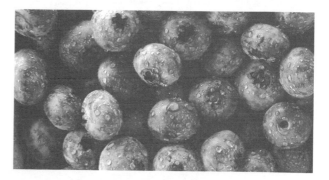

Simple Syrup Alternatives

Deliciously sweet syrups add that crowning touch to pancakes, waffles, and French toast. While all syrups are fat-free, they are generally almost pure sugar, and add up to 60 calories for each tablespoon used. Instead of the usual refined, sugary syrups, try any of the following toppings over pancakes, waffles, and other breakfast treats. As low in calories as most reduced-calorie brands, these syrups are more natural, wholesome, and economical.

Honey-Orange Syrup

YIELD: 1½ CUPS

1 tablespoon cornstarch

1 cup orange juice

½ cup honey

1. Place the cornstarch and 2 tablespoons of the orange juice in a 1-quart saucepan, and stir until the cornstarch is dissolved. Stir in first the remaining orange juice and then the honey.

2. Place the pan over medium heat, and cook, stirring constantly, for about 3 minutes, or until the mixture is bubbly and slightly thickened.

3. Serve warm over pancakes, French toast, or waffles. Store any leftovers in the refrigerator for up to 3 days.

NUTRITIONAL FACTS (PER 2-TABLESPOON SERVING)
Cal: 55   Carbs: 13.5 g   Chol: 0 mg   Fat: 0 g
Fiber: 0 g   Protein: 0.2 g   Sodium: 1 mg

Fast and Easy Fruit Sauce

YIELD: 1¾ CUPS

1 can (1 pound) peaches or apricots in juice or light syrup, undrained

2–3 tablespoons sugar

1. Place the peaches or apricots, including the juice, and the sugar in a blender, and process until smooth.

2. Pour the mixture into a 1-quart pot, place over medium heat, and cook until heated through.

3. Serve warm over pancakes, French toast, or waffles. Store any leftover sauce in the refrigerator for up to 3 days.

NUTRITIONAL FACTS (PER ¼-CUP SERVING)
Cal: 42   Carbs: 10 g   Chol: 0 mg   Fat: 0 g
Fiber: 0.9 g   Protein: 0.5 g   Sodium: 2 mg

Blueberry-Yogurt Pancakes

YIELD: 14 PANCAKES

1½ cups whole wheat pastry flour

1 tablespoon baking powder

¾ cup skim or low-fat milk

1 cup nonfat or low-fat vanilla yogurt

2 egg whites, lightly beaten, or ¼ cup fat-free egg substitute

1¼ cups fresh or frozen (unthawed) blueberries

1. Place the flour and baking powder in a large bowl, and stir to mix well. Add the milk, yogurt, and egg whites or egg substitute, and mix with a wire whisk to blend well. Fold in the blueberries.

2. Coat a griddle or large nonstick skillet with nonstick cooking spray, and preheat over medium heat until a drop of water sizzles when it hits the surface. (If using an electric griddle, preheat the griddle according to the manufacturer's directions.)

3. For each pancake, pour ¼ cup of batter onto the griddle, and spread into a 4-inch circle. Cook for

Warm Apple Topping

YIELD: 2 CUPS

1 cup apple juice, divided

1 tablespoon cornstarch

3 cups sliced peeled apples (about 4 medium)

1/4 cup light brown sugar

1/4 teaspoon ground cinnamon

Pinch ground nutmeg

1. Place 1 tablespoon of the apple juice and all of the cornstarch in a small bowl. Stir to dissolve the cornstarch, and set aside.

2. Place the apples, the remaining juice, and the brown sugar, cinnamon, and nutmeg in a 1-quart saucepan. Stir to mix well, and bring to a boil over high heat. Reduce the heat to low, cover, and simmer, stirring occasionally, for about 5 minutes, or until the apples are tender.

3. Stir the cornstarch mixture, and add it to the pot. Cook, stirring constantly, for another minute or 2, or until the mixture is thickened and bubbly.

4. Serve warm over pancakes, French toast, or waffles. Store any leftover sauce in the refrigerator for up to 3 days.

NUTRITIONAL FACTS (PER 1/4-CUP SERVING)
Cal: 59   Carbs: 15 g   Chol: 0 mg   Fat: 0.1 g
Fiber: 0.8 g   Protein: 0.1 g   Sodium: 3 mg

Berry Fresh Fruit Sauce

YIELD: 1 1/2 CUPS

3/4 cup white grape juice, divided

1 tablespoon cornstarch

2 cups fresh or frozen blueberries,
blackberries, raspberries,
or sliced strawberries

1/4 cup sugar

1. Place 2 tablespoons of the juice and all of the cornstarch in a small bowl. Stir to dissolve the cornstarch, and set aside.

2. Place the berries, the remaining juice, and the sugar in a 1 1/2-quart saucepan. Stir to mix well, and bring to a boil over medium-high heat. Reduce the heat to low, cover, and simmer, stirring occasionally, for about 5 minutes, or until the fruit is very soft.

3. Stir the cornstarch mixture, and add it to the pot. Cook, stirring constantly, for another minute or 2, or until the mixture is thickened and bubbly.

4. Serve warm over pancakes, French toast, or waffles. Store any leftover sauce in the refrigerator for up to 3 days.

NUTRITIONAL FACTS (PER 1/4-CUP SERVING)
Cal: 83   Carbs: 21 g   Chol: 0 mg   Fat: 0.2 g
Fiber: 1.4 g   Protein: 0.5 g   Sodium: 5 mg

about 1 minute and 30 seconds, or until the top is bubbly and the edges are dry. Turn and cook for an additional minute, or until the second side is golden brown. As the pancakes are done, transfer them to a serving plate and keep warm in a preheated oven.

4. Serve hot, topped with honey, maple syrup, or Fast and Easy Fruit Sauce (page 34).

NUTRITIONAL FACTS (PER PANCAKE)
Cal: 65   Carbs: 13 g   Chol: 1 mg   Fat: 0.4 g
Fiber: 1.9 g   Protein: 3 g   Sodium: 122 mg

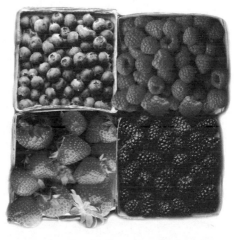

Applesauce Pancakes

YIELD: 12 PANCAKES

1½ cups whole wheat pastry flour

1 tablespoon baking powder

¾ cup unsweetened applesauce

1 cup nonfat or low-fat buttermilk

¼ cup fat-free egg substitute, or 2 egg whites, lightly beaten

1. Place the flour and baking powder in a medium-sized bowl, and stir to mix well. Stir in the applesauce, buttermilk, and egg substitute or egg whites.

2. Coat a griddle or large skillet with nonstick cooking spray, and preheat over medium heat until a drop of water sizzles when it hits the surface. (If using an electric griddle, heat the griddle according to the manufacturer's directions.)

3. For each pancake, pour ¼ cup of batter onto the griddle, and spread into a 4-inch circle. Cook for 1 minute and 30 seconds, or until the top is bubbly and the edges are dry. Turn and cook for an additional minute, or until the second side is golden brown. As the pancakes are done, transfer them to a serving plate and keep warm in a preheated oven.

4. Serve hot, topped with Warm Apple Topping (page 35), Berry Fresh Fruit Sauce (page 35), or maple syrup.

NUTRITIONAL FACTS (PER PANCAKE)
Cal: 69   Carbs: 13 g   Chol: 1 mg   Fat: 0.5 g
Fiber: 2 g   Protein: 3.2 g   Sodium: 122 mg

VARIATION

To make Applesauce Buckwheat Cakes, substitute ½ cup of buckwheat flour for ½ cup of the whole wheat pastry flour.

NUTRITIONAL FACTS (PER PANCAKE)
Cal: 69   Carbs: 13 g   Chol: 1 mg   Fat: 0.5 g
Fiber: 2 g   Protein: 3.2 g   Sodium: 122 mg

VARIATION

To make Applesauce Flax Cakes, substitute ¼ cup of flax meal (page 23) for ¼ cup of the whole wheat pastry flour.

NUTRITIONAL FACTS (PER PANCAKE)
Cal: 71   Carbs: 12 g   Chol: 1 mg   Fat: 1.4 g
Fiber: 2.4 g   Protein: 3.4 g   Sodium: 122 mg

Apple-Oatmeal Pancakes

YIELD: 16 PANCAKES

1½ cups quick-cooking oats

2¼ cups nonfat or low-fat buttermilk

½ cup whole wheat pastry flour or unbleached flour

1 tablespoon sugar

1 teaspoon baking soda

¼ teaspoon ground cinnamon

½ cup fat-free egg substitute

2 cups chopped peeled apple (about 2½ medium)

1. Place the oats and buttermilk in a large bowl. Stir to mix well, and set aside for 10 minutes.

2. Place the flour, sugar, baking soda, and cinnamon in a small bowl. Stir to mix well, and set aside.

3. Add the egg substitute to the oat mixture, and stir to mix well. Add the flour mixture, and stir to mix well. Fold in the apple.

4. Coat a griddle or large skillet with nonstick cooking spray, and preheat over medium heat until a drop of water sizzles when it hits the surface. (If using an electric griddle, heat the griddle according to the manufacturer's directions.)

5. For each pancake, pour ¼ cup of batter onto the griddle, and spread into a 4-inch circle. Cook for 1 minute and 30 seconds, or until the top is bubbly and the edges are dry. Turn and cook for an additional minute, or until the second side is golden brown. As the pancakes are done, transfer them to a serving plate and keep warm in a preheated oven.

6. Serve hot, topped with Berry Fresh Fruit Sauce (page 35), honey, or maple syrup.

NUTRITIONAL FACTS (PER PANCAKE)
Cal: 72   Carbs: 12 g   Chol: 1 mg   Fat: 0.8 g
Fiber: 1.5 g   Protein: 3.6 g   Sodium: 123 mg

Light and Fluffy Oatcakes

YIELD: 12 PANCAKES

¾ cup quick-cooking oats

1¾ cups nonfat or low-fat buttermilk

2 egg whites

1 cup whole wheat pastry flour

1 tablespoon sugar

2 teaspoons baking powder

1. Place the oats and buttermilk in a medium-sized bowl. Stir to mix well, and set aside for 10 minutes.

2. Place the egg whites in the bowl of an electric mixer, and beat on high until stiff peaks form. Set aside.

3. Combine the flour, sugar, and baking powder in a large bowl, and stir to mix well. Add the oat mixture to the flour mixture, and stir to mix well. Gently fold in the egg whites.

4. Coat a griddle or large skillet with nonstick cooking spray, and preheat over medium heat until a drop of water sizzles when it hits the surface. (If using an electric griddle, heat the griddle according to the manufacturer's directions.)

5. For each pancake, pour ¼ cup of batter onto the griddle, and spread into a 4-inch circle. Cook for 1 minute and 30 seconds, or until the top is bubbly and the edges are dry. Turn and cook for an additional minute, or until the second side is golden brown. As the pancakes are done, transfer them to a serving plate and keep warm in a preheated oven.

6. Serve hot, topped with Warm Apple Topping (page 35), Berry Fresh Fruit Sauce (page 35), or Honey-Orange Syrup (page 34).

NUTRITIONAL FACTS (PER PANCAKE)
Cal: 75   Carbs: 13 g   Chol: 1 mg   Fat: 0.8 g
Fiber: 1.8 g   Protein: 3.9 g   Sodium: 108 mg

VARIATION

To make Blueberry Oatcakes, fold ¾ cup of fresh or frozen (unthawed) blueberries into the batter.

NUTRITIONAL FACTS (PER PANCAKE)
Cal: 80   Carbs: 14 g   Chol: 1 mg   Fat: 0.8 g
Fiber: 2 g   Protein: 4 g   Sodium: 108 mg

Cottage Cheese Pancakes

YIELD: 16 PANCAKES

1 cup whole wheat pastry flour

1 teaspoon dried grated orange rind

1½ teaspoons baking powder

1 cup skim or low-fat milk

1 cup nonfat or low-fat cottage cheese

½ cup fat-free egg substitute, or 4 egg whites, lightly beaten

1. Place the flour, orange rind, and baking powder in a medium-sized bowl, and stir to mix well. Add the milk, cottage cheese, and egg substitute or egg whites, and stir to mix well.

2. Coat a griddle or large skillet with nonstick cooking spray, and preheat over medium heat until a drop of water sizzles when it hits the surface. (If using an electric griddle, heat the griddle according to the manufacturer's directions.)

3. For each pancake, pour 3 tablespoons of batter onto the griddle, and spread into a 3-inch circle. Cook for 1 minute and 30 seconds, or until the top is bubbly and the edges are dry. Turn and cook for an additional minute, or until the second side is golden brown. As the pancakes are done, transfer them to a serving plate and keep warm in a preheated oven.

4. Serve hot, topped with Berry Fresh Fruit Sauce (page 35) or Honey-Orange Syrup (page 34).

NUTRITIONAL FACTS (PER PANCAKE)
Cal: 45   Carbs: 7 g   Chol: 1 mg   Fat: 0.2 g
Fiber: 1 g   Protein: 4 g   Sodium: 100 mg

New England Corncakes

YIELD: 16 PANCAKES
1 cup whole wheat pastry flour
1 cup yellow cornmeal
1 teaspoon baking soda
2 cups nonfat or low-fat buttermilk
1/4 cup fat-free egg substitute, or 2 egg whites, lightly beaten
1 cup frozen (thawed) whole kernel corn, or 1 can (8 ounces) whole kernel corn, drained
1/2 cup finely chopped ham, at least 97% lean, or 5 slices extra-lean turkey bacon, cooked, drained, and crumbled

1. Place the flour, cornmeal, and baking soda in a medium-sized bowl, and stir to mix well. Add the buttermilk and egg substitute or egg whites, and stir to mix well. Fold in the corn and the ham or bacon.

2. Coat a griddle or large skillet with nonstick cooking spray, and preheat over medium heat until a drop of water sizzles when it hits the surface. (If using an electric griddle, heat the griddle according to the manufacturer's directions.)

3. For each pancake, pour 1/4 cup of batter onto the griddle, and spread into a 4-inch circle. Cook for 1 minute and 30 seconds, or until the top is bubbly and the edges are dry. Turn and cook for an additional minute, or until the second side is golden brown. As the pancakes are done, transfer them to a serving plate and keep warm in a preheated oven.

4. Serve hot, topped with maple syrup.

NUTRITIONAL FACTS (PER PANCAKE)
Cal: 79   Carbs: 14 g   Chol: 3 mg   Fat: 0.9 g   Fiber: 1.7 g   Protein: 4 g   Sodium: 165 mg

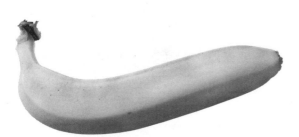

Banana French Toast

Like Cinnamon-Vanilla French Toast (page 39), this dish is just as delicious when made with English muffin halves or presliced bread.

YIELD: 12 SLICES
1 1/4 cups fat-free egg substitute
1 cup sliced banana (about 1 large)
1/2 cup evaporated skim milk
1 1/2 teaspoons vanilla extract
1/4 teaspoon ground nutmeg
1 oblong loaf multigrain or oatmeal bread (about 6-x-12 inches, or 1 pound), unsliced

1. Place the egg substitute, banana, milk, vanilla extract, and nutmeg in a blender, and process until smooth. Pour the mixture into a shallow bowl, and set aside.

2. Slice twelve 3/4-inch-thick pieces of bread from the loaf. (You will need only about three-fourths of the loaf.) Dip each bread slice in the egg mixture, turning to coat both sides and to thoroughly soak the bread.

3. Coat a griddle or large nonstick skillet with nonstick cooking spray, and preheat over medium heat until a drop of water sizzles when it hits the surface. (If using an electric griddle, preheat the griddle to 375°F.)

4. Arrange the bread slices on the griddle, and cook for about 2 minutes on each side, or until golden brown. As the slices are done, transfer them to a serving plate and keep warm in a preheated oven.

5. Serve hot, topped with maple syrup or honey. Garnish with a few banana slices and a sprinkling of pecans, if desired.

NUTRITIONAL FACTS (PER SLICE)
Cal: 97   Carbs: 16 g   Chol: 0 mg   Fat: 0.7 g   Fiber: 2 g   Protein: 6 g   Sodium: 180 mg

Cinnamon-Vanilla French Toast

For variety, substitute 12 oat bran or whole wheat English muffin halves or 12 pieces of presliced multigrain, oatmeal, or whole wheat bread for the bread called for in this recipe.

YIELD: 12 SLICES
1¼ cups fat-free egg substitute
1 cup evaporated skim milk
2 tablespoons maple syrup
½ teaspoon ground cinnamon
½ teaspoon vanilla extract
1 oblong loaf multigrain or oatmeal bread (about 6-x-12-inches, or 1 pound), unsliced

1. Place the egg substitute, milk, maple syrup, cinnamon, and vanilla extract in a blender, and process until well mixed. Pour the mixture into a shallow bowl, and set aside.

2. Slice twelve ¾-inch-thick pieces of bread from the loaf. (You will need only about three-fourths of the loaf.) Dip each bread slice in the egg mixture, turning to coat both sides and to thoroughly soak the bread.

3. Coat a griddle or large nonstick skillet with nonstick cooking spray, and preheat over medium heat until a drop of water sizzles when it hits the surface. (If using an electric griddle, preheat the griddle to 375°F.)

4. Arrange the bread slices on the griddle, and cook for about 2 minutes on each side, or until golden brown. As the slices are done, transfer them to a serving plate and keep warm in a preheated oven.

5. Serve hot, topped with Berry Fresh Fruit Sauce (page 35), Warm Apple Topping (page 35), maple syrup, or honey.

NUTRITIONAL FACTS (PER SLICE)
Cal: 106   Carbs: 18 g   Chol: 0 mg   Fat: 0.7g
Fiber: 2 g   Protein: 6.4 g   Sodium: 203 mg

Getting the Fat Out of Your Waffle Recipes

To make your favorite waffles light, crisp, and fat-free:

- Replace the oil in the recipe with three-fourths as much buttermilk, applesauce, or other liquid.

- Substitute 3 egg whites for every 2 whole eggs in the recipe, and whip the egg whites to soft peaks before folding them into the batter.

- For an extra-crisp texture, substitute cornmeal or brown rice flour for up to half of the wheat flour. These flours add a pleasing crunch to baked goods.

Crispy Cornmeal Waffles

Waffles are great for people with busy lifestyles, as they may be made in advance, placed in plastic zip-type bags, and frozen until needed. At breakfast time, heat the frozen waffles in the toaster, and serve.

YIELD: 12 WAFFLES
1 cup whole wheat pastry flour
1 cup yellow cornmeal
2 tablespoons sugar
2 teaspoons baking powder
¾ teaspoon baking soda
4 egg whites
1½ cups nonfat or low-fat buttermilk
¼ cup honey crunch wheat germ (optional)

1. Coat a waffle iron with nonstick cooking spray, and preheat according to the manufacturer's directions.

2. Place the flour, cornmeal, sugar, baking powder, and baking soda in a large bowl, and stir to mix well. Set aside.

3. Place the egg whites in the bowl of an electric mixer, and beat on high until soft peaks form. Set aside.

4. Add the buttermilk to the flour mixture, and stir to mix well. Fold in the wheat germ, if desired. Gently fold in the egg whites.

5. Spoon 1¼ cups of batter (or the amount stated by the manufacturer) onto the prepared waffle iron. Bake for 5 to 7 minutes, or until the iron has stopped steaming and the waffle is crisp and brown.

6. Serve hot, topped with Berry Fresh Fruit Sauce (page 35) or Honey-Orange Syrup (page 34).

NUTRITIONAL FACTS (PER WAFFLE)
Cal: 97   Carbs: 18 g   Chol: 1 mg   Fat: 0.7 g
Fiber: 2 g   Protein: 4.3 g   Sodium: 194 mg

VARIATION

To make Three Grain Waffles, substitute ½ cup of quick-cooking oats for ½ cup of the cornmeal.

NUTRITIONAL FACTS (PER WAFFLE)
Cal: 86   Carbs: 16 g   Chol: 1 mg   Fat: 0.8 g
Fiber: 1.9 g   Protein: 3.3 g   Sodium: 194 mg

VARIATION

To make Crispy Flax Waffles, substitute ¼ cup of flax meal (page 23) for ¼ cup of the cornmeal.

NUTRITIONAL FACTS (PER WAFFLE)
Cal: 98   Carbs: 17 g   Chol: 1 mg   Fat: 1.7 g
Fiber: 2.4 g   Protein: 4.6 g   Sodium: 193 mg

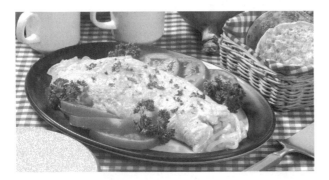

Country Morning Omelette

YIELD: 1 SERVING
1 tablespoon chopped green bell pepper
1 tablespoon chopped onion
3 tablespoons diced smoked sausage or kielbasa, at least 97% lean
1 tablespoon chopped tomato
½ cup fat-free egg substitute
3 tablespoons shredded nonfat or reduced fat Cheddar cheese
Ground paprika (garnish)

1. Coat an 8-inch nonstick skillet with nonstick cooking spray, and preheat over medium heat. Add the green pepper, onion, and sausage or kielbasa; cover; and cook, stirring frequently, for about 2 minutes, or until the vegetables start to soften and the sausage or kielbasa is lightly browned.

2. Add the tomato to the skillet, cover, and cook for about 15 seconds, or just until the tomato is heated through. Transfer the mixture to a warm bowl, and cover to keep warm.

3. Respray the skillet, and place over medium-low heat. Add the egg substitute, and cook without stirring for about 2 minutes, or until the eggs are set around the edges.

4. Use a spatula to lift the edges of the omelette, and allow the uncooked egg to flow below the cooked portion. Cook for another minute or 2, or until the eggs are almost set.

5. Arrange first the sausage mixture and then the cheese over half of the omelette. Fold the other half over the filling, and cook for another minute or 2, or until the cheese is melted and the eggs are completely set.

6. Slide the omelette onto a plate, sprinkle with the paprika, and serve hot.

NUTRITIONAL FACTS (PER SERVING)
Cal: 134   Carbs: 8 g   Chol: 11 mg   Fat: 0.8 g
Fiber: 0.5 g   Protein: 22 g   Sodium: 602 mg

Southwestern Omelette

YIELD: 1 SERVING

3 tablespoons diced ham, at least 97% lean

1 tablespoon chopped green bell pepper

1 tablespoon chopped onion

1/2 cup fat-free egg substitute

3 tablespoons shredded nonfat
or reduced-fat Cheddar cheese,
or 1 slice nonfat or reduced-fat Cheddar cheese

2 tablespoons chopped tomato
or picante sauce (garnish)

1. Coat an 8-inch nonstick skillet with nonstick cooking spray, and preheat over medium heat. Add the ham, green pepper, and onion; cover; and cook, stirring frequently, for about 2 minutes, or until the pepper and onion start to soften and the ham is lightly browned. Transfer the mixture to a warm bowl, and cover to keep warm.

2. Respray the skillet, and place over medium-low heat. Add the egg substitute, and let the eggs cook without stirring for about 2 minutes, or until set around the edges.

3. Use a spatula to lift the edges of the omelette, and allow the uncooked egg to flow below the cooked portion. Cook for another minute or 2, or until the eggs are almost set.

4. Arrange first the ham mixture and then the cheese over half of the omelette. Fold the other half over the filling, and cook for another minute or 2, or until the cheese is melted and the eggs are completely set.

5. Slide the omelette onto a plate, top with the tomatoes or picante sauce, and serve hot.

NUTRITIONAL FACTS (PER SERVING)
Cal: 132   Carbs: 7 g   Chol: 9 mg   Fat: 0.8 g
Fiber: 0.5 g   Protein: 23 g   Sodium: 626 mg

Glazed Onion Omelette

YIELD: 1 SERVING

1 small yellow onion, very thinly sliced

1/8 teaspoon dried thyme

Pinch salt

Pinch ground black pepper

1/2 cup fat-free egg substitute

1 1/2 teaspoons grated nonfat
or regular Parmesan cheese

1 slice extra-lean turkey bacon,
cooked, drained, and crumbled

2 tablespoons shredded nonfat or reduced-fat
mozzarella cheese

2 teaspoons finely chopped fresh parsley
or chives (garnish)

1. Coat an 8-inch nonstick skillet with olive oil cooking spray, and preheat over medium heat. Add the onion, thyme, salt, and pepper; cover; and cook, stirring occasionally, for about 3 minutes, or until the onions are wilted and just starting to brown. (If the skillet becomes too dry, add a few drops of water as needed.) Transfer the onion mixture to a warm bowl, and cover to keep warm.

2. Respray the skillet, and place over medium-low heat. Add the egg substitute, and cook without stirring for about 2 minutes, or until set around the edges.

3. Use a spatula to lift the edges of the omelette, and allow the uncooked egg to flow beneath the cooked portion. Cook for another minute or 2, or until the eggs are almost set.

4. Sprinkle the Parmesan over the top of the omelette. Then spread the onions over half of the omelette. Cover the onions with first the bacon and then the mozzarella. Fold the other half over the filling and cook for another minute or 2, or until the eggs are set and the cheese is melted.

5. Slide the omelette onto a plate, top with the parsley or chives, and serve hot.

NUTRITIONAL FACTS (PER SERVING)
Cal: 130   Carbs: 8 g   Chol: 24 mg   Fat: 0.6 g
Fiber: 1 g   Protein: 21 g   Sodium: 616 mg

Spinnaker Omelette

YIELD: 1 SERVING

2 tablespoons thinly sliced scallions

¼ cup (about 1½ ounces) cooked lump crab meat

½ cup fat-free egg substitute

3 tablespoons shredded nonfat or reduced-fat
Swiss cheese

Paprika (garnish)

1. Coat an 8-inch nonstick skillet with nonstick cooking spray, and heat over medium heat. Add the scallions, cover, and cook, stirring frequently, for a minute or 2, or until crisp-tender. (If the skillet becomes too dry, add a few drops of water as needed.)

2. Add the crab meat to the skillet, and cook uncovered for another minute, or until heated through. Transfer the scallion and crab mixture to a warm bowl, and cover to keep warm.

3. Respray the skillet, and place over medium-low heat. Add the egg substitute, and cook without stirring for about 2 minutes, or until the eggs are set around the edges.

4. Use a spatula to lift the edges of the omelette, and allow the uncooked egg to flow below the cooked portion. Cook for another minute or 2, or until the eggs are almost set.

5. Arrange first the the crab meat mixture and then the cheese over half of the omelette. Fold the other half over the filling, and cook for another minute or 2, or until the cheese is melted and the eggs are completely set.

6. Slide the omelette onto a plate, sprinkle with the paprika, and serve hot.

NUTRITIONAL FACTS (PER SERVING)
Cal: 130   Carbs: 4 g   Chol: 24 mg   Fat: 0.4 g
Fiber: 0.4 g   Protein: 25 g   Sodium: 496 mg

Bacon and Tomato Omelette

YIELD: 1 SERVING

½ cup fat-free egg substitute

Pinch ground black pepper

¼ cup chopped seeded plum tomato (about 1 medium)

1 slice extra-lean turkey bacon, cooked,
drained, and crumbled

3 tablespoons shredded nonfat or reduced-fat
mozzarella cheese

1 tablespoon finely chopped fresh parsley (garnish)

1. Coat an 8-inch nonstick skillet with nonstick cooking spray, and preheat over medium-low heat. Add the egg substitute, and cook without stirring for about 2 minutes, or until set around the edges. Sprinkle with the pepper.

2. Use a spatula to lift the edges of the omelette, and allow the uncooked egg to flow beneath the cooked portion. Cook for another minute or 2, or until the eggs are almost set.

3. Spread first the tomato and then the bacon and mozzarella over half of the omelette. Fold the other half over the filling and cook for another minute or 2, or until the eggs are set and the cheese is melted.

4. Slide the omelette onto a plate, sprinkle with the parsley, and serve hot.

NUTRITIONAL FACTS (PER SERVING)
Cal: 124   Carbs: 6 g   Chol: 22 mg   Fat: 0.7 g
Fiber: 0.5 g   Protein: 22 g   Sodium: 518 mg

Ham and Egg Scramble

YIELD: 4 SERVINGS

⅔ cup (about 3 ounces) diced ham, at least 97% lean

2 cups fat-free egg substitute

¼ cup plus 2 tablespoons shredded nonfat or
reduced-fat Cheddar cheese

1. Coat a 10-inch nonstick skillet with nonstick cooking spray, and preheat over medium-high heat. Add the ham and cook for 1 to 2 minutes, or until nicely browned.

2. Reduce the heat to medium-low, and pour the egg substitute over the ham. Cook without stirring for 3 to 4 minutes, or until the eggs are partially set. Stirring gently to scramble and continue to cook for another minute or 2, or until the eggs are almost set.

3. Sprinkle the cheese over the eggs, and cook and stir gently for 1 minute, or until the eggs are cooked but not dry and the cheese is melted. Serve hot.

NUTRITIONAL FACTS (PER SERVING)		
Cal: 100 Carbs: 3 g Chol: 7 mg Fat: 0.6 g		
Fiber: 0 g Protein: 19.6 g Sodium: 484 mg		

Artichoke and Roasted Red Pepper Omelette

YIELD: 1 SERVING

1/2 cup fat-free egg substitute

Pinch ground black pepper

Pinch dried Italian seasoning

1 1/2 teaspoons grated nonfat or regular Parmesan cheese

1/4 cup chopped frozen (thawed) or canned (drained) artichoke hearts

2 tablespoons chopped commercial roasted red pepper

2 tablespoons shredded nonfat or reduced-fat mozzarella or provolone cheese

1. Coat an 8-inch nonstick skillet with nonstick cooking spray, and preheat over medium-low heat. Add the egg substitute, and cook without stirring for about 2 minutes, or until set around the edges. Sprinkle with the pepper and Italian seasoning.

2. Use a spatula to lift the edges of the omelette, and allow the uncooked egg to flow beneath the cooked portion. Cook for another minute or 2, or until the eggs are almost set.

3. Sprinkle the Parmesan over the top of the omelette. Then spread first the artichokes and then the roasted pepper and cheese over half of the omelette. Fold the other half over the filling and cook for another minute or 2, or until the eggs are set and the cheese is melted.

4. Slide the omelette onto a plate, and serve hot.

NUTRITIONAL FACTS (PER SERVING)		
Cal: 113 Carbs: 8 g Chol: 3 mg Fat: 0.2 g		
Fiber: 2.8 g Protein: 19 g Sodium: 372 mg		

Ham and Mushroom Omelette

YIELD: 1 SERVING

3 tablespoons diced ham, at least 97% lean

1/2 cup sliced fresh mushrooms

1/2 cup fat-free egg substitute

Pinch ground black pepper

3 tablespoons shredded nonfat or reduced-fat mozzarella or Swiss cheese

1 tablespoon finely chopped fresh Italian parsley (garnish)

1. Coat an 8-inch nonstick skillet with olive oil cooking spray, and preheat over medium heat. Add the ham and mushrooms, and cook, stirring frequently, for about 3 minutes, or until nicely browned. Cover the skillet periodically if it begins to dry out. (The steam from the cooking mushrooms will moisten the skillet.) Transfer the ingredients to a warm bowl, and cover to keep warm.

2. Respray the skillet, and place over medium-low heat. Add the egg substitute, and cook without stirring for about 2 minutes, or until set around the edges. Sprinkle the pepper over the eggs.

3. Use a spatula to lift the edges of the omelette, and allow the uncooked egg to flow beneath the cooked portion. Cook for another minute or 2, or until the eggs are almost set.

4. Spread first the ham mixture and then the cheese over half of the omelette. Fold the other half over the filling and cook for another minute or 2, or until the eggs are set and the cheese is melted.

5. Slide the omelette onto a plate, sprinkle with the parsley, and serve hot.

NUTRITIONAL FACTS (PER SERVING)		
Cal: 132 Carbs: 5 g Chol: 9 mg Fat: 0.9 g		
Fiber: 0.5 g Protein: 25 g Sodium: 636 mg		

Mushroom and Mozzarella Frittata

YIELD: 4 SERVINGS

2 cups fat-free egg substitute

1/4 cup grated nonfat or regular Parmesan cheese

3 cups sliced fresh mushrooms

1/4 teaspoon dried thyme

1/4 teaspoon ground black pepper

3/4 cup shredded nonfat or reduced-fat mozzarella cheese

1. Place the egg substitute and Parmesan in a medium-sized bowl. Stir to mix well, and set aside.

2. Coat a 10-inch oven-proof skillet with olive oil cooking spray, and preheat over medium-high heat. Add the mushrooms, thyme, and pepper, and cook, stirring frequently, for about 4 minutes, or until the mushrooms start to brown and begin to release their juices. Cover the skillet periodically if it begins to dry out. (The steam from the cooking vegetables will moisten the skillet.) Spread the mushrooms evenly over the bottom of the skillet.

3. Reduce the heat to low, and pour the egg mixture over the mushrooms. Cook without stirring for 10 to 12 minutes, or until the eggs are almost set.

4. Place the skillet under a preheated broiler, and broil for about 3 minutes, or until the eggs are set but not dry.

5. Sprinkle the mozzarella over the frittata, and broil for an additional minute, or until the cheese has melted. Cut the frittata into wedges, and serve hot.

NUTRITIONAL FACTS (PER SERVING)
Cal: 128   Carbs: 9 g   Chol: 6 mg   Fat: 0.2 g
Fiber: 0.7 g   Protein: 22 g   Sodium: 441 mg

Potato Frittata

YIELD: 4 SERVINGS

1/3 cup chopped green bell pepper

1/3 cup chopped onion

1 teaspoon crushed fresh garlic

1 teaspoon dried Italian seasoning or fines herbes*

1/8 teaspoon ground black pepper

2 cups sliced cooked potatoes (about 2 medium)

2 cups fat-free egg substitute

1 tablespoon plus 1 teaspoon grated nonfat or regular Parmesan cheese

3/4 cup shredded nonfat or reduced-fat mozzarella cheese

* A blend of thyme, oregano, sage, rosemary, marjoram, and basil, fines herbes can be found in the dried spice section of most grocery stores.

1. Coat a 10-inch oven-proof skillet with nonstick cooking spray, and preheat over medium heat. Add the green pepper, onion, garlic, Italian seasoning or fines herbes, and pepper; cover; and cook, stirring occasionally, for about 2 minutes, or just until the vegetables are crisp-tender. Cover the skillet periodically if it begins to dry out. (The steam from the cooking vegetables will moisten the skillet.)

2. Add the potatoes to the skillet, and stir to mix well. Spread the mixture out to form an even layer over the bottom of the skillet.

3. Reduce the heat to low, and pour the egg substitute over the potato mixture. Cook for 10 to 12 minutes without stirring, or until the eggs are almost set.

4. Place the skillet under a preheated broiler, and broil for about 3 minutes, or until the eggs are set but not dry. Sprinkle first the Parmesan and then the mozzarella over the top, and broil for an additional minute, or until the cheese is melted and the top is nicely browned.

5. Cut the frittata into wedges, and serve hot.

NUTRITIONAL FACTS (PER SERVING)
Cal: 181   Carbs: 22 g   Chol: 3 mg   Fat: 0.3 g
Fiber: 2.2 g   Protein: 22 g   Sodium: 382 mg

Spring Vegetable Frittata

YIELD: 4 SERVINGS

1 cup 1-inch pieces fresh asparagus spears

1/3 cup chopped red bell pepper

1/3 cup chopped onion

1 teaspoon dried fines herbes* or dried thyme

1/4 teaspoon ground black pepper

1 cup diced cooked new potatoes (about 5 medium)

2 cups fat-free egg substitute

2 tablespoons grated nonfat
or regular Parmesan cheese

1 cup shredded nonfat or reduced-fat mozzarella
or provolone cheese

* A blend of thyme, oregano, sage, rosemary, marjoram, and basil, fines herbes can be found in the dried spice section of most grocery stores.

1. Coat a 10-inch oven-proof skillet with nonstick cooking spray, and preheat over medium heat. Add the asparagus, red pepper, onion, fines herbs or thyme, and pepper. Cover and cook, stirring occasionally, for about 3 minutes, or until the vegetables are crisp-tender. Add a few teaspoons of water if the skillet becomes too dry.

2. Add the potatoes to the skillet, and stir to mix. Cover and cook over medium heat for 1 minute, or until the mixture is heated through. Add a little water if the skillet becomes too dry.

3. Reduce the heat to low, and pour the egg substitute over the potato mixture. Cook without stirring for about 12 minutes, or until the eggs are almost set.

4. Place the skillet under a preheated broiler, and broil for about 3 minutes, or until the eggs are set but not dry. Sprinkle first the Parmesan and then the mozzarella or provolone over the top, and broil for another minute, or until the cheese is melted and lightly browned.

5. Cut the frittata into wedges, and serve hot.

NUTRITIONAL FACTS (PER SERVING)
Cal: 162   Carbs: 16 g   Chol: 5 mg   Fat: 0.3 g
Fiber: 1.9 g   Protein: 24 g   Sodium: 425 mg

Zucchini and Tomato Frittata

YIELD: 4 SERVINGS

2 cups fat-free egg substitute

1/4 cup grated nonfat or regular
Parmesan cheese

1 medium zucchini, halved lengthwise
and sliced 1/4-inch thick

1 medium yellow onion, cut into thin wedges

2 plum tomatoes, seeded and chopped

1 teaspoon dried basil

1/4 teaspoon ground black pepper

3/4 cup shredded nonfat
or reduced-fat mozzarella cheese

1. Place the egg substitute and Parmesan in a medium-sized bowl. Stir to mix well, and set aside.

2. Coat a 10-inch oven-proof skillet with nonstick cooking spray, and preheat over medium heat. Add the zucchini, onion, tomatoes, basil, and pepper, and stir-fry for about 4 minutes, or until the zucchini and onion are crisp-tender. Spread the mixture evenly over the bottom of the skillet.

3. Reduce the heat to low, and pour the egg mixture over the vegetables. Cook without stirring for 10 to 12 minutes, or until the eggs are almost set.

4. Place the skillet under a preheated broiler, and broil for about 3 minutes, or until the eggs are set but not dry. Sprinkle the mozzarella over the frittata, and broil for an additional minute, or until the cheese is melted and the top is nicely browned.

5. Cut the frittata into wedges, and serve hot.

NUTRITIONAL FACTS (PER SERVING)
Cal: 131   Carbs: 10 g   Chol: 6 mg   Fat: 0.2 g
Fiber: 1 g   Protein: 22 g   Sodium: 443 mg

Sausage, Pepper, and Onion Frittata

YIELD: 4 SERVINGS

2 cups fat-free egg substitute

3/4 cup shredded nonfat
or reduced-fat mozzarella cheese

8 ounces Turkey Italian Sausage (page 251)

1 small yellow onion, cut into thin wedges

1/2 medium red bell pepper, cut into thin strips

1/2 medium green bell pepper, cut into thin strips

1. Place the egg substitute and mozzarella in a medium-sized bowl. Stir to mix well, and set aside.

2. Coat a 10-inch oven-proof skillet with olive oil cooking spray, and preheat over medium heat. Add the sausage and cook, stirring to crumble, until the meat is no longer pink. (If the meat is very lean, there should be no fat to drain off.)

3. Add the onion and bell peppers to the skillet, and cook for 3 additional minutes, or until the vegetables are crisp-tender. Spread the mixture evenly over the bottom of the skillet.

4. Reduce the heat to low, and pour the egg mixture over the vegetables. Cook without stirring for 10 to 12 minutes, or until the eggs are almost set.

5. Place the skillet under a preheated broiler, and broil for about 3 minutes, or until the eggs are set but not dry and the top is nicely browned.

6. Cut the frittata into wedges, and serve hot.

NUTRITIONAL FACTS (PER SERVING)
Cal: 186   Carbs: 7 g   Chol: 37 mg   Fat: 2.2 g
Fiber: 1 g   Protein: 32 g   Sodium: 559 mg

Cottage Frittata

YIELD: 4 SERVINGS

1 1/2 cups fat-free egg substitute

3/4 cup nonfat or low-fat cottage cheese

1/8 teaspoon ground black pepper

1 small yellow onion, cut into thin wedges

1 teaspoon crushed fresh garlic

2 cups (packed) chopped fresh spinach

1/2 teaspoon dried thyme

1 1/2 cups diced cooked potato (about 1 large)

3/4 cup shredded nonfat or reduced-fat
mozzarella cheese or reduced-fat provolone cheese

1. Place the egg substitute, cottage cheese, and pepper in a medium-sized bowl. Stir to mix well, and set aside.

2. Coat a 10-inch oven-proof skillet with olive oil cooking spray, and preheat over medium heat. Add the onions, cover, and cook, stirring frequently, for about 2 minutes, or until the onions are crisp-tender.

3. Add the garlic, spinach, and thyme to the skillet, and stir-fry for about 1 minute, or until the spinach wilts. Add the potatoes, and stir to mix well. Spread the mixture evenly over the bottom of the skillet.

4. Reduce the heat to low, and pour the egg mixture over the potato mixture. Cook without stirring for about 12 minutes, or until the eggs are almost set.

5. Place the skillet under a preheated broiler, and broil for about 3 minutes, or until the eggs are set but not dry.

6. Sprinkle the cheese over the frittata, and broil for an additional minute, or until the cheese has melted. Let the frittata sit at room temperature for 5 minutes before cutting into wedges and serving.

NUTRITIONAL FACTS (PER SERVING)
Cal: 173   Carbs: 20 g   Chol: 5 mg   Fat: 0.3 g
Fiber: 2 g   Protein: 22 g   Sodium: 321 mg

Shrimp and Bacon Frittata

YIELD: 4 SERVINGS

2 cups fat-free egg substitute

¾ cup grated nonfat
or reduced-fat mozzarella cheese

1 medium yellow onion, cut into thin wedges

½ teaspoon dried Italian seasoning

⅛ teaspoon ground black pepper

5 ounces diced cooked shrimp (about 1 cup)

3 strips extra-lean turkey bacon, cooked,
drained, and crumbled

1. Place the egg substitute and mozzarella in a medium-sized bowl. Stir to mix well, and set aside.

2. Coat a 10-inch oven-proof skillet with olive oil cooking spray, and preheat over medium heat. Add the onion, Italian seasoning, and pepper; cover; and cook, stirring frequently, for about 4 minutes, or until the onion is crisp-tender.

3. Add the shrimp and bacon to the skillet. Stir to mix well, and spread the mixture evenly over the bottom of the skillet.

4. Reduce the heat to low, and pour the egg mixture over the onion mixture. Cook without stirring for 10 to 12 minutes, or until the eggs are almost set.

5. Place the skillet under a preheated broiler, and broil for about 3 minutes, or until the eggs are set but not dry and the top is nicely browned.

6. Cut the frittata into wedges, and serve hot.

NUTRITIONAL FACTS (PER SERVING)
Cal: 150   Carbs: 5 g   Chol: 86 mg   Fat: 0.8 g
Fiber: 0.3 g   Protein: 28 g   Sodium: 560 mg

Spinach and Ham Frittata

YIELD: 4 SERVINGS

2 cups fat-free egg substitute

2 teaspoons Dijon mustard

1 teaspoon crushed fresh garlic

2 cups (packed) chopped fresh spinach

4 ounces ham, at least 97% lean,
or Canadian bacon, diced

1 cup shredded nonfat
or reduced-fat mozzarella cheese

1. Place the egg substitute in a small bowl. Whisk in the mustard, and set aside.

2. Coat a 10-inch oven-proof skillet with olive oil cooking spray, and preheat over medium heat. Add the garlic, and stir-fry for about 30 seconds, or just until the garlic begins to turn color.

3. Add the spinach and ham to the skillet, and stir-fry for about 1 minute, or until the spinach begins to wilt. Spread the mixture evenly over the bottom of the skillet.

4. Reduce the heat to low, and pour the egg mixture over the spinach mixture. Cook without stirring for 10 to 12 minutes, or until the eggs are almost set.

5. Place the skillet under a preheated broiler, and broil for about 3 minutes, or until the eggs are set but not dry.

6. Sprinkle the mozzarella over the frittata, and broil for an additional minute, or until the cheese has melted. Cut the frittata into wedges, and serve hot.

NUTRITIONAL FACTS (PER SERVING)
Cal: 141   Carbs: 5.5 g   Chol: 20 mg   Fat: 0.9 g
Fiber: 0.8 g   Protein: 26.5 g   Sodium: 641 mg

Zucchini-Wild Rice Quiche

YIELD: 6 SERVINGS

2 cups zucchini sliced 1/4-inch thick
(about 2 medium)

1/3 cup chopped red bell pepper

1 teaspoon crushed fresh garlic

1 teaspoon dried Italian seasoning

1/8 teaspoon ground black pepper

1 cup shredded nonfat or reduced-fat
mozzarella cheese

1 cup fat-free egg substitute

1 cup evaporated skim milk

2 tablespoons unbleached flour

1 tablespoon nonfat Parmesan cheese*

CRUST

1 1/2 cups cooked wild rice

2 tablespoons grated Parmesan cheese*

1 tablespoon fat-free egg substitute

* In this recipe, use regular Parmesan cheese, not a fat-free product.

1. Coat a large nonstick skillet with nonstick cooking spray, and preheat over medium heat. Add the zucchini, red pepper, garlic, Italian seasoning, and black pepper. Cover, and, stirring occasionally, cook for about 5 minutes, or until the vegetables are crisp-tender. Add a little water if the skillet gets too dry. Remove the skillet from the heat, and let the vegetables cool slightly. Drain off any liquid, and set aside.

2. To make the crust, place the rice, Parmesan cheese, and egg substitute in a medium-sized bowl, and stir to mix well. Coat a 9-inch deep dish pie pan with nonstick cooking spray, and place the mixture in the pan. Using the back of a spoon, pat the mixture over the bottom and sides of the pan, forming an even crust.

3. Add the mozzarella to the zucchini mixture, and toss to mix well. Spread the mixture evenly over the crust.

4. Place the egg substitute, evaporated milk, and flour in a blender, and process until well mixed. Pour the egg mixture over the vegetables, and sprinkle with the Parmesan cheese.

5. Bake uncovered at 375°F for 45 minutes, or until the top is golden brown and a sharp knife inserted in the center of the quiche comes out clean. Allow to cool at room temperature for 10 minutes before cutting into wedges and serving.

NUTRITIONAL FACTS (PER SERVING)
Cal: 156   Carbs: 18 g   Chol: 6 mg   Fat: 1.2 g
Fiber: 1.5 g   Protein: 17 g   Sodium: 343 mg

Sausage and Potato Strata

YIELD: 6 SERVINGS

3 cups sliced cooked potatoes (about 3 medium)

1 1/4 cups shredded nonfat
or reduced-fat Cheddar cheese

1 cup (about 6 ounces) diced smoked sausage
or kielbasa, at least 97% lean,
or 8 ounces Turkey Breakfast Sausage
(page 56), cooked, crumbled, and drained

1 1/4 cups evaporated skim milk

1 1/4 cups fat-free egg substitute

1. Coat an 8-inch (2-quart) square baking pan with nonstick cooking spray, and arrange half of the potatoes over the bottom of the pan, slightly overlapping the slices. Sprinkle half of the cheese and then half of the sausage over the potatoes.

2. Place the evaporated milk and egg substitute in a medium-sized bowl, and whisk to mix well. Pour half of the egg mixture over the potato, cheese, and sausage layers. Repeat all of the layers.

3. Bake uncovered at 350°F for about 1 hour, or until the top is nicely browned and a sharp knife inserted in the center of the dish comes out clean. Remove the dish from the oven, and let sit for 15 minutes before cutting into squares and serving.

NUTRITIONAL FACTS (PER SERVING)
Cal: 196   Carbs: 24 g   Chol: 17 mg   Fat: 0.9 g
Fiber: 1 g   Protein: 22.3 g   Sodium: 557 mg

Spinach and Bacon Quiche

YIELD: 6 SERVINGS

4 slices extra-lean turkey bacon

1/2 cup chopped onion

2 cups (packed) chopped fresh spinach

1 1/4 cups shredded nonfat or reduced-fat mozzarella cheese

1 tablespoon plus 1 teaspoon unbleached flour

1/8 teaspoon ground black pepper

1 1/4 cups fat-free egg substitute

1 cup evaporated skim milk

2 medium baking potatoes, scrubbed

1 tablespoon grated Parmesan cheese*

Nonstick cooking spray

* In this recipe, use regular Parmesan cheese, not a fat-free product.

1. Arrange the bacon slices in a large nonstick skillet, and cook for 2 minutes over medium heat. Turn and cook for 2 or 3 additional minutes, or until crisp and brown. Transfer the bacon to paper towels, and set aside to drain.

2. Place the same skillet over medium heat, and add the onion. Cover and cook, stirring frequently, for about 3 minutes, or until the onion is crisp-tender. Add a little water if the skillet becomes too dry. Add the spinach, and stir-fry for another minute or 2, or until the spinach is wilted. Remove the skillet from the heat, and set aside to cool slightly.

3. Place the cheese, flour, and pepper in a large bowl, and toss to mix well. Add the egg substitute and evaporated milk, and stir to mix well. Stir in the spinach and onion. Crumble the bacon, and add to the egg mixture. Set aside.

4. Coat a 9-inch deep dish pie pan with nonstick cooking spray. Slice the unpeeled potatoes 1/4-inch thick, and arrange the slices in a single layer over the bottom and sides of the pan to form a crust. Pour the egg mixture into the crust, and sprinkle with the Parmesan cheese. Spray the exposed edges of the potatoes lightly with cooking spray.

5. Bake uncovered at 375°F for 45 to 50 minutes, or until the top is golden brown and a sharp knife inserted in the center of the quiche comes out clean. Allow to cool at room temperature for 10 minutes before cutting into wedges and serving.

NUTRITIONAL FACTS (PER SERVING)
Cal: 175   Carbs: 21 g   Chol: 18 mg   Fat: 0.9 g
Fiber: 1.9 g   Protein: 20 g   Sodium: 429 mg

Creamy Richness Without the Cream

To make creamy quiches, casseroles, sauces, custards, puddings, and other dishes without the usual cream, simply replace this high-fat ingredient with an equal amount of evaporated skim milk. Or use 7/8 cup of regular skim milk mixed with 1/3 cup of instant nonfat dry milk powder for each cup of cream. In many quiches and casseroles, you can also replace cream with nonfat or low-fat cottage cheese. For a firmer, richer texture, add a tablespoon of flour to the filling for each cup of cream substitute that you use.

Replacing just one cup of heavy cream with any of these healthful nonfat dairy products saves you over 600 calories and 88 grams of fat. As a bonus, the substitute ingredients add calcium and other nutrients to your dish.

Shrimp and Asparagus Quiche

YIELD: 6 SERVINGS

1 cup (about 5 ounces) diced cooked shrimp or crab meat

1 cup shredded nonfat or reduced-fat mozzarella or Swiss cheese

1 tablespoon unbleached flour

1 cup fat-free egg substitute

1 cup evaporated skim milk

1½ teaspoons Dijon mustard

12 fresh asparagus spears, each 4 inches long

1 tablespoon grated Parmesan cheese*

CRUST

1½ cups cooked brown rice

2 tablespoons grated Parmesan cheese*

1 tablespoon fat-free egg substitute

* In this recipe, use regular Parmesan cheese, not a fat-free product.

1. To make the crust, place the rice, Parmesan cheese, and egg substitute in a medium-sized bowl, and stir to mix well. Coat a 9-inch deep dish pie pan with nonstick cooking spray, and place the mixture in the pan. Using the back of a spoon, pat the mixture over the bottom and sides of the pan, forming an even crust. Set aside.

2. Place the shrimp or crab meat, mozzarella or Swiss cheese, and flour in a large bowl, and stir to mix well. Add the egg substitute, milk, and mustard, and stir to mix well. Pour the egg mixture into the crust.

3. Arrange the asparagus spears on top of the quiche like the spokes of a wheel, with the tips pointing outward. Sprinkle with the Parmesan cheese.

4. Bake uncovered at 375°F for 50 minutes, or until the top is golden brown and a sharp knife inserted in the center of the quiche comes out clean. Allow to cool at room temperature for 10 minutes before cutting into wedges and serving.

NUTRITIONAL FACTS (PER SERVING)
Cal: 188   Carbs: 20 g   Chol: 52 mg   Fat: 1.9 g
Fiber: 1.7 g   Protein: 22 g   Sodium: 428 mg

Broccoli Quiche in Potato Crust

YIELD: 5 SERVINGS

1 package (10 ounces) frozen chopped broccoli, thawed and squeezed dry

1 cup shredded nonfat or reduced-fat Cheddar or Swiss cheese

1 cup nonfat or low-fat cottage cheese

1 cup fat-free egg substitute

¼ cup finely chopped onion

1½ teaspoons Dijon mustard

1 tablespoon unbleached flour

⅛ teaspoon ground black pepper

2 medium potatoes, scrubbed

Nonstick cooking spray

1. Place all of the ingredients except for the potatoes and cooking spray in a large bowl, and stir to mix well. Set aside.

2. Coat a 9-inch deep dish pie pan with nonstick cooking spray. Slice the potatoes ¼-inch thick, and arrange the slices in a single layer over the bottom and sides of the pan to form a crust. Pour the broccoli mixture into the crust. Spray the exposed edges of the potatoes lightly with cooking spray.

3. Bake at 375°F for about 45 minutes, or until the top is golden brown and a sharp knife inserted in the center of the quiche comes out clean. Allow to cool at room temperature for 5 minutes before cutting into wedges and serving.

NUTRITIONAL FACTS (PER SERVING)
Cal: 175   Carbs: 21 g   Chol: 6 mg   Fat: 0.9 g
Fiber: 3 g   Protein: 19 g   Sodium: 458 mg

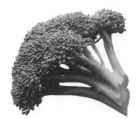

Potato-Crusted Sausage Quiche

YIELD: 5 SERVINGS

1½ cups fat-free egg substitute

1 cup nonfat or low-fat cottage cheese

1 tablespoon unbleached flour

⅛ teaspoon ground black pepper

½ teaspoon Tabasco pepper sauce

1 cup shredded nonfat
or reduced-fat Cheddar cheese

1 cup (about 6 ounces) diced smoked sausage
or kielbasa, at least 97% lean,
or 8 ounces Turkey Breakfast Sausage
(page 56), cooked, crumbled, and drained

2 scallions, finely chopped

2 medium potatoes, scrubbed

Nonstick cooking spray

1. Place the egg substitute, cottage cheese, flour, pepper, and Tabasco sauce in a large bowl, and stir to mix well. Stir in the cheese, sausage, and scallions. Set aside.

2. Coat a 9-inch deep dish pie pan with nonstick cooking spray. Slice the unpeeled potatoes ¼ inch thick, and arrange the slices in a single layer over the bottom and sides of the pan to form a crust. Pour the egg mixture into the crust. Spray the exposed edges of the potatoes lightly with cooking spray.

3. Bake uncovered at 375°F for 45 to 50 minutes, or until a sharp knife inserted in the center of the quiche comes out clean. Allow to cool at room temperature for 5 minutes before cutting into wedges and serving.

NUTRITIONAL FACTS (PER SERVING)
Cal: 203   Carbs: 20 g   Chol: 18 mg   Fat: 1 g
Fiber: 1.8 g   Protein: 27 g   Sodium: 720 mg

Ham and Swiss Quiche

YIELD: 6 SERVINGS

1 cup shredded nonfat or reduced-fat Swiss cheese

1 cup (about 5 ounces) diced ham,
at least 97% lean

3 tablespoons finely chopped onion

2 tablespoons finely chopped fresh parsley

1 tablespoon plus 1 teaspoon unbleached flour

⅛ teaspoon ground black pepper

Pinch ground nutmeg

1¼ cups fat-free egg substitute

1 cup nonfat or low-fat cottage cheese

1 tablespoon grated Parmesan cheese*

CRUST
1½ cups cooked brown rice

2 tablespoons grated Parmesan cheese*

1 tablespoon fat-free egg substitute

* In this recipe, use regular Parmesan cheese, not a fat-free product.

1. To make the crust, place the rice, Parmesan cheese, and egg substitute in a medium-sized bowl, and stir to mix well. Coat a 9-inch deep dish pie pan with nonstick cooking spray, and place the mixture in the pan. Using the back of a large spoon, pat the mixture over the bottom and sides of the pan, forming an even crust. Set aside.

2. Place the Swiss cheese, ham, onion, parsley, flour, pepper, and nutmeg in a large bowl, and toss to mix well. Add the egg substitute and cottage cheese, and stir to mix well. Pour the egg mixture into the crust, and sprinkle with the Parmesan cheese.

3. Bake uncovered at 375°F for 45 minutes, or until the top is golden brown and a sharp knife inserted in the center of the quiche comes out clean. Allow to cool at room temperature for 10 minutes before cutting into wedges and serving.

NUTRITIONAL FACTS (PER SERVING)
Cal: 178   Carbs: 17 g   Chol: 14 mg   Fat: 2 g
Fiber: 1.1 g   Protein: 22 g   Sodium: 640 mg

Sicilian Mushroom and Onion Quiche

YIELD: 6 SERVINGS

1¾ cups sliced fresh mushrooms

1 medium yellow onion, sliced into thin wedges

1 cup shredded nonfat or reduced-fat mozzarella cheese

1 tablespoon unbleached flour

1 cup fat-free egg substitute

1 cup evaporated skim milk

1 tablespoon grated Parmesan cheese*

CRUST

1½ cups cooked orzo pasta (about ½ cup dry)

2 tablespoons grated Parmesan cheese*

1 tablespoon fat-free egg substitute

* In this recipe, use regular Parmesan cheese, not a fat-free brand.

1. Coat a large nonstick skillet with nonstick cooking spray, and preheat over medium heat. Add the mushrooms and onion. Cover the skillet, and cook over medium heat, stirring occasionally, for about 5 minutes, or until the vegetables are tender. (Add a few teaspoons of water if the skillet becomes too dry.) Remove the skillet from the heat, and let the vegetables cool slightly. Drain off any liquid, and set aside.

2. To make the crust, place the orzo, Parmesan cheese, and egg substitute in a medium-sized bowl, and stir to mix well. Coat a 9-inch deep dish pie pan with nonstick cooking spray, and place the mixture in the pan. Using the back of a spoon, pat the mixture over the bottom and sides of the pan, forming an even crust. Set aside.

3. Place the mozzarella cheese and flour in a large bowl, and toss to mix well. Add the mushroom mixture, and toss to mix well. Add the egg substitute and evaporated milk, and stir to mix well. Spread the mixture evenly over the crust, and sprinkle with the Parmesan cheese.

4. Bake uncovered at 375°F for 45 minutes, or until the top is golden brown and a sharp knife inserted in the center of the quiche comes out clean. Allow to cool at room temperature for 10 minutes before cutting into wedges and serving.

NUTRITIONAL FACTS (PER SERVING)

Cal: 185   Carbs: 24 g   Chol: 6 mg   Fat: 1.4 g
Fiber: 1.3 g   Protein: 18 g   Sodium: 342 mg

Chili-Cheese Quiche

YIELD: 6 SERVINGS

2 cans (4 ounces each) whole mild green chilies, drained

1 cup shredded nonfat or reduced-fat Cheddar or Monterey jack cheese

1 cup fat-free egg substitute

1 cup evaporated skim milk

1 tablespoon unbleached flour

½ teaspoon ground cumin

⅛ teaspoon ground black pepper

CRUST

2 cups cooked brown rice

2 tablespoons fat-free egg substitute

1. To make the crust, place the rice and egg substitute in a medium-sized bowl, and stir to mix well. Coat a 10-inch pie pan with nonstick cooking spray, and place the mixture in the pan. Using the back of a spoon, pat the mixture over the bottom and sides of the pan, forming an even crust. Set aside.

2. Cut the chilies open, lay them flat, and arrange half of them in a single layer over the rice crust. Sprinkle half of the cheese over the chilies. Arrange the remaining chilies over the cheese, and finish with a layer of the remaining cheese.

3. Place the egg substitute, evaporated milk, flour, cumin, and pepper in a blender, and process until well mixed. Pour the egg mixture over the chili-cheese layers.

4. Bake uncovered at 375°F for 40 minutes, or until the top is golden brown and a sharp knife inserted in the center of the quiche comes out clean. Allow to cool at room temperature for 10 minutes before cutting into wedges and serving.

NUTRITIONAL FACTS (PER SERVING)

Cal: 172   Carbs: 25 g   Chol: 3 mg   Fat: 0.7 g
Fiber: 2.3 g   Protein: 15.5 g   Sodium: 362 mg

Breakfast Burritos

YIELD: 4 SERVINGS

¼ cup finely chopped onion
½ cup (about 2½ ounces) diced ham, at least 97% lean
3 tablespoons drained canned chopped green chilies
1¼ cups fat-free egg substitute
4 flour tortillas (8-inch rounds)
¼ cup plus 2 tablespoons fat-free or reduced-fat Cheddar cheese
¼ cup picante sauce (optional)

1. Coat a large nonstick skillet with nonstick cooking spray, and preheat over medium heat. Add the onion and ham, cover, and cook, stirring frequently, for about 2 minutes, or until the onion is crisp-tender. Add the chilies, and stir to mix well.

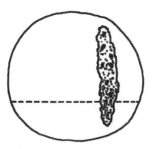

a. Arrange the filling along the right side of the tortilla.

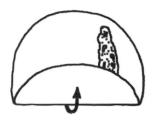

b. Fold up the bottom edge of the tortilla.

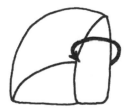

c. Fold the right side over the filling.

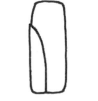

d. Continue folding to form a roll.

MAKING BREAKFAST BURRITOS

2. Pour the egg substitute over the onion mixture, and reduce the heat to medium-low. Cook uncovered without stirring for about 5 minutes, or until the eggs are almost set. Stirring gently to scramble, continue to cook for another minute or 2, or until the eggs are cooked but not dry.

3. While the eggs are cooking, warm the tortillas according to the manufacturer's directions.

4. Arrange the warm tortillas on a flat surface. Place a quarter of the egg mixture along the right side of each tortilla, stopping 1½ inches from the bottom. Top the eggs with 1½ tablespoons of the cheese and, if desired, 1 tablespoon of the picante sauce.

5. Fold the bottom edge of each tortilla up about 1 inch. (This fold will prevent the filling from falling out.) Then, beginning at the right edge, roll each tortilla up jelly-roll style. Serve hot.

NUTRITIONAL FACTS (PER SERVING)
Cal: 208   Carbs: 28 g   Chol: 6 mg   Fat: 2.5 g
Fiber: 2 g   Protein: 17 g   Sodium: 595 mg

Polenta Porridge

YIELD: 4 SERVINGS

2½ cups water
2½ cups skim or low-fat milk
1 cup polenta, coarsely ground cornmeal, or yellow corn grits
½ cup golden raisins

1. Place the water and milk in a 3-quart pot. Stir in the polenta, cornmeal, or grits, and bring to a boil over medium heat, stirring frequently.

2. Reduce the heat to low, cover, and simmer, stirring every few minutes, for about 15 minutes, or until the mixture is thick and creamy. Add the raisins during the last few minutes of cooking.

3. Serve hot, topped with honey or maple syrup, if desired.

NUTRITIONAL FACTS (PER 1⅛-CUP SERVING)
Cal: 252   Carbs: 52.4 g   Chol: 2 mg   Fat: 0.8 g
Fiber: 5.1 g   Protein: 9.3 g   Sodium: 81 mg

Southern Breakfast Bake

YIELD: 5 SERVINGS
$1/2$ cup water
$1/3$ cup quick-cooking yellow grits
1 can (12 ounces) evaporated skim milk
$3/4$ cup fat-free egg substitute
1 teaspoon dry mustard
$1/2$ teaspoon Tabasco pepper sauce
1 cup (about 5 ounces) diced ham, at least 97% lean
1 cup fat-free or reduced-fat shredded Cheddar cheese
2 tablespoons finely chopped scallions

1. Place the water in a $1^1/2$-quart pot, and bring to a boil over high heat. Reduce the heat to low, and whisk in the grits. Cook and stir for 2 minutes, or until the mixture is very thick.

2. Remove the pot from the heat, and slowly whisk in the evaporated milk. Whisk in the egg substitute, mustard, and Tabasco sauce. Stir in the ham, cheese, and scallions.

3. Coat a 9-inch deep dish pie pan with nonstick cooking spray, and pour the mixture into the pan. Bake uncovered at 375°F for 40 to 45 minutes, or until a sharp knife inserted in the center of the dish comes out clean.

4. Remove the dish from the oven, and let sit for 10 minutes before cutting into wedges and serving.

NUTRITIONAL FACTS (PER SERVING)
Cal: 176   Carbs: 19 g   Chol: 12 mg   Fat: 1 g
Fiber: 0.5 g   Protein: 23 g   Sodium: 583 mg

Baked Breakfast Polenta

YIELD: 16 SLICES
3 cups water
3 cups skim or low-fat milk
2 cups polenta, coarsely ground yellow cornmeal, or yellow corn grits
$1/2$ teaspoon salt
Nonstick butter-flavored cooking spray
$1/2$ cup fat-free egg substitute
$3/4$ cup plus 2 tablespoons toasted wheat germ

1. Place the water, milk, polenta, and salt in a 4-quart pot, and bring to a boil over high heat, stirring frequently. Reduce the heat to low, cover, and simmer, stirring every few minutes, for about 15 minutes, or until the polenta is very thick and begins to pull away from the sides of the pan when stirred.

2. Coat a 9-x-4-inch loaf pan with nonstick butter-flavored cooking spray, and spread the hot polenta evenly in the pan. Cover and refrigerate for several hours or overnight, or until the polenta is firm enough to slice.

3. When ready to prepare the dish, unmold the polenta onto a cutting board, and slice into eighteen $1/2$-inch-thick slices. Place the egg substitute in a shallow bowl, and place the wheat germ in another shallow bowl.

4. Dip each polenta slice first in the egg substitute, and then in the wheat germ, turning to coat each side. Coat a large baking sheet with the cooking spray, and arrange the slices on the sheet. Spray the tops lightly with the cooking spray.

5. Bake at 400°F for 15 to 20 minutes, or until the polenta is hot on the inside and golden brown on the outside. Serve hot, topped with Honey-Orange Syrup (page 34), maple syrup, or honey.

NUTRITIONAL FACTS (PER SLICE)
Cal: 116   Carbs: 21 g   Chol: 0 mg   Fat: 0.9 g
Fiber: 3.1 g   Protein: 5.8 g   Sodium: 103 mg

California Crunch Granola

2 cups old-fashioned oats*

1/2 cup oat bran

3/4 teaspoon ground cinnamon

1/2 cup chopped almonds, hazelnuts, or pecans (optional)

1/4 cup honey

3 tablespoons frozen (thawed) white grape juice concentrate

2 tablespoons light brown sugar

1/4 cup plus 2 tablespoons golden raisins or chopped dates

1/4 cup plus 2 tablespoons chopped dried apricots or dried cherries

* Look for oats that cook in 5 minutes.

1. Place the oats, oat bran, cinnamon, and nuts, if desired, in a medium-sized bowl, and stir to mix well. In a small bowl, stir together the honey, juice concentrate, and brown sugar. Add the honey mixture to the oat mixture, and stir until moist and crumbly.

2. Coat a nonstick 9-x-13-inch pan with nonstick cooking spray, and spread the mixture evenly in the pan. Bake at 325°F for about 30 minutes, or until the mixture is golden brown. Stir after the first 15 minutes of baking, and then every 5 minutes until done.

3. Remove the pan from the oven, stir in the dried fruits, and allow the granola to cool to room temperature. (As the granola cools, it will become crisp.) Transfer the mixture to an airtight container, and store for up to 1 month.

NUTRITIONAL FACTS (PER 1/2-CUP SERVING)
Cal: 176   Carbs: 39 g   Chol: 0 mg   Fat: 1.7 g
Fiber: 3.8 g   Protein: 4.8 g   Sodium: 3 mg

Cinnamon Apple-Raisin Granola

1 1/2 cups old-fashioned oats*

1/4 cup plus 2 tablespoons wheat bran

1/4 cup plus 2 tablespoons oat bran

1 teaspoon ground cinnamon

1/2 cup chopped pecans or walnuts (optional)

1/4 cup frozen (thawed) apple juice concentrate

3 tablespoons maple syrup or honey

2 tablespoons light brown sugar

3/4 cup dark raisins

* Look for oats that cook in 5 minutes.

1. Place the oats, wheat bran, oat bran, cinnamon, and nuts, if desired, in a medium-sized bowl, and stir to mix well. In a small bowl, stir together the juice concentrate, maple syrup or honey, and brown sugar. Add the apple juice mixture to the oat mixture, and stir until moist and crumbly.

2. Coat a nonstick 9-x-13-inch pan with nonstick cooking spray, and spread the mixture evenly in the pan. Bake at 325°F for about 30 minutes, or until the mixture is golden brown. Stir after the first 15 minutes of baking, and then after every 5 minutes until done.

3. Remove the pan from the oven, stir in the raisins, and allow the granola to cool to room temperature. (As the granola cools, it will become crisp.) Transfer the mixture to an airtight container, and store for up to 1 month.

NUTRITIONAL FACTS (PER 1/2-CUP SERVING)
Cal: 184   Carbs: 40 g   Chol: 0 mg   Fat: 1.6 g
Fiber: 4.4 g   Protein: 4.6 g   Sodium: 6 mg

Buttermilk Biscuits With Country Sausage Gravy

YIELD: 5 SERVINGS
2 cups skim or low-fat milk, divided
1/4 cup unbleached flour
1/4 cup instant nonfat dry milk powder
8 ounces Turkey Breakfast Sausage (below)
1/4 teaspoon salt
Pinch ground white pepper
5 Buttermilk Drop Biscuits (page 70)

1. Place 1/2 cup of the milk and all of the flour and dry milk powder in a jar with a tight-fitting lid. Shake until smooth, and set aside.

2. Coat a large nonstick skillet with nonstick cook-ing spray, and preheat over medium heat. Add the sausage, and cook, stirring to crumble, until the meat is no longer pink.

3. Add the remaining 1 1/2 cups of milk to the skillet, and stir in the salt and pepper. Cook, stirring frequently, until the milk begins to boil. Slowly stir in the flour mixture, and continue to cook, stirring constantly, for another minute or 2, or until the mixture is thickened and bubbly.

4. To serve, split each biscuit open, and arrange 2 biscuit halves on each of 5 individual serving plates, cut sides up. Spoon some of the gravy over the biscuits, and serve hot.

NUTRITIONAL FACTS
(PER 1 BISCUIT AND 1/2 CUP GRAVY)
Cal: 236   Carbs: 28 g   Chol: 31 mg   Fat: 4.5 g
Fiber: 0.4 g   Protein: 18.7 g   Sodium: 461 mg

Making Your Own Breakfast Sausage

For many people, the best part of breakfast is the spicy sausage patty that accompanies their eggs, waffles, or pancakes. Usually, though, that innocent-looking patty is packed with fat and calories. Is there a solution to this dilemma? The following mixture—which is so versatile, yet so low in fat—can be formed into delicious breakfast patties, used to make a creamy country-style gravy, or stirred into a tantalizing quiche. You'll never miss the extra calories!

Turkey Breakfast Sausage

YIELD: 6 SERVINGS
1 pound ground turkey, 96%–93% lean, or ground pork sirloin
2 teaspoons dried sage
1 1/2 teaspoons ham-flavored bouillon granules
1/2 teaspoon dried thyme
1/4 teaspoon ground black pepper
1/8 teaspoon cayenne pepper or crushed red pepper (optional)

1. Place all of the ingredients in a medium-sized bowl, and mix well. Cover and refrigerate for several hours to blend the flavors.

2. To make breakfast patties, shape the mixture into 6 (3-inch) patties. Coat a large skillet with nonstick cooking spray, and preheat over medium-low heat. Arrange the patties in the skillet and cook for 4 minutes on each side, or until browned and no longer pink inside. To precook before adding to other dishes, coat a large skillet with nonstick cooking spray, and preheat over medium heat. Add the sausage, and cook, stirring to crumble, until the meat is no longer pink. Then drain on paper towels and use as desired.

NUTRITIONAL FACTS (PER SERVING)
Cal: 101   Carbs: 0 g   Chol: 46 mg   Fat: 2.8 g
Fiber: 0 g   Protein: 17.6 g   Sodium: 226 mg

Creamy Rice Cereal

*This hearty breakfast cereal is a nutritious
alternative to refined cereals like farina or cream of
wheat. For variety, substitute millet for the rice.*

YIELD: 4 SERVINGS
1 cup brown rice
2 cups skim or low-fat milk
2 cups water

1. Place the rice in a blender or food processor, and
process at medium speed for 1 minute, or until it has
the texture of cornmeal.

2. Place the processed rice, milk, and water in a 2-
quart pot, and cook over medium heat, stirring frequently, until the mixture begins to boil. Reduce the
heat to low, cover, and simmer, stirring every couple
of minutes, for about 10 minutes, or until the mixture
is thick and creamy. Add a little more water or milk
during the last few minutes of cooking if necessary.

3. Serve hot, topped with a little honey, brown
sugar, or maple syrup and a sprinkling of raisins or
chopped dried fruit, if desired.

NUTRITIONAL FACTS (PER 1-CUP SERVING)
Cal: 213   Carbs: 42 g   Chol: 2 mg   Fat: 1.5 g
Fiber: 1.7 g   Protein: 7.9 g   Sodium: 66 mg

Cinnamon-Apple
Oatmeal

YIELD: 4 SERVINGS
2 cups old-fashioned oats*
3 cups water
1 cup unsweetened apple juice
1 cup chopped peeled apple (about 1 large)
1/4 cup dark raisins
3/4 teaspoon ground cinnamon

* Look for oats that cook in 5 minutes.

1. Place all of the ingredients in a 2-quart pot, and
stir to mix well. Bring to a boil over high heat. Then
reduce the heat to low, cover, and simmer, stirring
occasionally, until the oats are tender and the liquid
has been absorbed. (Depending on the thickness of
the oats, this will take from 5 to 15 minutes.)

2. Serve hot, topped with a little maple syrup or
brown sugar and some skim or low-fat milk, if
desired.

NUTRITIONAL FACTS (PER 1-CUP SERVING)
Cal: 234   Carbs: 50 g   Chol: 0 mg   Fat: 2.6 g
Fiber: 5.2 g   Protein: 6.8 g   Sodium: 5 mg

Fruit Muesli

*This supernutritious breakfast cereal
is a snap to make.*

YIELD: 6 CUPS
2 1/2 cups old-fashioned oats*
3/4 cup barley nugget cereal
3/4 cup honey crunch wheat germ
1/2 cup dark raisins or chopped dates
1/2 cup chopped dried apricots
1/2 cup chopped dried peaches or cranberries
1/2 cup chopped pecans, hazelnuts, walnuts, or almonds (optional)

* Look for oats that cook in 5 minutes.

1. Place all of the ingredients in a large bowl, and
stir to mix well. Transfer to an airtight container, and
store for up to 4 weeks.

2. To serve, place 1/2 cup of muesli in an individual
serving bowl, and add 3/4 cup of low-fat milk, nonfat
vanilla or plain yogurt, or applesauce. Stir, and let sit
for 5 minutes before serving.

NUTRITIONAL FACTS
(PER 1/2-CUP SERVING, CEREAL ONLY)
Cal: 159   Carbs: 30 g   Chol: 0 mg   Fat: 1.7 g
Fiber: 4.4 g   Protein: 6 g   Sodium: 49 mg

3. The Healthy Bread Basket

Bread is often called the staff of life. Acknowledging the goodness of this food, nutritionists recommend six to eleven servings of breads and other grain products daily. Unfortunately, most muffins, quick breads, biscuits, and other baked goods do nothing to promote good health. Why? Most are made with unhealthy amounts of butter, oil, and other high-fat ingredients. To make matters worse, most contain only nutrient-poor refined flours. The good news is that baked goods can be prepared with little or no fat, and can contain a wide range of wholesome, high-nutrient ingredients, as well, making them as healthful as they are tempting.

As the recipes in this chapter show, it is a simple matter to boost the nutritional value of your favorite muffins and quick breads by using a variety of whole grain flours, and by reducing the amount of sugar used. In fact, most of the baked goods recipes in this book contain 25 to 50 percent less sugar than traditional recipes. Naturally sweet and flavorful ingredients like fruit juices, fruit purées, and oats reduce the need for sugar while enhancing the taste and aroma of your home-baked treats.

Will your baked goods be dry if you leave out all that oil and butter? Not if you replace the fat with fruit purées, fruit juices, nonfat and low-fat buttermilk and yogurt, and other healthful fat substitutes. The recipes in this chapter artfully combine these naturally flavorful substitutes with a variety of whole grain flours, fresh and dried fruits, and other wholesome ingredients to produce an array of super-moist, super-tempting breads. From Buttermilk Cornbread and Apricot-Oat Scones to Apple Butter Bran Muffins and Golden Pumpkin Bread, you'll find breads that are perfect for every meal of the day or for a wholesome snack. You'll even learn how to modify your own recipes so that you and your family can enjoy healthful versions of old family favorites.

So take out your baking pans, preheat your oven, and get ready to create some of the healthiest, most flavorful breads you've ever tasted! It's easy—once you know the secrets of healthy cooking.

Cranberry Almond Muffins

YIELD: 12 MUFFINS

1⅓ cups whole wheat pastry flour
or unbleached flour

⅔ cup yellow cornmeal

½ cup sugar

1 tablespoon baking powder

1 cup plus 2 tablespoons nonfat
or low-fat buttermilk

¼ cup reduced-fat margarine
or light butter, melted

2 egg whites, lightly beaten

1 teaspoon almond extract

½ cup dried cranberries

TOPPING

1 tablespoon finely ground almonds

1 tablespoon sugar

1. To make the topping, place the almonds and sugar in a small bowl, and stir to mix well. Set aside.

2. Place the flour, cornmeal, sugar, and baking powder in a large bowl, and stir to mix well. Add the buttermilk, margarine, egg whites, and almond extract, and stir just until the dry ingredients are moistened. Fold in the cranberries.

3. Coat the bottoms only of muffin cups with nonstick cooking spray, and fill three-fourths full with the batter. Sprinkle the topping over the batter, and bake at 350°F for about 15 minutes, or just until a wooden toothpick inserted in the center of a muffin comes out clean. Be careful not to overbake.

4. Remove the muffin tins from the oven, and allow to sit for 5 minutes before removing the muffins. Serve warm or at room temperature, refrigerating any leftovers not eaten within 24 hours.

NUTRITIONAL FACTS (PER MUFFIN)
Cal: 155   Carbs: 29 g   Chol: 0 mg   Fat: 2.9 g
Fiber: 2.6 g   Protein: 3.8 g   Sodium: 181 mg

Cocoa Banana Muffins

YIELD: 12 MUFFINS

1¼ cups whole wheat pastry flour
or unbleached flour

½ cup oat bran

½ cup sugar

¼ cup plus 2 tablespoons Dutch
processed cocoa powder

1 tablespoon baking powder

1 cup very ripe mashed banana
(about 2 large)

½ cup skim or low-fat milk

⅓ cup reduced-fat margarine
or light butter, melted

2 egg whites, lightly beaten

1 teaspoon vanilla extract

½ cup chopped walnuts (optional)

TOPPING

4 teaspoons sugar

1. Place the flour, oat bran, sugar, cocoa, and baking powder in a large bowl, and stir to mix well. Add the banana, milk, margarine or butter, egg whites, and vanilla extract, and stir just until the dry ingredients are moistened. Fold in the walnuts, if desired.

2. Coat the bottoms only of muffin cups with nonstick cooking spray, and fill three-fourths full with the batter. Sprinkle the sugar over the batter, and bake at 350°F for about 16 minutes, or just until a wooden toothpick inserted in the center of a muffin comes out clean. Be careful not to overbake.

3. Remove the muffin tins from the oven, and allow to sit for 5 minutes before removing the muffins. Serve warm or at room temperature, refrigerating any leftovers not eaten within 24 hours.

NUTRITIONAL FACTS (PER MUFFIN)
Cal: 141   Carbs: 28 g   Chol: 0 mg   Fat: 3.3 g
Fiber: 3.4 g   Protein: 4 g   Sodium: 162 mg

Baking With Reduced-Fat Margarine and Light Butter

Contrary to popular belief, you can bake with reduced-fat margarine and light butter. These products make it possible to reduce fat by more than half and still enjoy light, tender, buttery-tasting muffins, quick breads, cakes, scones, biscuits, and other goodies that are not easily made fat-free.

The secret to using these reduced-fat products successfully in your baked goods is to substitute three-fourths as much of the light product for the full-fat butter or margarine. This will compensate for the extra water that the reduced-fat products contain. For example, if a cake recipe calls for 1 cup of butter, substitute ³⁄₄ cup of light butter. And be sure to choose brands that contain 5 to 6 grams of fat and 50 calories per tablespoon. (Full-fat brands contain 11 grams of fat and 100 calories per tablespoon.) Brands with less fat than this generally do not work well in baking.

Be careful not to overbake your reduced-fat creations, as they can become dry. Bake cakes, muffins, and quick breads at 325°F to 350°F, and biscuits and scones at 375°F to 400°F. Check the product for doneness a few minutes before the end of the usual baking time. Then enjoy!

Honey Oat Bran Muffins

YIELD: 12 MUFFINS

2¹⁄₂ cups oat bran

2 teaspoons baking powder

¹⁄₄ teaspoon baking soda

1¹⁄₂ cups nonfat or low-fat buttermilk

¹⁄₂ cup honey

2 egg whites, lightly beaten, or ¹⁄₄ cup fat-free egg substitute

1 teaspoon vanilla extract

¹⁄₂ cup dark raisins, walnuts, or toasted pecans (page 348), or ³⁄₄ cup fresh or frozen (unthawed) blueberries (optional)

1. Place the oat bran, baking powder, and baking soda in a large bowl, and stir to mix well. Add the buttermilk, honey, egg whites or egg substitute, and vanilla extract, and stir just until the dry ingredients are moistened. Fold in the raisins, nuts, or blueberries, if desired.

2. Coat the bottoms only of muffin cups with non-stick cooking spray, and fill three-fourths full with the batter. Bake at 350°F for about 14 minutes, or just until a wooden toothpick inserted in the center of a muffin comes out clean. Be careful not to overbake.

3. Remove the muffin tins from the oven, and allow to sit for 5 minutes before removing the muffins. Serve warm or at room temperature, refrigerating any leftovers not eaten within 24 hours.

NUTRITIONAL FACTS (PER MUFFIN)			
Cal: 107	Carbs: 18 g	Chol: 1 mg	Fat: 1.6 g
Fiber: 3.1 g	Protein: 5.1 g	Sodium: 150 mg	

VARIATION

To make Applesauce Oat Bran Muffins, substitute ¹⁄₂ cup of unsweetened applesauce for ¹⁄₂ cup of the buttermilk, and add ¹⁄₂ to 1 teaspoon of ground cinnamon to the dry ingredients.

NUTRITIONAL FACTS (PER MUFFIN)			
Cal: 107	Carbs: 18.5 g	Chol: 0 mg	Fat: 1.5 g
Fiber: 3.2 g	Protein: 4.8 g	Sodium: 140 mg	

VARIATION

To make Banana Oat Bran Muffins, substitute ¹⁄₂ cup of very ripe mashed banana (about 1 large) for ¹⁄₂ cup of the buttermilk, and add ¹⁄₄ teaspoon of ground nutmeg to the dry ingredients.

NUTRITIONAL FACTS (PER MUFFIN)			
Cal: 111	Carbs: 19.5 g	Chol: 0 mg	Fat: 1.6 g
Fiber: 3.3 g	Protein: 4.8 g	Sodium: 139 mg	

Fresh Pear Muffins

YIELD: 12 MUFFINS

1½ cups whole wheat pastry flour
or unbleached flour

¾ cup oat bran

⅓ cup sugar

1 tablespoon baking powder

¼ teaspoon ground cinnamon

¼ teaspoon ground nutmeg

1 cup pear nectar

¾ cup finely chopped peeled pear
(about 1 medium)

2 tablespoons walnut or vegetable oil

2 egg whites, lightly beaten

½ cup dark raisins or chopped walnuts

1. Place the flour, oat bran, sugar, baking powder, cinnamon, and nutmeg in a large bowl, and stir to mix well. Add the nectar, chopped pear, oil, and egg whites, and stir just until the dry ingredients are moistened. Fold in the raisins or walnuts.

2. Coat the bottoms only of muffin cups with nonstick cooking spray, and fill three-fourths full with the batter. Bake at 350°F for about 15 minutes, or just until a wooden toothpick inserted in the center of a muffin comes out clean. Be careful not to overbake.

3. Remove the muffin tins from the oven, and allow to sit for 5 minutes before removing the muffins. Serve warm or at room temperature, refrigerating any leftovers not eaten within 24 hours.

NUTRITIONAL FACTS (PER MUFFIN)
Cal: 145　Carbs: 29 g　Chol: 0 mg　Fat: 3 g
Fiber: 3.4 g　Protein: 3.8 g　Sodium: 133 mg

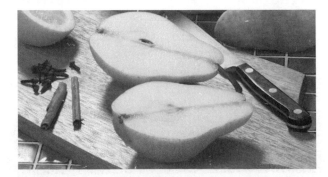

Poppy Seed Muffins

YIELD: 12 MUFFINS

1¼ cups whole wheat pastry flour
or unbleached flour

1 cup oat bran

½ cup sugar

3–4 teaspoons poppy seeds

1 tablespoon baking powder

1¼ cups vanilla or lemon nonfat or low-fat yogurt

¼ cup reduced-fat margarine
or light butter, melted

2 egg whites, lightly beaten

1 teaspoon vanilla or almond extract

¼ cup chopped almonds (optional)

TOPPING

1 tablespoon plus 1 teaspoon sugar

1. Place the flour, oat bran, sugar, poppy seeds, and baking powder in a large bowl, and stir to mix well. Set aside.

2. Place the yogurt, margarine or butter, egg whites, and vanilla or almond extract in a small bowl, and stir to mix well. Add the yogurt mixture to the flour mixture, and stir just until the dry ingredients are moistened. Fold in the almonds, if desired.

3. Coat the bottoms only of muffin cups with nonstick cooking spray, and fill two-thirds full with the batter. Sprinkle some of the sugar over the top of each muffin. Bake at 350°F for about 15 minutes, or just until a wooden toothpick inserted in the center of a muffin comes out clean. Be careful not to overbake.

4. Remove the muffin tins from the oven, and allow to sit for 5 minutes before removing the muffins. Serve warm or at room temperature, refrigerating any leftovers not eaten within 24 hours.

NUTRITIONAL FACTS (PER MUFFIN)
Cal: 147　Carbs: 28 g　Chol: 0 mg　Fat: 2.8 g
Fiber: 2.8 g　Protein: 4.6 g　Sodium: 172 mg

Fruit and Nut Muffins

YIELD: 12 MUFFINS

1⅓ cups whole wheat pastry flour
or unbleached flour

1 cup oat bran

¼ cup plus 2 tablespoons sugar

2 teaspoons baking powder

½ teaspoon baking soda

¾ cup nonfat or low-fat vanilla yogurt

¾ cup applesauce

¼ cup reduced-fat margarine
or light butter, melted

2 egg whites, lightly beaten

½ cup dried cherries, blueberries, cranberries,
or dark raisins

⅓ cup chopped toasted almonds, pecans,
or walnuts (page 348)

1. Place the flour, oat bran, sugar, baking powder, and baking soda in a large bowl, and stir to mix well. Set aside.

2. Place the yogurt, applesauce, margarine or butter, and egg whites in a small bowl, and stir to mix well. Add the yogurt mixture to the flour mixture, and stir just until the dry ingredients are moistened. Fold in the dried fruit and nuts.

3. Coat the bottoms only of muffin cups with non-stick cooking spray, and fill three-fourths full with the batter. Bake at 350°F for about 15 minutes, or just until a wooden toothpick inserted in the center of a muffin comes out clean. Be careful not to overbake.

4. Remove the muffin tins from the oven, and allow to sit for 5 minutes before removing the muffins. Serve warm or at room temperature, refrigerating any leftovers not eaten within 24 hours.

NUTRITIONAL FACTS (PER MUFFIN)
Cal: 158   Carbs: 28 g   Chol: 0 mg   Fat: 4.5 g
Fiber: 3.7 g   Protein: 5.4 g   Sodium: 175 mg

Honey Bran Muffins

YIELD: 12 MUFFINS

1¼ cups wheat bran

1¼ cups nonfat or low-fat buttermilk

1½ cups whole wheat pastry flour
or unbleached flour

1 teaspoon baking soda

½ cup honey

2 tablespoons walnut or vegetable oil

2 egg whites, lightly beaten

1 teaspoon vanilla extract

½ cup chopped dried apricots or prunes

1. Place the bran and buttermilk in a medium-sized bowl. Stir to mix well, and set aside for 15 minutes.

2. Place the flour and baking soda in a large bowl, and stir to mix well. Add the bran mixture and the honey, oil, egg whites, and vanilla extract, and stir just until the dry ingredients are moistened. Fold in the apricots or prunes.

3. Coat the bottoms only of muffin cups with non-stick cooking spray, and fill three-fourths full with the batter. Bake at 350°F for about 15 minutes, or just until a wooden toothpick inserted in the center of a muffin comes out clean. Be careful not to overbake.

4. Remove the muffin tins from the oven, and allow to sit for 5 minutes before removing the muffins. Serve warm or at room temperature, refrigerating any leftovers not eaten within 24 hours.

NUTRITIONAL FACTS (PER MUFFIN)
Cal: 152   Carbs: 30 g   Chol: 0 mg   Fat: 3 g
Fiber: 4.6 g   Protein: 4.5 g   Sodium: 145 mg

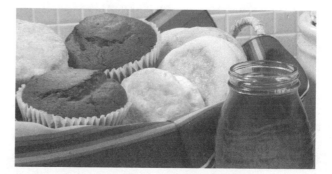

Cranberry Apple Muffins

YIELD: 12 MUFFINS
1½ cups whole wheat pastry flour or unbleached flour
½ cup oat bran
¼ cup plus 2 tablespoons sugar
1 tablespoon baking powder
½ teaspoon ground cinnamon
1 cup finely chopped peeled apple (about 1½ medium)
¾ cup plus 2 tablespoons apple juice
1 egg white, lightly beaten
2 tablespoons walnut or vegetable oil
½ cup dried cranberries

1. Place the flour, oat bran, sugar, baking powder, and cinnamon in a large bowl, and stir to mix well. Add the chopped apple, apple juice, egg white, and oil, and stir just until the dry ingredients are moistened. Fold in the cranberries.

2. Coat the bottoms only of muffin cups with nonstick cooking spray, and fill three-fourths full with the batter. Bake at 350°F for about 15 minutes, or just until a wooden toothpick inserted in the center of a muffin comes out clean. Be careful not to overbake.

3. Remove the muffin tins from the oven, and allow to sit for 5 minutes before removing the muffins. Serve warm or at room temperature, refrigerating any leftovers not eaten within 24 hours.

NUTRITIONAL FACTS (PER MUFFIN)
Cal: 136   Carbs: 27 g   Chol: 0 mg   Fat: 2.9 g
Fiber: 3.1 g   Protein: 3.3 g   Sodium: 131 mg

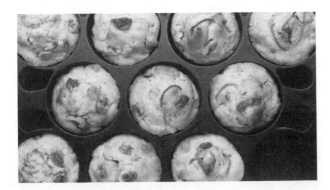

Very Blueberry Muffins

For variety, substitute coarsely chopped raspberries, blackberries, or sweet pitted cherries for the blueberries.

YIELD: 12 MUFFINS
1 cup oat flour
1¼ cups whole wheat pastry flour or unbleached flour
⅓ cup sugar
1 tablespoon baking powder
1 teaspoon dried grated orange rind, or 1 tablespoon fresh
¾ cup nonfat or low-fat vanilla yogurt
½ cup orange juice
¼ cup reduced-fat margarine or light butter, melted
2 egg whites, lightly beaten
¾ cup fresh or frozen (unthawed) blueberries

TOPPING
1 tablespoon sugar

1. Place the flours, sugar, baking powder, and orange rind in a large bowl, and stir to mix well. Add the yogurt, orange juice, margarine or butter, and egg whites, and stir just until the dry ingredients are moistened. Fold in the blueberries.

2. Coat the bottoms only of muffin cups with nonstick cooking spray, and fill three-fourths full with the batter. Sprinkle ¼ teaspoon of sugar over the top of each muffin, and bake at 350°F for about 16 minutes, or just until a wooden toothpick inserted in the center of a muffin comes out clean. Be careful not to overbake.

3. Remove the muffin tins from the oven, and allow to sit for 5 minutes before removing the muffins. Serve warm or at room temperature, refrigerating any leftovers not eaten within 24 hours.

NUTRITIONAL FACTS (PER MUFFIN)
Cal: 141   Carbs: 26 g   Chol: 0 mg   Fat: 2.6 g
Fiber: 2.8 g   Protein: 4.4 g   Sodium: 165 mg

Applesauce Maple Muffins

YIELD: 12 MUFFINS

1½ cups whole wheat pastry flour
or unbleached flour

½ cup plus 1 tablespoon oat bran

1 tablespoon baking powder

1¼ cups unsweetened applesauce

½ cup maple syrup

2 tablespoons walnut or vegetable oil

1 egg white, lightly beaten

1 teaspoon vanilla extract

½ cup dark raisins or chopped walnuts

1. Place the flour, oat bran, and baking powder in a large bowl, and stir to mix well. Add the applesauce, maple syrup, oil, egg white, and vanilla extract, and stir just until the dry ingredients are moistened. Fold in the raisins or walnuts.

2. Coat the bottoms only of muffin cups with non-stick cooking spray, and fill three-fourths full with the batter. Bake at 350°F for about 15 minutes, or just until a wooden toothpick inserted in the center of a muffin comes out clean. Be careful not to overbake.

3. Remove the muffin tins from the oven, and allow to sit for 5 minutes before removing the muffins. Serve warm or at room temperature, refrigerating any leftovers not eaten within 24 hours.

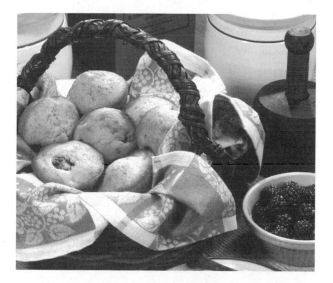

NUTRITIONAL FACTS (PER MUFFIN)			
Cal: 147	Carbs: 30 g	Chol: 0 mg	Fat: 2.9 g
Fiber: 3.2 g	Protein: 3.3 g	Sodium: 133 mg	

Mandarin Blueberry Muffins

YIELD: 12 MUFFINS

1 can (11 ounces) mandarin orange sections
in light syrup, undrained

1½ cups whole wheat pastry flour
or unbleached flour

¾ cup oat bran

½ cup sugar

1 tablespoon baking powder

2 egg whites, lightly beaten

¼ cup reduced-fat margarine
or light butter, melted

1 teaspoon vanilla or almond extract

¼ cup plus 2 tablespoons dried blueberries,
cherries, or cranberries

1. Drain the oranges, reserving ¼ cup plus 1 table-spoon of the syrup. Set aside.

2. Place the flour, oat bran, sugar, and baking powder in a large bowl, and stir to mix well. Crush the orange sections into small bits, and add the oranges and the reserved syrup, the egg whites, the margarine or butter, and the vanilla or almond extract to the flour mixture. Stir just until the dry ingredients are moistened. Fold in the blueberries, cherries, or cranberries.

3. Coat the bottoms only of muffin cups with non-stick cooking spray, and fill two-thirds full with the batter. Bake at 350°F for about 15 minutes, or just until a wooden toothpick inserted in the center of a muffin comes out clean. Be careful not to overbake.

4. Remove the muffin tins from the oven, and allow to sit for 5 minutes before removing the muffins. Serve warm or at room temperature, refrigerating any leftovers not eaten within 24 hours.

NUTRITIONAL FACTS (PER MUFFIN)			
Cal: 138	Carbs: 28 g	Chol: 0 mg	Fat: 2.6 g
Fiber: 3.3 g	Protein: 3.8 g	Sodium: 155 mg	

Cherry Vanilla Muffins

*For variety, substitute fresh or
frozen blueberries for the cherries.*

YIELD: 12 MUFFINS
1 1/2 cups whole wheat pastry flour or unbleached flour
1/2 cup yellow or white cornmeal
1/2 cup sugar
2 teaspoons baking powder
1/4 teaspoon baking soda
1 cup plain nonfat or low-fat vanilla yogurt
1/4 cup reduced-fat margarine or light butter, melted
2 egg whites, lightly beaten
3/4 cup halved frozen (unthawed) pitted cherries

TOPPING
1 tablespoon sugar

1. Place the flour, cornmeal, sugar, baking powder, and baking soda in a large bowl, and stir to mix well. Set aside.

2. Place the yogurt, margarine or butter, and egg whites in a small bowl, and stir to mix well. Add the yogurt mixture to the flour mixture, and stir just until the dry ingredients are moistened. Fold in the cherries.

3. Coat the bottoms only of muffin cups with non-stick cooking spray, and fill three-fourths full with the batter. Sprinkle some of the sugar over the top of each muffin. Bake at 350°F for about 15 minutes, or just until a wooden toothpick inserted in the center of a muffin comes out clean. Be careful not to overbake.

4. Remove the muffin tins from the oven, and allow to sit for 5 minutes before removing the muffins. Serve warm or at room temperature, refrigerating any leftovers not eaten within 24 hours.

NUTRITIONAL FACTS (PER MUFFIN)
Cal: 151   Carbs: 29 g   Chol: 0 mg   Fat: 2.3 g
Fiber: 2.5 g   Protein: 4.1 g   Sodium: 155 mg

Moist Cornmeal Muffins

*For muffins that are light and tender,
be sure to use only finely ground cornmeal.*

YIELD: 12 MUFFINS
2 cups finely ground yellow or white cornmeal
2 teaspoons baking powder
1/2 teaspoon baking soda
3 egg whites, lightly beaten, or 2 eggs, lightly beaten
2 cups nonfat or low-fat buttermilk
2–3 tablespoons honey

1. Place the cornmeal, baking powder, and baking soda in a large bowl, and stir to mix well. Add the egg whites or eggs, buttermilk, and honey, and stir just until the dry ingredients are moistened.

2. Coat the bottoms only of muffin cups with non-stick cooking spray, and fill three-fourths full with the batter. Bake at 350° about 16 minutes, or just until a wooden toothpick inserted in the center of a muffin comes out clean. Be careful not to overbake.

3. Remove the muffin tins from the oven, and allow to sit for 5 minutes before removing the muffins. Serve warm or at room temperature, refrigerating any leftovers not eaten within 24 hours.

NUTRITIONAL FACTS (PER MUFFIN)
Cal: 115   Carbs: 22 g   Chol: 1 mg   Fat: 0.9 g
Fiber: 2 g   Protein: 4 g   Sodium: 189 mg

Orange Marmalade Muffins

YIELD: 12 MUFFINS

1¼ cups whole wheat pastry flour
or unbleached flour

1 cup oat bran or wheat bran

2 tablespoons sugar

1 tablespoon baking powder

¾ cup skim or low-fat milk

½ cup orange marmalade

¼ cup reduced-fat margarine
or light butter, melted

2 egg whites, lightly beaten

1 teaspoon vanilla extract

½ cup chopped toasted pecans (page 348),
or ¾ cup fresh or frozen (unthawed)
blueberries (optional)

1. Place the flour, bran, sugar, and baking powder in a large bowl, and stir to mix well. Set aside.

2. Place the milk, marmalade, margarine or butter, egg whites, and vanilla extract in a small bowl, and stir to mix well. Add the milk mixture to the flour mixture, and stir just until the dry ingredients are moistened. Fold in the pecans or blueberries, if desired.

3. Coat the bottoms only of muffin cups with non-stick cooking spray, and fill three-fourths full with the batter. Bake at 350°F for about 15 minutes, or just until a wooden toothpick inserted in the center of a muffin comes out clean. Be careful not to overbake.

4. Remove the muffin tins from the oven, and allow to sit for 5 minutes before removing the muffins. Serve warm or at room temperature, refrigerating any leftovers not eaten within 24 hours.

NUTRITIONAL FACTS (PER MUFFIN)
Cal: 127   Carbs: 26 g   Chol: 0 mg   Fat: 2.6 g
Fiber: 2.8 g   Protein: 4.2 g   Sodium: 169 mg

Rise and Shine Muffins

YIELD: 12 MUFFINS

2 cups raisin bran cereal

1¼ cups skim or low-fat milk

3 tablespoons fat-free egg substitute,
or 1 egg, lightly beaten

2 tablespoons walnut or vegetable oil

1 teaspoon vanilla extract

1¼ cups whole wheat pastry flour
or unbleached flour

½ cup sugar

1 tablespoon baking powder

¼ teaspoon ground cinnamon

⅓ cup chopped dried apricots or prunes

¼ cup hulled sunflower seeds (optional)

1. Place the cereal and milk in a medium-sized bowl. Stir to mix well, and set aside for 10 minutes.

2. Add the egg substitute or egg, oil, and vanilla extract to the cereal mixture. Stir to mix well, and set aside.

3. Place the flour, sugar, baking powder, and cinnamon in a large bowl, and stir to mix well. Add the cereal mixture, and stir just until the dry ingredients are moistened. Fold in the apricots or prunes and, if desired, the sunflower seeds.

4. Coat the bottoms only of muffin cups with non-stick cooking spray, and fill three-fourths full with the batter. Bake at 350°F for about 16 minutes, or just until a wooden toothpick inserted in the center of a muffin comes out clean. Be careful not to overbake.

5. Remove the muffin tins from the oven, and allow to sit for 5 minutes before removing the muffins. Serve warm or at room temperature, refrigerating any leftovers not eaten within 24 hours.

NUTRITIONAL FACTS (PER MUFFIN)
Cal: 143   Carbs: 28 g   Chol: 0 mg   Fat: 2.7 g
Fiber: 3.2 g   Protein: 4.1 g   Sodium: 164 mg

Molasses Bran Muffins

YIELD: 12 MUFFINS

1¼ cups whole wheat pastry flour
or unbleached flour

1½ cups wheat bran

1 teaspoon baking soda

¾ cup nonfat or low-fat buttermilk

½ cup plus 2 tablespoons applesauce

¼ cup plus 2 tablespoons molasses

2 egg whites, lightly beaten

2 tablespoons walnut or vegetable oil

½ cup dark raisins, chopped pitted prunes,
or chopped dried apricots

¼ cup chopped walnuts (optional)

1. Place the flour, bran, and baking soda in a large bowl, and stir to mix well. Set aside.

2. Place the buttermilk, applesauce, molasses, egg whites, and oil in a small bowl, and stir to mix well. Add the buttermilk mixture to the flour mixture, and stir just until the dry ingredients are moistened. Fold in the raisins, prunes, or apricots, and, if desired, the walnuts.

3. Coat the bottoms only of muffin cups with nonstick cooking spray, and fill three-fourths full with the batter. Bake at 350°F for about 16 minutes, or just until a wooden toothpick inserted in the center of a muffin comes out clean. Be careful not to overbake.

4. Remove the muffin tins from the oven, and allow to sit for 5 minutes before removing the muffins. Serve warm or at room temperature, refrigerating any leftovers not eaten within 24 hours.

NUTRITIONAL FACTS (PER MUFFIN)
Cal: 131   Carbs: 26 g   Chol: 0 mg   Fat: 2.9 g
Fiber: 4 g   Protein: 3.6 g   Sodium: 135 mg

VARIATION

To make Flax Bran Muffins, substitute ¼ to ½ cup of flax meal (page 23) for an equal amount of wheat bran.

NUTRITIONAL FACTS (PER MUFFIN)
Cal: 140   Carbs: 26 g   Chol: 0 mg   Fat: 3.8 g
Fiber: 4.4 g   Protein: 4.4 g   Sodium: 135 mg

Three-Grain Muffins

YIELD: 12 MUFFINS

1½ cups wheat bran

¾ cup plus 2 tablespoons oat bran

½ cup yellow cornmeal

1 teaspoon baking soda

½ cup dark brown sugar

1 cup nonfat or low-fat buttermilk

¾ cup apple or orange juice

2 egg whites, lightly beaten

1 teaspoon vanilla extract

½ cup dark raisins or chopped dried apricots

1. Place the wheat bran, oat bran, cornmeal, and baking soda in a large bowl, and stir to mix well. Add the brown sugar, and stir to mix well. Using the back of a wooden spoon, press out any lumps in the brown sugar.

2. Add all of the remaining ingredients to the bran mixture, and stir just until the dry ingredients are moistened. Cover and refrigerate at least overnight. (This batter may be refrigerated for up to a week.)

3. Coat the bottoms only of muffin cups with nonstick cooking spray, and fill two-thirds full with the batter. Bake at 350°F for about 16 minutes, or just until a wooden toothpick inserted in the center of a muffin comes out clean. Be careful not to overbake.

4. Remove the muffin tins from the oven, and allow to sit for 5 minutes before removing the muffins. Serve warm or at room temperature, refrigerating any leftovers not eaten within 24 hours.

NUTRITIONAL FACTS (PER MUFFIN)
Cal: 121   Carbs: 29 g   Chol: 0 mg   Fat: 1.2 g
Fiber: 4.7 g   Protein: 4.1 g   Sodium: 141 mg

Apple Butter Bran Muffins

YIELD: 12 MUFFINS

1 cup whole wheat pastry flour or unbleached flour
1 cup wheat bran
1/2 cup oat bran
1 teaspoon baking soda
1/2 teaspoon ground cinnamon
1 cup apple butter
1 cup nonfat or low-fat buttermilk
2 egg whites, lightly beaten
2 tablespoons walnut or vegetable oil
1/2 cup dark raisins

1. Place the flour, wheat bran, oat bran, baking soda, and cinnamon in a large bowl, and stir to mix well. Add the apple butter, buttermilk, egg whites, and oil, and stir just until the dry ingredients are moistened. Fold in the raisins.

2. Coat the bottoms only of muffin cups with non-stick cooking spray, and fill three-fourths full with the batter. Bake at 350°F for about 15 minutes, or just until a wooden toothpick inserted in the center of a muffin comes out clean. Be careful not to overbake.

3. Remove the muffin tins from the oven, and allow to sit for 5 minutes before removing the muffins. Serve warm or at room temperature, refrigerating any leftovers not eaten within 24 hours.

NUTRITIONAL FACTS (PER MUFFIN)
Cal: 146   Carbs: 30 g   Chol: 0 mg   Fat: 3.2 g
Fiber: 4.4 g   Protein: 4 g   Sodium: 136 mg

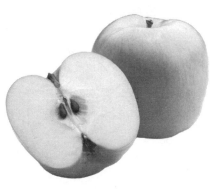

Pumpkin Praline Pecan Muffins

YIELD: 12 MUFFINS

1 1/2 cups whole wheat pastry flour or unbleached flour
1/2 cup oat bran
1 tablespoon baking powder
1/2 cup light brown sugar
2/3 cup mashed cooked or canned pumpkin
3/4 cup skim or low-fat milk
1/4 cup reduced-fat margarine or light butter, melted
2 egg whites, lightly beaten
1 teaspoon vanilla extract

TOPPING

1 tablespoon finely ground pecans
1 tablespoon light brown sugar

1. To make the topping, place the pecans and brown sugar in a small bowl, and stir until crumbly. Set aside.

2. Place the flour, oat bran, and baking powder in a large bowl, and stir to mix well. Add the brown sugar, and stir to mix well. Using the back of a wooden spoon, press out any lumps in the brown sugar. Set aside.

3. Place the pumpkin, milk, margarine or butter, egg whites, and vanilla extract in a small bowl, and whisk to mix well. Add the pumpkin mixture to the flour mixture, and stir just until the dry ingredients are moistened.

4. Coat the bottoms only of muffin cups with non-stick cooking spray, and fill two-thirds full with the batter. Sprinkle the topping over the batter. Bake at 350°F for about 15 minutes, or just until a wooden toothpick inserted in the center of a muffin comes out clean. Be careful not to overbake.

5. Remove the muffin tins from the oven, and allow to sit for 5 minutes before removing the muffins. Serve warm or at room temperature, refrigerating any leftovers not eaten within 24 hours.

NUTRITIONAL FACTS (PER MUFFIN)
Cal: 133   Carbs: 25 g   Chol: 0 mg   Fat: 2.8 g
Fiber: 2.9 g   Protein: 4 g   Sodium: 167 mg

Buttermilk Drop Biscuits

YIELD: 12 BISCUITS

2 cups unbleached flour

2 tablespoons sugar

1 tablespoon baking powder

$1/4$ teaspoon baking soda

$1/8$ teaspoon salt

2 tablespoons vegetable oil

1 cup plus 2 tablespoons nonfat or low-fat buttermilk

1. Place the flour, sugar, baking powder, baking soda, and salt in a medium-sized bowl, and stir to mix well. Add the oil and just enough of the buttermilk to make a thick batter, and stir just until the dry ingredients are moistened.

2. Coat a large baking sheet with nonstick cooking spray, and drop heaping tablespoons of the batter onto the sheet. For crusty biscuits, space the biscuits 1 inch apart. For soft biscuits, space the biscuits so that they are barely touching.

3. Bake at 375°F for 12 to 15 minutes, or just until the tops are lightly browned. Be careful not to overbake. Serve hot.

NUTRITIONAL FACTS (PER BISCUIT)
Cal: 103   Carbs: 17 g   Chol: 1 mg   Fat: 2.5 g
Fiber: 0.4 g   Protein: 2.7 g   Sodium: 193 mg

VARIATION

To make Whole Wheat-Buttermilk Drop Biscuits, substitute $3/4$ cup of whole wheat pastry flour for $3/4$ cup of the unbleached flour.

NUTRITIONAL FACTS (PER BISCUIT)
Cal: 105   Carbs: 17 g   Chol: 1 mg   Fat: 2.6 g
Fiber: 1.2 g   Protein: 2.9 g   Sodium: 193 mg

VARIATION

To make Cornmeal-Buttermilk Drop Biscuits, substitute $1/2$ cup of yellow or white cornmeal for $1/2$ cup of the unbleached flour.

NUTRITIONAL FACTS (PER BISCUIT)
Cal: 105   Carbs: 17 g   Chol: 1 mg   Fat: 2.6 g
Fiber: 0.7 g   Protein: 2.6 g   Sodium: 196 mg

VARIATION

To make Oatmeal-Buttermilk Drop Biscuits, substitute $1/2$ cup of quick-cooking rolled oats or oat bran for $1/2$ cup of the unbleached flour.

NUTRITIONAL FACTS (PER BISCUIT)
Cal: 100   Carbs: 16 g   Chol: 1 mg   Fat: 2.7 g
Fiber: 0.7 g   Protein: 2.7 g   Sodium: 194 mg

Sweet Corn Muffins

YIELD: 14 MUFFINS

1 cup whole wheat pastry flour or unbleached flour

1 cup yellow cornmeal

1 tablespoon baking powder

1 cup plus 2 tablespoons nonfat or low-fat buttermilk

$1/4$ cup plus 2 tablespoons molasses or honey

$1/4$ cup reduced-fat margarine or light butter, melted

2 egg whites, lightly beaten

$1/2$ cup chopped dates

1. Place the flour, cornmeal, and baking powder in a large bowl, and stir to mix well. Set aside.

2. Place the buttermilk, molasses or honey, margarine or butter, and egg whites in a small bowl, and stir to mix well. Add the buttermilk mixture to the flour mixture, and stir just until the dry ingredients are moistened. Fold in the dates.

3. Coat the bottoms only of muffin cups with nonstick cooking spray, and fill two-thirds full with the batter. Bake at 350°F for about 14 minutes, or just until a wooden toothpick inserted in the center of a muffin comes out clean. Be careful not to overbake.

4. Remove the muffin tins from the oven, and allow to sit for 5 minutes before removing the muffins. Serve warm or at room temperature, refrigerating any leftovers not eaten within 24 hours.

NUTRITIONAL FACTS (PER MUFFIN)
Cal: 147   Carbs: 29 g   Chol: 0 mg   Fat: 2.6 g
Fiber: 2.5 g   Protein: 3.6 g   Sodium: 185 mg

Zucchini Spice Muffins

YIELD: 12 MUFFINS

1 cup whole wheat pastry flour
or unbleached flour

1 cup oat bran

1½ teaspoons ground cinnamon

2 teaspoons baking powder

¼ teaspoon baking soda

¾ cup nonfat or low-fat buttermilk

½ cup dark brown sugar

2 egg whites, lightly beaten

2 tablespoons walnut or vegetable oil

1 cup (packed) shredded zucchini
(about 1 medium-large)

½ cup dark raisins

⅓ cup chopped walnuts (optional)

1. Place the flour, oat bran, cinnamon, baking powder, and baking soda in a large bowl, and stir to mix well. Set aside.

2. Place the buttermilk, brown sugar, egg whites, and oil in a small bowl, and whisk until smooth. Add the buttermilk mixture and the zucchini to the flour mixture, and stir just until the dry ingredients are moistened. Fold in the raisins, and, if desired, the walnuts.

3. Coat the bottoms only of muffin cups with nonstick cooking spray, and fill three-fourths full with the batter. Bake at 350°F for about 16 minutes, or just until a wooden toothpick inserted in the center of a muffin comes out clean. Be careful not to overbake.

4. Remove the muffin tins from the oven, and allow to sit for 10 minutes before removing the muffins. Serve warm or at room temperature, refrigerating any leftovers not eaten within 24 hours.

NUTRITIONAL FACTS (PER MUFFIN)
Cal: 132   Carbs: 24 g   Chol: 0 mg   Fat: 2.9 g
Fiber: 2.6 g   Protein: 3.9 g   Sodium: 135 mg

Applesauce-Bran Bread

YIELD: 16 SLICES

1¾ cups whole wheat pastry flour

½ cup wheat bran

2 teaspoons baking powder

¾ teaspoon baking soda

¾ teaspoon ground cinnamon

1 cup unsweetened applesauce

½ cup maple syrup or molasses

2 tablespoons vegetable oil

1 egg white, lightly beaten

1 teaspoon vanilla extract

½ cup dark raisins, dried cranberries,
or chopped prunes

½ cup chopped walnuts or pecans (optional)

1. Place the flour, wheat bran, baking powder, baking soda, and cinnamon in a large bowl, and stir to mix well. Add the applesauce, maple syrup or molasses, oil, egg white, and vanilla extract, and stir just until the dry ingredients are moistened. Fold in the dried fruits, and, if desired, the nuts.

2. Coat an 8-x-4-inch loaf pan with nonstick cooking spray. Spread the batter evenly in the pan, and bake at 325°F for about 50 minutes, or just until a wooden toothpick inserted in the center of the loaf comes out clean. Be careful not to overbake.

3. Remove the loaf from the oven, and let sit for 15 minutes. Invert the loaf onto a wire rack, turn right side up, and cool to room temperature. Wrap the loaf in plastic wrap or aluminum foil, and allow to sit for several hours before slicing and serving. (This will give the loaf a softer, moister crust.) Refrigerate any leftovers not eaten within 24 hours.

NUTRITIONAL FACTS (PER SLICE)
Cal: 109   Carbs: 22 g   Chol: 0 mg   Fat: 2 g
Fiber: 2.5 g   Protein: 2.3 g   Sodium: 121 mg

Raisin Bran Bread

YIELD: 16 SLICES

1²/₃ cups whole wheat pastry flour

1¹/₄ cups wheat bran

1 teaspoon baking soda

1¹/₃ cups skim or low-fat milk

¹/₂ cup molasses

2 tablespoons walnut or vegetable oil

1 tablespoon lemon juice

¹/₂ cup dark raisins

1. Place the flour, wheat bran, and baking soda in a large bowl, and stir to mix well. Set aside.

2. Place the milk, molasses, oil, and lemon juice in a medium-sized bowl, and stir to mix well. Add the milk mixture to the flour mixture, and stir just until the dry ingredients are moistened. Fold in the raisins.

3. Coat an 8-x-4-inch loaf pan with nonstick cooking spray. Spread the batter evenly in the pan, and bake at 325°F for about 50 minutes, or just until a wooden toothpick inserted in the center of the loaf comes out clean. Be careful not to overbake.

4. Remove the loaf from the oven, and let sit for 15 minutes. Invert the loaf onto a wire rack, turn right side up, and cool to room temperature. Wrap the loaf in plastic wrap or aluminum foil, and allow to sit for several hours before slicing and serving. (This will give the loaf a softer, moister crust.) Refrigerate any leftovers not eaten within 24 hours.

NUTRITIONAL FACTS (PER SLICE)
Cal: 115   Carbs: 23 g   Chol: 0 mg   Fat: 2.2 g
Fiber: 3.6 g   Protein: 3.3 g   Sodium: 93 mg

Brown Sugar Banana Bread

YIELD: 16 SLICES

2 cups whole wheat pastry flour

2 teaspoons baking powder

³/₄ teaspoon baking soda

¹/₂ teaspoon ground nutmeg

1³/₄ cups mashed very ripe banana (about 3¹/₂ large)

²/₃ cup light brown sugar

2 tablespoons walnut or vegetable oil

1 teaspoon vanilla extract

¹/₂ cup chopped toasted walnuts or pecans (page 348)

1. Place the flour, baking powder, baking soda, and nutmeg in a large bowl, and stir to mix well. Set aside.

2. Place the banana and brown sugar in a medium-sized bowl, and stir until the brown sugar has dissolved. Add the banana mixture, oil, and vanilla extract to the flour mixture, and stir just until the dry ingredients are moistened. Fold in the walnuts or pecans.

3. Coat an 8-x-4-inch loaf pan with nonstick cooking spray. Spread the batter evenly in the pan, and bake at 325°F for 50 to 55 minutes, or just until a wooden toothpick inserted in the center of the loaf comes out clean. Be careful not to overbake.

4. Remove the loaf from the oven, and let sit for 15 minutes. Invert the loaf onto a wire rack, turn right side up, and cool to room temperature. Wrap the loaf in plastic wrap or aluminum foil, and allow to sit for several hours before slicing and serving. (This will give the loaf a softer, moister crust.) Refrigerate any leftovers not eaten within 24 hours.

NUTRITIONAL FACTS (PER SLICE)
Cal: 146   Carbs: 26 g   Chol: 0 mg   Fat: 4.3 g
Fiber: 2.6 g   Protein: 3.3 g   Sodium: 123 mg

Mocha Banana Bread

YIELD: 16 SLICES

2 teaspoons vanilla extract
1/2 teaspoon instant coffee granules
1 3/4 cups whole wheat pastry flour
1/4 cup Dutch processed cocoa powder
2/3 cup sugar
2 teaspoons baking powder
3/4 teaspoon baking soda
1/2 teaspoon ground cinnamon
1 3/4 cups mashed very ripe banana (about 3 1/2 large)
2 tablespoons vegetable oil
1/2 cup chopped toasted pecans, almonds, or macadamia nuts (page 348)

1. Place the vanilla extract and coffee granules in a small bowl, and stir to mix well. Set aside.

2. Place the flour, cocoa powder, sugar, baking powder, baking soda, and cinnamon in a large bowl, and stir to mix well. Add the banana, oil, and vanilla extract mixture, and stir just until the dry ingredients are moistened. Fold in the nuts.

3. Coat an 8-x-4-inch loaf pan with nonstick cooking spray. Spread the batter evenly in the pan, and bake at 325°F for 50 to 55 minutes, or just until a wooden toothpick inserted in the center of the loaf comes out clean. Be careful not to overbake.

4. Remove the loaf from the oven, and let sit for 15 minutes. Invert the loaf onto a wire rack, turn right side up, and cool to room temperature. Wrap the loaf in plastic wrap or aluminum foil, and allow to sit for several hours before slicing and serving. (This will give the loaf a softer, moister crust.) Refrigerate any leftovers not eaten within 24 hours.

NUTRITIONAL FACTS (PER SLICE)
Cal: 141   Carbs: 25 g   Chol: 0 mg   Fat: 4.4 g
Fiber: 2.8 g   Protein: 3.3 g   Sodium: 121 g

Apple Butter Bread

YIELD: 16 SLICES

2 cups whole wheat pastry flour
2 teaspoons baking powder
3/4 teaspoon baking soda
1/4 teaspoon ground nutmeg
1 1/4 cups apple butter
1/2 cup plus 2 tablespoons apple juice
2 tablespoons walnut or vegetable oil
1 teaspoon vanilla extract
1/2 cup dark raisins or currants
1/4 cup chopped walnuts (optional)

1. Place the flour, baking powder, baking soda, and nutmeg in a large bowl, and stir to mix well. Add the apple butter, apple juice, oil, and vanilla extract, and stir just until the dry ingredients are moistened. Fold in the raisins or currants and, if desired, the walnuts.

2. Coat an 8-x-4-inch loaf pan with nonstick cooking spray. Spread the batter evenly in the pan, and bake at 325°F for 45 to 50 minutes, or just until a wooden toothpick inserted in the center of the loaf comes out clean. Be careful not to overbake.

3. Remove the loaf from the oven, and let sit for 15 minutes. Invert the loaf onto a wire rack, turn right side up, and cool to room temperature. Wrap the loaf in plastic wrap or aluminum foil, and allow to sit for several hours before slicing and serving. (This will give the loaf a softer, moister crust.) Refrigerate any leftovers not eaten within 24 hours.

NUTRITIONAL FACTS (PER SLICE)
Cal: 125   Carbs: 26 g   Chol: 0 mg   Fat: 2.1 g
Fiber: 2.3 g   Protein: 2.2 g   Sodium: 121 mg

Fresh Pear Bread

Make sure that the fresh pears you use for this recipe are perfectly ripe and sweet.

YIELD: 16 SLICES
2 cups whole wheat pastry flour
1/2 cup sugar
2 teaspoons baking powder
3/4 teaspoon baking soda
1/4 teaspoon ground nutmeg
1/4 teaspoon ground cinnamon
1/2 cup plus 1 tablespoon pear nectar
2 tablespoons walnut or vegetable oil
1 egg white, lightly beaten
1 teaspoon vanilla extract
1 1/3 cups finely chopped peeled pears (about 1 1/2 medium)
1/2 cup dried currants or dark raisins
1/3 cup chopped toasted walnuts (page 348) (optional)

1. Place the flour, sugar, baking powder, baking soda, nutmeg, and cinnamon in a large bowl, and stir to mix well. Add the nectar, oil, egg white, vanilla extract, and chopped pear, and stir just until the dry ingredients are moistened. Fold in the currants or raisins and, if desired, the walnuts.

2. Coat an 8-x-4-inch loaf pan with nonstick cooking spray. Spread the batter evenly in the pan, and bake at 325°F for 45 to 50 minutes, or just until a wooden toothpick inserted in the center of the loaf comes out clean. Be careful not to overbake.

3. Remove the loaf from the oven, and let sit for 15 minutes. Invert the loaf onto a wire rack, turn right side up, and cool to room temperature. Wrap the loaf in plastic wrap or aluminum foil, and allow to sit for several hours before slicing and serving. (This will give the loaf a softer, moister crust.) Refrigerate any leftovers not eaten within 24 hours.

NUTRITIONAL FACTS (PER SLICE)
Cal: 126   Carbs: 26 g   Chol: 0 mg   Fat: 2 g
Fiber: 2.5 g   Protein: 2.5 g   Sodium: 121 mg

Applesauce-Oatmeal Bread

YIELD: 16 SLICES
1 3/4 cups whole wheat pastry flour
1/2 cup quick-cooking oats
1/2 cup sugar
2 teaspoons baking powder
3/4 teaspoon baking soda
1/2 teaspoon ground cinnamon
1 1/4 cups unsweetened applesauce
2 tablespoons vegetable oil
1 egg white, lightly beaten
1 1/2 teaspoons vanilla extract
1/2 cup dark raisins or chopped dates
1/3 cup chopped toasted walnuts or pecans (page 348) (optional)

1. Place the flour, oats, sugar, baking powder, baking soda, and cinnamon in a large bowl, and stir to mix well. Add the applesauce, oil, egg white, and vanilla extract, and stir just until the dry ingredients are moistened. Fold in the raisins or dates and, if desired, the nuts.

2. Coat an 8-x-4-inch loaf pan with nonstick cooking spray. Spread the mixture evenly in the pan, and bake at 325°F for 50 to 55 minutes, or just until a wooden toothpick inserted in the center of the loaf comes out clean. Be careful not to overbake.

3. Remove the loaf from the oven, and let sit for 15 minutes. Invert the loaf onto a wire rack, turn right side up, and cool to room temperature. Wrap the loaf in plastic wrap or aluminum foil, and allow to sit for several hours before slicing and serving. (This will give the loaf a softer, moister crust.) Refrigerate any leftovers not eaten within 24 hours.

NUTRITIONAL FACTS (PER SLICE)
Cal: 115   Carbs: 23 g   Chol: 0 mg   Fat: 2.1 g
Fiber: 2.3 g   Protein: 2.6 g   Sodium: 121 mg

Golden Pumpkin Bread

YIELD: 16 SLICES
2 cups whole wheat pastry flour
2 teaspoons baking powder
3/4 teaspoon baking soda
2 teaspoons pumpkin pie spice
1 cup mashed cooked or canned pumpkin
3/4 cup apple or orange juice
1/2 cup plus 2 tablespoons light brown sugar
2 tablespoons vegetable oil
1 1/2 teaspoons vanilla extract
1/2 cup chopped toasted pecans or walnuts (page 348)

1. Place the flour, baking powder, baking soda, and pumpkin pie spice in a large bowl, and stir to mix well. Set aside.

2. Place the pumpkin, juice, brown sugar, oil, and vanilla extract in a medium-sized bowl, and stir to mix well and to dissolve the brown sugar. Add the pumpkin mixture to the flour mixture, and stir just until the dry ingredients are moistened. Fold in the nuts.

3. Coat an 8-x-4-inch loaf pan with nonstick cooking spray. Spread the batter evenly in the pan, and bake at 325°F for about 50 minutes, or just until a wooden toothpick inserted in the center of the loaf comes out clean. Be careful not to overbake.

4. Remove the loaf from the oven, and let sit for 15 minutes. Invert the loaf onto a wire rack, turn right side up, and cool to room temperature. Wrap the loaf in plastic wrap or aluminum foil, and allow to sit for several hours before slicing and serving. (This will give the loaf a softer, moister crust.) Refrigerate any leftovers not eaten within 24 hours.

NUTRITIONAL FACTS (PER SLICE)
Cal: 134   Carbs: 22 g   Chol: 0 mg   Fat: 4.5 g
Fiber: 2.7 g   Protein: 2.6 g   Sodium: 125 mg

Apricot-Pecan Bread

For variety, substitute prunes for the apricots, and walnuts for the pecans.

YIELD: 16 SLICES
1 cup chopped dried apricots
1 teaspoon baking soda
3/4 cup boiling water
2 cups whole wheat pastry flour
1/2 cup sugar
1/4 cup instant nonfat dry milk powder
1 teaspoon baking powder
1/2 cup applesauce
2 tablespoons vegetable oil
2 teaspoons vanilla extract
2/3 cup chopped toasted pecans (page 348)

1. Place the apricots in a medium-sized bowl. Stir the baking soda into the boiling water; then pour the water over the apricots. Set aside to cool to room temperature.

2. Place the flour, sugar, milk powder, and baking powder in a large bowl, and stir to mix well. Add the applesauce, oil, vanilla extract, and undrained cooled apricots, and stir just until the dry ingredients are moistened. Fold in the pecans.

3. Coat an 8-x-4-inch loaf pan with nonstick cooking spray. Spread the mixture evenly in the pan, and bake at 300°F for 55 to 60 minutes, or just until a wooden toothpick inserted in the center of the loaf comes out clean. Be careful not to overbake.

4. Remove the loaf from the oven, and let sit for 15 minutes. Invert the loaf onto a wire rack, turn right side up, and cool to room temperature. Wrap the loaf in plastic wrap or aluminum foil, and allow to sit for several hours before slicing and serving. (This will give the loaf a softer, moister crust.) Refrigerate any leftovers not eaten within 24 hours.

NUTRITIONAL FACTS (PER SLICE)
Cal: 149   Carbs: 23 g   Chol: 0 mg   Fat: 5.3 g
Fiber: 3 g   Protein: 3.2 g   Sodium: 117 mg

Carrot Raisin Bread

YIELD: 16 SLICES

2 cups whole wheat pastry flour

1/2 cup sugar

2 teaspoons baking powder

3/4 teaspoon baking soda

1 teaspoon ground cinnamon

3/4 cup apple or orange juice

2 tablespoons vegetable oil

1 egg white, lightly beaten

1 cup (packed) finely grated carrots
(about 2 medium)

1/2 cup dark or golden raisins

1/4 cup toasted wheat germ

1/3 cup chopped toasted walnuts
or pecans (page 348)

1. Place the flour, sugar, baking powder, baking soda, and cinnamon in a large bowl, and stir to mix well. Add the juice, oil, egg white, and carrots, and stir just until the dry ingredients are moistened. Fold in the raisins, wheat germ, and nuts.

2. Coat an 8-x-4-inch loaf pan with nonstick cooking spray. Spread the batter evenly in the pan, and bake at 325°F for 45 to 50 minutes, or just until a wooden toothpick inserted in the center of the loaf comes out clean. Be careful not to overbake.

3. Remove the loaf from the oven, and let sit for 15 minutes. Invert the loaf onto a wire rack, turn right side up, and cool to room temperature. Wrap the loaf in plastic wrap or aluminum foil, and allow to sit for several hours before slicing and serving. (This will give the loaf a softer, moister crust.) Refrigerate any leftovers not eaten within 24 hours.

NUTRITIONAL FACTS (PER SLICE)
Cal: 135   Carbs: 24 g   Chol: 0 mg   Fat: 3.6 g
Fiber: 2.6 g   Protein: 3.6 g   Sodium: 124 mg

Zucchini-Spice Bread

YIELD: 16 SLICES

2 cups whole wheat pastry flour

2/3 cup sugar

2 1/2 teaspoons baking powder

1/2 teaspoon baking soda

1 teaspoon ground cinnamon

1 teaspoon dried grated lemon rind,
or 1 tablespoon fresh

1/2 teaspoon ground nutmeg

1 1/4 cups (packed) shredded unpeeled zucchini
(about 1 medium-large)

1/2 cup skim or low-fat milk

2 tablespoons vegetable oil

1 egg white, lightly beaten

1 1/2 teaspoons vanilla extract

1/2 cup dark raisins or chopped walnuts,
or 1/4 cup each raisins and walnuts

1. Place the flour, sugar, baking powder, baking soda, cinnamon, lemon rind, and nutmeg in a large bowl, and stir to mix well. Add the zucchini, milk, oil, egg white, and vanilla extract, and stir just until the dry ingredients are moistened. Fold in the raisins or walnuts.

2. Coat an 8-x-4-inch loaf pan with nonstick cooking spray. Spread the batter evenly in the pan, and bake at 325°F for 45 to 50 minutes, or just until a wooden toothpick inserted in the center of the loaf comes out clean. Be careful not to overbake.

3. Remove the loaf from the oven, and let sit for 15 minutes. Invert the loaf onto a wire rack, turn right side up, and cool to room temperature. Wrap the loaf in plastic wrap or aluminum foil, and allow to sit for several hours before slicing and serving. (This will give the loaf a softer, moister crust.) Refrigerate any leftovers not eaten within 24 hours.

NUTRITIONAL FACTS (PER SLICE)
Cal: 116   Carbs: 23 g   Chol: 0 mg   Fat: 2 g
Fiber: 2.2 g   Protein: 2.8 g   Sodium: 123 mg

Pear-Cranberry Bread

YIELD: 16 SLICES

1 can (1 pound) pear halves in juice, undrained

$1/3$ cup oat bran

$1^3/4$ cups whole wheat pastry flour

$1/2$ cup sugar

2 teaspoons baking powder

$3/4$ teaspoon baking soda

2 tablespoons vegetable oil

1 egg white, lightly beaten

2 teaspoons vanilla extract

$1/2$ cup dried cranberries

$1/3$ cup chopped toasted walnuts or almonds (page 348) (optional)

1. Drain the pears, reserving the juice. Place the drained pears in a blender or food processor, and process until smooth. Pour the pear purée into a 2-cup measuring cup, and add enough of the reserved juice to bring the volume to $1^1/3$ cups.

2. Place the oat bran in a medium-sized bowl, and add the pear purée. Stir with a wire whisk until well mixed, and set the mixture aside for at least 15 minutes to allow the oat bran to soften.

3. Place the flour, sugar, baking powder, and baking soda in a large bowl, and stir to mix well. Add the pear mixture, oil, egg white, and vanilla extract, and stir just until the dry ingredients are moistened. Fold in the cranberries and, if desired, the walnuts or almonds.

4. Coat an 8-x-4-inch loaf pan with nonstick cooking spray. Spread the batter evenly in the pan, and bake at 325°F for about 45 minutes, or just until a wooden toothpick inserted in the center of the loaf comes out clean. Be careful not to overbake.

5. Remove the loaf from the oven, and let sit for 15 minutes. Invert the loaf onto a wire rack, turn right side up, and cool to room temperature. Wrap the loaf in plastic wrap or aluminum foil, and allow to sit for several hours before slicing and serving. (This will give the loaf a softer, moister crust.) Refrigerate any leftovers not eaten within 24 hours.

NUTRITIONAL FACTS (PER SLICE)
Cal: 113   Carbs: 23 g   Chol: 0 mg   Fat: 2.1 g
Fiber: 2.6 g   Protein: 2.4 g   Sodium: 122 mg

Prune and Walnut Bread

YIELD: 16 SLICES

2 cups whole wheat pastry flour

$1/2$ cup sugar

2 teaspoons baking powder

$3/4$ teaspoon baking soda

$1/2$ teaspoon ground cinnamon

$1^1/4$ cups plus 2 tablespoons unsweetened applesauce

2 tablespoons walnut or vegetable oil

1 teaspoon vanilla extract

1 cup chopped prunes

$1/2$ cup chopped toasted walnuts (page 348)

1. Place the flour, sugar, baking powder, baking soda, and cinnamon in a large bowl, and stir to mix well. Add the applesauce, oil, and vanilla extract, and stir just until the dry ingredients are moistened. Fold in the prunes and walnuts.

2. Coat an 8-x-4-inch loaf pan with nonstick cooking spray. Spread the mixture evenly in the pan, and bake at 325°F for 50 to 55 minutes, or just until a wooden toothpick inserted in the center of the loaf comes out clean. Be careful not to overbake.

3. Remove the loaf from the oven, and let sit for 15 minutes. Invert the loaf onto a wire rack, turn right side up, and cool to room temperature. Wrap the loaf in plastic wrap or aluminum foil, and allow to sit for several hours before slicing and serving. (This will give the loaf a softer, moister crust.) Refrigerate any leftovers not eaten within 24 hours.

NUTRITIONAL FACTS (PER SLICE)
Cal: 148   Carbs: 26 g   Chol: 0 mg   Fat: 4.2 g
Fiber: 3.1 g   Protein: 3.3 g   Sodium: 121 mg

Pumpkin-Orange Bread

YIELD: 16 SLICES

2 cups whole wheat pastry flour

1/3 cup sugar

2 teaspoons baking powder

3/4 teaspoon baking soda

3/4 cup mashed cooked or canned pumpkin

2/3 cup orange juice

2 tablespoons vegetable oil

1/3 cup orange marmalade

1 teaspoon vanilla extract

1/2 cup chopped dates, golden raisins, or dried cranberries

1/3 cup honey crunch wheat germ or toasted chopped pecans (page 348)

1. Place the flour, sugar, baking powder, and baking soda in a large bowl, and stir to mix well. Set aside.

2. Place the pumpkin, orange juice, oil, marmalade, and vanilla extract in a small bowl, and stir to mix well. Add the pumpkin mixture to the flour mixture, and stir just until the dry ingredients are moistened. Fold in the dates, raisins, or cranberries and the wheat germ or pecans.

3. Coat an 8-x-4-inch loaf pan with nonstick cooking spray. Spread the batter evenly in the pan, and bake at 325°F for about 50 minutes, or just until a wooden toothpick inserted in the center of the loaf comes out clean. Be careful not to overbake.

4. Remove the loaf from the oven, and let sit for 15 minutes. Invert the loaf onto a wire rack, turn right side up, and cool to room temperature. Wrap the loaf in plastic wrap or aluminum foil, and allow to sit for several hours before slicing and serving. (This will give the loaf a softer, moister crust.) Refrigerate any leftovers not eaten within 24 hours.

NUTRITIONAL FACTS (PER SLICE)
Cal: 131   Carbs: 27 g   Chol: 0 mg   Fat: 2.3 g
Fiber: 2.7 g   Protein: 2.9 g   Sodium: 106 mg

Orange Date-Nut Bread

YIELD: 16 SLICES

1 1/4 cups orange juice

1 cup chopped pitted dates

2 cups whole wheat pastry flour

1/4 cup sugar

1 teaspoon baking soda

1 teaspoon baking powder

2 tablespoons vegetable oil

1 1/2 teaspoons vanilla extract

2/3 cup chopped toasted walnuts or pecans (page 348)

1. Place the orange juice in a 1-quart pot, and bring to a boil over high heat. Place the dates in a medium-sized heatproof bowl, and pour the orange juice over the dates. Set aside to cool to room temperature.

2. Place the flour, sugar, baking soda, and baking powder in a large bowl, and stir to mix well. Set aside.

3. Stir the oil and vanilla extract into the cooled date mixture. Add the date mixture to the flour mixture, and stir just until the dry ingredients are moistened. Fold in the walnuts or pecans.

4. Coat an 8-x-4-inch loaf pan with nonstick cooking spray. Spread the batter evenly in the pan, and bake at 300°F for 45 to 50 minutes, or just until a wooden toothpick inserted in the center of the loaf comes out clean. Be careful not to overbake.

5. Remove the loaf from the oven, and let sit for 15 minutes. Invert the loaf onto a wire rack, turn right side up, and cool to room temperature. Wrap the loaf in plastic wrap or aluminum foil, and allow to sit for several hours before slicing and serving. (This will give the loaf a softer, moister crust.) Refrigerate any leftovers not eaten within 24 hours.

NUTRITIONAL FACTS (PER SLICE)
Cal: 148   Carbs: 25 g   Chol: 0 mg   Fat: 4.9 g
Fiber: 3 g   Protein: 3.7 g   Sodium: 111 mg

Fruitful Fat Substitutes

Looking for a healthful and delicious way to trim some fat from your baked goods? Think fruit. By now, everyone has heard about using applesauce as a fat substitute, but a variety of other products—including puréed canned pears, peaches, apricots, and plums; a purée made from one part prunes and two parts water; baby food fruit purées; and mashed bananas—can also replace part or all of the fat in baked goods.

How do fruit purées work? Fat performs many vital functions in baking, some of which can be duplicated by fruit purées. For instance, fat adds moistness and flavor, promotes browning, and imparts tenderness. Fruit purées reduce the need for fat because their fibers and naturally occurring sugars hold moisture into baked goods. These same fruit sugars also promote browning. Fruit purées also help tenderize baked goods, though not nearly to the extent that fat does.

Some recipes are better candidates for fat reduction than others. Which baked goods are most suited to the use of fruitful fat substitutes? Quick breads and muffins, dense cakes such as carrot cakes and fudgy chocolate cakes, and brownies and chewy cookies are some of the most easily slimmed-down recipes. Packaged muffin, quick bread, and cake mixes are also easily prepared with little or no fat. Baked goods that are meant to have a very light, tender texture are more difficult to make without fat. However, you can often eliminate 25 to 50 percent of the fat in these recipes, too.

How do you go about substituting fruit purées and other ingredients for the fat in recipes? Replace the desired amount of butter, margarine, or other solid shortening with half as much fat substitute. For instance, if you are omitting ½ cup of butter from a recipe, replace it with ¼ cup of fruit purée. (If the recipe calls for oil, substitute three-fourths as much purée.) Mix up the batter. If it seems too dry, add a little more fruit purée. To insure the greatest success when trimming the fat from your favorite recipes, also keep the following tips in mind.

• **At first, eliminate only half the fat in a recipe.** The next time you make the recipe, try replacing even more fat. Continue reducing the fat until you find the lowest amount that will give you the results you desire.

• **Use low-gluten flours.** Wheat flour contains proteins that when mixed with liquid into a batter, form tough strands called gluten. Fat tenderizes baked goods by interfering with this process. This is why removing the fat from baked goods often makes them tough or rubbery. Since sugar also interferes with gluten formation, many fat-free and low-fat recipes solve this problem by adding extra sugar. Unfortunately, this also means extra calories and an overly sweet product. What's a better solution? Use low-gluten flours like whole wheat pastry flour and oat flour in your lighter baking. Oat bran, rolled oats, and cornmeal are also low in gluten, making these products ideal ingredients for low-fat baking. Read more about these products in Chapter 1.

• **Minimize mixing.** Stirring batter excessively develops gluten and toughens the texture of baked goods. Stir only enough to mix well.

• **Avoid overbaking.** Reduced-fat baked goods tend to bake more quickly than do those made with fat, and if left in the oven too long, they can become dry. To prevent this, reduce oven temperatures by 25°F, and check the product for doneness a few minutes before the end of the usual baking time.

Buttermilk Cornbread

Be sure to use only finely ground cornmeal for the lightest, most tender texture possible.

YIELD: 12 SERVINGS
2 cups finely ground yellow or white cornmeal
2 tablespoons sugar
2 teaspoons baking powder
1/2 teaspoon baking soda
2 cups nonfat or low-fat buttermilk
3 egg whites, or 2 eggs, lightly beaten

1. Place the cornmeal, sugar, baking powder, and baking soda in a medium-sized bowl, and stir to mix well. Add the buttermilk and egg whites or eggs, and stir with a wire whisk to mix well.

2. Coat a 10-inch cast iron skillet with nonstick cooking spray, and spread the batter evenly in the pan. Bake at 375°F for 25 to 28 minutes, or just until a wooden toothpick inserted in the center of the bread comes out clean. Be careful not to overbake. Cut into wedges and serve hot, refrigerating any leftovers not eaten within 24 hours.

NUTRITIONAL FACTS (PER SERVING)
Cal: 102   Carbs: 19 g   Chol: 1 mg   Fat: 0.9 g
Fiber: 1.5 g   Protein: 3.8 g   Sodium: 195 mg

VARIATION

For a change of pace, after whisking in the buttermilk and eggs, fold one or more of the following ingredients into the batter:

❑ 3/4 to 1 cup frozen (thawed) whole kernel corn, or 1 can (8 ounces) whole kernel corn, drained.

❑ 3/4 to 1 cup shredded nonfat or reduced-fat Cheddar cheese.

❑ 2 to 4 tablespoons finely chopped pickled jalapeño peppers.

❑ 1 can (4 ounces) chopped green chilies, drained.

❑ 1/4 cup cooked crumbled turkey bacon.

Anadama Quick Bread

YIELD: 16 SLICES
2 cups whole wheat pastry flour
1/2 cup finely ground yellow or white cornmeal
2 teaspoons baking powder
3/4 teaspoon baking soda
1 1/2 cups nonfat or low-fat buttermilk
1/2 cup molasses
2 tablespoons vegetable oil

1. Place the flour, cornmeal, baking powder, and baking soda in a large bowl, and stir to mix well. Add the buttermilk, molasses, and oil, and stir just until the dry ingredients are moistened.

2. Coat an 8-x-4-inch loaf pan with nonstick cooking spray. Spread the batter evenly in the pan, and bake at 325°F for about 45 minutes, or just until a wooden toothpick inserted in the center of the loaf comes out clean. Be careful not to overbake.

3. Remove the loaf from the oven, and let sit for 15 minutes. Invert the loaf onto a wire rack, turn right side up, and cool to room temperature. Wrap the loaf in plastic wrap or aluminum foil, and allow to sit for several hours before slicing and serving. (This will give the loaf a softer, moister crust.) Refrigerate any leftovers not eaten within 24 hours.

NUTRITIONAL FACTS (PER SLICE)
Cal: 118   Carbs: 22 g   Chol: 1 mg   Fat: 2.3 g
Fiber: 2.2 g   Protein: 3.2 g   Sodium: 149 mg

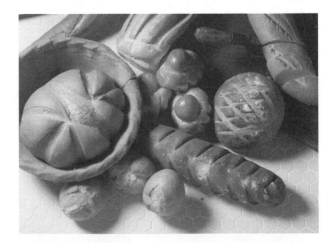

Pumpkin Gingerbread

YIELD: 32 SLICES

3 cups whole wheat pastry flour

1/2 cup sugar

1 teaspoon baking soda

2 teaspoons ground ginger

3/4 teaspoon ground allspice

3/4 teaspoon ground cinnamon

1 cup mashed cooked or canned pumpkin

1/4 cup apple or orange juice

1/4 cup vegetable oil

3/4 cup molasses

3/4 cup dark raisins or chopped dates

1. Place the flour, sugar, baking soda, ginger, allspice, and cinnamon in a large bowl, and stir to mix well. Add the pumpkin, apple or orange juice, oil, and molasses, and stir just until the dry ingredients are moistened. Fold in the raisins or dates.

2. Coat four 1-pound cans* with nonstick cooking spray. Divide the batter evenly among the cans, and tap each can onto a flat surface to smooth out the batter. Bake at 300°F for about 45 minutes, or just until a wooden toothpick inserted in the center of a loaf comes out clean.

3. Remove the bread from the oven, and let sit for 15 minutes. Invert the loaves onto a wire rack, turn right side up, and cool to room temperature. Wrap the loaves in plastic wrap or aluminum foil, and let sit for several hours before slicing and serving. (This will give the loaves a softer, moister crust.) Refrigerate any leftovers not eaten within 24 hours.

* Use only cans from foods produced in the United States, as cans from imported foods may contain lead.

NUTRITIONAL FACTS (PER SLICE)
Cal: 99   Carbs: 20 g   Chol: 0 mg   Fat: 1.9 g
Fiber: 1.7 g   Protein: 1.7 g   Sodium: 43 mg

Boston Brown Bread

YIELD: 32 SLICES

2 cups whole wheat pastry flour

1 cup finely ground yellow or white cornmeal

1 teaspoon baking soda

2 cups nonfat or low-fat buttermilk

3/4 cup molasses

1 cup dark raisins

1. Place the flour, cornmeal, and baking soda in a large bowl, and stir to mix well. Add the buttermilk and molasses, and stir to mix well. Fold in the raisins.

2. Coat four 1-pound cans* with nonstick cooking spray. Divide the batter evenly among the cans, and tap each can onto a flat surface to smooth out the batter. Bake at 300°F for about 45 minutes, or just until a wooden toothpick inserted in the center of a loaf comes out clean.

3. Remove the bread from the oven, and let sit for 15 minutes. Invert the loaves onto a wire rack, turn right side up, and cool to room temperature. Wrap the loaves in plastic wrap or aluminum foil, and let sit for several hours before slicing and serving. (This will give the loaves a softer, moister crust.) Refrigerate any leftovers not eaten within 24 hours.

* Use only cans from foods produced in the United States, as cans from imported foods may contain lead.

NUTRITIONAL FACTS (PER SLICE)
Cal: 80   Carbs: 18 g   Chol: 0 mg   Fat: 0.4 g
Fiber: 1.7 g   Protein: 2 g   Sodium: 60 mg

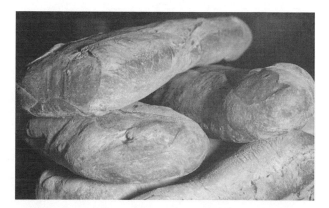

Prune-Filled Tea Bread

For variety, substitute chopped dried apricots for the prunes.

YIELD: 12 SLICES

1 recipe Whole Wheat Sweet Dough (page 85)
1½ teaspoons skim or low-fat milk

FILLING

¾ cup chopped prunes
¾ cup white grape juice

GLAZE

½ cup confectioner's sugar
2½ teaspoons skim or low-fat milk
¼ teaspoon almond extract

1. To make the filling, place the prunes and juice in a 1-quart saucepan, stir to mix, and bring to a boil over high heat. Reduce the heat to low, cover, and simmer for 15 to 20 minutes, or until the prunes have absorbed the liquid. Remove the pot from the heat, and let the mixture cool to room temperature.

2. Place the dough on a lightly floured surface, and, using a rolling pin, roll it into a 11-x-12-inch rectangle. Spread the cooled filling over the dough to within ½ inch of the edges. Roll the rectangle up jelly-roll style, beginning at the long end.

3. Coat a 12-inch round pizza pan or a large baking sheet with nonstick cooking spray, and place the roll on the pan, bringing the ends around to form a circle. Using scissors, cut almost all of the way through the dough at 1-inch intervals. Twist each 1-inch segment to turn the cut side up. (See the figure on page 88.) Cover with a clean kitchen towel, and let rise in a warm place for about 1 hour, or until doubled in size.

4. Lightly brush the top of the ring with the milk, and bake at 350°F for about 15 minutes, or until lightly browned. Remove from the oven, and allow to cool for 3 minutes.

5. To make the glaze, place all of the glaze ingredients in a small bowl, and stir until smooth. Drizzle the glaze over the warm ring, and serve immediately.

NUTRITIONAL FACTS (PER SERVING)
Cal: 144　Carbs: 31 g　Chol: 0 mg　Fat: 1.2 g
Fiber: 1.7 g　Protein: 2.7 g　Sodium: 69 mg

Cinnamon-Apple Chop Bread

YIELD: 10 SERVINGS

1 recipe Whole Wheat Sweet Dough (page 85)

FILLING

1 cup chopped peeled apples (about 1 large)
⅓ cup dark raisins or chopped toasted pecans or walnuts (page 348)
1 tablespoon sugar
½ teaspoon ground cinnamon

GLAZE

½ cup powdered sugar
2½ teaspoons skim or low-fat milk
½ teaspoon vanilla extract

1. To make the filling, place all of the filling ingredients in a small bowl, and toss to mix well. Set aside.

2. Place the dough on a large floured cutting board, and pat it into a 10-inch circle. Pile the apple mixture on top of the dough, and draw the dough up and around the apple mixture so that the edges of the dough meet in the middle, completely covering the apple filling. Flatten the dough into an 8-inch circle.

3. Using a large sharp knife, slice the mound 5 times in one direction, cutting through to the board. Then slice 5 times in the other direction to form pieces of dough that are about 1½ inches square. Use the knife to gently mix the dough and apple mixture by lifting the mixture from the bottom and piling it back on top.

4. Coat a medium-sized baking sheet with nonstick cooking spray, and gently mound the dough onto the sheet. (For best results, use a shiny baking sheet rather than a dark one.) Using your hands, gently shape the dough into an 8-inch circle, making sure that most of the apple mixture is touching pieces of dough. (This will insure that the dough holds together as it bakes.)

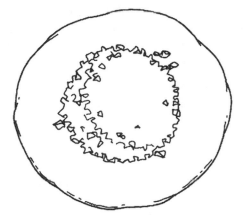

a. Pile the filling on the circle of dough.

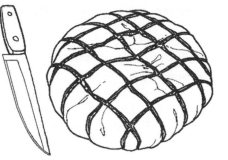

c. Slice the dough-wrapped mound
5 times in each direction.

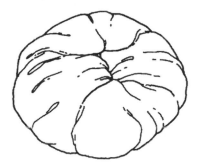

b. Draw the dough up and around
the filling.

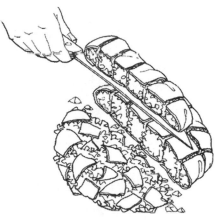

d. Use a knife to gently mix the dough
and the filling.

MAKING CINNAMON-APPLE CHOP BREAD

5. Cover the dough with a clean kitchen towel, and let rise in a warm place for about 1 hour, or until doubled in size. Bake at 350°F for about 20 minutes, or until the bread is light golden brown and puffy. Cover the bread loosely with aluminum foil during the last few minutes of baking if it begins to brown too quickly. Remove the bread from the oven, and allow to cool for 3 minutes.

6. To make the glaze, place all of the glaze ingredients in a small bowl, and stir until smooth. Drizzle the glaze over the warm loaf. Immediately cut into wedges, or simply pull off chunks and serve warm.

NUTRITIONAL FACTS (PER SERVING)
Cal: 157   Carbs: 33 g   Chol: 0 mg   Fat: 1.3 g
Fiber: 1.5 g   Protein: 3 g   Sodium: 82 mg

Cinnamon Apple Bread

YIELD: 16 SLICES

2 cups whole wheat pastry flour

²⁄₃ cup sugar

1 teaspoon ground cinnamon

1 teaspoon baking soda

²⁄₃ cup apple juice

2 tablespoons walnut or vegetable oil

1 teaspoon vanilla extract

1 egg white, lightly beaten

1½ cups finely chopped peeled
red Delicious apples (about 2 medium)

½ cup dark raisins or chopped dates or walnuts

1. Place the flour, sugar, cinnamon, and baking soda in a large bowl, and stir to mix well. Add the apple juice, oil, vanilla extract, egg white, and apples, and stir just until the dry ingredients are moistened. Fold in the raisins, dates, or walnuts.

2. Coat an 8-x-4-inch loaf pan with nonstick cooking spray. Spread the batter evenly in the pan, and bake at 325°F for 50 to 55 minutes, or just until a wooden toothpick inserted in the center of the loaf comes out clean.

3. Remove the loaf from the oven, and let sit for 15 minutes. Invert the loaf onto a wire rack, turn right side up, and cool to room temperature. Wrap the loaf in plastic wrap or aluminum foil, and allow to sit for several hours before slicing and serving. (This will give the loaf a softer, moister crust.) Refrigerate any leftovers not eaten within 24 hours.

NUTRITIONAL FACTS (PER SLICE)			
Cal: 123	Carbs: 25 g	Chol: 0 mg	Fat: 2 g
Fiber: 2.2 g	Protein: 2.4 g	Sodium: 82 mg	

Sunday Morning Scones

YIELD: 12 SCONES

1 cup whole wheat pastry flour
1 cup unbleached flour
1/3 cup sugar
1 tablespoon baking powder
1/4 teaspoon baking soda
1/2 cup dark raisins
2 tablespoons vegetable oil
1 cup nonfat or low-fat buttermilk

1. Place the flours, sugar, baking powder, and baking soda in a medium-sized bowl, and stir to mix well. Add the raisins, the oil, and just enough of the buttermilk to form a thick batter, and stir just until the dry ingredients are moistened.

2. Coat a large baking sheet with nonstick cooking spray, and drop heaping tablespoons of the batter onto the sheet, spacing them 1 inch apart. Bake at 375°F for 12 to 15 minutes, or just until the tops are lightly browned. Be careful not to overbake. Serve hot.

NUTRITIONAL FACTS (PER SCONE)			
Cal: 134	Carbs: 25 g	Chol: 0 mg	Fat: 2.6 g
Fiber: 1.7 g	Protein: 3.2 g	Sodium: 168 mg	

Apricot-Oat Scones

YIELD: 12 SCONES

1 2/3 cups unbleached flour
1/2 cup quick-cooking oats
1/3 cup sugar
1 tablespoon baking powder
1/4 teaspoon baking soda
1/2 cup chopped dried apricots, cranberries, cherries, or golden raisins
2 tablespoons vegetable oil
1 cup nonfat or low-fat buttermilk

1. Place the flour, oats, sugar, baking powder, and baking soda in a medium-sized bowl, and stir to mix well. Add the fruit, the oil, and just enough of the buttermilk to form a thick batter, and stir just until the dry ingredients are moistened.

2. Coat a large baking sheet with nonstick cooking spray, and drop heaping tablespoons of the batter onto the sheet, spacing them 1 inch apart. Bake at 375°F for 12 to 15 minutes, or just until the tops are lightly browned. Be careful not to overbake. Serve hot.

NUTRITIONAL FACTS (PER SCONE)			
Cal: 129	Carbs: 23 g	Chol: 0 mg	Fat: 2.6 g
Fiber: 1.2 g	Protein: 2.9 g	Sodium: 164 mg	

A Dough for All Seasons

Warm, fragrant, and delicious, sweet yeast breads, cakes, and buns are always a special treat. And with just one recipe, you can make an infinite number of tantalizing baked goods. Use Whole Wheat Sweet Dough to prepare some of the yeast dessert breads presented in this chapter, or draw upon your imagination to create your own cinnamon rolls, coffee cakes, buns, and breads.

If the thought of making yeast dough from scratch scares you, fear not. This recipe is easily mixed by hand. Or, if you own a bread machine, follow the simple instructions provided at the end of the recipe to prepare this versatile dough with a minimum of fuss.

Whole Wheat Sweet Dough

YIELD: ABOUT 12 OUNCES, OR 12 SERVINGS

3 tablespoons warm water (105°F–115°F)

1 1/2 teaspoons Rapid Rise yeast

1/4 cup sugar, divided

1 1/2 cups unbleached flour

1/2 cup whole wheat pastry flour

1/4 teaspoon salt

1/3 cup nonfat or low-fat buttermilk, warmed to room temperature

2 tablespoons reduced-fat margarine or light butter, melted

1. Place the water, the yeast, and 1 teaspoon of the sugar in a small bowl, and stir to dissolve the yeast. Set aside.

2. Place the remaining sugar, 1/2 cup of the unbleached flour, and all of the whole wheat flour and salt in a large bowl, and stir to mix well.

3. Add the yeast mixture, the buttermilk, and the margarine or butter to the flour mixture, and stir for 1 minute. Stir in enough of the remaining unbleached flour, 2 tablespoons at a time, to form a soft dough.

4. Sprinkle 2 tablespoons of the remaining unbleached flour over a dry surface, and turn the dough onto the surface. Knead the dough for 5 minutes, gradually adding just enough of the remaining flour to form a smooth, satiny ball.

5. Cover the dough with a clean kitchen towel, and set aside for 10 minutes. Then proceed to shape, fill, and bake the dough according to recipe directions.

NUTRITIONAL FACTS (PER SERVING)

Cal: 89   Carbs: 18 g   Chol: 0 mg   Fat: 1 g
Fiber: 0.9 g   Protein: 2.3 g   Sodium: 67 mg

TIME-SAVING TIP

To make Whole Wheat Sweet Dough in a bread machine, simply place all of the dough ingredients except for 3 tablespoons of the flour in the machine's bread pan. (Do not heat the water or melt the margarine or butter.) Turn the machine to the "rise," "dough," "manual," or equivalent setting so that the machine will mix, knead, and let the dough rise once.

Check the dough about 5 minutes after the machine has started. If the dough seems too sticky, add more of the remaining flour, a tablespoon at a time, until a smooth satiny dough is formed. When the dough is ready, remove it from the bread machine and proceed to shape, fill, and bake it as directed in the recipe of your choice.

Cherry-Almond Ring

For variety, substitute blueberries for the cherries.

YIELD: 12 SERVINGS

1 recipe Whole Wheat Sweet Dough (page 85)

1½ teaspoons skim or low-fat milk

1 tablespoon sliced toasted almonds (page 348)

FILLING

¾ cup chopped pitted fresh
or frozen (unthawed) cherries

2 tablespoons sugar

2 tablespoons plus 1 teaspoon white
grape juice, divided

2½ teaspoons cornstarch

GLAZE

½ cup powdered sugar

2½ teaspoons skim or low-fat milk

¼ teaspoon vanilla extract

¼ teaspoon almond extract

1. To make the filling, place the cherries, sugar, and 1 tablespoon plus 1 teaspoon of the juice in a 1-quart pot, and bring to a boil over medium-high heat, stirring constantly. Reduce the heat to low, cover, and simmer for about 4 minutes, or until the cherries are soft.

2. Place the remaining tablespoon of juice and the cornstarch in a small bowl, and stir to dissolve the cornstarch. Add the cornstarch mixture to the cherries, and cook and stir for another minute or 2, or until the mixture is thick and bubbly. Remove the pot from the heat, and allow the mixture to cool to room temperature.

3. Place the dough on a lightly floured surface, and, using a rolling pin, roll it into an 11-x-12-inch rectangle. Spread the cherry filling over the dough to within ½ inch of the edges. Roll the rectangle up jelly roll-style, beginning at the long end.

4. Coat a 12-inch pizza pan or a large nonstick baking sheet with nonstick cooking spray, and place the roll on the pan, bringing the ends around to form a circle. Using scissors, cut almost all of the way through the dough at 1-inch intervals. Twist each 1-inch segment to turn the cut side up. (See the figure on page 88.) Cover with a clean kitchen towel, and let rise in a warm place for about 1 hour, or until doubled in size.

5. Lightly brush the top of the ring with the milk, and bake at 350°F for about 15 minutes, or until lightly browned. Remove from the oven, and allow to cool for 3 minutes.

6. To make the glaze, place all of the glaze ingredients in a small bowl, and stir until smooth. Drizzle the glaze over the warm ring, sprinkle the almonds over the top, and serve immediately.

NUTRITIONAL FACTS (PER SERVING)

Cal: 132   Carbs: 27 g   Chol: 0 mg   Fat: 1.3 g
Fiber: 1.2 g   Protein: 2.5 g   Sodium: 68 mg

Apple Streusel Loaf

YIELD: 10 SERVINGS

1 recipe Whole Wheat Sweet Dough (page 85)

1 cup canned apple pie filling

1½ teaspoons skim or low-fat milk

STREUSEL TOPPING

2 tablespoons whole wheat pastry flour

2 tablespoons light brown sugar

¼ teaspoon ground cinnamon

1½ teaspoons tub-style nonfat margarine,
or 2¼ teaspoons reduced-fat margarine
or light butter, softened to room temperature

3 tablespoons honey crunch wheat germ or finely
chopped toasted pecans or walnuts (page 348)

GLAZE

⅓ cup powdered sugar

1½ teaspoons skim or low-fat milk

¼ teaspoon vanilla extract

⅛ teaspoon ground cinnamon

1. Place the dough on a lightly floured surface, and, using a rolling pin, roll it into a 10-x-10-inch square. Coat a large baking sheet with nonstick cooking spray, and transfer the dough to the sheet. (For best results, use a shiny baking sheet rather than a dark one.)

2. Using a sharp knife, make 3-inch-long cuts at 1-inch intervals on both the left and right sides of the square. Spread the pie filling down the center third of the dough. Fold the strips diagonally over the filling, overlapping them to create a braided look. (See the figure on page 89.)

3. Cover the loaf with a clean kitchen towel, and let rise in a warm place for about 1 hour, or until doubled in size.

4. To make the streusel topping, place the flour, brown sugar, and cinnamon in a small bowl, and stir to mix well. Add the margarine or butter, and stir until the mixture is moist and crumbly. If the mixture seems too dry, add more margarine or butter, $1/4$ teaspoon at a time, until the proper consistency is reached. Stir in the wheat germ or the nuts.

5. Lightly brush the top of the loaf with the milk. Sprinkle with the streusel topping.

6. Bake at 350°F for about 22 minutes, or until the loaf is lightly browned and no longer doughy in the center. Cover the bread loosely with aluminum foil during the last few minutes of baking if it begins to brown too quickly. Remove the loaf from the oven, and allow to cool for 3 minutes.

7. To make the glaze, place all of the glaze ingredients in a small bowl, and stir until smooth. Drizzle the glaze over the loaf. Let sit for 5 minutes before slicing and serving warm.

NUTRITIONAL FACTS (PER SERVING)			
Cal: 171	Carbs: 36 g	Chol: 0 mg	Fat: 1.5 g
Fiber: 1.5 g	Protein: 3.6 g	Sodium: 91 mg	

Maple Sticky Buns

YIELD: 12 BUNS

1 recipe Whole Wheat Sweet Dough (page 85)

FILLING

$1^1/2$ tablespoons sugar

$1^1/2$ tablespoons tub-style nonfat or reduced fat margarine or light butter, softened to room temperature

$1/4$ teaspoon ground cinnamon

$1/4$ cup plus 2 tablespoons dark raisins

3 tablespoons chopped toasted walnuts or pecans (page 348) (optional)

GLAZE

$1/4$ cup plus 2 tablespoons maple syrup or honey

1. Place the dough on a lightly floured surface, and, using a rolling pin, roll it into a 10-x-12-inch rectangle. Place the sugar, margarine or butter, and cinnamon in a small dish, stir to mix well, and spread the mixture over the dough to within $1/2$ inch of the edges. Sprinkle the raisins and, if desired, the nuts over the margarine mixture, and roll the rectangle up jelly-roll style, beginning at the long end.

2. Coat a 10-inch round pan with nonstick cooking spray, and pour the maple syrup or honey over the bottom of the pan. Cut the rolled-up dough into 1-inch slices, and lay the slices in the pan, cut side up. Cover the pan with a clean kitchen towel, and let rise in a warm place for about 1 hour, or until doubled in size.

3. Bake at 350°F for 18 to 20 minutes, or until lightly browned. Remove the pan from the oven, and run a knife around the edge to loosen the buns. Immediately invert the buns onto a serving plate, and serve warm.

NUTRITIONAL FACTS (PER BUN)			
Cal: 156	Carbs: 34 g	Chol: 0 mg	Fat: 1.2 g
Fiber: 1.1 g	Protein: 2.5 g	Sodium: 81 mg	

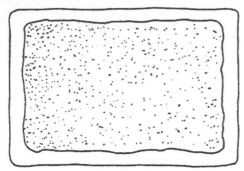

a. Spread the filling over the dough.

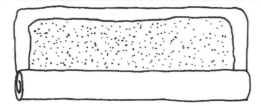

b. Roll the dough up jelly-roll style.

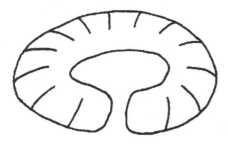

c. Bend the roll into a ring, and cut almost all the way through at 1-inch intervals.

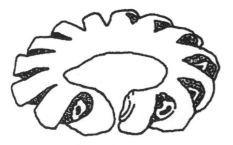

d. Twist each 1-inch segment to turn the cut side up.

MAKING CINNAMON-RAISIN RING

Cinnamon-Raisin Ring

YIELD: 12 SERVINGS

1 recipe Whole Wheat Sweet Dough (page 85)
1½ teaspoons skim or low-fat milk

FILLING

1½ tablespoons tub-style nonfat or reduced-fat margarine or light butter, softened to room temperature
1½ tablespoons sugar
½ teaspoon ground cinnamon
¼ cup plus 2 tablespoons dark raisins
3 tablespoons chopped toasted pecans or walnuts (page 348) (optional)

GLAZE

½ cup powdered sugar
⅛ teaspoon ground cinnamon
2½ teaspoons skim or low-fat milk
½ teaspoon vanilla extract

1. Place the dough on a lightly floured surface, and, using a rolling pin, roll it into an 11-x-12-inch rectangle. Place the margarine, sugar, and cinnamon in a small dish, stir to mix well, and spread the mixture over the dough to within ¼ inch of the edges. Sprinkle the raisins and, if desired, the nuts over the margarine mixture. Roll the rectangle up jelly roll-style, beginning at the long end.

2. Coat a 12-inch pizza pan or a large nonstick baking sheet with nonstick cooking spray, and place the roll on the pan, bringing the ends around to form a circle. Using scissors, cut almost all of the way through the dough at 1-inch intervals. Twist each 1-inch segment to turn the cut side up. Cover with a clean kitchen towel, and let rise in a warm place for about 1 hour, or until doubled in size.

3. Lightly brush the top of the ring with the milk, and bake at 350°F for about 15 minutes, or until lightly browned. Remove from the oven, and allow to cool for 3 minutes.

4. To make the glaze, place all of the glaze ingredients in a small bowl, and stir until smooth. Drizzle the glaze over the warm ring, and serve immediately.

NUTRITIONAL FACTS (PER SERVING)
Cal: 130   Carbs: 27 g   Chol: 0 mg   Fat: 1.1 g
Fiber: 1.1 g   Protein: 2.5 g   Sodium: 80 mg

Cherry-Cheese Loaf

YIELD: 10 SLICES

1 recipe Whole Wheat Sweet Dough (page 85)
1½ teaspoons skim or low-fat milk
1 tablespoon chopped toasted almonds, pecans, walnuts, or hazelnuts (page 348)

FILLING

4 ounces nonfat or reduced-fat cream cheese, softened to room temperature
2 tablespoons sugar
1 tablespoon fat-free egg substitute
1 tablespoon unbleached flour
¼ teaspoon vanilla extract
½ cup canned light (reduced-sugar) cherry pie filling

GLAZE

½ cup powdered sugar
2½ teaspoons skim or low-fat milk
½ teaspoon vanilla extract

1. To make the filling, place the cream cheese and sugar in a small bowl, and beat with an electric mixer until smooth. Add the egg substitute, flour, and vanilla extract, and beat until smooth. (If using reduced-fat cream cheese, omit the flour.) Set aside.

2. Place the dough on a lightly floured surface, and, using a rolling pin, roll it into a 10-x-10-inch square. Coat a large baking sheet with nonstick cooking spray, and transfer the dough to the sheet. (For best results, use a shiny baking sheet rather than a dark one.)

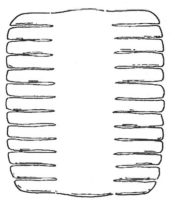

a. Make 3-inch-long cuts at 1-inch intervals on each side of the dough.

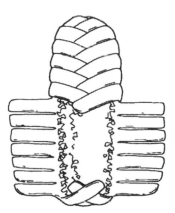

b. Fold the dough strips diagonally over the filling.

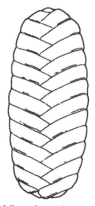

c. Continue folding the strips to create a "braided" loaf.

MAKING CHERRY CHEESE LOAF

3. Using a sharp knife, make 3-inch-long cuts at 1-inch intervals on both the left and right sides of the square. Spread the cheese filling down the center third of the dough; then dot the cheese mixture with the cherry pie filling. Fold the strips diagonally over the filling, overlapping them to create a braided look.

4. Cover the loaf with a clean kitchen towel, and let rise in a warm place for about 1 hour, or until doubled in size.

5. Lightly brush the top of the loaf with the milk. Bake at 350°F for 20 to 22 minutes, or until the loaf is lightly browned and no longer doughy in the center.

Cover the bread loosely with aluminum foil during the last few minutes of baking if it begins to brown too quickly. Remove the loaf from the oven, and set aside while you prepare the glaze.

6. To make the glaze, place all of the glaze ingredients in a small bowl, and stir until smooth. Drizzle the glaze over the loaf, and sprinkle with the nuts. Let sit for 10 minutes before slicing and serving warm.

NUTRITIONAL FACTS (PER SERVING)

Cal: 155   Carbs: 31 g   Chol: 1 mg   Fat: 1.4 g

Fiber: 1.2 g   Protein: 4.8 g   Sodium: 140 mg

4. *Party Perfect Hors D'Oeuvres and Appetizers*

For most of us, party foods spell fun, festivity—and an overdose of fat and calories. Creamy dips, fried chips, and other high-fat finger foods make most special occasions a nightmare for anyone who's trying to eat healthfully.

Fortunately, adopting a light and healthy lifestyle does not mean giving up your favorite party foods. For just about any high-fat ingredient you can think of, there is a substantially lower-fat alternative. No- and low-fat cheeses, nonfat sour cream and mayonnaise, ultra-lean lunchmeats, and a host of other products can help trim fat and calories from your celebrations and get-togethers. You'll be amazed by the big fat difference a few simple ingredient substitutions can make in traditional party favorites. For instance, a bowl of dip made with a cup of full-fat mayonnaise gets 1,582 calories and 186 fat grams from the mayonnaise alone. Prepare the same dip with a light or nonfat mayonnaise, and you will cut the fat and calories by 50 to 90 percent!

This chapter uses these and other healthful ingredients to create a wide range of hot and cold hors d'oeuvres, both plain and fancy. The following pages first present recipes for hot treats—meatballs, kabobs, quesadillas, potato skins, chicken fingers, and other savory snacks that can be passed around on platters or placed in a chafing dish for fuss-free serving. This is followed by a tempting variety of finger sandwiches and other cold pick-up snacks. Finally, you'll find a tantalizing collection of recipes for perhaps the most popular and versatile party foods of all, dips and spreads.

Whether you are planning to have a few people over for light hors d'oeuvres or an open house for fifty, this chapter is sure to meet your needs with a wealth of ideas for light and healthy finger foods that are so delicious, no one will guess that they're also good for you. So send out the invitations, and get ready to treat friends and family to a menu that's high on satisfaction, yet remarkably low in fat and calories. Your guests will appreciate this more than you know.

Bruschetta Florentine

YIELD: 48 APPETIZERS

1 package (10 ounces) frozen chopped spinach, thawed and squeezed dry

1¼ cups shredded nonfat or reduced-fat mozzarella cheese

¼ cup grated Parmesan cheese*

1 cup finely chopped plum tomatoes (about 3 medium)

2 tablespoons finely chopped onion

1 teaspoon dried Italian seasoning

4 whole wheat submarine-sandwich rolls, each 6 inches long, or 1 long, thin loaf French bread (24 x 2 inches)

Nonstick garlic-flavored cooking spray

* In this recipe, use regular Parmesan cheese, not a fat-free product.

1. Place the spinach, mozzarella and Parmesan cheeses, tomatoes, onion, and Italian seasoning in a medium-sized bowl, and stir to mix well. Set aside.

2. Slice each roll crosswise into 12 (½-inch) slices. If you're using French bread instead of rolls, slice the French bread into 48 (½-inch) slices. Arrange the slices on a baking sheet, and spray both sides lightly with the cooking spray. Bake at 400°F for 3 minutes. Turn the slices, and bake for 3 to 5 additional minutes, or until lightly browned and crisp.

3. Top each slice with 1 tablespoon of the spinach mixture, and return the appetizers to the oven for 5 minutes, or until the cheese is melted. Arrange the appetizers on a serving platter, and serve hot.

NUTRITIONAL FACTS (PER APPETIZER)
Cal: 28   Carbs: 4 g   Chol: 0 mg   Fat: 0.4 g
Fiber: 0.5 g   Protein: 1.9 g   Sodium: 76 mg

Corn and Pepper Quesadillas

YIELD: 16 APPETIZERS

4 flour tortillas (8-inch rounds), warmed to room temperature

1 cup shredded nonfat or reduced-fat Monterey jack cheese

½ cup well-drained diced commercial roasted red pepper (half of a 7-ounce jar)

½ cup frozen (thawed) whole kernel corn

Nonstick butter-flavored cooking spray

TOPPINGS

⅓ cup nonfat or light sour cream

3 tablespoons sliced scallions

1. Place the sour cream and scallions in separate serving dishes, and set aside.

2. Lay a tortilla on a flat surface, and spread 2 table-spoons of the cheese over the *bottom half only* of the tortilla. Top the cheese with 2 tablespoons of the roasted pepper, 2 tablespoons of the corn, and 2 more tablespoons of the cheese. Fold the top half of the tortilla over to enclose the filling. Repeat with the remaining ingredients to make 4 filled tortillas.

3. Coat a large baking sheet with nonstick cooking spray, and arrange the folded tortillas on the sheets in a single layer. Spray the tops lightly with the cooking spray.

4. Bake at 425°F for 5 minutes. Turn the quesadillas over, and bake for 4 additional minutes, or until the tortillas are lightly browned and the cheese is melted.

5. To serve, place each quesadilla on a cutting board, and cut into 4 wedges. Arrange the wedges on a serving platter, and serve hot, accompanied by the dishes of sour cream and scallions.

NUTRITIONAL FACTS (PER APPETIZER)
Cal: 52   Carbs: 8 g   Chol: 0 mg   Fat: 0.8 g
Fiber: 0.2 g   Protein: 3.4 g   Sodium: 178 mg

Crunchy Crab Crostini

YIELD: 24 APPETIZERS
5 ounces (about 1 cup) flaked cooked crab meat or drained canned crab meat
1/4 cup finely chopped red bell pepper
1/4 cup finely chopped green bell pepper
1/4 cup finely chopped scallions
1 teaspoon dried oregano
1/4 cup nonfat or reduced-fat mayonnaise
2 whole wheat submarine-sandwich rolls, each 6 inches long
Nonstick garlic-flavored cooking spray
2 tablespoons grated Parmesan cheese*

* In this recipe, use regular Parmesan cheese, not a fat-free product.

1. Place the crab meat, peppers, scallions, and oregano in a medium-sized bowl, and stir to mix well. Add the mayonnaise, and stir to mix well. Set aside.

2. Slice each roll crosswise into 12 (1/2-inch) slices. Arrange the slices on a baking sheet, and spray both sides lightly with the cooking spray. Bake at 400°F for 3 minutes. Turn the slices, and bake for 3 to 5 additional minutes, or until lightly browned and crisp.

3. Spread each slice with 1 tablespoon of the crab meat mixture. Top with 1/4 teaspoon of the Parmesan cheese, and return the appetizers to the oven for 5 minutes, or until the cheese is lightly browned. Arrange the appetizers on a serving platter, and serve hot.

NUTRITIONAL FACTS (PER APPETIZER)
Cal: 29   Carbs: 4 g   Chol: 4 mg   Fat: 0.5 g
Fiber: 0.4 g   Protein: 2.1 g   Sodium: 86 mg

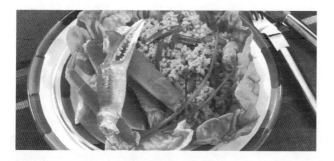

Florentine Stuffed Mushrooms

YIELD: 24 APPETIZERS
24 medium-large fresh mushroom caps
4 cups (packed) chopped fresh spinach
1/2 teaspoon dried thyme or oregano
1/2 teaspoon crushed fresh garlic
2 scallions, finely chopped
1/4 cup grated nonfat or regular Parmesan cheese
2 cups soft bread crumbs*
2 tablespoons fat-free egg substitute
Nonstick butter-flavored cooking spray
Lemon wedges (garnish)

* To make soft bread crumbs, tear about 3 slices of bread into chunks, place the chunks in a food processor or blender, and process into crumbs.

1. Wash the mushroom caps, pat dry, and set aside.

2. Coat a large nonstick skillet with cooking spray. Place the spinach, thyme or oregano, garlic, and scallions in the skillet, and sauté over medium heat just until the spinach is wilted. Add a tablespoon of white wine or broth if the skillet is too dry. Remove the skillet from the heat, and set aside for a few minutes to cool slightly.

3. Add the Parmesan cheese and bread crumbs to the skillet mixture, and toss gently to mix well. Add the egg substitute, and toss again. The mixture should be moist but not wet, and should hold together nicely. Add a little broth or water if the mixture seems too dry.

4. Coat a 9-x-13-inch pan with nonstick cooking spray. Place a heaping teaspoonful of stuffing in each mushroom cap, and arrange the mushrooms in the pan. Spray the tops lightly with the cooking spray.

5. Cover the pan with aluminum foil, and bake at 400°F for 15 minutes. Remove the foil and bake for 5 additional minutes, or until the mushrooms are tender and the stuffing is lightly browned. Serve hot, accompanied by the lemon wedges.

NUTRITIONAL FACTS (PER APPETIZER)
Cal: 22   Carbs: 3 g   Chol: 1 mg   Fat: 0.3 g
Fiber: 0.7 g   Protein: 1.5 g   Sodium: 43 mg

Clam-Stuffed Mushrooms

YIELD: 24 APPETIZERS

24 medium-large fresh mushroom caps

2 cans (6½ ounces each) chopped clams, undrained

½ cup finely chopped onion

½ cup finely chopped celery
(include the leaves)

1 teaspoon crushed fresh garlic

¾ teaspoon dried oregano

⅛ teaspoon ground black pepper

1 cup soft whole wheat bread crumbs*

¼ cup grated nonfat or regular Parmesan cheese

2 tablespoons fat-free egg substitute

Nonstick olive oil cooking spray

Lemon wedges (garnish)

* To make soft bread crumbs, tear about 1⅓ slices of bread into chunks, place the chunks in a food processor or blender, and process into crumbs.

1. Wash the mushroom caps, pat dry, and set aside. Drain the clams, reserving the juice, and set aside.

2. Coat a large nonstick skillet with olive oil cooking spray, and preheat over medium-high heat. Add the onion, celery, garlic, oregano, and pepper; cover; and cook, stirring frequently, for about 3 minutes, or until the onion and celery begin to soften. Add a little of the reserved clam juice to the skillet if it becomes too dry. Remove the skillet from the heat, and set aside for a few minutes to cool slightly.

3. Add the bread crumbs and Parmesan to the skillet mixture, and toss to mix well. Gently toss in first the drained clams, and then the egg substitute. The mixture should be moist but not wet, and should hold together nicely. Add a little of the reserved clam juice if the mixture seems too dry.

4. Coat a 9-x-13-inch pan with nonstick cooking spray. Place a heaping teaspoonful of the stuffing in each mushroom cap, and arrange the mushrooms in the pan. Spray the tops lightly with the cooking spray.

5. Cover the pan with aluminum foil, and bake at 400°F for 15 minutes. Remove the foil and bake for 5 additional minutes, or until the mushrooms are tender and the stuffing is lightly browned. Serve hot, accompanied by the lemon wedges.

NUTRITIONAL FACTS (PER APPETIZER)
Cal: 28   Carbs: 3.1 g   Chol: 5 mg   Fat: 0.6 g
Fiber: 0.6 g   Protein: 3.2 g   Sodium: 40 mg

Sausage and Artichoke Bruschetta

YIELD: 48 APPETIZERS

1 cup plus 2 tablespoons finely chopped frozen (thawed) or canned (drained) artichoke hearts

¾ cup finely chopped plum tomatoes
(about 2½ medium)

6 ounces Turkey Italian Sausage (page 251),
cooked, finely crumbled, and drained

1¼ cups shredded nonfat or reduced-fat
mozzarella cheese

2 tablespoons grated Parmesan cheese*

1 long, thin loaf sourdough French bread
(24 x 2 inches)

Nonstick garlic-flavored cooking spray

* In this recipe, use regular Parmesan cheese, not a fat-free product.

1. Place the artichoke hearts, tomatoes, sausage, mozzarella, and Parmesan cheese in a medium-sized bowl, and stir to mix well. Set aside.

2. Slice the bread into 48 (½-inch) slices. Arrange the slices on a baking sheet, and spray both sides lightly with the cooking spray. Bake at 400°F for 3 minutes. Turn the slices, and bake for 3 to 5 additional minutes, or until lightly browned and crisp.

3. Top each slice with 1 tablespoon of the artichoke mixture, and return the appetizers to the oven for 5 minutes, or until the cheese is melted. Arrange the appetizers on a serving platter, and serve hot.

NUTRITIONAL FACTS (PER APPETIZER)
Cal: 34   Carbs: 4.5   Chol: 3 mg   Fat: 0.7 g
Fiber: 0.4 g   Protein: 2.4 g   Sodium: 72 mg

Oven-Fried Mushrooms

YIELD: 20 APPETIZERS

20 medium whole fresh mushrooms
(about 8 ounces)

Nonstick olive oil cooking spray

BATTER COATING

¼ cup unbleached flour

¼ cup fat-free egg substitute,
or 2 egg whites, lightly beaten

3 tablespoons skim or low-fat milk

CRUMB COATING

½ cup plain dried bread crumbs

¾ teaspoon dried thyme

¾ teaspoon ground paprika

DIPPING SAUCE

½ cup nonfat or light sour cream

2 tablespoons nonfat or reduced-fat mayonnaise

1½ tablespoons finely chopped onion

1–2 teaspoons prepared horseradish

1. Wash the mushrooms, pat dry, and set aside.

2. To make the batter coating, place all of the batter ingredients in a shallow bowl, and stir with a wire whisk until smooth. Set aside.

3. To make the crumb coating, place all of the crumb coating ingredients in a shallow bowl, and stir to mix well. Set aside.

4. Coat a large baking sheet with nonstick cooking spray. Dip each mushroom first in the batter coating, and then in the crumb coating. Arrange the mushrooms in a single layer on the prepared pan.

5. Spray the mushrooms lightly with the olive oil cooking spray, and bake at 400°F for 8 minutes. Turn the mushrooms over, and bake for 7 to 9 additional minutes, or until nicely browned.

6. While the mushrooms are baking, place all of the dipping sauce ingredients in a small bowl, and stir to mix well. Arrange the mushrooms on a serving platter, and serve hot, accompanied by the dish of sauce. Be aware that the centers of the mushrooms will be

very hot when they first come out of the oven, so bite carefully.

NUTRITIONAL FACTS (PER APPETIZER)
Cal: 23   Carbs: 4 g   Chol: 0 mg   Fat: 0.1 g
Fiber: 0.3 g   Protein: 1.2 g   Sodium: 36 mg

Pita Party Pizzas

YIELD: 24 APPETIZERS

4 whole wheat or oat bran pita pockets
(6-inch rounds)

¾ cup bottled marinara sauce

2 tablespoons grated nonfat or regular
Parmesan cheese

1 cup shredded reduced-fat mozzarella cheese

¼ cup thinly sliced fresh mushrooms

2 thin slices onion, separated into rings

1 teaspoon dried Italian seasoning

1. Arrange the pita pockets on a flat surface. Spread 3 tablespoons of the marinara sauce on top of each pita pocket. Top with a quarter of the Parmesan cheese followed by a quarter of the mozzarella cheese, a quarter of the mushrooms, and a few onion rings. Sprinkle with a quarter of the Italian seasoning.

2. Arrange the pita pizzas on a baking sheet, and bake at 400°F for about 12 minutes, or until the cheese is melted and lightly browned. Cut each pizza into 6 pieces, transfer to a serving platter, and serve hot.

NUTRITIONAL FACTS (PER APPETIZER)
Cal: 39   Carbs: 4 g   Chol: 1 mg   Fat: 0.8 g
Fiber: 0.8 g   Protein: 2 g   Sodium: 86 mg

VARIATIONS
In addition to or instead of the cheese, mushrooms, and onions, top the pizzas with thinly sliced yellow squash, broccoli florets, diced Canadian bacon, or cooked turkey Italian sausage.

Broccoli Baked Potato Skins

YIELD: 12 APPETIZERS

6 small baking potatoes (each about 3 inches long)

3/4 cup frozen chopped broccoli, thawed and squeezed dry

3/4 cup shredded nonfat or reduced-fat Cheddar cheese

Nonstick butter-flavored cooking spray

3/4 cup nonfat or light sour cream

1/4 cup thinly sliced scallions

1. If using a conventional oven, wrap the potatoes in aluminum foil, and bake at 400°F for about 35 minutes, or until tender. If using a microwave oven, pierce each potato in several places with a fork and microwave on high power for about 12 minutes, or until tender. Set aside to cool.

2. Cut the potatoes in half lengthwise. Scoop out and discard the pulp, leaving a 1/4-inch-thick shell. Place 1 tablespoon of broccoli in each skin, and top with 1 tablespoon of cheese. Spray the tops of the stuffed potatoes lightly with the cooking spray.

3. Arrange the potato skins on a baking sheet, and bake at 450°F for about 12 minutes, or until the cheese is bubbly. Transfer the skins to a serving platter, top each with 1 tablespoon of sour cream and a sprinkling of scallions, and serve hot.

NUTRITIONAL FACTS (PER APPETIZER)
Cal: 58　Carbs: 10 g　Chol: 1 mg　Fat: 0.2 g
Fiber: 1 g　Protein: 3.7 g　Sodium: 70 mg

VARIATION

To make Spicy Chicken Skins, combine 3/4 cup of shredded cooked chicken breast, 2 tablespoons of picante sauce, and 1 teaspoon of chili powder. Substitute this mixture for the broccoli, top with the cheese, and bake.

NUTRITIONAL FACTS (PER APPETIZER)
Cal: 72　Carbs: 10 g　Chol: 8 mg　Fat: 0.5 g
Fiber: 0.7 g　Protein: 6.3 g　Sodium: 89 mg

Chili-Cheese Potato Skins

YIELD: 12 APPETIZERS

6 small baking potatoes (each about 3 inches long)

3/4 cup Fiesta Chili (page 177) or canned low-fat chili

1/2 cup shredded nonfat or reduced-fat Cheddar or Monterey jack cheese

Nonstick olive oil cooking spray

1/2 cup nonfat or light sour cream

1/4 cup thinly sliced scallions

1. If using a conventional oven, wrap the potatoes in aluminum foil and bake at 400°F for about 35 minutes, or until tender. If using a microwave oven, pierce each potato in several places with a fork and microwave on high power for about 12 minutes, or until tender. Set aside to cool.

2. Cut the potatoes in half lengthwise. Scoop out and discard the pulp, leaving a 1/4-inch-thick shell. Place 1 tablespoon of chili in each skin, and top with 2 teaspoons of cheese. Spray the tops of the stuffed potatoes lightly with the cooking spray.

3. Arrange the potato skins on a baking sheet, and bake at 450°F for about 12 minutes, or until the filling is hot and the cheese is bubbly. Transfer the skins to a serving platter, top each with 2 teaspoons of sour cream and a sprinkling of scallions, and serve hot.

NUTRITIONAL FACTS (PER APPETIZER)
Cal: 75　Carbs: 13 g　Chol: 1 mg　Fat: 0.6 g
Fiber: 1.8 g　Protein: 5 g　Sodium: 88 mg

Mini Reuben Melts

YIELD: 24 APPETIZERS

6 slices (1 ounce each) reduced-fat Swiss cheese

1/2 cup bottled nonfat Thousand Island salad dressing

24 slices cocktail rye bread

24 thin slices (about 8 ounces) corned beef or turkey pastrami, at least 97% lean

3/4 cup well-drained sauerkraut

1. Cut each slice of cheese into 4 squares, and set aside. Spread 1 teaspoon of Thousand Island dressing on each piece of bread, and top with 1 slice of corned beef or pastrami, folding the slice as necessary to accommodate the shape of the bread. Top with 1/2 tablespoon of sauerkraut and 1 square of cheese.

2. Place the Reubens on a baking sheet, and bake at 350°F for 10 minutes, or until the cheese is melted and the Reubens are hot. Transfer to a serving platter, and serve hot.

NUTRITIONAL FACTS (PER APPETIZER)			
Cal: 56	Carbs: 6 g	Chol: 5 mg	Fat: 1.3 g
Fiber: 0.7 g	Protein: 5 g	Sodium: 267 mg	

Hot Artichoke Appetizers

YIELD: 40 APPETIZERS

3 packages (10 ounces each) frozen artichoke hearts, thawed, or 3 cans (14 ounces each) artichoke hearts, drained

Five 4-inch square slices (1 ounce each) ham, at least 97% lean

MARINADE

1/3 cup Dijon mustard

1/3 cup water

1/4 cup finely chopped onion

2 tablespoons sugar or honey

1. If the artichoke hearts are large, cut them into quarters. If they are small, cut them in half. You should have about 40 pieces.

2. Place all of the marinade ingredients in a blender, and process for 30 seconds, or until smooth. Place the artichoke hearts in a shallow dish, and pour the marinade over them. Cover and refrigerate for several hours or overnight.

3. Cut each ham slice into eight 1/2-inch strips. Drain the artichoke hearts, and discard the marinade. Wrap a ham strip around each artichoke piece, and secure with a wooden toothpick.

4. Arrange the wrapped artichokes in a shallow baking dish, and bake at 350°F for 10 to 15 minutes, or

until thoroughly heated. Transfer to a serving platter, and serve hot.

NUTRITIONAL FACTS (PER APPETIZER)			
Cal: 12	Carbs: 1.2 g	Chol: 2 mg	Fat: 0.3 g
Fiber: 1 g	Protein: 1.1 g	Sodium: 49 mg	

Chicken Tortilla Crisps

YIELD: 32 APPETIZERS

4 flour tortillas (8-inch rounds)

1 cup shredded cooked chicken breast (about 5 ounces)

1/2 cup bottled chunky salsa

2 teaspoons chili powder

1 1/2 cups shredded nonfat or reduced-fat Cheddar or Monterey jack cheese

1/4 cup sliced black olives

1/4 cup sliced scallions

1/2 cup plus 2 tablespoons nonfat or light sour cream

1. Coat 2 large baking sheets with nonstick cooking spray, and arrange 2 tortillas on each sheet. Bake at 350°F for about 6 minutes, or until lightly browned.

2. While the tortillas are baking, place the chicken, salsa, and chili powder in a small bowl, and stir to mix well. Set aside.

3. Remove the tortillas from the oven, and sprinkle 1/4 cup of the cheese over each tortilla. Top each tortilla with a quarter of the chicken mixture, 1 tablespoon of olives, and 1 tablespoon of scallions. Sprinkle with 2 tablespoons of the cheese.

4. Return the tortillas to the oven for 5 to 7 minutes, or until the cheese is melted and the tortillas are crisp. While the tortillas are baking, place the sour cream in a small serving bowl. Cut each tortilla into 8 wedges, and arrange the wedges on a serving platter accompanied by the sour cream. Serve hot.

NUTRITIONAL FACTS (PER APPETIZER)			
Cal: 36	Carbs: 3.8 g	Chol: 4 mg	Fat: 0.4 g
Fiber: 0.3 g	Protein: 4.3 g	Sodium: 95 mg	

Flaky Spinach Pies

YIELD: 40 APPETIZERS

1 package (10 ounces) frozen chopped spinach, thawed and squeezed dry

1 cup nonfat or low-fat ricotta cheese

¾ cup shredded nonfat or reduced-fat mozzarella cheese

¼ cup grated nonfat or regular Parmesan cheese

½ teaspoon dried oregano

20 sheets (12 x 18 inches) phyllo pastry (about 1 pound)

Nonstick olive oil cooking spray

1. Place the spinach, ricotta, mozzarella, Parmesan, and oregano in a medium-sized bowl, and stir to mix well. Set aside.

2. Spread the phyllo dough out on a clean dry surface. You should have a 12-x-18-inch sheet that is 20 layers thick. Cut the phyllo dough lengthwise into 4 long strips. Cover the phyllo dough with plastic wrap to prevent it from drying out as you work. (Remove strips as you need them, being sure to re-cover the remaining dough.)

3. Remove 1 strip of phyllo dough, and lay it flat on a clean dry surface. Spray the strip lightly with cooking spray. Top with another phyllo strip, and spray lightly with cooking spray. Spread 1 tablespoon of filling over the bottom right-hand corner of the double phyllo strip. Fold the filled corner up and over to the left, so that the corner meets the left side of the strip. Continue folding in this manner until you form a triangle of dough. Repeat with the remaining dough and filling to make 40 triangles.

4. Coat a large baking sheet with nonstick cooking spray. Place the appetizers seam side down on the sheet, and bake at 375°F for about 15 minutes, or until nicely browned. Allow to cool for 5 to 10 minutes before serving warm.

TIME-SAVING TIP
To speed last-minute party preparations, prepare the pies in advance to the point of baking, and arrange them in single layers in airtight plastic containers, separating the layers with sheets of waxed paper. Freeze until the day of the party. Then arrange the frozen pies on a coated baking sheet, and allow them to sit at room temperature for 45 minutes before baking.

NUTRITIONAL FACTS (PER APPETIZER)
Cal: 43   Carbs: 6 g   Chol: 1 mg   Fat: 0.7 g
Fiber: 0.4 g   Protein: 2.8 g   Sodium: 69 mg

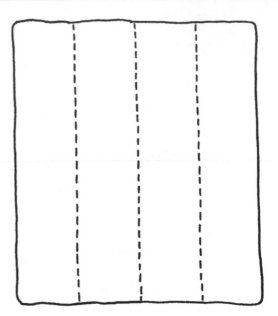

a. Cut the dough into 4 strips.

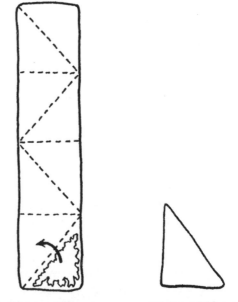

b. Fold the filled corner up and over.

c. Continue folding to form a triangle.

MAKING FLAKY SPINACH PIES

Zesty Barbecue Meatballs

YIELD: 60 APPETIZERS

MEATBALLS

1½ pounds 95% lean ground beef

¾ cup quick-cooking oats

2 egg whites

1 cup finely chopped onion

1 tablespoon plus 1 teaspoon spicy mustard

1½ teaspoons crushed fresh garlic

¼ cup minced fresh parsley, or 1 tablespoon
plus 1 teaspoon dried

1 teaspoon dried oregano

1½ teaspoons instant beef bouillon granules

½ teaspoon ground black pepper

⅓ cup skim or low-fat milk

SAUCE

1½ cups bottled barbecue sauce

1. Place all of the meatball ingredients in a medium-sized bowl, and mix thoroughly. Coat a large baking sheet with nonstick cooking spray. Shape the meatball mixture into 60 (1-inch) balls, and arrange the meatballs on the baking sheet.

2. Bake at 350°F for about 25 minutes, or until thoroughly cooked. (At this point, the meatballs can be frozen for later use. See the Time-Saving Tip on page 100.) Transfer the meatballs to a chafing dish or Crock-Pot electric casserole to keep warm.

3. Place the barbecue sauce in a small saucepan, and cook over medium heat, stirring frequently, just until hot. Pour the sauce over the meatballs, toss gently to mix, and serve.

NUTRITIONAL FACTS (PER APPETIZER)
Cal: 25   Carbs: 1.8 g   Chol: 6 mg   Fat: 0.6 g
Fiber: 0.2 g   Protein: 2.7 g   Sodium: 76 mg

Meatball Makeovers

When prepared in the usual way, meatballs are among the fattiest of party fare. But these tasty morsels need not blow your fat budget, for there are plenty of ways to give these appetizers a slimming makeover and, at the same time, greatly boost nutritional value. Here are some ideas for giving your favorite meatball recipes a healthful makeover.

- Add lots of finely chopped vegetables—such as onions, mushrooms, and green peppers—to the meatball mixture. As the meatballs cook, the chopped vegetables will release their juices into the meat, keeping your ultra-lean appetizers moist and flavorful.

- Add some rolled oats or oat bran as a meat extender. During cooking, the oats will soak up the juices released from the meat and from any chopped vegetables in the mixture, and will hold in the moisture.

- Replace part of the ground beef with meatless recipe crumbles, TVP, or tofu hamburger. You can easily replace up to a third of the ground meat in your recipe with these products with no detectable difference. (Read more about these fat-saving products in Chapter 1.)

- Add ingredients like cooked brown rice, cooked bulgur wheat, chopped cooked spinach, and chopped water chestnuts to the meatball mixture. These ingredients add texture and flavor, while making a little bit of meat go a long way.

Aloha Meatballs

YIELD: 45 APPETIZERS

MEATBALLS

1 pound 95% lean ground beef or ground turkey

1 cup cooked brown rice

2 egg whites

1 can (8 ounces) crushed pineapple in juice, drained

1 can (8 ounces) sliced water chestnuts, drained and chopped

½ cup chopped scallions

1 tablespoon reduced-sodium soy sauce

1 teaspoon ground ginger

SAUCE

¾ cup unsalted chicken broth, divided

2½ teaspoons cornstarch

⅓ cup ketchup or chili sauce

3 tablespoons seasoned rice wine vinegar

2 tablespoons dark brown sugar

½ teaspoon ground ginger

1. Place all of the meatball ingredients in a medium-sized bowl, and mix thoroughly. Coat a large baking sheet with nonstick cooking spray. Shape the meatball mixture into 45 (1-inch) balls, and arrange the meatballs on the baking sheet.

2. Bake at 350°F for about 25 minutes, or until thoroughly cooked. Transfer the meatballs to a chafing dish or Crock-Pot electric casserole to keep warm.

3. To make the sauce, place 2 tablespoons of the broth and all of the cornstarch in a small saucepan, and stir until the cornstarch is dissolved. Add the remaining broth and all of the remaining sauce ingredients, and stir to mix well. Cook over medium heat, stirring frequently, until the mixture comes to a boil. Reduce the heat to low, and cook and stir for another minute, or until the mixture thickens slightly. Pour the sauce over the meatballs, toss gently to mix, and serve.

NUTRITIONAL FACTS (PER APPETIZER)
Cal: 27   Carbs: 3.5 g   Chol: 5 mg   Fat: 0.5 g
Fiber: 0.4 g   Protein: 2.2 g   Sodium: 60 mg

TIME-SAVING TIP
To avoid a last-minute rush, make the meatballs in advance. Just cook them as directed—without the sauce—and freeze them in freezer bags. The day before the party, thaw the meatballs in the refrigerator. The next day, simply make the sauce and heat it along with the meatballs.

Curried Meatballs

YIELD: 45 APPETIZERS

MEATBALLS

1 pound ground turkey breast or 95% lean ground beef

¾ cup quick-cooking oats

1 cup finely chopped fresh mushrooms

2 egg whites

1 cup finely chopped onion

1 tablespoon curry paste

1 teaspoon ground ginger

¼ teaspoon ground black pepper

SAUCE

¼ cup plus 2 tablespoons honey

¼ cup plus 2 tablespoons Dijon mustard

2 teaspoons curry paste

1. Place all of the meatball ingredients in a medium-sized bowl, and mix thoroughly. Coat a large baking sheet with nonstick cooking spray. Shape the meatball mixture into 45 (1-inch) balls, and arrange the meatballs on the baking sheet.

2. Bake at 350°F for about 25 minutes, or until thoroughly cooked. (At this point, the meatballs can be frozen for later use. See the Time-Saving Tip above. Transfer the meatballs to a chafing dish or Crock-Pot heated casserole to keep warm.

3. To make the sauce, place all of the sauce ingredients in a small saucepan, and cook over medium heat, stirring frequently, just until hot. Pour the sauce over the meatballs, toss gently to mix, and serve.

NUTRITIONAL FACTS (PER APPETIZER)
Cal: 31   Carbs: 4 g   Chol: 5 mg   Fat: 0.7 g
Fiber: 0.3 g   Protein: 2.8 g   Sodium: 85 mg

Oven-Fried Zucchini Fingers

YIELD: 32 APPETIZERS

4 medium zucchini (about 1½ pounds)

Nonstick olive oil cooking spray

1½ cups bottled marinara sauce

BATTER

¼ cup plus 2 tablespoons unbleached flour

¼ cup plus 2 tablespoons fat-free egg substitute,
or 3 egg whites, lightly beaten

¼ cup skim or low-fat milk

CRUMB COATING

3¼ cups corn flakes

¼ cup plus 1 tablespoon grated Parmesan cheese*

1¼ teaspoons dried Italian seasoning

¼ teaspoon ground black pepper

* In this recipe, use regular Parmesan cheese, not a fat-free product.

1. Rinse the zucchini, pat dry, and trim and discard the ends. Quarter each zucchini lengthwise; then cut each piece in half crosswise. You should now have 32 zucchini fingers, each about 3½ inches long.

2. To make the batter, place all of the batter ingredients in a shallow dish, and stir with a wire whisk to mix well. Set aside.

3. To make the coating, place the corn flakes in a food processor or blender, and process into crumbs. (You should have about ¾ cup plus 2 tablespoons of crumbs. Adjust the amount if necessary.) Transfer the crumbs to a shallow dish, and stir in the remaining coating ingredients. Set aside.

4. Coat a large baking sheet with olive oil cooking spray. Dip the zucchini fingers, 1 at a time, first in the batter and then in the crumb coating mixture, turning to coat all sides. Arrange the zucchini fingers in a single layer on the prepared sheet.

5. Spray the zucchini fingers lightly with the cooking spray, and bake at 400°F for about 15 minutes, or until the zucchini is golden brown and crisp.

6. While the zucchini is baking, place the sauce in a small pot and cook over medium heat until heated through. Arrange the zucchini on a serving platter, and serve hot, accompanied by the bowl of hot sauce.

NUTRITIONAL FACTS
(PER APPETIZER, WITH 2 TEASPOONS OF SAUCE)
Cal: 30　Carbs: 5 g　Chol: 0 mg　Fat: 0.5 g
Fiber: 0.6 g　Protein: 1.4 g　Sodium: 74 mg

Stuffed Finger Sandwiches

YIELD: 18 APPETIZERS

1 long, thin loaf French bread (about 24 x 2 inches)

½ cup plus 2 tablespoons nonfat or reduced-fat
cream cheese, softened to room temperature

½ teaspoon dried Italian seasoning

¾ teaspoon crushed fresh garlic

4 ounces thinly sliced cooked turkey breast

8–10 fresh tender spinach leaves

½ medium red bell pepper, cut in thin strips

½ cup chopped frozen (thawed) artichoke hearts, or
½ cup drained and chopped canned artichoke hearts

1. Using a serrated knife, slice the French bread lengthwise, cutting off the top third of the loaf. Using your fingers, remove and discard enough of the soft inner bread to leave only a ½-inch-thick shell.

2. Place the cream cheese, Italian seasoning, and garlic in a small bowl, and stir to mix well. Spread half of this mixture evenly over the inside of the bottom shell. Roll up the turkey slices, and arrange them in an even layer over the cream cheese mixture. Lay the spinach leaves over the turkey, and top with a layer of pepper strips. Finish with a layer of artichokes.

3. Spread the remaining cream cheese mixture over the inside of the top shell. Place the top shell over the bottom shell to reform the loaf, and wrap the loaf tightly in aluminum foil or plastic wrap. Chill for several hours or overnight.

4. When ready to serve, unwrap the loaf, and use a serrated knife to cut the loaf diagonally into 1-inch slices. Secure each piece with a wooden toothpick, arrange on a platter, and serve.

NUTRITIONAL FACTS (PER APPETIZER)
Cal: 60　Carbs: 9 g　Chol: 8 mg　Fat: 0.2 g
Fiber: 0.7 g　Protein: 5.5 g　Sodium: 179 mg

Chicken Fingers With Honey Mustard Sauce

YIELD: 20 APPETIZERS

1 pound boneless skinless chicken breasts
(about 4 breast halves)

3 cups corn flakes

1/2 teaspoon poultry seasoning

1/4 teaspoon ground black pepper

3 tablespoons fat-free egg substitute,
or 1 egg, lightly beaten

3 tablespoons skim or low-fat milk

Nonstick cooking spray

SAUCE

1/2 cup nonfat or reduced-fat mayonnaise

3 tablespoons spicy mustard

3 tablespoons honey

1. Rinse the chicken with cool water, and pat it dry with paper towels. Cut each piece into 5 long strips, and set aside.

2. Place the corn flakes in a blender or food processor, and process into crumbs. (You should have about 3/4 cup of crumbs. Adjust the amount if necessary.) Transfer the crumbs to a shallow dish, and stir in the poultry seasoning and pepper. Set aside.

3. Place the egg substitute or egg and the milk in another shallow dish. Stir to mix well, and set aside.

4. Coat a large baking sheet with nonstick cooking spray. Dip each chicken strip first in the egg mixture and then in the crumb mixture, turning to coat each side with crumbs. Arrange the strips in a single layer on the prepared sheet.

5. Spray the tops of the chicken strips lightly with the cooking spray, and bake at 400°F for 15 minutes, or until the strips are golden brown and no longer pink inside.

6. While the chicken is baking, place all of the sauce ingredients in a small dish, and stir to mix well. Arrange the chicken strips on a serving platter, and serve hot, accompanied by the bowl of sauce.

NUTRITIONAL FACTS
(PER APPETIZER, WITH 2 TEASPOONS OF SAUCE)
Cal: 53   Carbs: 6 g   Chol: 13 mg   Fat: 0.4 g
Fiber: 0.1 g   Protein: 5.8 g   Sodium: 127 mg

Cashew Chicken Salad Finger Sandwiches

YIELD: 32 APPETIZERS

1 1/2 cups finely chopped cooked chicken
or turkey breast, or 1 can (12 ounces)
chicken or turkey breast, drained

1/2 cup finely chopped celery

1/2 cup chopped roasted cashews

2 tablespoons finely chopped red bell pepper

2 tablespoons finely chopped scallion

1/4 cup nonfat or reduced-fat mayonnaise

1/4 cup nonfat or light sour cream

16 slices firm multigrain, oatmeal,
or whole wheat bread

1. Place the chicken or turkey, celery, cashews, red pepper, and scallion in a medium-sized bowl, and toss to mix well. Add the mayonnaise and sour cream, and stir to mix well, adding a little more mayonnaise if the filling seems too dry.

2. Spread 1/4 cup of the filling over each of 8 slices of bread. Top each slice with 1 of the remaining slices, making 8 sandwiches. Trim the crusts from the bread, and cut each sandwich into 4 rectangles, squares, or triangles. Arrange the sandwiches on a platter and serve immediately, or cover with plastic wrap and refrigerate for up to 3 hours before serving.

NUTRITIONAL FACTS (PER APPETIZER)
Cal: 59   Carbs: 7 g   Chol: 5 mg   Fat: 1.7 g
Fiber: 1 g   Protein: 3.9 g   Sodium: 91 mg

Submarine Finger Sandwiches

YIELD: 14 APPETIZERS

1 loaf French bread (14 x 2½ inches)

2 tablespoons nonfat or reduced-fat mayonnaise

1 tablespoon plus 1 teaspoon spicy mustard

1½ cups shredded romaine lettuce, divided

2 ounces thinly sliced roasted turkey breast

2 ounces thinly sliced honey ham, at least 97% lean

2 ounces thinly sliced nonfat or reduced-fat provolone or Cheddar cheese

1 plum tomato, thinly sliced

3 very thin onion slices, separated into rings

6 very thin green bell pepper rings

3 tablespoons canned hot banana pepper rings

1 tablespoon plus 1 teaspoon bottled nonfat Italian salad dressing

1. Using a serrated knife, slice the bread in half lengthwise. Using your fingers, remove and discard the top ½ inch of bread from the center of each half to form a slight depression.

2. Spread the mayonnaise over the bottom piece of bread, and the mustard over the top piece. Lay the bottom of the loaf on a flat surface, and arrange ½ cup of the lettuce over the bread. Layer the turkey, ham, and cheese over the lettuce. Top with the tomato, onion, green pepper, and banana pepper, and the remaining lettuce. Drizzle the Italian dressing over the lettuce, and replace the top of the loaf.

3. Cut the sandwich into 1-inch slices, and secure each piece with a toothpick. Arrange the appetizers on a platter and serve immediately, or cover with plastic wrap and refrigerate for up to 3 hours before serving.

NUTRITIONAL FACTS (PER APPETIZER)
Cal: 62   Carbs: 10 g   Chol: 6 mg   Fat: 0.6 g
Fiber: 0.7 g   Protein: 4.2 g   Sodium: 204 mg

Dilly Chicken Salad Finger Sandwiches

YIELD: 32 APPETIZERS

1½ cups finely chopped cooked chicken or turkey breast, or 1 can (12 ounces) chicken or turkey breast, drained

½ cup finely chopped celery

¼ cup grated carrot

2 tablespoons finely chopped onion

1 tablespoon minced fresh dill, or 1 teaspoon dried

¼ cup nonfat or reduced-fat mayonnaise

¼ cup nonfat or light sour cream

16 slices firm whole wheat, rye, or pumpernickel bread

1. Place the chicken or turkey, celery, carrot, and onion in a medium-sized bowl, and stir to mix well. Add all of the remaining ingredients except for the bread, and stir to mix well, adding more mayonnaise if the filling seems dry.

2. Spread ¼ cup of the filling over each of 8 slices of bread. Top each slice with 1 of the remaining slices, making 8 sandwiches. Trim the crusts from the bread, and cut each sandwich into 4 rectangles, squares, or triangles. Arrange the sandwiches on a platter and serve immediately, or cover with plastic wrap and refrigerate for up to 3 hours before serving.

NUTRITIONAL FACTS (PER APPETIZER)
Cal: 48   Carbs: 7.5 g   Chol: 5 mg   Fat: 0.6 g
Fiber: 1.2 g   Protein: 3.2 g   Sodium: 108 mg

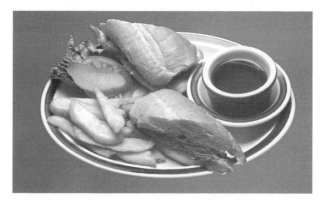

Chicken Fingers With Tangy Apricot Sauce

YIELD: 20 APPETIZERS

1 pound boneless skinless chicken breasts (about 4 halves)

3 cups corn flakes

1/4 teaspoon poultry seasoning

1/4 teaspoon ground ginger

1/4 teaspoon ground white pepper

2 tablespoons sesame seeds

1/2 cup fat-free egg substitute, or 2 eggs plus 1 egg white, lightly beaten

Nonstick cooking spray

SAUCE

1/2 cup apricot spread or jam

1/4 cup chicken broth

1 tablespoon plus 1 teaspoon seasoned rice wine vinegar

1/8 teaspoon ground ginger

1. Rinse the chicken with cool water, and pat it dry with paper towels. Cut each piece into 5 long strips, and set aside.

2. Place the corn flakes in a blender or food processor, and process into crumbs. (You should have about 3/4 cup of crumbs. Adjust the amount if necessary.) Transfer the crumbs to a shallow dish, and stir in the poultry seasoning, ginger, white pepper, and sesame seeds. Set aside.

3. Place the egg substitute or eggs in another shallow dish, and set aside.

4. Coat a large baking sheet with nonstick cooking spray. Dip each chicken strip first in the egg and then in the crumb mixture, turning to coat each side with crumbs. Arrange the strips in a single layer on the prepared sheet.

5. Spray the tops of the chicken strips lightly with the cooking spray, and bake at 400°F for 15 minutes, or until the strips are golden brown and no longer pink inside.

6. While the chicken is baking, place all of the sauce ingredients in a blender, and process until smooth. Pour the mixture into a small saucepan, and cook over medium heat for several minutes, or just until heated through. Transfer the sauce to a small dish.

7. Arrange the chicken strips on a serving platter, and serve hot, accompanied by the dish of warm sauce.

NUTRITIONAL FACTS
(PER APPETIZER, WITH 2 TEASPOONS OF SAUCE)
Cal: 67   Carbs: 7 g   Chol: 13 mg   Fat: 0.8 g
Fiber: 0.2 g   Protein: 6.3 g   Sodium: 76 mg

Veggie-Cheese Finger Sandwiches

YIELD: 32 APPETIZERS

2 blocks (8 ounces each) nonfat or reduced fat cream cheese, softened to room temperature

1/4 cup finely chopped onion

1/4 cup finely chopped green bell pepper

1/4 cup grated carrot

2 tablespoons finely chopped fresh parsley

1–2 teaspoons prepared horseradish or spicy mustard (optional)

16 slices firm whole wheat, rye, or pumpernickel bread

1. Place the softened cream cheese in a medium-sized bowl. Place the vegetables, parsley, and, if desired, the horseradish or mustard in a small bowl, and stir to mix well. Stir the vegetable mixture into the softened cream cheese, cover, and chill for several hours to allow the flavors to blend.

2. Spread 1/4 cup of the filling over each of 8 slices of bread. Top each slice with 1 of the remaining slices, making 8 sandwiches. Trim the crusts from the bread, and cut each sandwich into 4 fingers. Arrange the sandwiches on a platter and serve immediately, or cover with plastic wrap and refrigerate for up to 3 hours before serving.

NUTRITIONAL FACTS (PER APPETIZER)
Cal: 51   Carbs: 7 g   Chol: 2 mg   Fat: 0.4 g
Fiber: 1.1 g   Protein: 4.5 g   Sodium: 169 mg

Italian Roll-Ups

YIELD: 48 APPETIZERS

8 flour tortillas (10-inch rounds)

1½ cups nonfat or reduced-fat cream cheese
(plain or garlic-and-herb flavor)

1 pound thinly sliced roasted turkey breast,
or 1 pound thinly sliced ham, at least 97% lean

8 ounces thinly sliced nonfat or reduced-fat
mozzarella cheese or reduced-fat provolone cheese

½ cup bottled nonfat creamy Italian
or roasted garlic salad dressing

48 fresh tender spinach or arugula leaves

½ cup coarsely chopped black olives

32 ¼-inch-thick strips commercial roasted red pepper
(about one 7-ounce jar)

4 thin slices red onion, separated into rings

9 ounces frozen (thawed) artichoke hearts,
chopped, or 1 can (14 ounces) artichoke hearts,
drained and chopped

1. Arrange the tortillas on a flat surface, and spread each with 3 tablespoons of cream cheese, extending the cheese to the outer edges. Lay 2 ounces of sliced turkey or ham over the *bottom half only* of each tortilla, leaving a 1-inch margin on each outer edge. Place 1 ounce of sliced cheese over the meat, and spread with 1 tablespoon of the dressing. Arrange 6 spinach or arugula leaves over the cheese, and sprinkle with 1 tablespoon of olives. Arrange 4 red pepper strips and a few onion rings over the olive layer, and top with 3 tablespoons of artichoke hearts.

2. Starting at the bottom, roll each tortilla up tightly. Cut a 1¼-inch piece off each end, and discard. Slice the remainder of each tortilla into six 1¼-inch pieces. Arrange the rolls on a platter and serve immediately, or cover with plastic wrap and refrigerate for up to 8 hours before serving.

NUTRITIONAL FACTS (PER APPETIZER)
Cal: 61   Carbs: 6.6 g   Chol: 8 mg   Fat: 0.9 g
Fiber: 0.9 g   Protein: 6.2 g   Sodium: 159 mg

Fiesta Roll-Ups

YIELD: 48 APPETIZERS

¼ cup nonfat or light sour cream

¼ cup bottled picante sauce

8 flour tortillas (10-inch rounds)

1½ cups nonfat or reduced-fat cream cheese

1 pound thinly sliced roasted turkey breast,
or 1 pound thinly sliced ham, at least 97% lean

8 ounces thinly sliced nonfat or reduced-fat
Cheddar cheese

8 large fresh lettuce leaves

½ cup chopped black olives

24 very thin slices tomato

½ cup sliced scallions

1. Place the sour cream and picante sauce in a small bowl. Stir to mix well, and set aside.

2. Arrange the tortillas on a flat surface, and spread each with 3 tablespoons of cream cheese, extending the cheese to the outer edges. Lay 2 ounces of sliced turkey or ham over the *bottom half only* of each tortilla, leaving a 1-inch margin on each outer edge. Place 1 ounce of Cheddar over the turkey, and spread with 1 tablespoon of the sour cream-picante mixture. Arrange 1 lettuce leaf over the cheese, and sprinkle with 1 tablespoon of olives. Arrange 3 tomato slices over the olive layer, and top with 1 tablespoon of scallions.

3. Starting at the bottom, roll each tortilla up tightly. Cut a 1¼-inch piece off each end, and discard. Slice the remainder of each tortilla into six 1¼-inch pieces. Arrange the rolls on a platter and serve immediately, or cover with plastic wrap and refrigerate for up to 8 hours before serving.

NUTRITIONAL FACTS (PER APPETIZER)
Cal: 55   Carbs: 6 g   Chol: 9 mg   Fat: 0.7 g
Fiber: 0.6 g   Protein: 6 g   Sodium: 136 mg

Spinach, Ham, and Swiss Strudels

YIELD: 28 APPETIZERS

3 cups (packed) chopped fresh spinach

1 cup shredded nonfat or reduced-fat Swiss cheese

3/4 cup (about 3 1/2 ounces) finely chopped ham, at least 97% lean

1 1/2 teaspoons spicy mustard

1/4 cup fat-free egg substitute

12 sheets (12 x 18 inches) phyllo pastry (about 10 ounces)

Nonstick butter-flavored cooking spray

1. Coat a medium-sized nonstick skillet with nonstick cooking spray, and preheat over medium heat. Add the spinach, and stir-fry for about 2 minutes, or just until wilted. Remove the skillet from the heat, and allow the spinach to cool to room temperature.

2. Add the cheese and ham to the cooled spinach, and toss to mix well. Combine the mustard and egg substitute in a small bowl, and add to the spinach mixture, tossing to mix well. Set aside.

3. Spread the phyllo dough out on a clean dry surface. You should have a 12-x-18-inch sheet that is 12

layers thick. Cover the phyllo dough with plastic wrap to prevent it from drying out as you work. (Remove sheets as you need them, being sure to re-cover the remaining dough.)

4. Remove 1 sheet of phyllo dough, and lay it flat on a clean dry surface with the short end near you. Spray the strip lightly with the cooking spray. Top with another phyllo sheet, and spray lightly with cooking spray. Repeat with a third sheet.

5. Spread a fourth of the filling over the lower third of the stacked sheets, leaving a 3-inch margin on each side. Fold the left and right edges inward to enclose the filling, and roll the sheet up from the bottom, jelly-roll style. Repeat with the remaining dough and filling to make 4 rolls.

6. Coat a large baking sheet with nonstick cooking spray. Place the rolls seam side down on the sheet, and spray the tops lightly with the cooking spray. Score the rolls with a sharp knife at 1-inch intervals, cutting through just the outer layer of phyllo. (This will keep the baked phyllo from shattering when you slice it.)

7. Bake at 350°F for 25 minutes, or until light golden brown. Remove the rolls from the oven, and allow to cool for 5 minutes. Slice along the score lines, and serve hot.

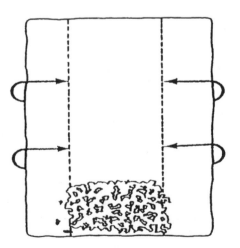

a. Spread the filling over the dough, and fold the left and right edges inward over the filling.

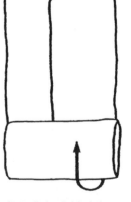
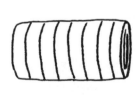

b. Roll the folded sheet up.

c. Score each roll at 1-inch intervals.

MAKING SPINACH, HAM, AND SWISS STRUDELS

NUTRITIONAL FACTS (PER APPETIZER)
Cal: 38   Carbs: 5 g   Chol: 1 mg   Fat: 0.8 g
Fiber: 0.2 g   Protein: 3 g   Sodium: 99 mg

VARIATION

To make Sensational Broccoli Strudels, combine 1 package (10 ounces) of frozen chopped broccoli (thawed and squeezed dry) with 1 cup of shredded nonfat or reduced-fat mozzarella or Swiss cheese, 1½ teaspoons of Dijon mustard, and ¼ cup of fat-free egg substitute. Stir to mix well, and use as a substitute for the spinach filling.

NUTRITIONAL FACTS (PER APPETIZER)
Cal: 33   Carbs: 14.5 g   Chol: 0 mg   Fat: 0.6 g
Fiber: 0.3 g   Protein: 2.3 g   Sodium: 80 mg

Strawberry-Cheese Bites

YIELD: 24 SERVINGS

1 block (8 ounces) nonfat or reduced-fat
cream cheese

3–4 tablespoons sugar

¾ teaspoon vanilla extract

24 reduced-fat vanilla or chocolate wafers
or lemon snaps

12 medium strawberries, halved

1. Place the cream cheese, sugar, and vanilla extract in a medium-sized bowl, and beat with an electric mixer until smooth.

2. Place 1 rounded teaspoonful of the cheese mixture in the center of each cookie, and press a strawberry half into the cheese. Arrange on a serving plate and serve immediately.

NUTRITIONAL FACTS (PER SERVING)
Cal: 31   Carbs: 5 g   Chol: 1 mg   Fat: 0.4 g
Fiber: 0.2 g   Protein: 1.7 g   Sodium: 58 mg

Chutney Chicken Kabobs

YIELD: 18 APPETIZERS

1 pound boneless skinless chicken breasts
(about 4 halves)

1 can (15 ounces) unsweetened pineapple chunks
in juice, undrained

¼ cup mango chutney

2 tablespoons reduced-sodium soy sauce

1½ teaspoons crushed fresh garlic

36 one-inch scallion pieces (white and light green parts only), or 36 green bell pepper strips (each 1-x-½ inch)

1. Rinse the chicken with cool water, and pat it dry with paper towels. Cut the chicken breasts lengthwise into ⅓-inch-thick strips. (This will be easiest to do if the meat is partially frozen.) Place the strips in a shallow nonmetal container, and set aside.

2. Drain the pineapple, and place ¼ cup plus 2 tablespoons of the juice in a blender. Refrigerate the pineapple chunks until ready to assemble the kabobs.

3. To make the marinade, add the chutney, soy sauce, and garlic to the pineapple juice, and process for about 1 minute, or until smooth. Remove ¼ cup of the marinade, and refrigerate until ready to cook the kabobs. Pour the remaining marinade over the chicken strips, and toss to mix well. Cover the chicken and refrigerate for at least 3 hours, and for up to 24 hours.

4. Just before making the kabobs, place 18 six-inch bamboo skewers in a shallow dish, and cover with water. Allow the skewers to soak for 20 minutes. (This will prevent them from burning.)

5. Loosely weave 1 long and 1 short chicken strip, 2 pineapple chunks, and 2 pieces of scallion or green pepper onto each skewer. Grill the skewers over medium coals or broil 6 inches under a preheated broiler for about 3 minutes on each side, or until almost done. Baste the kabobs with the reserved marinade and cook for another minute or 2 on each side, or until the meat is nicely browned and no longer pink inside. Serve hot.

NUTRITIONAL FACTS (PER APPETIZER)
Cal: 42   Carbs: 3.4 g   Chol: 15 mg   Fat: 0.3 g
Fiber: 0.3 g   Protein: 6 g   Sodium: 48 mg

Crispy Shrimp

For variety, substitute bite-sized pieces of chicken breast for the shrimp.

YIELD: 40 APPETIZERS

40 large raw shrimp (about 1 pound), peeled and deveined

1/4 cup plus 2 tablespoons unbleached flour

1/4 cup plus 2 tablespoons fat-free egg substitute, or 3 egg whites, lightly beaten

1/4 cup orange juice

4 cups corn flakes

1/4 cup toasted wheat germ or finely ground pecans

1/2 teaspoon coarsely ground black pepper

Nonstick cooking spray

SAUCE

1/2 cup nonfat or reduced-fat mayonnaise

1 tablespoon plus 1 teaspoon spicy mustard

1 tablespoon honey

3 tablespoons orange juice

1. Rinse the shrimp with cool water, and pat them dry with paper towels. Set aside.

2. Place the flour, egg substitute or egg whites, and orange juice in a shallow bowl, and stir with a wire whisk until smooth. Set aside.

3. Place the corn flakes in a blender or food processor, and process into crumbs. (You should have about 1 cup of crumbs. Adjust the amount if necessary.) Transfer the crumbs to a shallow dish, and stir in the wheat germ or pecans and the pepper. Set aside.

4. Coat a large baking sheet or Crispy Crust pizza pan with nonstick cooking spray. Dip the shrimp first in the crumb mixture, then in the egg mixture, and once again in the crumb mixture, turning to coat well. Arrange the shrimp in a single layer on the prepared pan.

5. Spray the shrimp lightly with the cooking spray, and bake at 400°F for about 12 minutes, or until the

shrimp are nicely browned on the outside and opaque on the inside.

6. While the shrimp are baking, place the mayonnaise, mustard, and honey in a small dish, and stir to mix well. Stir in the orange juice. Arrange the shrimp on a serving platter, and serve hot, accompanied by the dish of sauce.

> **NUTRITIONAL FACTS**
> **(PER APPETIZER, WITH 1 TEASPOON OF SAUCE)**
> Cal: 29   Carbs: 4 g   Chol: 11 mg   Fat: 0.2 g
> Fiber: 0.2 g   Protein: 2.2 g   Sodium: 71 mg

Shrimp-Stuffed Artichokes

YIELD: 12 APPETIZERS

1/2 cup finely chopped onion

1/3 cup finely chopped green bell pepper

1/3 cup finely chopped red bell pepper

1 teaspoon crushed fresh garlic

1/2 teaspoon dried Italian seasoning

1/8 teaspoon ground black pepper

3/4 cup finely diced cooked shrimp or crab meat (about 4 ounces)

1 cup soft whole wheat or Italian bread crumbs*

3 tablespoons grated nonfat or regular Parmesan cheese

2 tablespoons nonfat or reduced-fat mayonnaise

12 canned artichoke bottoms (about two 14-ounce cans, drained)

Nonstick olive oil cooking spray

Lemon wedges (garnish)

* To make soft bread crumbs, tear about 1 1/3 slices of bread into chunks, place the chunks in a food processor or blender, and process into crumbs.

1. Coat a large nonstick skillet with olive oil cooking spray, and preheat over medium heat. Add the onion, green and red pepper, garlic, Italian seasoning, and pepper, and stir to mix well. Cover and cook, stirring frequently, for about 4 minutes, or until the vegetables are soft. Remove the skillet from the heat, and allow to cool for several minutes.

2. Add first the shrimp or crab meat and then the bread crumbs and Parmesan to the skillet mixture, and toss to mix well. Add the mayonnaise, and toss gently to mix. The mixture should be moist, but not wet, and should hold together nicely. Add a little more mayonnaise if the mixture seems too dry.

3. Place a heaping tablespoonful of stuffing in the hollow of each artichoke bottom. Coat a 9-x-9-inch pan with nonstick cooking spray, and arrange the artichokes in the pan. Spray the tops of the stuffing lightly with the cooking spray.

4. Cover the pan with aluminum foil, and bake at 400°F for 15 minutes. Remove the foil, and bake for 5 additional minutes, or until the stuffing is lightly browned. Serve hot, accompanied by the lemon wedges.

NUTRITIONAL FACTS (PER APPETIZER)
Cal: 52   Carbs: 8.1 g   Chol: 19 mg   Fat: 0.6 g
Fiber: 2.9 g   Protein: 4.8 g   Sodium: 157 mg

Shrimp Wrapped in Snow Peas

YIELD: 64 APPETIZERS

64 large fresh snow peas (about 8 ounces)

64 large shrimp (about 1¾ pounds), peeled and cooked

DIPPING SAUCE

½ cup nonfat or light sour cream

½ cup nonfat or reduced-fat mayonnaise

3 tablespoons honey

3 tablespoons Dijon mustard

1. To make the sauce, place all of the sauce ingredients in a small bowl, and stir to mix well. Set aside.

2. Rinse the snow peas with cool running water, and arrange in a microwave or conventional steamer. Cover and cook on high power or over medium-high heat for about 3 minutes, or just until the pods are bright green and pliable. Rinse with cool water, dry, and set aside.

3. Wrap a snow pea around each shrimp, and secure with a wooden toothpick. Arrange on a serving platter and serve, accompanied by the bowl of dipping sauce.

NUTRITIONAL FACTS
(PER APPETIZER, WITH ½ TEASPOON SAUCE)
Cal: 14   Carbs: 2 g   Chol: 11 mg   Fat: 0.1 g
Fiber: 0.2 g   Protein: 1.4 g   Sodium: 41 mg

Asparagus Roll-Ups

YIELD: 30 APPETIZERS

30 fresh asparagus spears (about 1 pound)

30 thin slices (about 6 ounces) honey roasted turkey breast

DIPPING SAUCE

½ cup nonfat or reduced-fat mayonnaise

½ cup nonfat or light sour cream

3 tablespoons Dijon mustard

2–3 tablespoons honey

1. To make the sauce, place all of the sauce ingredients in a small bowl, and stir to mix well. Set aside.

2. Rinse the asparagus with cool running water, and snap off the tough stem ends. Arrange the asparagus spears in a microwave or conventional steamer. Cover and cook on high power or over medium-high heat for about 3 minutes, or just until the spears are crisp-tender.

3. Drain the asparagus, and plunge them into a large bowl of ice water to stop the cooking process. Drain the spears, and pat dry.

4. Lay 1 slice of turkey on a flat surface, and place 1 asparagus spear on the lower end of the slice. Roll the asparagus spear up in the turkey slice, and secure with a wooden toothpick. Repeat with the remaining turkey slices and asparagus spears.

5. Arrange the roll-ups on a serving platter and serve, accompanied by the bowl of dipping sauce.

NUTRITIONAL FACTS (PER APPETIZER WITH SAUCE)
Cal: 23   Carbs: 3.3 g   Chol: 2 mg   Fat: 0.3 g
Fiber: 0.4 g   Protein: 1.8 g   Sodium: 133 mg

Super Stuffed Veggies

It takes a matter of minutes to turn fresh vegetables and any of the dips or sandwich fillings presented in this book into delicious stuffed veggies. Serve these veggies as healthy hors d'oeuvres, or use them to decorate platters of finger sandwiches and canapés. The following ideas should get you started, but do experiment with other vegetables and dips to find the combination that you like best.

- Slice off the tops of cherry tomatoes, scoop out the seeds, and fill with Light Blue Cheese Dip (page 114) or Dilled Shrimp Dip (page 117).

- Cut peeled cucumbers into ¾- to 1-inch-thick slices. Scoop out some of the seeds, creating a cucumber cup with a ¼-inch-thick shell. Fill with Smoked Salmon Spread (page 118) or Onion Dill Dip (page 117).

- Cut celery into 2- or 3-inch lengths, and fill with Pimento Cheese Spread (page 120) or Bacon, Cheddar, and Pecan Spread (page 119).

- Boil new potatoes until tender but firm. Cut a thin slice off the bottom of each potato so that it will sit upright, and scoop out some of the flesh, leaving a ½-inch-thick shell. Fill with Onion Dill Dip (page 117) or Light Blue Cheese Dip (page 114).

High Rollers

Simple to prepare and festive in appearance, these appetizers go fast, so be sure to make plenty.

YIELD: 48 APPETIZERS
8 flour tortillas (10-inch rounds)
1½ cups nonfat or reduced-fat cream cheese (plain or garlic-and-herb flavor)
1 pound thinly sliced roasted turkey breast
8 ounces thinly sliced nonfat or reduced-fat Swiss cheese
½ cup bottled nonfat ranch salad dressing
48 tender fresh spinach leaves
½ cup finely chopped black olives (optional)
48 very thin slices red bell pepper or tomato
1 can (14 ounces) artichoke hearts, drained and chopped

1. Arrange the tortillas on a flat surface, and spread each with 3 tablespoons of cream cheese, extending the cheese to the outer edges. Lay 2 ounces of sliced turkey over the *bottom half only* of each tortilla, leaving a 1-inch margin on each outer edge. Place 1 ounce of sliced Swiss cheese over the turkey, and spread with 1 tablespoon of ranch dressing. Arrange 6 spinach leaves over the cheese, and sprinkle with 1 tablespoon of olives, if desired. Arrange 6 red pepper or tomato slices over the olive layer, and top with ¼ cup of artichoke hearts.

2. Starting at the bottom, roll each tortilla up tightly. Cut a 1¼-inch piece off each end, and discard. Slice the remainder of each tortilla into six 1¼-inch pieces. Arrange the rolls on a platter and serve immediately, or cover with plastic wrap and refrigerate for up to 8 hours before serving.

NUTRITIONAL FACTS (PER APPETIZER)			
Cal: 55	Carbs: 6 g	Chol: 6 mg	Fat: 0.8 g
Fiber: 0.7 g	Protein: 6 g	Sodium: 122 mg	

Parmesan Pita Crisps

YIELD: 12 SERVINGS

6 whole wheat or oat bran pita pockets (6-inch rounds)

1/4 cup plus 2 tablespoons grated Parmesan cheese*

1 1/2 teaspoons dried Italian seasoning

* In this recipe, use regular Parmesan cheese, not a fat-free product.

1. Using a sharp knife, cut each piece of pita bread around the entire outer edge to separate the bread into 2 rounds.

2. Arrange the pita rounds on a flat surface with the inside of the bread facing up. Sprinkle each round first with 1 1/2 teaspoons of the Parmesan, and then with 1/8 teaspoon of the Italian seasoning.

3. Cut each round into 6 wedges. Arrange the wedges in a single layer on a large ungreased baking sheet, and bake at 375°F for 4 to 6 minutes, or until lightly browned and crisp. Cool to room temperature.

4. Serve the crisps with dips and spreads, or as an accompaniment to soups and salads.

NUTRITIONAL FACTS (PER 6 CHIPS)
Cal: 84   Carbs: 15 g   Chol: 2 mg   Fat: 1.2 g
Fiber: 2 g   Protein: 4.3 g   Sodium: 218 mg

Garlic and Herb Bagel Chips

For variety, make these chips with other types of bagels, such as onion, sun-dried tomato, and spinach.

YIELD: 8 SERVINGS

4 large whole wheat or oat bran bagels
(about 4 ounces each)

Nonstick garlic-flavored cooking spray

2 teaspoons dried Italian seasoning

1. Slice the bagels diagonally into 1/4-inch-thick slices. Set aside.

2. Coat a large baking sheet with garlic-flavored cooking spray. Arrange the chips on the sheet in a single layer. Spray the tops of the chips lightly with the cooking spray, and sprinkle with half of the dried seasoning. Bake at 350°F for 5 minutes. Turn the chips over, spray again, and sprinkle with the remaining seasoning. Bake for 3 to 5 additional minutes, or until lightly browned and crisp. Cool to room temperature.

3. Serve the chips with dips and spreads, or as an accompaniment to soups and salads.

NUTRITIONAL FACTS (PER SERVING)
Cal: 151   Carbs: 32 g   Chol: 0 mg   Fat: 0.9 g
Fiber: 3.6 g   Protein: 6.2 g   Sodium: 278 mg

Mexican Bean Dip

YIELD: 2 1/2 CUPS

1 can (1 pound) pinto beans, rinsed and drained

1/4 cup nonfat or light sour cream

2–3 teaspoons chili powder

1/2 teaspoon ground cumin

1/2 cup shredded reduced-fat Cheddar cheese

1/4 cup thinly sliced scallions

1/4 cup sliced black olives

2 tablespoons finely chopped pickled
jalapeño peppers

1. Place the beans, sour cream, chili powder, and cumin in a food processor or blender, and process until smooth. Spread the mixture over the bottom of a 9-inch glass pie pan. Top with the cheese, followed by the scallions, olives, and jalapeños, in that order.

2. Serve at room temperature or hot. If using a microwave oven, heat uncovered on high power for 5 minutes, or until the edges are bubbly and the cheese is melted. If using a conventional oven, cover loosely with foil and bake at 350°F for 20 minutes. Serve with baked tortilla chips.

NUTRITIONAL FACTS (PER TABLESPOON)
Cal: 16   Carbs: 2 g   Chol: 0 mg   Fat: 0.3 g
Fiber: 0.7 g   Protein: 1.2 g   Sodium: 44 mg

Baked Spinach and Artichoke Spread

YIELD: 2½ CUPS

1 package (10 ounces) frozen chopped spinach, thawed and squeezed dry

1 package (9 ounces) frozen artichoke hearts, thawed, drained, and finely chopped, or 1 can (14 ounces) artichoke hearts, drained and finely chopped

⅔ cup nonfat or reduced-fat mayonnaise

1 tablespoon Dijon mustard

½ cup Parmesan cheese, divided*

* In this recipe, use regular Parmesan cheese, not a fat-free product.

1. Place all of the ingredients except for 2 tablespoons of the Parmesan cheese in a medium-sized bowl, and stir to mix well.

2. Coat a 1-quart casserole dish with nonstick cooking spray, and spread the mixture evenly in the dish. Sprinkle the remaining 2 tablespoons of Parmesan over the top.

3. Cover the dish with aluminum foil, and bake at 350°F for 25 minutes, or until the mixture is heated through. Remove the foil, and bake for 5 additional minutes, or until the top is lightly browned. Serve hot with a loaf of Italian bread, Garlic and Herb Bagel Chips (page 111), or Parmesan Pita Crisps (page 111).

NUTRITIONAL FACTS (PER TABLESPOON)
Cal: 13   Carbs: 1.6 g   Chol: 1 mg   Fat: 0.4 g
Fiber: 0.4 g   Protein: 0.8 g   Sodium: 58 mg

Spiced Artichoke Spread

YIELD: 1¼ CUPS

1 package (9 ounces) frozen artichoke hearts, thawed and drained, or 1 can (14 ounces) artichoke hearts, drained

1 tablespoon spicy mustard

¼ cup nonfat or reduced-fat mayonnaise

Pinch cayenne pepper

¼ cup grated Parmesan cheese, divided*

* In this recipe, use regular Parmesan cheese, not a fat-free product.

1. Place all of the ingredients except for 2 tablespoons of the Parmesan cheese in a food processor, and process until well mixed but still slightly chunky.

2. Coat a 2-cup casserole dish with nonstick cooking spray, and spread the mixture evenly in the dish. Sprinkle the remaining 2 tablespoons of Parmesan over the top.

3. Cover the dish with aluminum foil, and bake at 350°F for 20 minutes. Remove the foil, and bake for 5 additional minutes, or until the top is lightly browned. Serve hot with whole grain crackers, flatbread, French bread, or Parmesan Pita Crisps (page 111).

NUTRITIONAL FACTS (PER TABLESPOON)
Cal: 14   Carbs: 1.8 g   Chol: 1 mg   Fat: 0.4 g
Fiber: 0.8 g   Protein: 0.9 g   Sodium: 54 mg

Hot and Creamy Crab Dip

YIELD: 3¼ CUPS

1 large round loaf sourdough bread

2 blocks (8 ounces each) nonfat or reduced-fat cream cheese, softened to room temperature

2 tablespoons skim or low-fat milk

1 tablespoon lemon juice

1 tablespoon white wine Worcestershire sauce

1½ cups (about 8 ounces) flaked cooked crab meat or drained canned crab meat

2 tablespoons finely chopped onion

Ground paprika

1. Cut the top from the bread loaf, and set aside. Hollow out the bread, leaving a 1-inch-thick shell. Set aside.

2. Coat a baking sheet with nonstick cooking spray. Cut the removed bread into cubes, and arrange on the baking sheet. Bake at 350°F for 10 minutes, or until lightly toasted. Set aside.

3. Place the cream cheese, milk, lemon juice, and Worcestershire sauce in a large bowl, and beat with an electric mixer until smooth. Stir in the crab meat and onion. Evenly spread the mixture in the hollowed loaf, cover with the bread top, and wrap in aluminum foil.

4. Bake the filled loaf at 350°F for 1 hour and 10 minutes, or until the dip is hot and creamy. Place the loaf on a serving plate, remove and discard the top, and sprinkle the dip lightly with the paprika. Serve hot with whole grain crackers and the toasted bread cubes.

NUTRITIONAL FACTS (PER TABLESPOON)
Cal: 13   Carbs: 1.9 g   Chol: 4 mg   Fat: 0.1 g
Fiber: 0 g   Protein: 2.2 g   Sodium: 61 mg

Beef and Bean Dip

YIELD: 3⅓ CUPS

6 ounces 95% lean ground beef

1 medium onion, chopped

1 tablespoon chili powder, divided

1 can (1 pound) pinto beans, rinsed and drained

½ teaspoon ground cumin

½ cup bottled picante sauce or salsa

¾ cup shredded reduced-fat sharp
Cheddar cheese

¼ cup thinly sliced scallions

1. Place the ground beef in a medium-sized nonstick skillet, and brown over medium-high heat, stirring constantly. Drain off and discard any excess fat.

2. Add the onion and 2 teaspoons of the chili powder to the beef, and stir to mix. Cover and cook over medium heat until the onions are crisp-tender. Set aside.

3. Place the beans, the remaining teaspoon of chili powder, and the cumin in a food processor or blender, and process to the desired consistency. Spread the bean mixture over the bottom of a 9-inch deep dish pie pan. Top the beans with the ground meat mixture, followed by the picante sauce or salsa, Cheddar cheese, and scallions, in that order.

4. If using a microwave oven, heat uncovered on high power for about 5 minutes, or until the edges are bubbly and the cheese is melted. If using a con-

ventional oven, cover loosely with aluminum foil and bake at 350°F for about 20 minutes, or until the edges are bubbly. Serve with baked tortilla chips.

NUTRITIONAL FACTS (PER TABLESPOON)
Cal: 18   Carbs: 1.6 g   Chol: 2 mg   Fat: 0.4 g
Fiber: 0.6 g   Protein: 2 g   Sodium: 35 mg

Baked Clam Dip

YIELD: 3¼ CUPS

2 cans (10 ounces each) chopped clams, undrained

1 large round loaf sourdough bread

2 blocks (8 ounces each) nonfat or reduced-fat
cream cheese, softened to room temperature

1 tablespoon lemon juice

2 tablespoons finely chopped onion

2 teaspoons white wine Worcestershire sauce

1. Drain the clams, reserving 2 tablespoons of the liquid. Set aside.

2. Cut the top from the bread loaf, and set aside. Hollow out the bread, leaving a 1-inch-thick shell. Set aside.

3. Coat a baking sheet with nonstick cooking spray. Cut the removed bread into cubes, and arrange on the baking sheet. Bake at 350°F for 10 minutes, or until lightly toasted. Set aside.

4. Place the cream cheese, lemon juice, onion, Worcestershire sauce, and reserved clam juice in a large bowl, and beat with an electric mixer until smooth. Stir in the drained clams. Evenly spread the mixture in the hollowed loaf, cover with the bread top, and wrap in aluminum foil.

5. Bake the filled loaf at 350°F for 1 hour and 10 minutes, or until the dip is hot and creamy. Place the loaf on a serving plate, remove and discard the top, and serve hot with whole grain crackers and the toasted bread cubes.

NUTRITIONAL FACTS (PER TABLESPOON)
Cal: 17   Carbs: 0.9 g   Chol: 4 mg   Fat: 0.1 g
Fiber: 0 g   Protein: 2.8 g   Sodium: 59 mg

Great Garbanzo Dip

YIELD: 1³/₄ CUPS

| 1 tablespoon extra virgin olive oil |
| 1 tablespoon crushed fresh garlic |
| ¹/₂ cup chopped onion |
| ¹/₃ cup chopped red bell pepper |
| ¹/₃ cup chopped green bell pepper |
| ¹/₂ teaspoon dried oregano |
| 1 can (15 ounces) chickpeas, rinsed and drained, or 1³/₄ cups cooked chickpeas |
| 1 tablespoon lemon juice |
| 2 tablespoons chicken or vegetable broth |
| ¹/₄ teaspoon ground black pepper |

1. Place the olive oil in a large nonstick skillet, and preheat over medium-high heat. Add the garlic, onion, red and green peppers, and oregano, and stir to mix. Cover and cook, stirring frequently, for about 4 minutes, or until the vegetables begin to soften. Add a little broth if the skillet becomes too dry.

2. Place the chickpeas, lemon juice, broth, and black pepper in the bowl of a food processor. Add the vegetable mixture, and process, scraping down the sides occasionally, for about 2 minutes, or until the ingredients are well mixed and the dip has reached the desired consistency. Add a little more broth if needed.

3. Transfer the spread to a serving dish, and serve at room temperature with whole grain crackers, raw vegetables, Parmesan Pita Crisps (page 111), or Garlic and Herb Bagel Chips (page 111).

NUTRITIONAL FACTS (PER TABLESPOON)
Cal: 20   Carbs: 2.7 g   Chol: 0 mg   Fat: 0.6 g
Fiber: 0.8 g   Protein: 0.8 g   Sodium: 27 mg

Healthy Hummus

YIELD: 1 ³/₄ CUPS

| 1 can (19 ounces) chickpeas, rinsed and drained, or 2 cups cooked chickpeas |
| ¹/₄ cup plus 2 tablespoons plain nonfat yogurt |
| 3–4 tablespoons toasted sesame tahini |
| 3 tablespoons lemon juice |
| ¹/₂ teaspoon ground cumin |
| 1 teaspoon crushed fresh garlic |
| 3 tablespoons chopped fresh parsley |

1. Place the chickpeas, yogurt, tahini, lemon juice, cumin, and garlic in the bowl of a food processor, and process until smooth, scraping down the sides occasionally. Add the parsley, and process until the ingredients are well mixed and the parsley is finely chopped. Transfer the mixture to a serving dish, cover, and chill for several hours.

2. Serve with wedges of pita bread or whole grain crackers, or use as a sandwich filling.

NUTRITIONAL FACTS (PER TABLESPOON)
Cal: 29   Carbs: 3.4 g   Chol: 0 mg   Fat: 1.2 g
Fiber: 1.2 g   Protein: 1.2 g   Sodium: 28 mg

Light Blue Cheese Dip

YIELD: 2¹/₂ CUPS

| 2 cups nonfat or light sour cream |
| ¹/₂ cup crumbled blue cheese |

1. Place both of the ingredients in a medium-sized bowl, and stir to mix well. Transfer the dip to a serving dish, cover, and chill for several hours.

2. Serve with raw vegetables, apple and pear wedges dipped in pineapple juice to prevent browning, and whole grain crackers.

NUTRITIONAL FACTS (PER TABLESPOON)
Cal: 17   Carbs: 2.2 g   Chol: 1 mg   Fat: 0.4 g
Fiber: 0 g   Protein: 1.1 g   Sodium: 35 mg

Garden Artichoke Dip

YIELD: 4 CUPS

2 cups nonfat or light sour cream

$\frac{1}{2}$ cup nonfat or reduced-fat mayonnaise

1 package (1.4 ounces) dry vegetable soup mix

1 package (9 ounces) frozen (thawed) artichoke hearts, chopped, or 1 can (14 ounces) artichoke hearts, drained and chopped

1 can (8 ounces) sliced water chestnuts, drained and chopped

$\frac{1}{3}$ cup chopped red bell pepper

$\frac{1}{4}$ cup chopped scallions

1. Place the sour cream, mayonnaise, and vegetable soup mix in a large bowl, and stir to mix well. Add the artichokes, water chestnuts, red pepper, and scallions, and stir to mix well. Transfer the dip to a serving dish, cover, and chill for several hours.

2. Serve with whole grain crackers, thinly sliced bagels, and fresh-cut vegetables.

NUTRITIONAL FACTS (PER TABLESPOON)
Cal: 16   Carbs: 3 g   Chol: 0 mg   Fat: 0.2 g
Fiber: 0.3 g   Protein: 0.5 g   Sodium: 69 mg

Peanut Butter-Hot Fudge Dip

YIELD: 2$\frac{1}{4}$ CUPS

$\frac{3}{4}$ cup sugar

$\frac{1}{2}$ cup Dutch Processed cocoa powder

1 tablespoon plus 1 teaspoon cornstarch

1 cup skim or low-fat milk

$\frac{1}{2}$ cup evaporated skim milk

$\frac{1}{3}$ cup creamy peanut butter

2 teaspoons vanilla extract

1. Place the sugar, cocoa, and cornstarch in a 1$\frac{1}{2}$-quart pot, and stir to mix well. Using a wire whisk, slowly stir in the milk and the evaporated milk. Place the pot over medium heat, and cook, stirring constantly, for 5 minutes, or just until the mixture comes to a boil.

2. Reduce the heat to low, add the peanut butter, and cook and stir for 2 minutes, or until the peanut butter has melted into the chocolate mixture. Remove the pot from the heat, and stir in the vanilla extract.

3. Transfer the mixture to a small chafing dish or Crock-Pot electric casserole to keep warm, and serve with chunks of angel food cake, whole fresh strawberries, pineapple chunks, and chunks of banana, apple, and pear that have been dipped in pineapple juice to prevent browning.

NUTRITIONAL FACTS (PER TABLESPOON)
Cal: 38   Carbs: 6 g   Chol: 0 mg   Fat: 1.3 g
Fiber: 0.5 g   Protein: 1.3 g   Sodium: 14 mg

Guacamole Dip

YIELD: 2$\frac{1}{8}$ CUPS

2 cups diced peeled avocado (about 2 medium)

$\frac{2}{3}$ cup nonfat or light sour cream

3 tablespoons finely chopped onion

3 tablespoons finely chopped seeded plum tomato (about 1 small)

1 tablespoon plus 1 teaspoon minced fresh cilantro

1 tablespoon minced pickled jalapeño pepper

$\frac{3}{4}$ teaspoon crushed fresh garlic

$\frac{1}{8}$ teaspoon salt

1. Place the avocado in a medium-sized bowl, and mash with a potato masher, leaving it slightly chunky. Stir in all of the remaining ingredients. Transfer the dip to a serving dish, and serve immediately or cover and chill for several hours.

2. Serve with baked tortilla chips.

NUTRITIONAL FACTS (PER TABLESPOON)
Cal: 20   Carbs: 1.5 g   Chol: 0 mg   Fat: 1.4 g
Fiber: 0.5 g   Protein: 0.5 g   Sodium: 14 mg

Creamy Fruit Dip

YIELD: 1¼ CUPS

1 cup plain yogurt cheese (page 12),
nonfat or light sour cream, or nonfat
or reduced-fat cream cheese

¼–⅓ cup apricot, strawberry, or cherry preserves

1. Place both of the ingredients in a small bowl, and stir to mix well. (If you are using cream cheese, beat both ingredients together with an electric mixer.) Transfer the dip to a serving dish, cover, and chill for at least 2 hours.

2. Serve with fresh fruit, bagel slices, and whole grain crackers.

NUTRITIONAL FACTS (PER TABLESPOON)
Cal: 18   Carbs: 3.6 g   Chol: 0 mg   Fat: 0 g
Fiber: 0 g   Protein: 0.9 g   Sodium: 10 mg

Honey Mustard Dip

YIELD: 1⅛ CUPS

½ cup nonfat or light sour cream

½ cup nonfat or reduced-fat mayonnaise

2 tablespoons Dijon mustard

2 tablespoons honey

1. Place the sour cream and mayonnaise in a medium-sized bowl, and stir to mix well. Add the mustard and honey, and stir to mix well. Transfer the dip to a serving dish and serve immediately, or cover and chill until ready to serve.

2. Serve with fresh vegetables such as broccoli and cauliflower florets, carrot and celery sticks, red and green bell pepper strips, and blanched asparagus and snow peas. This dip is also delicious with cubes or rolled-up slices of turkey or lean ham, and cubes of low-fat Swiss cheese.

NUTRITIONAL FACTS (PER TABLESPOON)
Cal: 19   Carbs: 4 g   Chol: 0 mg   Fat: 0.1 g
Fiber: 1.7 g   Protein: 0.5 g   Sodium: 73 mg

Broccoli Cheese Dip

YIELD: 4 CUPS

2 cups nonfat or light sour cream

½ cup nonfat or reduced-fat mayonnaise

1 package (10 ounces) frozen chopped broccoli,
thawed and squeezed dry

1 cup shredded nonfat or reduced-fat
Cheddar cheese

1. Place the sour cream and mayonnaise in a medium-sized bowl, and stir to mix well. Fold in the broccoli and cheese. Transfer the dip to a serving dish, cover, and chill for at least 1 hour.

2. Serve with sliced bagels or vegetable crackers.

NUTRITIONAL FACTS (PER TABLESPOON)
Cal: 12   Carbs: 1.8 g   Chol: 0 mg   Fat: 0 g
Fiber: 0.1 g   Protein: 1.2 g   Sodium: 39 mg

Deviled Crab Dip

YIELD: 2½ CUPS

1¼ cups nonfat or light sour cream

¼ cup nonfat or reduced-fat mayonnaise

1–2 tablespoons spicy brown mustard

1 cup flaked cooked crab meat
or drained canned crab meat

¼ cup finely chopped onion

Paprika (garnish)

1. Place the sour cream, mayonnaise, and mustard in a medium-sized bowl, and stir to mix well. Fold in the crab meat and onion. Transfer the dip to a serving dish, cover, and chill for several hours.

2. Just before serving, sprinkle the dip with paprika. Serve with whole grain crackers or chunks of sourdough bread and raw vegetables.

NUTRITIONAL FACTS (PER TABLESPOON)
Cal: 13   Carbs: 1.7 g   Chol: 2 mg   Fat: 0.1 g
Fiber: 0 g   Protein: 1.1 g   Sodium: 32 mg

Spinach Dip

A party favorite made healthy. Serve in a hollowed-out loaf of pumpernickel with raw vegetables and whole grain crackers.

YIELD: 4 CUPS

1 package (10 ounces) frozen chopped spinach, thawed and squeezed dry
2 cups nonfat or light sour cream
1/2 cup nonfat or reduced-fat mayonnaise
1 can (8 ounces) water chestnuts, drained and chopped
1/2 cup thinly sliced scallions
1 package (1 1/2 ounces) dry vegetable soup mix

1. Place all of the ingredients in a large bowl, and stir to mix well. Transfer the dip to a serving dish, cover, and chill for several hours.

2. Serve with raw vegetables and whole grain crackers, or use as a filling for finger sandwiches or hollowed-out cherry tomatoes.

NUTRITIONAL FACTS (PER TABLESPOON)

Cal: 13   Carbs: 2.6 g   Chol: 0 mg   Fat: 0 g
Fiber: 0.2 g   Protein: 0.7 g   Sodium: 52 mg

Onion Dill Dip

YIELD: 2 CUPS

2 cups nonfat or light sour cream
2–3 tablespoons minced fresh dill
1/4 cup finely chopped onion

1. Place all of the ingredients in a medium-sized bowl, and stir to mix well. Transfer the dip to a serving dish, cover, and chill for several hours.

2. Serve with raw vegetables and whole grain crackers.

NUTRITIONAL FACTS (PER TABLESPOON)

Cal: 16   Carbs: 2.8 g   Chol: 0 mg   Fat: 0 g
Fiber: 0 g   Protein: 1 g   Sodium: 11 mg

Dilled Shrimp Dip

YIELD: 2 1/2 CUPS

1 1/4 cups nonfat or light sour cream
1/4 cup nonfat or reduced-fat mayonnaise
1–2 tablespoons minced fresh dill
5 ounces (about 1 cup) frozen (thawed) cooked small salad shrimp, or 5 ounces diced cooked shrimp
1/4 cup finely chopped onion

1. Place the sour cream, mayonnaise, and dill in a medium-sized bowl, and stir to mix well. Fold in the shrimp and onion. Transfer the dip to a serving dish, cover, and chill for at least 2 hours.

2. Serve with whole grain crackers and raw vegetables, or use as a filling for hollowed-out cherry tomatoes or cucumbers.

NUTRITIONAL FACTS (PER TABLESPOON)

Cal: 13   Carbs: 1.6 g   Chol: 7 mg   Fat: 0 g
Fiber: 0 g   Protein: 1.2 g   Sodium: 24 mg

Caramel Cream Cheese Dip

YIELD: 1 CUP

1 block (8 ounces) nonfat or reduced-fat cream cheese, softened to room temperature
1/4 cup light brown sugar
1/2 teaspoon vanilla extract

1. Place all of the ingredients in a medium-sized bowl, and beat with an electric mixer until smooth. Transfer the dip to a serving dish and serve immediately, or cover and chill until ready to serve.

2. Serve with apple and pear slices that have been dipped in pineapple juice to prevent browning, whole fresh strawberries, and fresh pineapple spears.

NUTRITIONAL FACTS (PER TABLESPOON)

Cal: 26   Carbs: 4 g   Chol: 1 mg   Fat: 0 g
Fiber: 0 g   Protein: 2.7 g   Sodium: 67 mg

Savannah Seafood Spread

YIELD: 12 SERVINGS

1 block (8 ounces) nonfat or
reduced-fat cream cheese

³/₄ cup (4–5 ounces) frozen (thawed) cooked small
salad shrimp, or ³/₄ cup diced cooked shrimp

³/₄ cup flaked cooked crab meat
or drained canned crab meat

SAUCE

³/₄ cup ketchup

2 tablespoons prepared horseradish

2 tablespoons lemon juice

1. Place the block of cheese in the center of a serving plate. Combine the shrimp and crab meat in a medium-sized bowl, and pile over the cheese. Combine the sauce ingredients in a small bowl, and pour over the seafood.

2. Serve with whole scallions, celery sticks, and whole grain crackers.

NUTRITIONAL FACTS (PER SERVING)
Cal: 57   Carbs: 5 g   Chol: 32 mg   Fat: 0.3 g
Fiber: 0.4 g   Protein: 8.2 g   Sodium: 329 mg

Smoked Salmon Spread

YIELD: 2 CUPS

12 ounces smoked salmon

1 block (8 ounces) nonfat or reduced-fat
cream cheese, softened to room temperature

1¹/₂ teaspoons lemon juice

¹/₄ cup finely chopped onion

¹/₄ cup minced fresh parsley, dill, or chives (garnish)

1. Place the salmon in a medium-sized bowl, and separate it into flakes. There should be 2 cups. Set aside.

2. Place the cream cheese and lemon juice in a medium-sized bowl, and beat with an electric mixer until smooth. Stir in the salmon and onion. Spread the

mixture evenly in a serving dish, cover, and chill for several hours.

3. Just before serving, sprinkle the parsley, dill, or chives over the top of the spread. Serve with whole grain crackers and carrot sticks.

NUTRITIONAL FACTS (PER TABLESPOON)
Cal: 17   Carbs: 0.6 g   Chol: 3 mg   Fat: 0.4 g
Fiber: 0 g   Protein: 2.6 g   Sodium: 99 mg

Roasted Eggplant Spread

YIELD: 2¹/₂ CUPS

2 large eggplants (1 pound each),
peeled and cut into ³/₄-inch chunks

4 plum tomatoes, seeded and chopped

2 tablespoons extra virgin olive oil

1 tablespoon balsamic vinegar

6 cloves garlic, coarsely chopped

1 teaspoon dried oregano

¹/₂ teaspoon salt

¹/₄ teaspoon coarsely ground black pepper

3 tablespoons vegetable or chicken broth

¹/₄ cup sliced black olives (garnish)

1. Place the eggplant, tomatoes, olive oil, vinegar, garlic, oregano, salt, and pepper in a large bowl, and toss to mix well.

2. Coat a large roasting pan with nonstick cooking spray, and spread the eggplant mixture over the bottom of the pan. Bake at 425°F, stirring every 15 minutes, for about 1 hour, or until the eggplant is very soft. Remove the pan from the oven, stir in the broth, and allow the mixture to cool to room temperature.

3. When ready to serve, mound the mixture in a serving bowl, and sprinkle with the olives. Serve at room temperature with whole grain crackers, fresh French or Italian bread, Garlic and Herb Bagel Chips (page 111), or Parmesan Pita Crisps (page 111).

NUTRITIONAL FACTS (PER TABLESPOON)
Cal: 14   Carbs: 1.8 g   Chol: 0 mg   Fat: 0.8 g
Fiber: 0.7 g   Protein: 0.3 g   Sodium: 45 mg

Bacon, Cheddar, and Pecan Spread

YIELD: 3 CUPS

1 block (8 ounces) nonfat or reduced-fat cream cheese

1 cup nonfat or low-fat cottage cheese

1/2 cup nonfat or reduced-fat mayonnaise

1/8 teaspoon ground white pepper

2 tablespoons finely chopped onion

1 cup shredded nonfat or reduced-fat Cheddar cheese

4 slices extra-lean turkey bacon, cooked, drained, and crumbled

1/4 cup chopped toasted pecans (page 348)

1. Place the cream cheese, cottage cheese, mayonnaise, and pepper in a food processor, and process until smooth. Add all of the remaining ingredients, and process just until well mixed. Transfer the spread to a serving dish, cover, and chill for several hours or overnight.

2. Serve with whole grain crackers, sliced bagels, and fresh-cut vegetables, or use as a stuffing for celery or as a filling for finger sandwiches.

NUTRITIONAL FACTS (PER TABLESPOON)
Cal: 19   Carbs: 1 g   Chol: 2 mg   Fat: 0.5 g
Fiber: 0 g   Protein: 2.5 g   Sodium: 85 mg

Dilly Cucumber Dip

YIELD: 2 1/4 CUPS

1 medium-large cucumber, peeled, seeded, and cut into chunks

1 1/2 cups nonfat or light sour cream

1/2 cup nonfat or reduced-fat mayonnaise

2 tablespoons finely chopped onion

1 tablespoon finely chopped fresh dill

Pinch ground white pepper

1. Place the cucumber in a food processor or blender, and process until finely chopped. Roll the cucumber in a clean kitchen towel, and squeeze out any excess moisture.

2. Place the sour cream and mayonnaise in a medium-sized bowl, and stir to mix well. Fold in the cucumber and all of the remaining ingredients. Transfer the dip to a serving dish, cover, and chill for several hours.

3. Serve with raw vegetables, whole grain crackers, chunks of pumpernickel or sourdough bread, and smoked salmon.

NUTRITIONAL FACTS (PER TABLESPOON)
Cal: 13   Carbs: 2 g   Chol: 0 mg   Fat: 0 g
Fiber: 0.1 g   Protein: 2.2 g   Sodium: 36 mg

Chutney Chicken Spread

YIELD: 2 1/4 CUPS

1 block (8 ounces) nonfat or reduced-fat cream cheese, softened to room temperature

1/4 cup plus 2 tablespoons finely chopped onion

1/4 cup plus 2 tablespoons finely chopped celery

1/4 cup mango chutney

3/4 cup finely chopped cooked chicken or turkey breast, or 1 can (6 ounces) white meat chicken or turkey, drained

3 tablespoons toasted sliced almonds (page 348) or chopped roasted peanuts

1. Place the cream cheese, onion, celery, and chutney in a medium-sized bowl, and stir to mix well. Add the chicken or turkey, and stir to mix well. Spread the mixture in a small bowl, and sprinkle the almonds or peanuts over the top. Cover and chill for at least 2 hours.

2. Serve with whole grain crackers, carrot sticks, and celery sticks, or use as a filling for finger sandwiches.

NUTRITIONAL FACTS (PER TABLESPOON)
Cal: 18   Carbs: 1 g   Chol: 3 mg   Fat: 0.4 g
Fiber: 0.1 g   Protein: 2.2 g   Sodium: 38 mg

Apple Cheddar Spread

YIELD: 3¼ CUPS

1 block (8 ounces) nonfat or reduced-fat cream cheese
1 cup nonfat or low-fat cottage cheese
1½ cups finely chopped peeled tart apples (about 2 medium)
¾ cup shredded nonfat or reduced-fat Cheddar cheese
⅓ cup chopped dates

1. Place the cream cheese and cottage cheese in a food processor, and process until smooth. Stir in the apples, Cheddar cheese, and dates. Transfer the spread to a serving dish, cover, and chill for several hours.

2. Serve with whole grain bagel slices, whole grain crackers, celery sticks, and apple wedges dipped in pineapple juice to prevent browning.

NUTRITIONAL FACTS (PER TABLESPOON)
Cal: 15   Carbs: 1.8 g   Chol: 1 mg   Fat: 0 g
Fiber: 0.1 g   Protein: 1.8 g   Sodium: 48 mg

Pimento Cheese Spread

YIELD: 1½ CUPS

⅔ cup nonfat or low-fat cottage cheese
¼ cup nonfat or reduced-fat mayonnaise
2 teaspoons spicy mustard
¼ teaspoon crushed fresh garlic
⅛ teaspoon ground white pepper
1 jar (4 ounces) chopped pimentos, well drained, divided
2 tablespoons finely chopped onion
1 cup shredded nonfat or reduced-fat Cheddar cheese

1. Place the cottage cheese, mayonnaise, mustard, garlic, pepper, and half of the pimentos in a food processor or blender, and process until smooth. Add

the onion and Cheddar cheese, and process to the desired consistency. Stir in the remaining pimentos. Transfer the spread to a serving dish, cover, and chill for several hours.

2. Serve with whole grain crackers, or use as a filling for finger sandwiches or celery.

NUTRITIONAL FACTS (PER TABLESPOON)
Cal: 15   Carbs: 1.1g   Chol: 1 mg   Fat: 0 g
Fiber: 0.1 g   Protein: 2.4 g   Sodium: 75 mg

Sun-Dried Tomato and Scallion Spread

YIELD: 1⅛ CUPS

2 tablespoons finely chopped sun-dried tomatoes (not packed in oil)
2 tablespoons water
1 block (8 ounces) nonfat or reduced-fat cream cheese, softened to room temperature
¼ teaspoon dried basil or Italian seasoning
¼ cup finely chopped scallions

1. Place sun-dried tomatoes and water in small pot, and bring to boil over high heat. Reduce the heat to low, cover, and simmer for 2 minutes, or just until the water has been absorbed and the tomatoes have plumped. Remove the pot from the heat, and set aside.

2. Place the cream cheese in a small bowl, and beat with an electric mixer until smooth. Add the tomatoes and the basil or Italian seasoning, and beat just until well mixed. Stir in the scallions. Transfer the spread to a serving dish, cover, and chill for several hours.

3. Serve with sliced bagels, wedges of pita bread, whole grain crackers, or celery sticks, or use as a filling for hollowed-out cherry tomatoes or finger sandwiches.

NUTRITIONAL FACTS (PER TABLESPOON)
Cal: 13   Carbs: 1 g   Chol: 1 mg   Fat: 0 g
Fiber: 0.1 g   Protein: 2 g   Sodium: 69 mg

5. *Sensational Sandwiches and Pizzas*

Versatile, portable, and fast and easy to make and eat, sandwiches are perhaps the most popular quick-meal choice of both active children and on-the-go adults. Unfortunately, this lunchtime favorite is often a nutritional nightmare, packing in a full day's worth of fat and far too many calories. Take the deli-style Reuben, for instance. Six ounces of fatty corned beef topped with a couple of ounces of full-fat cheese and a couple of tablespoons of Thousand Island dressing can add up to more than 900 calories and 50 grams of fat! Even a seemingly innocent chicken or tuna salad sandwich can contain over 500 calories and 30 grams of fat.

If you now fear that you must forever abandon your favorite sandwiches, take heart. Made properly, a sandwich can be the perfect meal, packed with complex carbohydrates, lean protein, calcium, and other important nutrients. And, as you will see, just about any sandwich can be easily slimmed down. New low-and no-fat ingredients provide a wealth of exciting sandwich possibilities. Add a few low-fat cooking tricks, and you'll find that even the Monte Cristo Sandwich can have a place in a low-fat lifestyle.

Though many sandwiches are uniquely American, many other cuisines feature their own variation of the sandwich. Pizzas and calzones from Italy; burritos and tacos from Mexico; and stuffed pitas from the Middle East are just some examples of hand-held meals that are loved the world over. Happily, even the richest of these ethnic favorites can be made light and healthy—without sacrificing the tastes that you love.

This chapter offers a selection of all-American favorites as well as many popular ethnic sandwiches that can be enjoyed without guilt. And from Salsa Burgers to Bean Burritos Supreme to Chicken Caesar Wraps, you will find creations as tantalizing as they are healthy. So whether you're looking for a quick snack to fight those afternoon hunger pangs or a fast but hearty entrée for a family dinner, you are sure to find a sensational sandwich that meets your needs deliciously.

Dilled Salmon Burgers

YIELD: 4 SERVINGS

Nonstick cooking spray

4 multigrain burger buns

4 slices tomato

4 leaves lettuce

BURGERS

1½ slices whole wheat or multigrain bread

2 cans (6½ ounces each) water-packed boneless skinless pink salmon

2 egg whites, or ¼ cup fat-free egg substitute

2 tablespoons finely chopped fresh parsley

2 tablespoons finely chopped onion

¼ teaspoon dried dill

¼ teaspoon coarsely ground black pepper

DRESSING

3 tablespoons nonfat or reduced-fat mayonnaise

2 tablespoons nonfat or light sour cream

¼ teaspoon dried dill

1. To make the dressing, place all of the dressing ingredients in a small bowl, and stir to mix well. Set aside.

2. To make the burgers, tear the bread slices into pieces, place in a blender or food processor, and process into fine crumbs. Measure the crumbs; there should be ¾ cup. (Adjust the amount if necessary.)

3. Place the bread crumbs and all of the remaining burger ingredients in a medium-sized bowl, and stir to mix well. Shape the mixture into 4 (4-inch) patties.

4. Coat a large nonstick skillet with nonstick cooking spray, and preheat over medium heat. Cook the burgers for about 3 minutes, or until the bottoms are nicely browned. Spray the tops of the burgers lightly with the cooking spray, turn, and cook for 3 additional minutes, or until the burgers are nicely browned on the second side.

5. Place each burger on the bottom half of a bun, and top with some of the dressing, a slice of tomato, a lettuce leaf, and a remaining bun half. Serve hot.

NUTRITIONAL FACTS (PER BURGER WITH BUN AND TOPPINGS)
Cal: 321   Carbs: 35 g   Chol: 65 mg   Fat: 5.3 g
Fiber: 4.4 g   Protein: 33 g   Sodium: 527 mg

Making Juicy Low-Fat Burgers

For flavorful, juicy low-fat burgers, add lots of finely chopped vegetables—such as onions, mushrooms, and green peppers—to the burger mixture. As the burgers cook, the chopped vegetables will release their juices into the meat, keeping your ultra-lean burgers moist and flavorful. Another great way to trim the fat from your burgers is to add some meatless recipe crumbles as a meat extender. In the burger recipes in this chapter, the addition of both chopped vegetables and recipe crumbles allows you to get six generous servings from a pound of meat instead of the usual four servings.

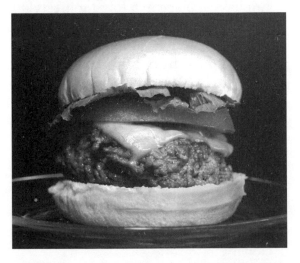

Salsa Burgers

YIELD: 6 SERVINGS
1 pound 95% lean ground beef
1 cup frozen (thawed) meatless recipe crumbles
1/2 cup finely chopped onion
1/2 cup bottled chunky salsa
2 teaspoons chili powder
6 multigrain burger buns

TOPPINGS

3/4 cup nonfat or reduced-fat shredded Cheddar cheese
1/3 cup nonfat or reduced-fat mayonnaise
1/3 cup bottled chunky salsa
6 thin slices tomato
6 thin slices onion
1 1/2 cups shredded romaine lettuce

1. Place the ground beef, recipe crumbles, onion, salsa, and chili powder in a large bowl, and use a potato masher to mix the ingredients thoroughly. Gently shape the mixture into 6 (4-inch) patties.

2. Coat a large nonstick skillet with nonstick cooking spray, and preheat over medium heat. Place the patties in the skillet, and cook for 4 to 5 minutes on each side, or until the meat is no longer pink inside. Alternatively, grill the burgers over medium heat for about 7 minutes on each side, or until the meat is thoroughly cooked. Sprinkle some of the cheese over each burger, cover the skillet or grill, and cook for another minute, or until the cheese melts.

3. Place the mayonnaise and salsa in a small bowl, and stir to mix well. Spread some of this mixture over both halves of each bun. Place each burger on the bottom half of a bun, and top with a slice of tomato, a slice of onion, some of the lettuce, and a remaining bun half. Serve hot.

NUTRITIONAL FACTS
(PER BURGER WITH BUN AND TOPPINGS)
Cal: 322   Carbs: 34 g   Chol: 42 mg   Fat: 5.4 g
Fiber: 5 g   Protein: 30 g   Sodium: 743 mg

Mushroom and Onion Burgers

While these burgers cook, the chopped mushrooms and onions release their juices into the meat, keeping these ultra-lean burgers moist and flavorful.

YIELD: 6 SERVINGS
1 pound 95% lean ground beef
1 1/2 cups finely chopped fresh mushrooms
1 cup frozen (thawed) meatless recipe crumbles
1/2 cup finely chopped onion
2 tablespoons Worcestershire sauce
6 multigrain burger buns

TOPPINGS

6 thin slices tomato
6 thin slices onion
6 lettuce leaves
1/4 cup plus 2 tablespoons nonfat or low-fat mayonnaise, mustard, or ketchup

1. Place the ground beef, mushrooms, recipe crumbles, onion, and Worcestershire sauce in a large bowl, and use a potato masher to mix the ingredients thoroughly. Gently shape the mixture into 6 (4-inch) patties.

2. Coat a large nonstick skillet with nonstick cooking spray, and preheat over medium heat. Place the patties in the skillet, and cook for 4 to 5 minutes on each side, or until the meat is no longer pink inside. Alternatively, grill the burgers over medium heat for about 7 minutes on each side, or until the meat is thoroughly cooked.

3. Place each burger on the bottom half of a bun, and top with a slice of tomato, a slice of onion, a lettuce leaf, your choice of condiments, and a remaining bun half. Serve hot.

NUTRITIONAL FACTS
(PER BURGER WITH BUN AND TOPPINGS)
Cal: 302   Carbs: 34 g   Chol: 40 mg   Fat: 5.5 g
Fiber: 4.1 g   Protein: 26 g   Sodium: 448 mg

Skinny Sloppy Joes

For even skinnier Sloppy Joes, substitute 1 cup of frozen meatless recipe crumbles, tofu hamburger, or TVP for half of the ground beef.

YIELD: 6 SERVINGS
1 pound 95% lean ground beef
1 cup chopped onion
3/4 cup chopped green bell pepper
1 can (1 pound) unsalted tomato sauce
1/4 cup tomato paste
2 tablespoons dark brown sugar
1 tablespoon spicy brown mustard
1 tablespoon Worcestershire sauce
2 teaspoons chili powder
1/2 teaspoon dried oregano
1/4 teaspoon salt
1/4 teaspoon ground black pepper
6 whole wheat or multigrain burger buns

1. Coat a large nonstick skillet with nonstick cooking spray, and preheat over medium heat. Add the ground meat, and cook, stirring to crumble, until the meat is no longer pink. Drain off and discard any excess fat.

2. Add the onion and green pepper to the skillet, and stir to mix. Cover and cook, stirring frequently, for about 4 minutes, or until the vegetables start to soften.

3. Add all of the remaining ingredients except for the buns to the skillet, and bring to a boil over medium-high heat. Reduce the heat to low, cover, and simmer, stirring occasionally, for about 15 minutes, or until the onions and peppers are soft and the flavors are well blended. Allow the mixture to simmer uncovered for a few minutes if the sauce seems too thin.

4. Spoon 1/2 cup of the mixture onto the bottom half of each bun, top with the remaining half, and serve hot.

NUTRITIONAL FACTS (PER SERVING)
Cal: 354   Carbs: 47 g   Chol: 49 mg   Fat: 5.6 g
Fiber: 5.2 g   Protein: 27 g   Sodium: 573 mg

Monte Cristo Sandwiches

YIELD: 4 SERVINGS
12 slices sourdough or firm multigrain bread
2 tablespoons Dijon mustard
4 slices (1 ounce each) roasted turkey breast
8 thin slices (1/2 ounce each) nonfat or reduced-fat Swiss cheese
4 slices (1 ounce each) ham, at least 97% lean
1/2 cup fat-free egg substitute
1/4 cup skim or low-fat milk
Pinch ground nutmeg
Nonstick cooking spray

1. Arrange 3 pieces of the bread on a flat surface, and spread each with 1/2 teaspoon of the mustard. Place 1 slice of turkey and 1 slice of cheese over the mustard on one bread slice. Top with a second bread slice, mustard side up, and lay 1 slice of ham and 1 slice of cheese on the second bread slice. Top with the remaining bread slice, mustard side down. Repeat this procedure with the remaining ingredients to make 4 sandwiches.

2. Place the egg substitute, milk, and nutmeg in a shallow dish, and stir to mix well. Dip both sides of each sandwich into the egg mixture.

3. Coat a large griddle or nonstick skillet with nonstick cooking spray, and preheat over medium heat until a drop of water sizzles when it hits the heated surface. Arrange the sandwiches on the griddle, and cook for 1 1/2 to 2 minutes, or until the bottoms are golden brown. Spray the tops of the sandwiches with cooking spray, turn them over, and cook for another couple of minutes, or until both sides are golden brown.

4. Coat a baking sheet with nonstick cooking spray, and transfer the sandwiches to the sheet. Bake at 450°F for 5 to 7 minutes, or until the sandwiches are heated through and the cheese is melted. Cut each sandwich in half diagonally, and serve hot.

NUTRITIONAL FACTS (PER SERVING)
Cal: 353   Carbs: 45 g   Chol: 38 mg   Fat: 4.7 g
Fiber: 3.2 g   Protein: 33 g   Sodium: 834 mg

Tuna Cheddar Melts

YIELD: 4 SERVINGS

1 can (12 ounces) water-packed chunk light
or albacore tuna, drained

1/2 cup finely chopped celery

1/2 cup finely chopped onion

1/4 cup plus 2 tablespoons nonfat
or reduced-fat mayonnaise

3–4 tablespoons sweet pickle relish

1/8 teaspoon ground black pepper

4 whole wheat or oat bran
English muffins, split

1 cup shredded reduced-fat Cheddar cheese

1. Place the tuna, celery, onion, mayonnaise, relish, and pepper in a small bowl, and stir to mix well. Set aside.

2. Toast the English muffins, and arrange on a baking sheet, split side up. Spread about 1/4 cup of the tuna mixture on each piece, and place under a preheated broiler for 2 to 3 minutes, or until the mixture is hot. Top each muffin half with 2 tablespoons of the cheese, and broil for another minute or 2, or until the cheese is melted. Serve hot.

NUTRITIONAL FACTS (PER SERVING)
Cal: 372   Carbs: 40 g   Chol: 39 mg   Fat: 6 g
Fiber: 3.4 g   Protein: 37 g   Sodium: 914 mg

Skinny Sandwich Secrets

When people decide to cut back on fat and calories, they often assume that sandwiches are out. And while it's true that sandwiches piled high with ingredients like fatty cold cuts, quarter-pound greasy burgers, bacon, full-fat cheeses, mayonnaise, and special sauces can be a nutritional nightmare, just about any sandwich can be slimmed down enough to be part of a healthy diet. As the recipes in this chapter show, a few simple ingredient substitutions can make a big fat—and calorie—difference in your favorite sandwiches. Here are some tips for trimming the fat and calories from your favorite sandwiches.

❑ Spread bread with mustard or nonfat or low-fat mayonnaise instead of full-fat mayonnaise. For a change of pace, try moistening your sandwiches with fat-free ranch salad dressing or other nonfat dressings.

❑ Substitute nonfat or reduced-fat cream cheese for regular cream cheese in sandwich fillings.

❑ Use nonfat or reduced-fat mayonnaise and sour cream in sandwich fillings.

❑ When making grilled cheese and other grilled sandwiches, spread the bread with a thin layer of reduced-fat margarine or light butter instead of regular margarine or butter. Or spray the bread lightly with butter-flavored nonstick cooking spray before grilling.

❑ Substitute water-packed tuna for oil-packed tuna.

❑ Substitute nonfat or reduced-fat Cheddar, Swiss, and other firm and hard cheeses for their full-fat counterparts.

❑ Douse subs with oil-free Italian dressing or a splash of vinegar instead of a full-fat dressing or oil.

❑ Replace fatty cold cuts with their lean counterparts.

❑ Limit meat to 2 to 3 ounces per sandwich, and make up the volume by piling on extra lettuce, tomato, cucumbers, grated carrots, sprouts, and other vegetables.

❑ Experiment with a wide variety of yeast breads, sub rolls, burger buns, English muffins, bagels, pita bread, and tortillas when making your sandwiches. Keep in mind that, with the exception of biscuits and croissants, most breads are quite low in fat. For maximum nutrients and fiber—and a heartier flavor—choose whole grain breads over refined white breads as often as possible.

Portabella Mushroom Sandwiches

YIELD: 4 SERVINGS

20 slices (each ¾-inch thick) Portabella mushroom (about 4 medium-large)

Nonstick olive oil cooking spray

⅛ teaspoon salt

⅛ teaspoon coarsely ground black pepper

½ teaspoon dried fines herbes* or dried Italian seasoning

4 sourdough rolls, onion rolls, or multigrain burger buns (2 ounces each)

4 ounces sliced nonfat or reduced-fat mozzarella or provolone cheese

TOPPINGS

¼ cup nonfat or reduced-fat mayonnaise

4 teaspoons Dijon mustard

4 slices red onion

4 slices tomato

12 fresh tender spinach or arugula leaves

* A blend of thyme, oregano, sage, rosemary, marjoram, and basil, fines herbes can be found in the dried spice section of most grocery stores.

1. Coat a large baking sheet with nonstick olive oil cooking spray, and arrange the mushrooms in a single layer on the sheet. Spray the tops of the mushrooms lightly with the cooking spray, and sprinkle with the salt, pepper, and herbs.

2. Bake uncovered at 450°F for 10 minutes. Turn the slices, and bake for 5 additional minutes, or until tender and nicely browned. Remove the mushrooms from the oven, and set aside.

3. While the mushrooms are cooking, place the mayonnaise and mustard in a small bowl, and stir to mix well. Set aside.

4. Split the rolls in half lengthwise, and arrange the halves on a large baking sheet, cut sides up. Place under a preheated broiler, and broil for a minute or 2, or until lightly toasted. Spread each of the cut sides with some of the mayonnaise mixture. Set the roll tops aside, leaving the bottoms on the baking sheet.

5. Place first a quarter of the mushroom slices and then a quarter of the cheese over the bottom half of each roll. Return to the broiler for about 1 minute, or until the cheese is melted.

6. Top the melted cheese on each roll with a slice of onion, a slice of tomato, 3 spinach or arugula leaves, and a roll half. Serve hot.

NUTRITIONAL FACTS (PER SERVING)
Cal: 264   Carbs: 44 g   Chol: 3 mg   Fat: 2.7 g
Fiber: 3.7 g   Protein: 16.6 g   Sodium: 834 mg

Veggie-Cheese Bagelwiches

YIELD: 4 SERVINGS

4 oat bran, whole wheat, or pumpernickel bagels, halved and toasted if desired

8 thin slices tomato

12 thin slices cucumber

1 cup alfalfa or spicy sprouts

VEGGIE-CHEESE SPREAD

1 block (8 ounces) nonfat or reduced-fat cream cheese, softened to room temperature

½ teaspoon crushed fresh garlic

2 tablespoons plus 1 teaspoon finely chopped scallions

2 tablespoons plus 1 teaspoon finely chopped green bell pepper

2 tablespoons plus 1 teaspoon grated carrot

1. To make the spread, place the cream cheese and garlic in a medium-sized bowl, and beat with an electric mixer until smooth. Stir in all of the remaining spread ingredients, and set aside.

2. Place half of the bagel halves on a flat surface, and spread each with ¼ cup of the cream cheese spread. Top with 2 slices of tomato, 3 slices of cucumber, and ¼ cup of sprouts.

3. Top each sandwich with 1 of the remaining bagel halves, cut each sandwich in half, and serve.

NUTRITIONAL FACTS (PER SERVING)
Cal: 344   Carbs: 64 g   Chol: 4 mg   Fat: 1.5 g
Fiber: 4.8 g   Protein: 21 g   Sodium: 837 mg

Cajun Chicken Sandwiches

YIELD: 4 SERVINGS

4 boneless skinless chicken breast halves
(about 4 ounces each)

2–3 tablespoons Cajun Spice Rub (page 137)

Nonstick cooking spray

1/2 cup shredded nonfat or reduced-fat
Swiss cheese

4 whole wheat or multigrain burger buns

4 slices tomato

4 slices red onion

4 leaves romaine lettuce

DRESSING

1/4 cup nonfat or low-fat mayonnaise

1 tablespoon mustard

1 tablespoon honey

1. Rinse the chicken with cool water, and pat it dry with paper towels. Using your fingers, rub both sides of each piece of chicken with some of the rub. If you have time, set the chicken aside for 15 to 30 minutes to allow the flavors to better penetrate the meat.

2. To make the dressing, place all of the dressing ingredients in a small bowl, and stir to mix well. Set aside.

3. Coat a broiler pan with nonstick cooking spray, and arrange the chicken on the pan. Spray the tops of the chicken lightly with the cooking spray, and broil 6 inches under a preheated broiler, turning occasionally, for 12 to 15 minutes, or until the meat is nicely browned and no longer pink inside. Alternatively, grill the chicken over medium coals for 12 to 15 minutes, or until done.

4. Sprinkle 2 tablespoons of cheese over the top of each piece of chicken, and return the chicken to the broiler or grill for 30 to 60 additional seconds, or until the cheese has melted. If you want toasted buns, split them open and place them on the broiler pan or grill along with the chicken during the last minute of cooking.

5. Spread the top and bottom of each bun with some of the dressing. Place a piece of chicken on the bottom half of each bun, and top with a slice of tomato, a slice of onion, a lettuce leaf, and the top half of the bun. Serve hot.

NUTRITIONAL FACTS (PER SERVING)			
Cal: 340	Carbs: 40 g	Chol: 67 mg	Fat: 4.8 g
Fiber: 2.2 g	Protein: 35 g	Sodium: 635 mg	

California Veggiewiches

YIELD: 4 SERVINGS

1/4 cup nonfat or reduced-fat mayonnaise

1/4 cup nonfat or light sour cream

8 slices firm wheatberry or multigrain bread,
toasted if desired

8 thin slices tomato

24 fresh spinach leaves

1/2 cup coarsely shredded carrot

16 thin slices cucumber

4 ounces thinly sliced nonfat or reduced-fat
Cheddar or Swiss cheese

8 thin rings green bell pepper

4 thin slices sweet onion, separated into rings

8 slices avocado, each 1/4-inch thick

1/2 cup alfalfa or spicy sprouts

1. Place the mayonnaise and sour cream in a small bowl, and stir to mix well.

2. Arrange the bread slices on a flat surface, and spread 1 tablespoon of the mayonnaise mixture on each slice of bread. On each of 4 of the slices, layer 2 tomato slices, 6 spinach leaves, 2 tablespoons of carrot, 4 cucumber slices, 1 ounce of cheese, 2 green pepper rings, and a quarter of the onion rings. Top with 2 slices of avocado and 2 tablespoons of sprouts.

3. Top each sandwich with another bread slice, and cut in half. Secure each half with a toothpick, and serve.

NUTRITIONAL FACTS (PER SERVING)			
Cal: 281	Carbs: 37 g	Chol: 2 mg	Fat: 7.8 g
Fiber: 5.6 g	Protein: 15.5 g	Sodium: 621 mg	

Italian Meatball Subs

YIELD: 5 SERVINGS

1 pound 95% lean ground beef

1 cup soft Italian bread crumbs*

2 egg whites

1/2 cup finely chopped onion

1 teaspoon dried Italian seasoning

1/4 teaspoon ground black pepper

1 1/4 cups bottled marinara sauce

1 medium green bell pepper,
cut into thin strips

1 medium onion, cut into thin wedges

5 whole wheat submarine-sandwich rolls,
each 6 inches long, or 5 pieces Italian bread,
each 6 inches long

1/2 cup plus 2 tablespoons shredded nonfat or
reduced-fat mozzarella cheese

* To make soft bread crumbs, tear about 1 1/3 slices of bread into chunks, place the chunks in a food processor or blender, and process into crumbs.

1. Place the ground beef, bread crumbs, egg whites, onion, Italian seasoning, and pepper in a large bowl, and mix thoroughly. Coat a baking sheet with non-stick cooking spray. Shape the meatball mixture into 15 (1 3/4-inch) balls, and arrange them on the baking sheet.

2. Bake the meatballs at 350°F for about 23 minutes, or until the meat is no longer pink inside. Remove the meatballs from the oven, and set aside.

3. Place the marinara sauce in a 2-quart saucepan, and simmer over medium heat just until hot. Add the meatballs, and toss to mix well. Cover the pot to keep warm, and set aside.

4. Coat a large nonstick skillet with nonstick cooking spray, and preheat over medium-high heat. Add the peppers and onions, and stir-fry for about 4 minutes, or until the vegetables are just tender. Cover the skillet periodically if it begins to dry out. (The steam from the cooking vegetables will moisten the skillet.) Add a little water if the skillet becomes too dry.

5. To assemble the subs, slice the rolls or Italian bread in half lengthwise, being careful to avoid cutting all the way through. Lay each of the rolls open on a plate, and arrange 3 meatballs and 1/4 cup of sauce in each one. Top with 1/4 cup of the peppers and onions and 2 tablespoons of the cheese. Serve hot.

NUTRITIONAL FACTS (PER SERVING)
Cal: 394   Carbs: 52 g   Chol: 64 mg   Fat: 6.5 g
Fiber: 5 g   Protein: 31.2 g   Sodium: 810 mg

Turkey BLTs

YIELD: 4 SERVINGS

12 slices extra-lean turkey bacon

8 slices whole wheat bread, toasted

1/4 cup nonfat or reduced-fat mayonnaise

8 thin slices tomato

4 leaves romaine lettuce

1. To microwave the bacon, place a paper towel on a large microwave-safe plate, and arrange the bacon in a single layer on the plate. Cover with another paper towel, and microwave on high power for about 1 minute per slice of bacon. (Note that depending on the size of your microwave, you will have to cook the bacon in 2 or 3 batches.) Alternatively, arrange the bacon on a large nonstick baking sheet, and bake at 400°F for 12 to 15 minutes, or until the bacon is nicely browned and crisp.

2. Arrange the bread slices on a flat surface, and spread each slice of toast with 1 1/2 teaspoons of mayonnaise. Arrange 3 slices of bacon on each of 4 slices of toast. Top the bacon with 2 slices of tomato, a lettuce leaf, and a remaining toast slice. Cut each sandwich in half, and serve.

NUTRITIONAL FACTS (PER SERVING)
Cal: 198   Carbs: 25 g   Chol: 45 mg   Fat: 2.6 g
Fiber: 2.5 g   Protein: 13.4 g   Sodium: 688 mg

Roasted Vegetable Sandwiches

YIELD: 4 SERVINGS

2 medium-large zucchini, each diagonally
cut into 8 (3/8-inch) slices

2 Portabella mushrooms,
each cut into 8 (1/2-inch) slices

2 medium red bell peppers,
each cut into 6 (1 1/2-inch) strips

1 medium-large Spanish or red onion,
cut into 8 (3/8-inch) slices

Nonstick olive oil cooking spray

1 teaspoon dried fines herbes*
or dried Italian seasoning

1/4 teaspoon salt

4 whole wheat submarine-sandwich rolls,
each 6 inches long

4 ounces nonfat or reduced-fat mozzarella
or provolone cheese, thinly sliced

1/4 cup crumbled nonfat or reduced-fat feta cheese

2 tablespoons plus 2 teaspoons bottled nonfat
or reduced-fat balsamic vinaigrette
or Italian salad dressing

* A blend of thyme, oregano, sage, rosemary, marjoram, and basil, fines herbes can be found in the dried spice section of most grocery stores.

1. Coat a large baking sheet with nonstick olive oil cooking spray, and arrange the vegetables in a single layer on the sheet. Spray the vegetables lightly with the cooking spray, and sprinkle with the herbs and salt.

2. Bake uncovered at 450°F degrees for 12 minutes. Turn the vegetables, and bake for 8 additional minutes, or until tender and nicely browned.

3. While the vegetables are cooking, split the rolls in half lengthwise, and arrange the halves on a large baking sheet, cut sides up. Place under a preheated broiler, and broil for a minute or 2, or until lightly toasted. Place the bottom half of each roll on an individual serving plate, and set aside. Lay 1 ounce of

the mozzarella or provolone cheese on the inside of the top half of each roll, and return the roll tops to the broiler for about 1 minute, or until the cheese is melted.

4. Layer 4 zucchini slices, 4 mushroom slices, 3 red pepper strips, and 2 onion slices on the bottom half of each roll. Sprinkle with 1 tablespoon of the feta cheese and 2 teaspoons of the dressing. Place the top half of the roll, cheese side down, over the vegetables, and serve hot.

NUTRITIONAL FACTS (PER SERVING)
Cal: 310   Carbs: 49 g   Chol: 0 mg   Fat: 2.9 g
Fiber: 6.1 g   Protein: 22 g   Sodium: 696 mg

Light Grilled Cheese Sandwiches

For variety, make these sandwiches with rye or pumpernickel bread and Swiss cheese.

YIELD: 4 SERVINGS

8 slices whole wheat or multigrain bread

Nonstick butter-flavored cooking spray, or
8 teaspoons reduced-fat margarine or light butter

6 ounces thinly sliced nonfat or reduced-fat
Cheddar or American cheese

1. Arrange the bread slices on a flat surface. Spray 1 side of each slice of bread with the cooking spray, or spread with 1 teaspoon of the margarine or butter.

2. Place 4 of the bread slices on a flat surface, with the sprayed or margarine sides down. Top each bread slice with a quarter of the cheese slices. Top with the remaining bread slices, with the sprayed or margarine sides up.

3. Preheat a large nonstick skillet or griddle over medium-low heat, and place the sandwiches in the skillet or griddle. Cook for about 3 minutes on each side, or until the bread is toasted and the cheese is melted. Cut each sandwich in half, and serve hot.

NUTRITIONAL FACTS (PER SERVING)
Cal: 198   Carbs: 27 g   Chol: 4 mg   Fat: 2.3 g
Fiber: 3.9 g   Protein: 17.5 g   Sodium: 629 mg

Fabulous French Dips

YIELD: 6 SERVINGS

| 2 cups sliced fresh mushrooms |
| 1 medium yellow onion, cut into thin wedges |
| 2 tablespoons dry sherry |
| 6 pieces French bread, each 6 inches long, or 6 whole wheat submarine-sandwich rolls, each 6 inches long |
| 1 pound 2 ounces thinly sliced cooked lean roast beef |
| 6 ounces thinly sliced nonfat or reduced-fat mozzarella or provolone cheese |

BROTH

| 1 can (14$\frac{1}{2}$ ounces) beef broth |
| $\frac{1}{2}$ teaspoon crushed fresh garlic |
| $\frac{1}{4}$ teaspoon coarsely ground black pepper |
| $\frac{1}{4}$ teaspoon dried marjoram |
| $\frac{1}{4}$ teaspoon dried thyme |
| 1 bay leaf |

1. To make the broth, place all of the broth ingredients in a 1-quart pot. Stir to mix, and bring to a boil over high heat. Reduce the heat to low, cover, and simmer for 15 minutes, or until the flavors are well blended.

2. While the broth is simmering, coat a medium-sized nonstick skillet with nonstick cooking spray, and preheat over medium heat. Add the mushrooms, onion, and sherry, and sauté, stirring occasionally, for 5 minutes, or until the vegetables are tender. Cover the skillet periodically if it begins to dry out. (The steam from the cooking vegetables will moisten the skillet.) Add a little more sherry if the skillet gets too dry.

3. Slice the French bread or rolls in half lengthwise, and lay the pieces open on a flat surface. Arrange 3 ounces of beef on the bottom half of each piece. Top with some of the sautéed mushrooms and onions and 1 ounce of the cheese. Replace the tops of the sandwiches, and cut each one in half.

4. Arrange the sandwiches on a microwave-safe platter. Cover with a paper towel, and microwave on high power for 2 minutes, or until the cheese is melt-

ed. Alternatively, wrap each sandwich in aluminum foil and bake at 400°F for 10 minutes, or until the cheese is melted. Place the sandwiches on serving plates, accompany each plate with a dish of the broth, and serve.

NUTRITIONAL FACTS (PER SERVING)
Cal: 365   Carbs: 37.3 g   Chol: 50 mg   Fat: 6.2 g
Fiber: 3.3 g   Protein: 40 g   Sodium: 833 mg

Curried Turkey Salad Sandwiches

YIELD: 4 SERVINGS

| 2 cups diced cooked turkey breast (about 10 ounces) |
| 1 cup chopped peeled tart apple (about 1 medium) |
| $\frac{1}{2}$ cup thinly sliced celery |
| $\frac{1}{4}$ cup golden raisins |
| $\frac{1}{4}$ cup plus 2 tablespoons nonfat or light sour cream |
| $\frac{1}{4}$ cup plus 2 tablespoons nonfat or reduced-fat mayonnaise |
| 3 tablespoons mango chutney |
| 1 teaspoon curry paste |
| 4 whole wheat pita pockets (6-inch rounds), cut in half |
| 1$\frac{1}{2}$ cups alfalfa sprouts or shredded romaine lettuce |

1. Place the turkey, apple, celery, and raisins in a medium-sized bowl, and toss to mix well. Place the sour cream, mayonnaise, chutney, and curry paste in a small bowl, and stir to mix well. Add the sour cream mixture to the turkey mixture, and toss to mix well. Cover the mixture, and chill for at least 2 hours.

2. To assemble the sandwiches, fill each pita half with a scant $\frac{1}{2}$ cup of the turkey mixture, and some of the sprouts or lettuce. Serve.

NUTRITIONAL FACTS (PER SERVING)
Cal: 336   Carbs: 50 g   Chol: 58 mg   Fat: 1.8 g
Fiber: 6.1 g   Protein: 30 g   Sodium: 553 mg

Greek Chicken Pitas

In a hurry? Substitute 1¼ cups of sliced store-bought rotisserie chicken for the grilled chicken.

YIELD: 4 SERVINGS

4 boneless skinless chicken breast halves
(about 4 ounces each)

2–3 tablespoons Lemon-Herb Rub (page 137)

Nonstick olive oil cooking spray

4 whole wheat or oat bran pita pockets
(6-inch rounds), cut in half

TOPPINGS

½ cup plus 2 tablespoons diced seeded peeled
cucumber (about 1 medium)

½ cup plus 2 tablespoons diced tomato
(about 1 medium)

⅓ cup diced red onion or sliced scallions

⅓ cup crumbled nonfat or reduced-fat feta cheese

1 cup shredded romaine lettuce

¼ cup bottled nonfat or reduced-fat red wine
vinaigrette, Caesar, or ranch salad dressing

1. Rinse the chicken with cool water, and pat it dry with paper towels. Using your fingers, rub both sides of each piece of chicken with some of the rub. If you have time, set the chicken aside for 15 to 30 minutes to allow the flavors to better penetrate the meat.

2. Coat a broiler pan with nonstick cooking spray, and arrange the chicken on the pan. Spray the tops of the chicken lightly with the cooking spray, and broil 6 inches under a preheated broiler, turning occasionally, for 12 to 15 minutes, or until the meat is nicely browned and no longer pink inside. Alternatively, grill the chicken over medium coals for 12 to 15 minutes, or until done.

3. While the chicken is cooking, place the cucumber, tomato, onion or scallion, and feta cheese in a medium-sized bowl, and toss to mix well. Set aside.

4. To heat the pita pockets, place them on a microwave-safe plate. Cover with a damp paper towel, and microwave on high power for about 45 seconds, or until warm.

5. Place the chicken on a cutting board, and thinly slice at an angle. Stuff each pita half with some of the chicken slices, a scant ¼ cup of the cucumber mixture, and 2 tablespoons of the lettuce. Drizzle 1½ teaspoons of dressing over the filling, and serve.

NUTRITIONAL FACTS (PER SERVING)
Cal: 336   Carbs: 42 g   Chol: 66 mg   Fat: 1.9 g
Fiber: 4.8 g   Protein: 35 g   Sodium: 759 mg

Italian Heroes

YIELD: 4 SERVINGS

4 whole wheat or Italian submarine-sandwich rolls,
each 6 inches long

¼ cup nonfat or reduced-fat mayonnaise

8 ounces thinly sliced ham,
at least 97% lean

24 slices turkey pepperoni

4 ounces thinly sliced nonfat or reduced-fat
mozzarella or provolone cheese

12 thin slices plum tomato

4 thin slices red onion, separated into rings

8 thin slices green bell pepper

1⅓ cups shredded romaine lettuce

¼ cup bottled nonfat or reduced-fat
Italian salad dressing

¼ cup sliced black olives (optional)

1. Place the bottom half of each roll on a flat surface, and spread with 1½ teaspoons of mayonnaise. Top with a quarter of the ham, pepperoni, and cheese, followed by 3 tomato slices, some of the onion rings, 2 rings of green pepper, and ⅓ cup of lettuce. Drizzle 1 tablespoon of Italian dressing over each sandwich, and sprinkle with a few olives, if desired.

2. Spread the top half of each roll with 1½ teaspoons of mayonnaise. Place each top on a sandwich, cut each sandwich in half, and serve.

NUTRITIONAL FACTS (PER SERVING)
Cal: 412   Carbs: 57 g   Chol: 45 mg   Fat: 5.6 g
Fiber: 3.6 g   Protein: 32 g   Sodium: 1,270 mg

Unfried Falafel Pockets

YIELD: 6 SERVINGS

Nonstick olive oil cooking spray

3 whole wheat or oat bran pita pockets
(6-inch rounds), cut in half

18 thin slices cucumber

6 slices tomato

1½ cups alfalfa sprouts or shredded
romaine lettuce

FALAFEL MIXTURE

1 can (19 ounces) chickpeas, rinsed and drained,
or 2 cups cooked chickpeas

1 cup diced cooked sweet potato
(about 1 medium)

4 scallions, chopped

¼ cup plus 2 tablespoons chopped fresh parsley

2 teaspoons crushed fresh garlic

1 teaspoon ground cumin

1 teaspoon ground coriander

½ teaspoon coarsely ground black pepper

⅓ cup toasted wheat germ

DRESSING

¼ cup plain nonfat yogurt

2–3 tablespoons toasted sesame tahini

2 tablespoons seasoned rice vinegar

½ teaspoon crushed fresh garlic

¼ teaspoon ground ginger

1. To make the dressing, place all of the dressing ingredients in a blender or mini-food processor, and blend until smooth. Set aside.

2. To make the falafel, place all of the falafel mixture ingredients except for the wheat germ in a food processor, and process until puréed, but still slightly chunky. Add a few teaspoons of plain yogurt or water if the mixture seems too dry to shape into patties.

3. Coat a large baking sheet with nonstick cooking spray, and set aside.

4. Place the wheat germ in a shallow dish. Shape the falafel mixture into 12 (2-inch) patties and, 1 at a time, lay the patties in the dish containing the wheat germ, turning to coat both sides. Arrange the patties in a single layer on the prepared baking sheet.

5. Spray the tops of the patties lightly with olive oil cooking spray, and bake at 400°F for 10 minutes. Turn the patties, and bake for 10 additional minutes, or until nicely browned.

6. To heat the pita pockets, place them on a microwave-safe plate. Cover with a damp paper towel, and microwave on high power for about 45 seconds, or until warm.

7. Place 2 falafel patties in each pita half. Add 3 slices of cucumber, 1 slice of tomato, and ¼ cup of sprouts or lettuce. Drizzle with the dressing, and serve.

NUTRITIONAL FACTS (PER SERVING)
Cal: 253   Carbs: 44 g   Chol: 0 mg   Fat: 5 g
Fiber: 8.9 g   Protein: 12 g   Sodium: 331 mg

Grilled Hummus Pitawiches

YIELD: 6 SERVINGS

6 whole wheat or oat bran pita pockets
(6-inch rounds)

18 fresh spinach leaves

3 medium plum tomatoes, thinly sliced

1½ cups shredded nonfat or reduced-fat
mozzarella cheese

Nonstick olive oil cooking spray

FILLING

1 can (1 pound) chickpeas, rinsed and drained,
or 1¾ cups cooked chickpeas

½ cup sliced scallions

¼ cup finely chopped fresh parsley

¼ cup plain nonfat or low-fat yogurt

2–3 tablespoons toasted sesame tahini

1½ teaspoons crushed fresh garlic

¼ teaspoon ground black pepper

1. To make the filling, place all of the filling ingredients in a food processor, and process until smooth. Set aside.

2. Using a sharp knife or scissors, cut each pita round about two-thirds of the way around the edges. Carefully open the pita bread round, and spread $1/4$ cup of the filling over the bottom layer. Arrange first 3 spinach leaves, then 3 slices of tomato, and finally $1/4$ cup of cheese over the filling.

3. Coat a large nonstick griddle or skillet with nonstick olive oil cooking spray, and preheat over medium heat. Lay the sandwiches on the griddle, and cook for about 2 minutes, or until the bottoms are lightly toasted. Spray the tops of the sandwiches with the cooking spray, turn them over, and cook for another couple of minutes, or until both sides are toasted, the filling is hot, and the cheese is melted.

4. Cut each sandwich into 4 wedges, and serve hot.

NUTRITIONAL FACTS (PER SERVING)		
Cal: 293 Carbs: 48 g Chol: 2 mg Fat: 4.5 g		
Fiber: 8.7 g Protein: 20 g Sodium: 661 mg		

Garden Stuffed Pitas

YIELD: 4 SERVINGS

3 cups mixed salad greens or torn romaine lettuce

$1/2$ cup sliced fresh mushrooms

1 small carrot, peeled and shredded
with a potato peeler

$1/4$ cup diced red bell pepper

$3/4$ cup shredded nonfat or reduced-fat
Cheddar or mozzarella cheese

4 whole wheat or oat bran pita pockets
(6-inch rounds), cut in half

$1/4$ cup bottled nonfat or reduced-fat ranch,
honey mustard, or Italian salad dressing

1. To make the filling, place the salad greens or lettuce, mushrooms, carrot, red pepper, and cheese in a large bowl, and toss to mix well. Set aside.

2. To heat the pita pockets, place them on a microwave-safe plate. Cover with a damp paper towel, and microwave on high power for about 45 seconds, or until warm.

3. Stuff each pita half with some of the salad mixture. Drizzle $1 1/2$ teaspoons of dressing over the filling in each pocket, and serve.

NUTRITIONAL FACTS (PER SERVING)		
Cal: 230 Carbs: 41 g Chol: 2 mg Fat: 0.6 g		
Fiber: 5.2 g Protein: 14 g Sodium: 530 mg		

Shrimp in a Pita Boat

YIELD: 4 SERVINGS

4 whole wheat or oat bran pita pockets
(6-inch rounds), cut in half

2 cups cooked peeled shrimp (about 12 ounces)

4 ounces thinly sliced nonfat or reduced-fat
Swiss cheese (optional)

2 cups shredded lettuce

8 slices tomato

4 thin slices red onion, separated into rings

$1/2$ cup bottled nonfat or reduced-fat
ranch salad dressing

1. Fill each pita half with $1/4$ cup of the shrimp and, if desired, $1/2$ ounce of the cheese.

2. To heat the sandwiches, arrange them on a large microwave-safe plate, cover with damp paper towels, and microwave on high power for 2 minutes, or just until the sandwiches are heated through.

3. Place some of the lettuce, 1 slice of tomato, and a few onion rings in each pita half. Drizzle some dressing over the filling, and serve.

NUTRITIONAL FACTS (PER SERVING)		
Cal: 269 Carbs: 41 g Chol: 269 mg Fat: 2.5 g		
Fiber: 4.9 g Protein: 21 g Sodium: 636 mg		

Tempting Soft Tacos

YIELD: 10 TACOS

1 pound 95% lean ground beef

1 medium yellow onion, chopped

1/2 cup bottled salsa

2 teaspoons chili powder

1/2 teaspoon ground cumin

10 flour tortillas (6-inch rounds)

1/2 cup plus 2 tablespoons shredded nonfat
or reduced-fat Cheddar cheese

1/2 cup plus 2 tablespoons nonfat or light sour cream

1/2 cup plus 2 tablespoons diced tomatoes

1 1/4 cups shredded romaine lettuce

1. To make the filling, coat a large nonstick skillet with nonstick cooking spray, and preheat over medium heat. Add the ground beef, and cook, stirring to crumble, until the meat is no longer pink. Drain off and discard any excess fat.

2. Stir the onion, salsa, chili powder, and cumin into the beef. Cover and cook, stirring frequently, for about 3 minutes, or until the onions are soft. Remove the cover and cook, stirring frequently, for a minute or 2, or until most of the liquid has evaporated. Cover the filling to keep warm, and set aside.

3. Heat the tortillas according to package directions. To assemble the tacos, lay a warm tortilla on a flat surface, and cover the *bottom half only* with 1/4 cup of the filling. Top the filling with 1 tablespoon of cheese, 1 tablespoon of sour cream, 1 tablespoon of tomatoes, and 2 tablespoons of lettuce. Fold the top half over to cover the bottom half. Repeat this procedure with the remaining ingredients to make 10 tacos, and serve hot.

NUTRITIONAL FACTS (PER TACO)
Cal: 190   Carbs: 23 g   Chol: 26 mg   Fat: 3.5 g
Fiber: 2 g   Protein: 16.4 g   Sodium: 297 mg

Bean Burritos Supreme

YIELD: 6 SERVINGS

1 3/4 cups cooked pinto beans, or 1 can (1 pound)
pinto beans, rinsed and drained

2 teaspoons chili powder

1/4 teaspoon ground cumin

1/2 cup finely chopped yellow onion

1/2 cup finely chopped tomato

6 flour tortillas (8- to 10-inch rounds)

1/2 cup nonfat or light sour cream

1/2 cup shredded nonfat or reduced-fat Cheddar cheese

3/4 cup shredded lettuce

1. Place the beans in a medium-sized bowl, and mash with a fork until slightly chunky. Stir in the chili powder and cumin, and set aside.

2. Coat a large skillet with nonstick cooking spray, and add the onion and tomato. Place the pan over medium heat, cover, and cook, stirring occasionally, for about 5 minutes, or until the vegetables are soft.

3. Add the beans to the skillet mixture, and cook uncovered, stirring constantly, until the beans are heated through and the mixture has the consistency of thick refried beans. Remove the skillet from the heat, cover to keep warm, and set aside.

4. Heat the tortillas according to package directions. To assemble the burritos, lay a warm tortilla on a flat surface, and spoon 1/4 cup of the warm bean mixture along the right side of the tortilla. Top the bean mixture with 1 tablespoon of the sour cream, 1 tablespoon of the cheese, and 2 tablespoons of the lettuce.

5. Fold the bottom edge of the tortilla up about 1 inch. (This fold will prevent the filling from falling out.) Then, beginning at the right edge, roll the tortilla up jelly-roll style.

6. Transfer the tortilla to a serving platter, cover with aluminum foil, and place in a 200°F oven to keep warm. Repeat with the remaining tortillas, and serve hot.

NUTRITIONAL FACTS (PER BURRITO)
Cal: 246   Carbs: 43 g   Chol: 1 mg   Fat: 2.5 g
Fiber: 6.6 g   Protein: 12 g   Sodium: 395 mg

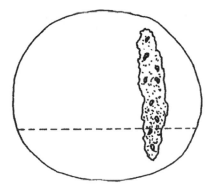

a. Arrange the filling along the right side of the tortilla.

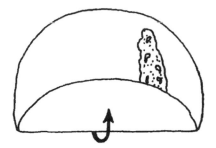

b. Fold the bottom edge of the tortilla up.

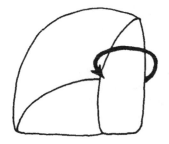

c. Fold the right side over the filling.

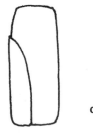

d. Continue folding to form a roll.

MAKING BEAN BURRITOS SUPREME

Southwestern Shrimp Wraps

YIELD: 8 SERVINGS

1 pound large raw shrimp, peeled and deveined
3 tablespoons Spicy Tex-Mex Rub (page 137)
Nonstick butter-flavored cooking spray
8 flour tortillas (8- to 10-inch rounds)
1/2 cup shredded nonfat or reduced-fat Cheddar cheese
1/2 cup nonfat or light sour cream
3/4 cup diced fresh tomatoes
1 1/2 cups shredded romaine lettuce

1. Rinse the shrimp with cool water, and pat them dry with paper towels. Place the shrimp in a large bowl, sprinkle with the rub mixture, and stir well to coat.

2. Thread a quarter of the shrimp on each of four 12-inch skewers. (If you use wooden rather than metal skewers, soak them in water for 30 minutes prior to using them to prevent them from burning.) Spray the skewered shrimp lightly with the cooking spray, and broil under a preheated broiler or grill over medium coals for 3 to 4 minutes on each side, or until the shrimp turn pink and are cooked through.

3. While the shrimp are cooking, heat the tortillas according to package directions. Arrange the warm tortillas on a flat surface. Place an eighth of the shrimp along the right side of each tortilla, stopping 1 1/2 inches from the bottom. Top the shrimp with 1 tablespoon of cheese, 1 tablespoon of sour cream, 1 1/2 tablespoons of tomatoes, and 3 tablespoons of the lettuce.

4. Fold the bottom edge of each tortilla up about 1 inch. (This fold will prevent the filling from falling out.) Then, beginning at the right edge, roll each tortilla up jelly-roll style. (See the figures at left.) Serve hot.

NUTRITIONAL FACTS (PER SERVING)
Cal: 216   Carbs: 30 g   Chol: 82 mg   Fat: 2.7 g
Fiber: 1.7 g   Protein: 16.3 g   Sodium: 361 mg

Chicken Caesar Wraps

In a hurry? Substitute 1¼ cups of diced store-bought rotisserie chicken for the grilled chicken.

YIELD: 4 SERVINGS
2 boneless skinless chicken breast halves (about 5 ounces each)
2 tablespoons Lemon-Herb Rub (page 137)
Nonstick cooking spray
4 cups torn romaine lettuce
3 tablespoons chopped red onion
¼ cup bottled nonfat or reduced-fat Caesar salad dressing
2 tablespoons grated nonfat or regular Parmesan cheese
4 flour tortillas (8- to 10-inch rounds)

1. Rinse the chicken with cool water, and pat it dry with paper towels. Using your fingers, rub both sides of each piece of chicken with some of the rub. If you have time, set the chicken aside for 15 to 30 minutes to allow the flavors to better penetrate the meat.

2. Coat a broiler pan with nonstick cooking spray, and arrange the chicken on the pan. Spray the tops of the chicken lightly with the cooking spray, and broil 6 inches under a preheated broiler, turning occasionally, for 12 to 15 minutes, or until the meat is nicely browned and no longer pink inside. Alternatively, grill the chicken over medium coals for 12 to 15 minutes, or until done. Transfer the chicken to a cutting board, and set aside.

3. Place the lettuce and onions in a large bowl. Add the salad dressing, and toss to mix well. Add the Parmesan, and toss again. Dice the chicken, add it to the lettuce mixture, and toss to mix well.

4. Heat the tortillas according to package directions. Arrange the warm tortillas on a flat surface. Place ¼ of the lettuce mixture along the right side of each tortilla, stopping 1½ inches from the bottom.

5. Fold the bottom edge of each tortilla up about 1 inch. (This fold will prevent the filling from falling out.) Then, beginning at the right edge, roll each tortilla up jelly-roll style, and serve. (See the figures on page 135.)

NUTRITIONAL FACTS (PER SERVING)
Cal: 248   Carbs: 31 g   Chol: 43 mg   Fat: 3 g
Fiber: 2.6 g   Protein: 22 g   Sodium: 480 mg

Turkey Tortilla Wraps

YIELD: 4 SERVINGS
4 flour tortillas (8- to 10-inch rounds)
8 ounces thinly sliced roasted turkey breast or lean ham
8 thin slices tomato
8 thin rings green bell pepper
1 cup shredded romaine lettuce
½ cup shredded nonfat or reduced-fat Cheddar, Swiss, or mozzarella cheese
¼ cup bottled nonfat or reduced-fat ranch or honey-mustard salad dressing

1. Heat the tortillas according to package directions. Arrange the warm tortillas on a flat surface, and top each tortilla with ¼ of the turkey or ham slices, covering the entire tortilla except for a 1-inch margin on the bottom. Top the turkey on each tortilla with 2 tomato slices, 2 green pepper rings, ¼ cup of lettuce, and 2 tablespoons of cheese. Drizzle with 1 tablespoon of dressing.

2. Fold the bottom edge of each tortilla up about 1 inch. (This fold will prevent the filling from falling out.) Then, beginning at the right edge, roll each tortilla up jelly-roll style, and serve. (See the figures on page 135.)

NUTRITIONAL FACTS (PER SERVING)
Cal: 264   Carbs: 33 g   Chol: 50 mg   Fat: 2.8 g
Fiber: 1.8 g   Protein: 26 g   Sodium: 639 mg

Fast and Flavorful Spice Rubs

Bursting with flavor, spice rubs can transform bland and boring meat, seafood, and poultry into delicious culinary creations—without adding a lot of fat or salt to your meal.

To apply the rub, rinse the food and pat it dry with paper towels. Then, using your fingers, rub the outside surface of the meat with the seasoning blend. If you have time, allow the food to stand at room temperature for fifteen to thirty minutes before cooking. This will enable the seasonings to permeate the food. (Refrigerate if you are going to set the food aside for more than an hour.) Spray the food lightly with nonstick cooking spray, and grill, broil, or roast as desired. Then enjoy great flavor without added fat!

The following rub mixtures will remain flavorful for several months, so make a double or triple batch of your favorite rubs, and store the mixtures in airtight containers so that you'll always have a supply on hand. Note that each of the following recipes will make enough rub to season two pounds of meat, seafood, or poultry.

Spicy Tex-Mex Rub

YIELD: ABOUT 5 TABLESPOONS

1 tablespoon chili powder

1 tablespoon ground paprika

1 tablespoon light brown sugar

2 teaspoons lemon pepper

1 teaspoon ground cumin

1/2 teaspoon garlic powder

1/4 teaspoon salt

1. Place all of the ingredients in a small bowl, and stir to mix well.

2. Apply the rub according to the directions given above, and grill, broil, or roast the meat as desired.

NUTRITIONAL FACTS (PER 2-TEASPOON SERVING)
Cal: 15   Carbs: 3.1 g   Chol: 0 mg   Fat: 0.2 g
Fiber: 0.5 g   Protein: 0.2 g   Sodium: 47 mg

Lemon-Herb Rub

YIELD: ABOUT 5 TABLESPOONS

2 tablespoons dried crushed oregano or thyme

1 tablespoon dried grated lemon rind

1 tablespoon light brown sugar

3/4 teaspoon coarsely ground black pepper

3/4 teaspoon garlic powder

1/2 teaspoon salt

1. Place all of the ingredients in a small bowl, and stir to mix well.

2. Apply the rub according to the directions given above, and grill, broil, or roast the meat as desired.

NUTRITIONAL FACTS (PER 2-TEASPOON SERVING)
Cal: 12   Carbs: 2.9 g   Chol: 0 mg   Fat: 0.1 g
Fiber: 0.6 g   Protein: 0.2 g   Sodium: 156 mg

Cajun Spice Rub

YIELD: ABOUT 5 TABLESPOONS

1 1/2 tablespoons ground paprika

1 tablespoon light brown sugar

1 1/2 teaspoons garlic powder

1 teaspoon onion powder

1 teaspoon dried thyme

1 teaspoon dried oregano

3/4 teaspoon ground black pepper

1/4–3/4 teaspoon ground cayenne pepper

1/2 teaspoon salt

1. Place all of the ingredients in a small bowl, and stir to mix well.

2. Apply the rub according to the directions given above, and grill, broil, or roast the meat as desired.

NUTRITIONAL FACTS (PER 2-TEASPOON SERVING)
Cal: 14   Carbs: 3.3 g   Chol: 0 mg   Fat: 0.2 g
Fiber: 0.5 g   Protein: 0.4 g   Sodium: 147 mg

Primavera Pan Pizza

YIELD: 8 SLICES

1 recipe Hearty Wheat Pizza Dough (page 140) or Oatmeal Pizza Dough (page 141)
1 teaspoon crushed fresh garlic
3 cups (moderately packed) chopped fresh spinach
1/2 cup Arrabbiata Sauce (page 233), Chunky Garden Marinara Sauce (page 235), or bottled marinara sauce
1 tablespoon grated nonfat or egular Parmesan cheese
1 cup shredded reduced-fat mozzarella cheese
1/2 cup fresh or frozen (thawed) cut broccoli florets
1/4 cup diced red bell pepper
1/4 cup thinly sliced fresh mushrooms
1/2 teaspoon dried Italian seasoning

1. Turn the dough onto a lightly floured surface. Using a rolling pin, roll the dough into a 10-x-14-inch rectangle. Coat a 9-x-13-inch pan with nonstick cooking spray, and press the dough over the bottom and 1/2-inch up the sides of the pan. Set the crust aside for 5 to 10 minutes.

2. Coat a large nonstick skillet with nonstick cooking spray, and preheat over medium heat. Add the garlic, and stir-fry for about 30 seconds, or until the garlic just begins to turn color. Add the spinach, and stir-fry for another minute, or just until the spinach is wilted. Remove the skillet from the heat, and set aside.

3. Spread the sauce over the bottom of the crust. Sprinkle the Parmesan over the sauce, and top with the spinach mixture. Follow with layers of the mozzarella, broccoli, red pepper, and mushrooms, and sprinkle with the Italian seasoning.

4. Bake at 425°F for about 12 minutes, or until the cheese is melted and the crust is lightly browned. Slice and serve immediately.

NUTRITIONAL FACTS (PER SLICE)
Cal: 144   Carbs: 21.4 g   Chol: 5 mg   Fat: 2.8 g
Fiber: 3 g   Protein: 8.3 g   Sodium: 230 mg

Black Bean Pizzas

YIELD: 6 SERVINGS

1 3/4 cups cooked black beans, or 1 can (1 pound) black beans, rinsed and drained
2 teaspoons chili powder
1/4 teaspoon ground cumin
1 1/2 cups chopped tomato, divided
6 flour tortillas (8-inch rounds)
1 1/2 cups shredded reduced-fat Cheddar or Monterey jack cheese
6 thin slices onion, separated into rings
6 large black olives, thinly sliced
2 tablespoons finely chopped pickled jalapeño peppers (optional)
1 cup shredded lettuce

1. Place the beans in a medium-sized bowl, and mash with a fork until slightly chunky. Stir in the chili powder and cumin, and set aside.

2. Coat a large skillet with nonstick cooking spray, and add 3/4 cup of the tomato. Place over medium heat, cover, and cook, stirring occasionally, for about 5 minutes, or until the tomatoes are soft.

3. Add the beans to the skillet, and cook uncovered, stirring constantly, until the beans are heated through and the mixture has the consistency of thick refried beans. Remove the skillet from the heat, and set aside.

4. Coat 2 large baking sheets with nonstick cooking spray, and lay the tortillas on the sheet. Spread 1/4 cup of the bean mixture over each tortilla, extending the mixture to within 1/2 inch of the edges. Top each tortilla with 1/4 cup of the cheese, a sixth of the onions, a sixth of the olives, and 2 teaspoons of the jalapeños, if desired.

5. Bake uncovered at 400°F for 7 to 9 minutes, or until the pizzas are lightly browned and crisp. Remove from the oven, top each pizza with some of the remaining chopped tomato and the shredded lettuce, and serve immediately.

NUTRITIONAL FACTS (PER PIZZA)
Cal: 270   Carbs: 35 g   Chol: 15 mg   Fat: 6.9 g
Fiber: 7.4 g   Protein: 17 g   Sodium: 505 mg

White Pizza

YIELD: 8 SLICES

1 recipe Oatmeal Pizza Dough (page 141)
or Hearty Wheat Pizza Dough (page 140)

3/4 cup nonfat or low-fat ricotta cheese

2 tablespoons grated nonfat or regular
Parmesan cheese

1/2 cup shredded reduced-fat mozzarella cheese

1/2 cup shredded reduced-fat provolone cheese

1/4 cup thinly sliced scallions

3 tablespoons sliced black olives (optional)

3/4 teaspoon dried Italian seasoning

1/2 teaspoon whole fennel seeds

1. Turn the dough onto a lightly floured surface. Using a rolling pin, roll the dough into a 14-inch circle. (For a thick crust, roll the dough into a 12-inch circle.) Coat a 14-inch (or 12-inch) pizza pan with nonstick cooking spray. Place the dough on the pan, forming a slight rim around the edges. Set the crust aside for 5 to 10 minutes.

2. Place the ricotta and Parmesan in a small bowl, and stir to mix well. Spread the cheese mixture over the crust to within 1/2 inch of the edges. Sprinkle the mozzarella and provolone over the ricotta. Sprinkle the cheeses with the scallions; the olives, if desired; and the Italian seasoning and fennel seeds.

3. Bake at 425°F for about 12 minutes, or until the cheese is melted and the crust is lightly browned. Slice and serve immediately.

NUTRITIONAL FACTS (PER SLICE)
Cal: 156   Carbs: 21.4 g   Chol: 7 mg   Fat: 2.7 g
Fiber: 1.2 g   Protein: 11.3 g   Sodium: 229 mg

Puttanesca Pizza

YIELD: 8 SLICES

1 can (14 1/2 ounces) unsalted
whole tomatoes, drained

1 recipe Hearty Wheat Pizza Dough (page 140)
or Oatmeal Pizza Dough (page 141)

1 tablespoon plus 1 1/2 teaspoons grated nonfat
or regular Parmesan cheese

1 cup shredded reduced-fat mozzarella cheese

1/4 cup sliced black olives

1 tablespoon small capers

3/4 teaspoon dried Italian seasoning

1/2 teaspoon crushed red pepper

1. Place the drained tomatoes in a small bowl, and mash with a fork until coarsely crushed. Drain off any liquid that has accumulated, and set aside.

2. Turn the dough onto a lightly floured surface. Using a rolling pin, roll the dough into a 14-inch circle. (For a thick crust, roll the dough into a 12-inch circle.) Coat a 14-inch (or 12-inch) pizza pan with nonstick cooking spray. Place the dough on the pan, forming a slight rim around the edges. Set the crust aside for 5 to 10 minutes.

3. Spread the tomatoes over the crust to within 1/2 inch of the edges. Sprinkle first the Parmesan and then the mozzarella over the tomatoes. Top with the olives and capers, and sprinkle with the Italian seasoning and red pepper.

4. Bake at 425°F for about 10 minutes, or until the cheese is melted and the crust is lightly browned. Slice and serve immediately.

NUTRITIONAL FACTS (PER SLICE)
Cal: 154   Carbs: 24.5 g   Chol: 5 mg   Fat: 2.9 g
Fiber: 1.7 g   Protein: 8.3 g   Sodium: 307 mg

Making Pizza Crusts

Few foods are as well-loved as the pizza. And, certainly, nothing compares to the fresh flavor of a homemade pie. Although many quick-and-easy options are available for pizza crusts (see the inset on page 143), for optimal nutrition and flavor, you may want to consider making your crusts from scratch. The following recipes will allow you to make both pizza and calzone crusts that are as delicious and satisfying as they are healthy. (For information on making these crusts in a bread machine, see the Time-Saving Tip below.)

Hearty Wheat Pizza Dough

**YIELD: ABOUT ³/₄ POUND DOUGH, ENOUGH FOR
A 14-INCH THIN CRUST OR A 12-INCH THICK CRUST**

1¼ cups plus 2 tablespoons bread flour

⅓ cup toasted wheat germ

1½ teaspoons Rapid Rise yeast

¼ teaspoon salt

½ cup plus 2 tablespoons water or skim
or low-fat milk

1 teaspoon honey

1. Place ³/₄ cup of the flour and all of the wheat germ, yeast, and salt in a large bowl, and stir to mix well. Place the water or milk and the honey in a small saucepan, and heat until very warm (125°F to 130°F). Add the water mixture to the flour mixture, and stir for 1 minute. Stir in enough of the remaining flour, 2 tablespoons at a time, to form a soft dough.

2. Sprinkle 2 tablespoons of the remaining flour over a flat surface, and turn the dough onto the surface. Knead the dough for 5 minutes, gradually adding just enough of the remaining flour to form a smooth, satiny ball. (Be careful not to make the dough too stiff, or it will be hard to roll out.)

3. Coat a large bowl with nonstick cooking spray, and place the ball of dough in the bowl. Cover the bowl with a clean kitchen towel, and let rise in a warm place for about 35 minutes, or until doubled in size.

4. When the dough has risen, punch it down, shape it into a ball, and turn it onto a lightly floured surface. The dough is now ready for shaping, topping, and baking.

TIME-SAVING TIP

To make Oatmeal Pizza Dough or Hearty Wheat Pizza Dough in a bread machine, place all of the dough ingredients except for 2 tablespoons of the bread flour in the machine's bread pan. (Do not heat the water or milk.) Turn the machine on to the "rise," "dough," "manual," or equivalent setting so that the machine will mix, knead, and let the dough rise once. Check the dough about 5 minutes after the machine has started. If the dough seems too sticky, add more of the remaining flour, a tablespoon at a time. When the dough is ready, remove it from the machine and proceed to shape, top, and bake it as directed in your recipe.

Oatmeal Pizza Dough

YIELD: ABOUT ¾ POUND DOUGH, ENOUGH FOR A 14-INCH THIN CRUST OR A 12-INCH THICK CRUST

1¼ cups plus 2 tablespoons bread flour

⅓ cup quick-cooking oats

1½ teaspoons Rapid Rise yeast

1 teaspoon sugar

¼ teaspoon salt

½ cup plus 2 tablespoons skim or low-fat milk or water

1. Place ¾ cup of the flour and all of the oats, yeast, sugar, and salt in a large bowl, and stir to mix well. Place the milk or water in a small saucepan, and heat until very warm (125°F to 130°F). Add the liquid to the flour mixture, and stir for 1 minute. Stir in enough of the remaining flour, 2 tablespoons at a time, to form a soft dough.

2. Sprinkle 2 tablespoons of the remaining flour over a flat surface, and turn the dough onto the surface. Knead the dough for 5 minutes, gradually adding just enough of the remaining flour to form a smooth, satiny ball. (Be careful not to make the dough too stiff, or it will be hard to roll out.)

3. Coat a large bowl with nonstick cooking spray, and place the ball of dough in the bowl. Cover the bowl with a clean kitchen towel, and let rise in a warm place for about 35 minutes, or until doubled in size.

4. When the dough has risen, punch it down, shape it into a ball, and turn it onto a lightly floured surface. The dough is now ready for shaping, topping, and baking.

Neapolitan Pizza

YIELD: 8 SLICES

1 can (14½ ounces) unsalted whole tomatoes, drained

1 teaspoon crushed fresh garlic

¼ teaspoon coarsely ground black pepper

1 recipe Oatmeal Pizza Dough (above) or Hearty Wheat Pizza Dough (page 140)

1 tablespoon plus 1½ teaspoons grated nonfat or regular Parmesan cheese

1 cup shredded reduced-fat mozzarella cheese

4 anchovy fillets, drained and coarsely chopped

1 tablespoon finely chopped fresh oregano, or 1 teaspoon dried

1. Place the drained tomatoes in a small bowl, and mash with a fork until coarsely crushed. Drain off any liquid that has accumulated, stir in the garlic and pepper, and set aside.

2. Turn the dough onto a lightly floured surface. Using a rolling pin, roll the dough into a 14-inch circle. (For a thick crust, roll the dough into a 12-inch circle.) Coat a 14-inch (or 12-inch) pizza pan with nonstick cooking spray. Place the dough on the pan, forming a slight rim around the edges. Set the crust aside for 5 to 10 minutes.

3. Spread the tomato mixture over the crust to within ½ inch of the edges. Sprinkle first the Parmesan and then the mozzarella over the tomatoes. Top with the anchovies, and sprinkle with the oregano.

4. Bake at 425°F for about 10 minutes, or until the cheese is melted and the crust is lightly browned. Slice and serve immediately.

NUTRITIONAL FACTS (PER SLICE)
Cal: 147   Carbs: 22.4 g   Chol: 5 mg   Fat: 2.7 g
Fiber: 1.5 g   Protein: 8.3 g   Sodium: 265 mg

Savory Sausage, Pepper, and Onion Pizza

YIELD: 8 SLICES

1 recipe Oatmeal Pizza Dough (page 141)
or Hearty Wheat Pizza Dough (page 140)

1 cup shredded reduced-fat mozzarella cheese

3/4 cup canned tomato purée or
Arrabbiata Sauce (page 233)

6 ounces Turkey Italian Sausage (page 251),
cooked, drained, and crumbled

8 thin rings green bell pepper

3–4 thin slices onion, separated into rings

1/2 teaspoon dried Italian seasoning

1. Turn the dough onto a lightly floured surface. Using a rolling pin, roll the dough into a 14-inch circle. (For a thick crust, roll the dough into a 12-inch circle.) Coat a 14-inch (or 12-inch) pizza pan with nonstick cooking spray. Place the dough on the pan, forming a slight rim around the edges. Set the crust aside for 5 to 10 minutes.

2. Spread the tomato purée or sauce over the crust to within 1/2 inch of the edges. Sprinkle the mozzarella over the sauce, and top with the sausage, green pepper, and onion. Sprinkle with the Italian seasoning.

3. Bake at 425°F for about 12 minutes, or until the cheese is melted and the crust is lightly browned. Slice and serve immediately.

NUTRITIONAL FACTS (PER SLICE)
Cal: 168   Carbs: 23.8 g   Chol: 13 mg   Fat: 3.5 g
Fiber: 2.1 g   Protein: 10.8 g   Sodium: 198 mg

Margherita Pizza

YIELD: 8 SLICES

1 can (14 1/2 ounces) unsalted
whole tomatoes, drained

1/2 teaspoon crushed fresh garlic

1 recipe Oatmeal Pizza Dough (page 141)
or Hearty Wheat Pizza Dough (page 140)

1/2 cup shredded reduced-fat mozzarella cheese

1/2 cup shredded reduced-fat provolone cheese

1 tablespoon chopped fresh basil, or 1 teaspoon dried

1. Place the drained tomatoes in a small bowl, and mash with a fork until coarsely crushed. Drain off any liquid that has accumulated, stir in the garlic, and set aside.

2. Turn the dough onto a lightly floured surface. Using a rolling pin, roll the dough into a 14-inch circle. (For a thick crust, roll the dough into a 12-inch circle.) Coat a 14-inch (or 12-inch) pizza pan with nonstick cooking spray. Place the dough on the pan, forming a slight rim around the edges. Set the crust aside for 5 to 10 minutes.

3. Spread the tomato mixture over the crust to within 1/2 inch of the edges. Sprinkle first the mozzarella and then the provolone over the tomatoes. Sprinkle with the basil.

4. Bake at 425°F for about 10 minutes, or until the cheese is melted and the crust is lightly browned. Slice and serve immediately.

NUTRITIONAL FACTS (PER SLICE)
Cal: 132   Carbs: 19.4 g   Chol: 5 mg   Fat: 2.7 g
Fiber: 1.2 g   Protein: 7.3 g   Sodium: 147 mg

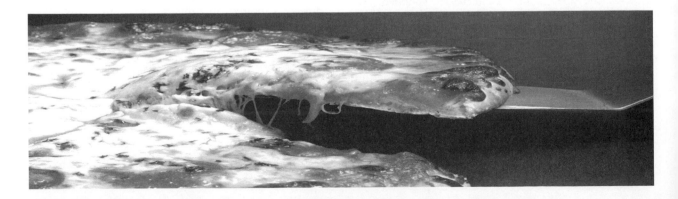

Pizza Crusts on the Run

Even when time is in short supply, you can enjoy the incomparable flavor and nutrition of a delicious homemade pizza. The pizza recipes in this chapter will give you some great ideas for toppings. And for the fastest and simplest of toppings, you can always purchase low-fat cheeses and ready-made sauces at your local supermarket. What about the crust? Following are some ideas for delicious ready-made crusts that you can purchase at your grocery store. Add just a little imagination, and you'll find that you can whip up a mouthwatering homemade pizza on any night of the week.

❏ For an excellent quick crust, use frozen bread dough. Simply thaw the dough—you'll need about 12 ounces—roll it out, add your favorite toppings,

and bake. Or try refrigerated pizza doughs and pizza dough mixes. All of these products are low in fat and easy to use.

❏ If you don't mind your pizzas being a bit unconventional, try one of a number of ready-made breads that, although not designed for pizza, make great crusts. For individual pizzas, try rounds of pita bread (choose oat bran or whole wheat), English muffin and bagel halves, or flour tortillas. For larger pizzas, horizontally slice a French or Italian bread.

❏ For the simplest quick-crust option of them all, use one of the prebaked foccacia breads or pizza shells that are now widely available. Be sure to read the labels, though, as calorie and fat counts can vary widely between brands.

Ground Beef and Onion Pizza

YIELD: 8 SLICES

8 ounces 95% lean ground beef
1 teaspoon crushed fresh garlic
¼ teaspoon ground black pepper
⅛ teaspoon salt
1 recipe Oatmeal Pizza Dough (page 141) or Hearty Wheat Pizza Dough (page 140)
¾ cup bottled marinara sauce or Arrabbiata Sauce (page 233)
1 cup shredded reduced-fat mozzarella cheese
1 medium yellow onion, cut into thin wedges and separated into pieces
½ teaspoon dried oregano

1. Coat a medium-sized nonstick skillet with nonstick cooking spray, and preheat over medium heat. Add the ground beef, garlic, pepper, and salt, and cook, stirring to crumble, until the meat is no longer pink. Drain off and discard any fat, and set aside.

2. Turn the dough onto a lightly floured surface. Using a rolling pin, roll the dough into a 14-inch circle. (For a thick crust, roll the dough into a 12-inch circle). Coat a 14-inch (or 12-inch) pizza pan with nonstick cooking spray. Place the dough on the pan, forming a slight rim around the edges. Set the crust aside for 5 to 10 minutes.

3. Spread the sauce over the crust to within ½ inch of the edges. Top with the ground beef mixture, followed by the mozzarella and onions. Sprinkle with the oregano.

4. Bake at 425°F for about 12 minutes, or until the cheese is melted and the crust is lightly browned. Slice and serve immediately.

NUTRITIONAL FACTS (PER SLICE)
Cal: 173   Carbs: 22.6 g   Chol: 20 mg   Fat: 3.7 g
Fiber: 2 g   Protein: 12 g   Sodium: 218 mg

Roasted Red Pepper Pizza

YIELD: 8 SLICES

1 recipe Oatmeal Pizza Dough (page 141)
or Hearty Wheat Pizza Dough (page 140)

1/2 cup bottled marinara sauce,
Chunky Garden Marinara Sauce (page 235),
or Arrabbiata Sauce (page 233)

2 tablespoons grated nonfat or regular
Parmesan cheese

2 medium commercial roasted red peppers,
cut into thin strips

1 cup shredded reduced-fat mozzarella cheese

1 small yellow onion, quartered and thinly sliced

1/4 cup sliced black olives (optional)

1/2 teaspoon dried basil

1/2 teaspoon dried oregano

1. Turn the dough onto a lightly floured surface. Using a rolling pin, roll the dough into a 14-inch circle. (For a thick crust, roll the dough into a 12-inch circle.) Coat a 14-inch (or 12-inch) pizza pan with nonstick cooking spray. Place the dough on the pan, forming a slight rim around the edges. Set the crust aside for 5 to 10 minutes.

2. Spread the sauce over the crust to within 1/2 inch of the edges. Sprinkle with the Parmesan, and arrange the roasted pepper strips in concentric circles over the sauce and cheese. Top first with the mozzarella, and then with the onions and, if desired, the olives. Sprinkle with the basil and oregano.

3. Bake at 425°F for about 12 minutes, or until the cheese is melted and the crust is lightly browned. Slice and serve immediately.

NUTRITIONAL FACTS (PER SLICE)
Cal: 141   Carbs: 22.6 g   Chol: 5 mg   Fat: 2.6 g
Fiber: 2 g   Protein: 7 g   Sodium: 238 mg

Artichoke and Sun-Dried Tomato Pizza

YIELD: 8 SLICES

1/4 cup plus 2 tablespoons diced sun-dried tomatoes
(not packed in oil)

1/4 cup plus 2 tablespoons water

1 package (9 ounces) frozen (thawed)
artichoke hearts, or 1 can (14 ounces)
artichoke hearts, drained

1 recipe Oatmeal Pizza Dough (page 141) or
Hearty Wheat Pizza Dough (page 140)

1/2 cup shredded reduced-fat mozzarella cheese

1/2 cup shredded reduced-fat provolone cheese

1 teaspoon dried Italian seasoning

1. Place the sun-dried tomatoes and the water in a small saucepan, and bring to a boil over high heat. Reduce the heat to low, cover, and simmer for 2 minutes, or just until the tomatoes have plumped. Remove the pot from the heat, drain off any excess water, and set aside.

2. Coarsely chop the artichoke hearts, and set aside.

3. Turn the dough onto a lightly floured surface. Using a rolling pin, roll the dough into a 14-inch circle. (For a thick crust, roll the dough into a 12-inch circle.) Coat a 14-inch (or 12-inch) pizza pan with nonstick cooking spray. Place the dough on the pan, forming a slight rim around the edges. Set the crust aside for 5 to 10 minutes.

4. Sprinkle first the mozzarella and then the provolone over the crust to within 1/2 inch of the edges. Top with the artichoke hearts and tomatoes, and sprinkle with the Italian seasoning.

5. Bake at 425°F for about 12 minutes, or until the cheese is melted and the crust is lightly browned. Slice and serve immediately.

NUTRITIONAL FACTS (PER SLICE)
Cal: 156   Carbs: 24 g   Chol: 5 mg   Fat: 2.9 g
Fiber: 3 g   Protein: 8.3 g   Sodium: 215 mg

Fresh Tomato and Herb Pizza

YIELD: 8 SLICES

1¼ cups chopped plum tomatoes (about 4 medium)

1 teaspoon crushed fresh garlic

¼ teaspoon ground black pepper

1 recipe Oatmeal Pizza Dough (page 141) or Hearty Wheat Pizza Dough (page 140)

2 tablespoons grated nonfat or regular Parmesan cheese

1 cup shredded reduced-fat mozzarella cheese

1½ teaspoons finely chopped fresh basil, or ½ teaspoon dried

1½ teaspoons finely chopped fresh oregano, or ½ teaspoon dried

1½ teaspoons finely chopped fresh rosemary, or ½ teaspoon dried

1. Place the tomatoes, garlic, and pepper in a medium-sized bowl, and stir to mix well. Set aside.

2. Turn the dough onto a lightly floured surface. Using a rolling pin, roll the dough into a 14-inch circle. (For a thick crust, roll the dough into a 12-inch circle.) Coat a 14-inch (or 12-inch) pizza pan with nonstick cooking spray. Place the dough on the pan, forming a slight rim around the edges. Set the crust aside for 5 to 10 minutes.

3. Spread the tomato mixture over the crust, extending it to within ½ inch of the edges. Sprinkle first the Parmesan and then the mozzarella over the tomatoes. Sprinkle with the herbs.

4. Bake at 425°F for about 12 minutes, or until the cheese is melted and the crust is lightly browned. Slice and serve immediately.

NUTRITIONAL FACTS (PER SLICE)
Cal: 143   Carbs: 21.5 g   Chol: 5 mg   Fat: 2.6 g
Fiber: 1.4 g   Protein: 8.3 g   Sodium: 198 mg

Pesto Pizza

YIELD: 8 SLICES

1 recipe Oatmeal Pizza Dough (page 141) or Hearty Wheat Pizza Dough (page 140)

2–3 medium plum tomatoes, thinly sliced

1 cup shredded reduced-fat mozzarella cheese

PESTO

½ cup (packed) chopped fresh spinach

¼ cup (packed) chopped fresh basil

¼ cup grated Parmesan cheese*

2 teaspoons crushed fresh garlic

* In this recipe, use regular Parmesan cheese, not a fat-free product.

1. To make the pesto, place all of the pesto ingredients in a blender or food processor, and process until the mixture is finely ground. Set aside.

2. Turn the dough onto a lightly floured surface. Using a rolling pin, roll the dough into a 14-inch circle. (For a thick crust, roll the dough into a 12-inch circle.) Coat a 14-inch (or 12-inch) pizza pan with nonstick cooking spray. Place the dough on the pan, forming a slight rim around the edges. Set the crust aside for 5 to 10 minutes.

3. Sprinkle the pesto over the crust, extending it to within ½ inch of the edges. Arrange the tomatoes over the pesto, and top with the mozzarella.

4. Bake at 425°F for about 12 minutes, or until the cheese is melted and the crust is lightly browned. Slice and serve immediately.

NUTRITIONAL FACTS (PER SLICE)
Cal: 144   Carbs: 19 g   Chol: 9 mg   Fat: 3.3 g
Fiber: 1.3 g   Protein: 9 g   Sodium: 225 mg

Spinach and Mushroom Calzones

YIELD: 4 CALZONES

1 recipe Oatmeal Pizza Dough (page 141)
or Hearty Wheat Pizza Dough (page 140)

3 tablespoons beaten egg white
or fat-free egg substitute

1 1/3 cups bottled marinara sauce or Chunky Garden
Marinara Sauce (page 235)

FILLING

1 teaspoon crushed fresh garlic

1 1/2 cups sliced fresh mushrooms

5 cups (packed) coarsely chopped fresh
spinach leaves (about 5 ounces)

1/4 teaspoon dried thyme

1/4 teaspoon coarsely ground black pepper

2 tablespoons grated nonfat
or regular Parmesan cheese

3/4 cup shredded reduced-fat mozzarella cheese

1. To make the filling, coat a large nonstick skillet with olive oil cooking spray, and preheat over medium-high heat. Add the garlic and mushrooms, and stir-fry for about 3 minutes, or until the mushrooms are tender and most of the liquid has evaporated. Add the spinach, thyme, and pepper, and stir-fry for 2 additional minutes, or until the spinach is wilted and any excess liquid has evaporated. Remove the skillet from the heat, and stir in the Parmesan. Set aside.

2. Divide the dough into 4 portions, and shape each portion into a ball. Working on a lightly floured surface, use a rolling pin to roll each ball into a 7-inch circle.

3. Spread a quarter of the spinach mixture over half of each crust to within 1/2 inch of the edges, and top with 3 tablespoons of mozzarella. Moisten the edges of the dough with water, and fold the circle in half to enclose the filling. Seal the edges by pressing with the tines of a fork.

4. Coat a baking sheet with nonstick cooking spray, and transfer the calzones to the sheet. Brush the tops lightly with the beaten egg white or egg substitute,

and prick the tops in a couple of places with a fork. Bake at 450°F for about 10 minutes, or until the crust is lightly browned.

5. While the calzones are baking, place the sauce in a small saucepan, and cook over medium heat until warmed through. Serve the calzones hot with a side dish of the warm dipping sauce.

NUTRITIONAL FACTS (PER CALZONE)
Cal: 306   Carbs: 50 g   Chol: 8 mg   Fat: 4.2 g
Fiber: 5.2 g   Protein: 17 g   Sodium: 288 mg

Ham and Mushroom Pizza

YIELD: 8 SLICES

1 recipe Hearty Wheat Pizza Dough (page 140)
or Oatmeal Pizza Dough (page 141)

3/4 cup Arrabbiata Sauce (page 233)
or bottled marinara sauce

1 cup shredded reduced-fat mozzarella cheese

3 ounces ham, at least 97% lean, thinly sliced
and cut into thin strips

3/4 cup thinly sliced fresh mushrooms

1/2 teaspoon dried Italian seasoning

1. Turn the dough onto a lightly floured surface. Using a rolling pin, roll the dough into a 14-inch circle. (For a thick crust, roll the dough into a 12-inch circle.) Coat a 14-inch (or 12-inch) pizza pan with nonstick cooking spray. Place the dough on the pan, forming a slight rim around the edges. Set the crust aside for 5 to 10 minutes.

2. Spread the sauce over the crust to within 1/2 inch of the edges. Sprinkle the mozzarella over the sauce. Arrange the ham strips in concentric circles over the sauce. Top with the mushrooms, and sprinkle with the Italian seasoning.

3. Bake at 425°F for about 12 minutes, or until the cheese is melted and the crust is lightly browned. Slice and serve immediately.

NUTRITIONAL FACTS (PER SLICE)
Cal: 149   Carbs: 21.5 g   Chol: 7 mg   Fat: 3 g
Fiber: 0.9 g   Protein: 9 g   Sodium: 248 mg

Greek Pizza

YIELD: 8 SLICES

1 recipe Oatmeal Pizza Dough (page 141)
or Hearty Wheat Pizza Dough (page 140)

1 cup finely chopped tomatoes (about 3 medium)

3/4 cup shredded reduced-fat mozzarella cheese

1/2 cup crumbled nonfat or reduced-fat feta cheese

1 tablespoon finely chopped fresh oregano,
or 1 teaspoon dried

3–4 slices red onion, separated into rings

1/4 cup sliced black olives

1. Turn the dough onto a lightly floured surface. Using a rolling pin, roll the dough into a 14-inch circle. (For a thick crust, roll the dough into a 12-inch circle.) Coat a 14-inch (or 12-inch) pizza pan with nonstick cooking spray. Place the dough on the pan, forming a slight rim around the edges. Set the crust aside for 5 to 10 minutes.

2. Spread the tomatoes over the crust to within 1/2 inch of the edges. Sprinkle first the mozzarella and then the feta over the tomatoes. Sprinkle with the oregano. Then spread the onion rings over the pizza, and top with the olives.

3. Bake at 425°F for about 12 minutes, or until the cheese is melted and the crust is lightly browned. Slice and serve immediately.

NUTRITIONAL FACTS (PER SLICE)
Cal: 137　Carbs: 19 g　Chol: 4 mg　Fat: 2.6 g
Fiber: 1.7 g　Protein: 9.5 g　Sodium: 333 mg

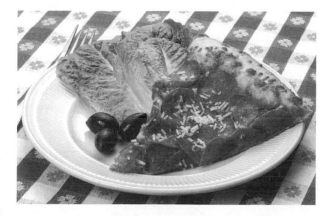

Ham and Cheese Calzones

YIELD: 4 CALZONES

1 recipe Oatmeal Pizza Dough (page 141)
or Hearty Wheat Pizza Dough (page 140)

3 tablespoons beaten egg white
or fat-free egg substitute

FILLING
3 ounces finely chopped ham (about 2/3 cup),
at least 97% lean

2/3 cup nonfat or reduced-fat ricotta cheese

2/3 cup shredded reduced-fat mozzarella cheese

1/2 teaspoon dried Italian seasoning

1. To make the filling, place all of the filling ingredients in a medium-sized bowl, and stir to mix well. Set aside.

2. Divide the dough into 4 portions, and shape each portion into a ball. Working on a lightly floured surface, use a rolling pin to roll each ball into a 7-inch circle.

3. Spread a quarter of the ham mixture over half of each crust to within 1/2 inch of the edges. Moisten the edges of the dough with water, and fold the circle in half to enclose the filling. Seal the edges by pressing with the tines of a fork.

4. Coat a baking sheet with nonstick cooking spray, and transfer the calzones to the sheet. Brush the tops lightly with the beaten egg white or egg substitute, and prick the tops in a couple of places with a fork. Bake at 450°F for about 10 minutes, or until the crust is lightly browned. Serve hot.

NUTRITIONAL FACTS (PER CALZONE)
Cal: 277　Carbs: 41 g　Chol: 17 mg　Fat: 3.9 g
Fiber: 2.6 g　Protein: 19 g　Sodium: 465 mg

6. Soups and Stews That Satisfy

There's nothing quite as warming and comforting as a steaming bowl of homemade soup or a thick and hearty stew. And soups and stews are naturals for healthy low-fat cooking. Lean meats and poultry, seafood, whole grains, pasta, beans, and vegetables can be combined to produce a variety of culinary creations that are filling but not fattening.

Watching your weight? Soups can be especially helpful. Soups take longer to eat than most foods, so that less food and fewer calories are consumed in the twenty-minute period it takes for the brain to realize that the stomach is full. This helps prevent overeating.

Because soups and stews are perhaps the most versatile of foods, they are as much a boon to the menu planner as they are to the calorie counter. A light soup is the perfect introduction to a full meal. A more substantial soup or a hearty stew needs only crusty whole grain bread and a salad to make a satisfying lunch or light supper.

Of course, homemade soups and stews have more than one advantage over store-bought versions. Made from fresh, wholesome ingredients, your soups and stews are bursting with nutrients and garden-fresh flavor. Just as important, while many commercially prepared products are loaded with fat and salt, your creations can easily be made with far less of both. Will your slimmed-down soups taste flat? Absolutely not! Herbs like oregano, thyme, marjoram, and bay leaf; lots of celery and onion; a clove or two of garlic; a splash of wine vinegar or sherry; and plenty of other flavorful ingredients will make your soups so savory, no will ever miss the extra salt or fat.

This chapter presents a variety of delectable soups and stews that minimize fat and salt while maximizing flavor and nutrition. Whether you are looking for a golden broth floating with chunks of chicken and tender noodles, a colorful minestrone brimming with fresh vegetables, or an old-fashioned beef stew, there's a dish that will meet your needs deliciously. So take out your kettle, and get ready to make soups and stews a healthful part of your menus.

Mama Mia Minestrone

YIELD: 10 SERVINGS

1 tablespoon extra virgin olive oil

2 teaspoons crushed fresh garlic

1 medium Spanish onion, chopped

1/2 cup thinly sliced celery (include the leaves)

4 cups unsalted beef broth or water

1 can (14 1/2 ounces) tomatoes, crushed

2 medium carrots, peeled, halved lengthwise,
and sliced 1/4-inch thick

2 cups coarsely shredded cabbage

2 1/2 teaspoons dried Italian seasoning

1 tablespoon instant beef bouillon granules

1/4 teaspoon ground black pepper

2 medium zucchini, quartered lengthwise and
sliced 1/4-inch thick

4 ounces elbow macaroni (about 7/8 cup)

1 can (1 pound) cannellini or navy beans, drained

3 tablespoons finely chopped fresh parsley

1/3 cup grated nonfat or regular
Parmesan cheese (garnish)

1. Place the olive oil in a 4-quart pot, and preheat over medium-high heat. Add the garlic, onion, and celery, and stir-fry for about 3 minutes, or until the vegetables are crisp-tender.

2. Add the broth or water, undrained tomatoes, carrots, cabbage, Italian seasoning, bouillon granules, and pepper to the pot, and bring to a boil. Stir the mixture, reduce the heat to low, cover, and simmer for 12 minutes, or until the vegetables are barely tender.

3. Add the zucchini, macaroni, and beans to the pot, and bring to a boil over high heat. Reduce the heat to low, cover, and simmer for about 8 minutes, or until the macaroni is al dente. (Be careful not to overcook, as the pasta will continue to soften in the hot soup.)

4. Remove the pot from the heat, and stir in the parsley. Ladle the soup into individual serving bowls, and serve hot, topping each serving with a rounded teaspoon of the Parmesan cheese.

NUTRITIONAL FACTS (PER 1-CUP SERVING)
Cal: 117   Carbs: 18 g   Chol: 2 mg   Fat: 1.9 g
Fiber: 4.4 g   Protein: 6.2 g   Sodium: 403 mg

Turkey Gumbo Soup

YIELD: 9 CUPS

4 cups unsalted chicken broth

1 medium yellow onion, chopped

1 medium green bell pepper, chopped

2 stalks celery, thinly sliced (include leaves)

1 can (14 1/2 ounces) stewed tomatoes, crushed

1 cup diced smoked sausage or kielbasa,
at least 97% lean (about 5 ounces)

2 bay leaves

1 1/2 teaspoons Cajun seasoning

1/2 teaspoon dried thyme

2 cups diced cooked turkey or chicken breast
(about 10 ounces)

2 cups fresh or frozen (unthawed) cut okra

1 cup quick-cooking brown rice

1. Place the broth, onion, green pepper, celery, tomatoes, sausage, bay leaves, Cajun seasoning, and thyme in a 3-quart pot, and bring to a boil over high heat. Stir the mixture, reduce the heat to low, cover, and simmer for 20 minutes, or until the vegetables are tender.

2. Add the turkey or chicken, okra, and rice to the pot, and bring to a boil over high heat. Reduce the heat to low, cover, and simmer for about 10 minutes, or until the rice and okra are tender.

3. Remove the bay leaves from the soup, and discard. Ladle the soup into individual serving bowls, and serve hot.

NUTRITIONAL FACTS (PER 1-CUP SERVING)
Cal: 142   Carbs: 18 g   Chol: 34 mg   Fat: 1.3 g
Fiber: 2.9 g   Protein: 14.4 g   Sodium: 348 mg

Flavorful Fat-Free
Soup Stocks

Whether you're making Chunky Chicken Noodle Soup or following your own treasured recipe, a rich-tasting, well-seasoned stock is sure to result in a more flavorful dish. And while many low- and no-fat stocks are now commercially available, the flavor of canned or made-from-mix brews simply can't compare with that of your own homemade stocks. Just as important, by preparing your stock from scratch, you can in-sure that your product is low in both fat and salt.

The following stocks can be used in any soup recipe that calls for unsalted beef, chicken, turkey, or vegetable stock or broth. These stocks are also a great way to enhance flavor when making rice or other grains, or when cooking vegetables. In fact, you can use these broths freely, as they are fat- and sodium-free, and con-tain only about 15 calories per cup!

Savory Chicken or Turkey Stock

YIELD: ABOUT 2½ QUARTS

3 roast-chicken carcasses, 1 roast-turkey carcass, or 3 pounds chicken or turkey backs and wings

3 medium onions, quartered

2 medium carrots, peeled and sliced

2 medium stalks celery, sliced (include the leaves)

4 cloves garlic, chopped

2 bay leaves

1 teaspoon dried crushed thyme or savory

¼ teaspoon ground black pepper, or 6 whole peppercorns

4 quarts water

1. Break up the chicken or turkey carcass, and place in a 6-quart stock pot. (If using backs and wings, rinse them with cool water and place them in the pot as is.) Add any defatted drippings left over from roasting the turkey or chicken. Add the vegetables, seasonings, and just enough of the water to cover the mixture by one inch.

2. Bring the mixture to a boil over high heat. Reduce the heat to low, and simmer uncovered for 5 minutes. Remove any froth that forms on the surface of the stock.

3. Cover the pot, leaving the lid slightly ajar to allow steam to escape. Simmer the mixture slowly for at least 2 hours, and for up to 5 hours. The longer you simmer the stock, the more it will con-dense and intensify its flavors.

4. Cool the stock to room temperature, and pour it through a strainer lined with cheesecloth. Trans-fer the stock to a covered pot or other container, and refrigerate overnight.

5. The next day, remove and discard any fat that has risen to the surface of the stock. Use the stock immediately, or pour it into freezer containers and freeze for up to 6 months. (Note that when freez-ing stock, you should always leave a little room in the container for expansion.)

Hearty Beef Stock

YIELD: ABOUT 2½ QUARTS

4 pounds beef bones

Nonstick cooking spray

3 medium yellow onions, quartered,
or 2 leeks, washed, trimmed, and coarsely chopped

3 medium stalks celery, coarsely chopped
(include the leaves)

6 cloves garlic, chopped

4 sprigs fresh parsley

1 teaspoon dried thyme

1 teaspoon dried marjoram

2 bay leaves

¼ teaspoon ground black pepper

4 quarts water

1. Coat a shallow roasting pan with nonstick cooking spray, and arrange the bones in a single layer in the pan. Spray the tops lightly with cooking spray, and roast at 425°F for 45 minutes to 1 hour, or until the bones are browned, turning them after 25 minutes.

2. Place the bones in a 6-quart stock pot, and add the vegetables and seasonings. Pour ½ cup of the water into the roasting pan, and scrape up any crusty browned bits from the bottom of the pan. Add this mixture to the stock pot. Then add just enough of the water to cover the mixture by 1 inch.

3. Bring the mixture to a boil over high heat. Reduce the heat to low, and simmer uncovered for 5 minutes. Remove any froth that forms on the surface of the stock.

4. Cover the pot, leaving the lid slightly ajar to allow steam to escape. Simmer the mixture slowly for at least 2 hours, and for up to 5 hours. The longer you simmer the stock, the more it will condense and intensify its flavors.

5. Cool the stock to room temperature, and pour it through a strainer lined with cheesecloth. Transfer the stock to a covered pot or other container, and refrigerate overnight.

6. The next day, remove and discard any fat that has risen to the surface of the stock. Use the stock immediately, or pour it into freezer containers and freeze for up to 6 months. (Note that when freezing stock, you should always leave a little room in the container for expansion.)

Mama's Meatball Soup

YIELD: 9 SERVINGS

6 cups unsalted beef broth or water

1 medium yellow onion, chopped

1 tablespoon instant beef bouillon granules

1 teaspoon dried Italian seasoning

¼ teaspoon ground black pepper

2 medium carrots, peeled, halved lengthwise,
and sliced, divided

2 medium stalks celery, sliced, divided

1 can (14½ ounces) unsalted tomatoes, crushed

1 cup fresh or frozen (unthawed) cut green beans

4 ounces ziti pasta (about 1½ cups)

MEATBALLS

12 ounces 95% lean ground beef

¼ cup grated nonfat or regular Parmesan cheese

1 egg white

1 teaspoon dried Italian seasoning

¼ teaspoon ground black pepper

1. To make the meatballs, place all of the meatball ingredients in a medium-sized bowl, and mix well. Shape the mixture into ¾-inch balls. Coat a baking sheet with nonstick cooking spray, and arrange the meatballs on the pan. Bake at 350°F for about 18 minutes, or until the meatballs are no longer pink inside. Set aside.

Garden Vegetable Stock

Don't hesitate to vary this stock to make use of any leftover vegetables you have on hand. Simply save up the vegetable peelings (of organic produce only); bits of herbs; and leftover bits of onion, celery, carrots, potatoes, mushrooms, parsnips, turnips, rutabagas, and other vegetables. Toss all of these items into a freezer container until you're ready to make the stock. Avoid using any strong-flavored vegetables like cabbage; collard, mustard, and other greens; broccoli; and peppers, as they can overwhelm the flavors of the other ingredients.

YIELD: ABOUT 2½ QUARTS

3 medium yellow onions, thinly sliced

3 medium stalks celery, thinly sliced (include the leaves)

3 medium carrots, peeled, halved lengthwise, and thinly sliced

3 medium tomatoes, chopped

1½ cups thinly sliced fresh mushrooms

4 sprigs fresh parsley

4 cloves garlic, chopped

1 teaspoon dried marjoram

1 teaspoon dried thyme

1 bay leaf

¼ teaspoon ground white pepper

3 quarts water

1. Place all of the ingredients except for the water in a 6-quart stock pot. Add just enough of the water to start the vegetables cooking (about 1 cup). Bring the mixture to a boil over high heat. Reduce the heat to medium, cover, and cook for about 15 minutes, or until the vegetables are wilted and tender.

2. Add the remaining water to the pot, and bring the mixture to a boil over high heat. Reduce the heat to low and cover, leaving the lid slightly ajar to allow steam to escape. Simmer the mixture slowly for at least 1 hour, and for up to 2 hours. The longer you simmer the stock, the more it will condense and intensify its flavors.

3. Cool the stock to room temperature and pour it through a strainer lined with cheesecloth, pressing as much liquid as possible from the vegetables before discarding them. Use the stock immediately, or pour it into freezer containers and freeze for up to 6 months. (Note that when freezing stock, you should always leave a little room in the container for expansion.)

2. Place the broth or water, onion, bouillon granules, Italian seasoning, and pepper in a 4-quart pot. Add half of the carrots and half of the celery, and bring to a boil over high heat. Reduce the heat to low, cover, and simmer for 20 minutes, or until the vegetables are tender.

3. Using a slotted spoon, transfer the vegetables to a blender. Add 1½ cups of the hot broth, and place the lid on the blender, leaving the top slightly ajar to allow steam to escape. Carefully blend at low speed until the mixture is smooth. Return the puréed mixture to the pot, and stir to mix well.

4. Add the remaining carrots and celery to the pot, along with the undrained tomatoes, and bring to a boil over high heat. Reduce the heat to low, cover, and simmer for 10 minutes, or until the vegetables are barely tender.

5. Add the meatballs, green beans, and pasta to the pot, and bring to a boil over high heat. Reduce the heat to medium-low, cover, and simmer for about 8 minutes, or until the pasta is al dente. (Be careful not to overcook, as the pasta will continue to soften in the hot soup.)

6. Ladle the soup into individual serving bowls, and serve hot.

NUTRITIONAL FACTS (PER 1-CUP SERVING)
Cal: 142   Carbs: 15.8 g   Chol: 25 mg   Fat: 2.1 g
Fiber: 2.4 g   Protein: 15 g   Sodium: 356 mg

Savory Italian Sausage Soup

YIELD: 11 SERVINGS

12 ounces Turkey Italian Sausage (page 251)

1 can (14$\frac{1}{2}$ ounces) unsalted
stewed tomatoes, crushed

1 can (1 pound) chickpeas, drained

6 cups unsalted chicken broth or water

1 medium onion, chopped

1 cup sliced fresh mushrooms

1 large carrot, peeled, halved lengthwise, and sliced

1 tablespoon instant chicken bouillon granules

1 teaspoon dried oregano

$\frac{1}{4}$ teaspoon ground black pepper

1 teaspoon crushed fresh garlic

1$\frac{1}{2}$ medium zucchini, halved lengthwise and sliced

6 ounces rotini pasta (about 2$\frac{1}{4}$ cups)

$\frac{1}{3}$ cup grated nonfat or regular
Parmesan cheese (garnish)

1. Coat a 4-quart pot with nonstick cooking spray, and preheat over medium heat. Add the sausage, and cook, stirring to crumble, until the meat is no longer pink. Drain off and discard any excess fat.

2. Add all of the remaining ingredients except for the zucchini, pasta, and cheese to the pot, and bring to a boil over high heat. Reduce the heat to low, cover, and simmer for 20 minutes, or until the vegetables are tender.

3. Add the zucchini and pasta to the pot, and bring to a boil. Reduce the heat to low, cover, and simmer for 10 minutes, or until the pasta is al dente. (Be careful not to overcook, as the pasta will continue to soften in the hot soup.)

4. Ladle the soup into individual serving bowls, and serve hot, topping each serving with a rounded teaspoon of the Parmesan cheese.

NUTRITIONAL FACTS (PER 1-CUP SERVING)
Cal: 160   Carbs: 22 g   Chol: 21 mg   Fat: 2.2 g
Fiber: 3 g   Protein: 13 g   Sodium: 416 mg

Golden Turkey Noodle Soup

YIELD: 8 SERVINGS

6$\frac{1}{2}$ cups unsalted chicken broth

1$\frac{1}{2}$ cups diced peeled sweet potatoes
(about 1$\frac{1}{2}$ medium)

1 medium onion, chopped

1 tablespoon instant chicken bouillon granules

$\frac{1}{8}$ teaspoon ground white pepper

1 medium carrot, peeled and diced

1 stalk celery, thinly sliced (include the leaves)

4 ounces medium no-yolk noodles

2 cups diced cooked turkey breast
or chicken breast

1. Place the broth, sweet potatoes, onion, bouillon granules, and pepper in a 3-quart pot, and bring to a boil over high heat. Reduce the heat to low, cover, and simmer for 15 minutes, or until the potatoes are tender.

2. Remove the pot from the heat. Using a slotted spoon, transfer the sweet potatoes to a blender. Add 1$\frac{1}{2}$ cups of the hot broth to the blender, and place the lid on the blender, leaving the top slightly ajar to allow steam to escape. Carefully blend the mixture at low speed until smooth.

3. Return the blended mixture to the pot, and place over high heat. Add the carrot and celery, and bring the mixture to a boil. Reduce the heat to low, cover, and simmer for 6 to 8 minutes, or until the vegetables are barely tender.

4. Add the noodles and the turkey or chicken to the pot, cover, and simmer, stirring occasionally, for about 8 minutes, or just until the noodles are al dente. (Be careful not to overcook, as the pasta will continue to soften in the hot soup.)

5. Ladle the soup into individual serving bowls, and serve hot.

NUTRITIONAL FACTS (PER 1-CUP SERVING)
Cal: 151   Carbs: 23 g   Chol: 30 mg   Fat: 0.9 g
Fiber: 1.7 g   Protein: 13 g   Sodium: 362 mg

Savory Vegetable-Beef Soup

YIELD: 11 CUPS

1¼ pounds beef top round or lean stew meat,
cut into ½-inch pieces

4 cups unsalted beef broth or water

3 cups canned vegetable juice,
like V-8 vegetable juice

1 tablespoon instant beef bouillon granules

1½ teaspoons dried oregano

1 teaspoon chili powder

2 bay leaves

¼ teaspoon ground black pepper

1½ cups diced unpeeled potatoes
(about 1½ medium)

1½ cups sliced carrots

1 medium-large yellow onion,
cut into thin wedges

1½ cups fresh cut green beans

1½ cups fresh or frozen (unthawed)
whole kernel corn

1. Trim any visible fat from the meat. Rinse the meat with cool water, and pat it dry with paper towels.

2. Coat a 4-quart nonstick pot with nonstick cooking spray, and preheat over medium-high heat. Add half of the beef at a time to the skillet, and stir-fry for about 4 minutes, or until nicely browned.

3. Add the broth or water, vegetable juice, bouillon granules, oregano, chili powder, bay leaves, and pepper to the pot, and bring the mixture to a boil. Reduce the heat to low, cover, and simmer, stirring occasionally, for 30 minutes.

4. Add the potatoes, carrots, onion, and green beans to the pot, and increase the heat slightly to return the mixture to a boil. Reduce the heat to low, cover, and simmer, stirring occasionally, for 20 additional minutes, or until the meat and vegetables are tender.

5. Add the corn to the pot, and increase the heat slightly to return the mixture to a boil. Reduce the heat to low, cover, and simmer for 10 minutes, or until the vegetables are tender.

6. Remove the bay leaves from the soup, and discard. Ladle the soup into individual serving bowls, and serve hot.

NUTRITIONAL FACTS (PER 1-CUP SERVING)
Cal: 128   Carbs: 14 g   Chol: 32 mg   Fat: 2.1 g
Fiber: 2.8 g   Protein: 14 g   Sodium: 389 mg

Beef and Barley Soup

YIELD: 6 SERVINGS

8 ounces coarsely ground top beef round
or 95% lean ground beef

3 cups water

1 can (10½ ounces) condensed beef broth

2 cups sliced fresh mushrooms

1 medium yellow onion, chopped

⅔ cup thinly sliced celery

1 bay leaf

½ teaspoon crushed dried thyme or marjoram

¼ teaspoon coarsely ground black pepper

¾ cup quick-cooking barley

1. Coat a 2½-quart pot with nonstick cooking spray, and preheat over medium heat. Add the ground meat, and cook, stirring to crumble, until the meat is no longer pink. Drain off and discard any excess fat.

2. Add all of the remaining ingredients except for the barley to the pot, and bring to boil over high heat. Reduce the heat to low, cover, and simmer for 20 minutes, or until the vegetables are tender.

3. Add the barley, and bring to boil over high heat. Reduce heat to low, cover, and simmer for 10 minutes, or until the barley is tender.

4. Remove the bay leaf from the soup, and discard. Ladle the soup into individual serving bowls, and serve hot.

NUTRITIONAL FACTS (PER 1-CUP SERVING)
Cal: 140   Carbs: 17 g   Chol: 26 mg   Fat: 2.4 g
Fiber: 2.7 g   Protein: 13 g   Sodium: 440 mg

Golden Chicken and Dumpling Soup

5 cups unsalted chicken broth or water

1 tablespoon plus 1 teaspoon instant chicken bouillon granules

1¾ cups diced peeled sweet potatoes (about 2 medium)

1 medium onion, chopped

⅛ teaspoon ground white pepper

2 medium carrots, peeled, halved lengthwise, and sliced

1 stalk celery, thinly sliced (include the leaves)

2 cups diced cooked chicken breast

DUMPLINGS

1¼ cups unbleached flour

1½ teaspoons baking powder

¾ cup nonfat or low-fat buttermilk

1. Place the broth or water, bouillon granules, sweet potatoes, onion, and pepper in a 3-quart pot, and bring to a boil over high heat. Reduce the heat to low, cover, and simmer for 15 minutes, or until the potatoes are tender.

2. Remove the pot from the heat. Using a slotted spoon, transfer the sweet potatoes and onion to a blender. Add 1½ cups of the hot broth, and place the lid on the blender, leaving the top slightly ajar to allow steam to escape. Carefully blend the mixture at low speed until smooth.

3. Return the blended mixture to the pot, and place over high heat. Add the carrots and celery, and bring the mixture to a boil. Reduce the heat to low, cover, and simmer for 6 to 8 minutes, or until the vegetables are barely tender. Stir in the chicken.

4. To make the dumplings, place the flour and baking powder in a medium-sized bowl, and stir to mix well. Add enough of the buttermilk to form a moderately thick batter, stirring just until the dry ingredients are moistened.

5. Drop rounded teaspoons of batter onto the simmering soup. Cover and simmer for 12 minutes, or until the dumplings are fluffy.

6. Ladle the soup into individual serving bowls, and serve hot.

> **NUTRITIONAL FACTS (PER 1-CUP SERVING)**
> Cal: 165   Carbs: 24 g   Chol: 27 mg   Fat: 1.4 g
> Fiber: 2.2 g   Protein: 13 g   Sodium: 424 mg

Golden Matzo Ball Soup

5 cups unsalted vegetable or chicken broth

1¼ cups diced peeled sweet potato or butternut squash

1 medium yellow onion, chopped

1 stalk celery, thinly sliced

1 tablespoon instant vegetable or chicken bouillon granules

1 recipe Fluffy Fat-Free Matzo Balls (page 157)

1. Place the broth, sweet potato or squash, onion, celery, and bouillon granules in a 2½-quart pot, and bring to a boil over high heat. Reduce the heat to low, cover, and simmer for about 30 minutes, or until the vegetables are very tender.

2. Using a slotted spoon, transfer the vegetables to a blender. Add 1 cup of the hot broth, and place the lid on the blender, leaving the top slightly ajar to allow steam to escape. Carefully blend at low speed until smooth. Return the puréed mixture to the pot, and stir to mix well.

3. Add the matzo balls to the soup, and simmer, covered, for 10 minutes. Ladle the soup into individual serving bowls, placing 2 matzo balls in each bowl, and serve hot.

> **NUTRITIONAL FACTS (PER ¾ CUP BROTH AND 2 MATZO BALLS)**
> Cal: 81   Carbs: 15 g   Chol: 0 mg   Fat: 0.4 g
> Fiber: 1.2 g   Protein: 4.4 g   Sodium: 424 mg

Making Fat-Free Matzo Balls

An essential part of a traditional Passover dinner, matzo balls are a great way to add substance to a simple chicken broth at any time of the year, special occasion or not. The problem has always been that most matzo balls are prepared with egg yolks and oil, which add unnecessary fat, cholesterol, and calories to your soup. But you'll be delighted to find that matzo balls can be made tender and satisfying without the usual fat. Try the foolproof recipe below, and enjoy these delicacies with your next meal.

Fluffy Fat-Free Matzo Balls

YIELD: 8 SERVINGS

6 egg whites, warmed to room temperature

$\frac{1}{2}$ teaspoon salt

1 cup plus 2 tablespoons matzo meal

$1\frac{1}{2}$ teaspoons instant chicken or vegetable bouillon granules, or $\frac{1}{2}$ teaspoon salt

1. Place the egg whites in the bowl of an electric mixer, and sprinkle with the salt. Beat at high speed until stiff peaks form when the beaters are removed. Remove the beaters, and gently fold in the matzo meal, 3 tablespoons at a time. Cover the mixture, and chill for 15 minutes.

2. Half fill a 6-quart stock pot with water, and bring to a rapid boil over high heat. Add the chicken bouillon granules or salt. Coat your hands with nonstick cooking spray, and gently shape the chilled matzo meal mixture into 16 ($1\frac{1}{4}$-inch) balls. Drop the balls into the boiling water, reduce the heat to medium-low, and cover the pot. Simmer for 20 minutes, or until the matzo balls are firm.

3. Remove the matzo balls with a slotted spoon and add immediately to your chicken soup, or store in a covered container for up to 2 days.

NUTRITIONAL FACTS (PER SERVING)
Cal: 48   Carbs: 8 g   Chol: 0 mg   Fat: 0 g
Fiber: 0.3 g   Protein: 3.6 g   Sodium: 175 mg

Chicken Soup With Matzo Balls

YIELD: 8 SERVINGS

6 cups unsalted chicken broth

1 medium Spanish onion, chopped

1 stalk celery, thinly sliced

1 tablespoon instant chicken bouillon granules

$\frac{1}{8}$ teaspoon ground white pepper

$\frac{1}{8}$ teaspoon ground nutmeg

2 tablespoons finely chopped fresh parsley, or 2 teaspoons dried

1 recipe Fluffy Fat-Free Matzo Balls (above)

1. Place the chicken broth, onion, celery, bouillon granules, pepper, and nutmeg in a $2\frac{1}{2}$-quart pot, and bring to a boil over high heat. Reduce the heat to low, cover, and simmer for 30 minutes, or until the vegetables are very tender.

2. Using a slotted spoon, transfer the vegetables to a blender. Add 1 cup of the hot broth, and place the lid on the blender, leaving the top slightly ajar to allow steam to escape. Carefully blend at low speed until smooth. Return the puréed mixture to the pot, and stir to mix well.

3. Add the parsley and matzo balls to the soup, and simmer, covered, for 10 minutes. Ladle the soup into individual serving bowls, placing 2 matzo balls in each bowl, and serve hot.

NUTRITIONAL FACTS (PER $\frac{3}{4}$ CUP BROTH AND 2 MATZO BALLS)
Cal: 62   Carbs: 64 g   Chol: 0 mg   Fat: 0.3 g
Fiber: 0.8 g   Protein: 4.2 g   Sodium: 424 mg

Chicken Capellini Soup

YIELD: 8 SERVINGS

7 cups unsalted chicken broth

1 medium-large yellow onion, chopped

4 cloves garlic, peeled

1 tablespoon instant chicken bouillon granules

1½ teaspoons dried Italian seasoning or dried rosemary

⅛ teaspoon ground white pepper

2 medium carrots, peeled, halved lengthwise,
and sliced, divided

2 medium stalks celery, sliced
(include the leaves), divided

2 cups diced cooked chicken breast

3 ounces capellini (angel hair) pasta,
broken into 2-inch pieces (about 1 cup)

2 tablespoons finely chopped fresh Italian parsley

1. Place the chicken broth, onion, garlic cloves, bouillon granules, Italian seasoning or rosemary, and pepper in a 4-quart pot. Add half of the carrots and half of the celery, and bring to a boil over high heat. Reduce the heat to low, cover, and simmer for 20 minutes, or until the vegetables are tender.

2. Using a slotted spoon, transfer the vegetables and garlic cloves to a blender. Add 1½ cups of the hot broth, and place the lid on the blender, leaving the top slightly ajar to allow steam to escape. Carefully blend at low speed until the mixture is smooth. Return the puréed mixture to the pot, and stir to mix well.

3. Add the remaining carrots and celery to the pot, and bring to a boil over high heat. Reduce the heat to low, cover, and simmer for 15 minutes, or until the vegetables are tender. Add the chicken, and simmer for 5 additional minutes.

4. Add the capellini to the pot, and bring to a boil over high heat. Reduce the heat to medium, cover, and simmer for about 3 minutes, or until the pasta is al dente. (Be careful not to overcook, as the pasta will continue to soften in the hot soup.)

5. Stir the parsley into the soup. Ladle the soup into individual serving bowls, and serve hot.

NUTRITIONAL FACTS (PER 1-CUP SERVING)
Cal: 131   Carbs: 18.7 g   Chol: 25 mg   Fat: 1.1 g
Fiber: 1.1 g   Protein: 19 g   Sodium: 364 mg

Hearty Chicken and Barley Soup

YIELD: 8 CUPS

2 bone-in skinless chicken breast halves
(about 8 ounces each)

5 cups water or unsalted chicken broth

½ cup hulled or pearled barley

1 tablespoon plus 1 teaspoon instant chicken
bouillon granules

1½ teaspoons crushed fresh garlic

1 teaspoon poultry seasoning

¼ teaspoon ground black pepper

2 cups sliced fresh mushrooms

2 cups diced unpeeled potatoes (about 2 medium)

¾ cup chopped yellow onion

¾ cup sliced carrots

¾ cup sliced celery (include the leaves)

1. Rinse the chicken with cool water, and place the chicken, water or broth, barley, bouillon granules, garlic, poultry seasoning, and pepper in a 3-quart pot. Bring the mixture to a boil over medium-high heat. Then reduce the heat to low, cover, and simmer for about 30 minutes, or until the chicken is tender and no longer pink inside.

2. Remove the chicken from the pot, and set aside. Add the mushrooms, potatoes, onion, carrots, and celery to the pot, and increase the heat to return the mixture to a boil. Reduce the heat to low, cover, and simmer, stirring occasionally, for 25 additional minutes, or until the barley and vegetables are tender and the flavors are well blended.

3. Pull the chicken meat from the bones, and tear or dice it into bite-sized pieces. Add the chicken to the soup, and simmer for 5 additional minutes. Ladle the soup into individual serving bowls, and serve hot.

NUTRITIONAL FACTS (PER 1-CUP SERVING)
Cal: 130   Carbs: 21 g   Chol: 18 mg   Fat: 0.7 g
Fiber: 3.4 g   Protein: 9 g   Sodium: 332 mg

Chunky Chicken Noodle Soup

YIELD: 7 CUPS

2 bone-in skinless chicken breast halves
(about 8 ounces each)

6$^{1}/_{2}$ cups unsalted chicken broth

1 tablespoon plus 1$^{1}/_{2}$ teaspoons instant chicken
bouillon granules

1 cup sliced fresh mushrooms

$^{3}/_{4}$ cup thinly sliced celery (include the leaves)

$^{3}/_{4}$ cup sliced carrots

1 medium yellow onion, chopped

1 teaspoon dried savory

$^{1}/_{2}$ teaspoon dried thyme

$^{1}/_{8}$ teaspoon ground white pepper

3 ounces medium no-yolk noodles

2 tablespoons chopped fresh parsley

1. Rinse the chicken with cool water, and place the chicken, broth, and bouillon granules in a 3-quart pot. Bring the broth to a boil over high heat. Reduce the heat to low, cover, and simmer for about 30 minutes, or until the chicken is tender and no longer pink inside.

2. Remove the chicken from the pot, and set aside. Add the mushrooms, celery, carrots, onion, savory, thyme, and pepper to the pot, and bring the mixture to a boil over high heat. Reduce the heat to low, cover, and simmer, stirring occasionally, for 15 additional minutes, or until the vegetables are tender.

3. Pull the chicken meat from the bones, and tear or dice it into bite-sized pieces. Add it to the soup along with the noodles.

4. Increase the heat slightly to return the mixture to a boil. Then reduce the heat to medium-low, cover, and simmer for about 5 minutes, or until the noodles are al dente. (Be careful not to overcook, as the noodles will continue to soften in the hot soup.) Stir the parsley into the soup, ladle the soup into individual serving bowls, and serve hot.

NUTRITIONAL FACTS (PER 1-CUP SERVING)
Cal: 115   Carbs: 15 g   Chol: 23 mg   Fat: 0.8 g
Fiber: 1.2 g   Protein: 11.8 g   Sodium: 463 mg

Chunky Clam Chowder

YIELD: 6 SERVINGS

2 cans (6$^{1}/_{2}$ ounces each) chopped clams, undrained

$^{1}/_{2}$ cup water

2 cups diced peeled Yukon Gold potatoes
(about 2 medium)

$^{1}/_{3}$ cup thinly sliced celery

$^{1}/_{3}$ cup chopped onion

$^{1}/_{2}$ teaspoon dried savory

$^{1}/_{8}$ teaspoon ground white pepper

2 cups fresh or frozen (thawed) whole kernel corn

1 cup skim or low-fat milk

$^{3}/_{4}$ cup evaporated skim milk, divided

1 tablespoon cornstarch

1. Drain the clams, reserving the juice, and set aside.

2. Place the water, potatoes, celery, onion, savory, pepper, and $^{1}/_{2}$ cup of the reserved clam juice in a 2$^{1}/_{2}$-quart pot, and bring to a boil over high heat. Reduce the heat to low, cover, and simmer for 5 to 7 minutes, or until the potatoes are almost tender.

3. Add the corn to the pot. Cover and simmer for 5 minutes, or until the potatoes and corn are tender. Add all of the milk and $^{1}/_{2}$ cup of the evaporated milk to the pot. Cook, stirring constantly, for about 5 minutes, or until the mixture is heated through.

4. Place 1 cup of the soup—including both broth and vegetables—in a blender, and place the lid on the blender, leaving the top slightly ajar to allow steam to escape. Carefully blend the mixture at low speed until smooth. Return the blended mixture to the pot.

5. Add the clams to the pot. Place the remaining $^{1}/_{4}$ cup of evaporated milk and the cornstarch in a small dish, and stir until the cornstarch is dissolved. Add the cornstarch mixture to the soup, and, stirring constantly, simmer the soup for 5 additional minutes, or until thickened and bubbly.

6. Ladle the soup into individual serving bowls, and serve hot.

NUTRITIONAL FACTS (PER 1-CUP SERVING)
Cal: 176   Carbs: 28 g   Chol: 21 mg   Fat: 0.8 g
Fiber: 2.2 g   Protein: 13.8 g   Sodium: 144 mg

Cool Gazpacho

YIELD: 5 CUPS

SOUP

3 cups diced tomatoes (about 4 medium)

1 cup diced peeled and seeded cucumber
(about 1 medium)

1 cup diced green bell pepper (about 1 medium)

1/2 cup plus 2 tablespoons chopped onion

1/3 cup sliced black olives

1 cup canned vegetable juice, like V-8 vegetable juice

3–4 tablespoons red wine vinegar

1 1/2 teaspoons crushed fresh garlic

1 teaspoon sugar

1 teaspoon chili powder

3/4 teaspoon dried oregano

1/4 teaspoon salt

TOPPINGS

1/2 cup nonfat or light sour cream (optional)

1/2 cup plus 2 tablespoons ready-made fat-free
or low-fat croutons (optional)

1. Place all of the vegetables and the olives in a large bowl. Stir to mix, and set aside.

2. Place all of the remaining soup ingredients in a medium-sized bowl, and stir to mix well. Pour the vegetable juice mixture over the vegetables, and toss to mix.

3. Transfer the vegetable mixture to a blender or food processor, and, working in batches as necessary, process for a few seconds, or just until the vegetables are finely chopped. Transfer the soup to a covered container, and chill for 2 to 6 hours.

4. When ready to serve, place 1 cup of the gazpacho in each of 5 serving bowls. Top each serving with a rounded tablespoon of the sour cream and 2 tablespoons of the croutons, if desired, and serve immediately.

NUTRITIONAL FACTS (PER 1-CUP SERVING)
Cal: 62   Carbs: 12 g   Chol: 0 mg   Fat: 1.4 g
Fiber: 3 g   Protein: 2 g   Sodium: 321 mg

Tuscan Tomato Soup

YIELD: 6 SERVINGS

1 1/2 teaspoons crushed fresh garlic

3 cups unsalted chicken or vegetable broth

2 cans (14 1/2 ounces each) tomatoes, crushed

1/2 cup chopped onion

1 teaspoon instant chicken or vegetable
bouillon granules

2 teaspoons dried Italian seasoning

1/4 teaspoon coarsely ground black pepper

3 ounces orzo or other small pasta (about 1/2 cup)

3 tablespoons grated nonfat or regular
Parmesan cheese (garnish)

1. Coat a 2-quart pot with nonstick cooking spray, and preheat over medium heat. Add the garlic, and sauté for about 30 seconds, or until the garlic starts to turn color.

2. Add the broth, undrained tomatoes, onion, bouillon granules, Italian seasoning, and pepper to the pot, and bring to a boil over high heat. Reduce the heat to low, cover, and simmer for about 20 minutes, or until the onions are soft.

3. Transfer 2 cups of the soup—including vegetables and hot broth—to a blender, and place the lid on the blender, leaving the top slightly ajar to allow steam to escape. Carefully blend the mixture at low speed until smooth. Repeat this procedure until all of the soup has been blended.

4. Return all of the puréed soup to the pot, and bring the mixture to a boil over medium-high heat. Add the orzo, and reduce the heat to medium-low. Cover and cook, stirring occasionally, for about 8 minutes, or until the orzo is al dente. (Be careful not to overcook, as the pasta will continue to soften in the hot soup.)

5. Ladle the soup into individual serving bowls, and serve hot, topping each serving with a rounded teaspoon of the Parmesan.

NUTRITIONAL FACTS (PER 1-CUP SERVING)
Cal: 101   Carbs: 18 g   Chol: 1 mg   Fat: 0.5 g
Fiber: 2 g   Protein: 7 g   Sodium: 370 mg

Tomato Florentine Soup

YIELD: 7 SERVINGS

1 tablespoon extra virgin olive oil

1 medium onion, chopped

1 can (14½ ounces) stewed tomatoes, crushed

4 cups unsalted vegetable broth or water

2 tablespoons tomato paste

¾ teaspoon salt

⅛ teaspoon ground black pepper

1 teaspoon dried Italian seasoning

4 ounces small seashell pasta (about 1⅓ cups)

2 cups (packed) chopped fresh spinach

½ cup grated nonfat or regular
Parmesan cheese (optional)

1. Coat a 3-quart pot with the olive oil, and place over medium heat. Add the onion, and sauté for 3 minutes, or until the onion is soft.

2. Add the tomatoes, broth or water, tomato paste, salt, pepper, and Italian seasoning to the pot. Increase the heat to high, and bring to a boil. Stir in the pasta, cover, and cook over medium-low heat for 8 minutes, or until the pasta is almost al dente.

3. Add the spinach to the pot, and simmer for 1 to 2 minutes, or just until the pasta is al dente and the spinach is wilted. (Be careful not to overcook, as the pasta will continue to soften in the hot soup.)

4. Ladle the soup into individual serving bowls, and serve hot, topping each serving with a tablespoon of cheese, if desired.

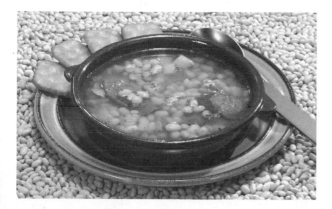

NUTRITIONAL FACTS (PER 1-CUP SERVING)			
Cal: 142	Carbs: 25 g	Chol: 0 mg	Fat: 2.6 g
Fiber: 3.4 g	Protein: 4.5 g	Sodium: 408 mg	

Tomato-Dill Soup

YIELD: 5 CUPS

2 cans (14½ ounces each) tomatoes, crushed

2½ cups unsalted vegetable or chicken broth

1 cup chopped yellow onion

¼ cup finely chopped celery (include the leaves)

2 teaspoons crushed fresh garlic

2 teaspoons dried thyme, or 2 tablespoons
finely chopped fresh

2 teaspoons light brown sugar

1 teaspoon instant chicken or vegetable
bouillon granules

½ teaspoon dried dill, or 1½ teaspoons finely
chopped fresh

⅛ teaspoon ground black pepper

1 teaspoon dried dill, or 1 tablespoon
finely chopped fresh (garnish)

1. Place all of the ingredients except for the dill garnish in a 3-quart pot, and bring to a boil over high heat. Reduce the heat to low, cover, and simmer, stirring occasionally, for about 30 minutes, or until the onion and celery are soft.

2. Transfer 2 cups of the soup to a blender and cover, leaving the lid slightly ajar to allow steam to escape. Carefully blend the mixture at low speed until smooth. Repeat this procedure until all of the soup has been blended.

3. Return all of the puréed soup to the pot, and cook over medium heat for a couple of minutes to reheat. Add a little more broth if the soup seems too thick.

4. Ladle the soup into individual serving bowls, and serve hot, topping each serving with a sprinkling of dill.

NUTRITIONAL FACTS (PER 1-CUP SERVING)			
Cal: 61	Carbs: 12 g	Chol: 0 mg	Fat: 0.4 g
Fiber: 3 g	Protein: 4 g	Sodium: 415 mg	

French Onion Soup

YIELD: 4 SERVINGS

1 large Spanish or sweet onion (about 1 pound)

2 tablespoons dry sherry

1¼ teaspoons instant beef bouillon granules

¼ teaspoon dried marjoram

⅛ teaspoon ground black pepper

3½ cups unsalted beef broth

1½ teaspoons balsamic vinegar

4 slices (each ¾-inch thick) French bread, lightly toasted

2 tablespoons grated nonfat or regular Parmesan cheese

¾ cup shredded reduced-fat provolone or Swiss cheese

1. Cut the onion in half, and slice each half into very thin wedges.

2. Place the onion, sherry, bouillon granules, marjoram, and pepper in a large nonstick skillet. Place the skillet over medium-high heat, and cook, stirring frequently, for about 5 minutes, or until the onions are wilted. Add a little more sherry if the skillet becomes too dry.

3. Add the broth to the skillet, and bring the mixture to a boil over high heat. Reduce the heat to low and cover, leaving the lid slightly ajar. Simmer, stirring occasionally, for about 20 minutes, or until the soup is reduced by about a quarter. Stir in the balsamic vinegar.

4. Divide the soup among four 12-ounce oven-proof bowls. Float a piece of French bread on top of each serving, and sprinkle the bread first with 1½ teaspoons of the Parmesan, and then with 3 tablespoons of the provolone or Swiss.

5. Place the soup bowls under a preheated broiler for about 1 minute, or until the cheese is melted and nicely browned. Serve hot.

NUTRITIONAL FACTS (PER ONE-CUP SERVING PLUS TOPPING)
Cal: 186   Carbs: 22 g   Chol: 14 mg   Fat: 3.6 g
Fiber: 2.4 g   Protein: 14 g   Sodium: 523 mg

Escarole and Orzo Soup

YIELD: 10 SERVINGS

8 cups unsalted chicken or vegetable broth

1 medium yellow onion, chopped

1 large carrot, peeled, halved lengthwise, and sliced

1 large stalk celery, thinly sliced (include the leaves)

1 tablespoon plus 1 teaspoon instant chicken bouillon granules

4 cloves garlic, peeled

⅛ teaspoon ground white pepper

3 ounces orzo pasta (about ½ cup)

1 head escarole (about 1 pound), rinsed well and torn into pieces

½ cup grated nonfat or regular Parmesan cheese (garnish)

1. Place the broth, onion, carrot, celery, bouillon granules, garlic cloves, and pepper in a 4-quart pot, and bring to a boil over high heat. Reduce the heat to low, cover, and simmer for 20 minutes, or until the vegetables are tender.

2. Using a slotted spoon, transfer the vegetables and garlic cloves to a blender. Add 1 cup of the hot broth, and place the lid on the blender, leaving the top slightly ajar to allow steam to escape. Carefully blend the mixture at low speed until smooth. Return the puréed mixture to the pot, and stir to mix well.

3. Add the orzo to the pot, and bring to a boil over high heat. Reduce the heat to medium, cover, and cook for about 8 minutes, or until the orzo is almost al dente. Add the escarole, and cook, uncovered, for 2 additional minutes, or until the orzo is al dente and the escarole is wilted. (Be careful not to overcook, as the pasta will continue to soften in the hot soup.)

4. Ladle the soup into individual serving bowls, and serve hot, topping each serving with a heaping teaspoon of the Parmesan.

NUTRITIONAL FACTS (PER 1-CUP SERVING)
Cal: 78   Carbs: 12 g   Chol: 2 mg   Fat: 0.3 g
Fiber: 2.3 g   Protein: 7.5 g   Sodium: 363 mg

Roasted Vegetable Soup

YIELD: 8 SERVINGS

6 cups unsalted beef broth

1 tablespoon instant beef bouillon granules

2 bay leaves

1/2 cup quick-cooking barley

ROASTED VEGETABLE MIXTURE

2 medium carrots, peeled
and sliced 1/2-inch thick

2 medium yellow onions,
cut into 1/2-inch-thick wedges

2 medium potatoes, unpeeled,
cut into 3/4-inch cubes

1 1/2 cups thickly sliced fresh mushrooms

10 cloves garlic, peeled

1 tablespoon plus 1 1/2 teaspoons balsamic vinegar

1 tablespoon unsalted beef broth

1 tablespoon fresh rosemary, or 1 teaspoon dried

1/4 teaspoon coarsely ground black pepper

1 tablespoon extra virgin olive oil

1. To make the roasted vegetables, place all of the vegetables, including the garlic, in a large bowl, and toss to mix well. Add the vinegar, broth, rosemary, pepper, and olive oil, and stir to mix well.

2. Coat a nonstick 9-x-13-inch pan with olive oil cooking spray, and spread the vegetables in an even layer in the pan. Bake uncovered at 450°F for 15 minutes. Then turn the vegetables with a spatula, and bake for 15 additional minutes, or until the vegetables are tender and nicely browned.

3. Remove the vegetables from the oven, and pick out the roasted garlic cloves. Using the blade of a large knife, smash the cloves. Transfer the garlic and the other roasted vegetables to a 4-quart pot.

4. Use part of the 6 cups of broth to "rinse out" the pan used for roasting the vegetables. Add this liquid and the remainder of the broth to the pot, along with the bouillon granules and bay leaves. Bring the mixture to a boil over high heat. Reduce the heat to low, cover, and simmer for 10 minutes.

5. Add the barley to the pot, cover, and simmer for 15 additional minutes, or until the barley is tender and the flavors are well blended.

6. Remove the bay leaves from the soup, and discard. Ladle the soup into individual serving bowls, and serve hot.

NUTRITIONAL FACTS (PER 1-CUP SERVING)
Cal: 122   Carbs: 22.3 g   Chol: 0 mg   Fat: 2.4 g
Fiber: 2.7 g   Protein: 2.8 g   Sodium: 266 mg

Summer Vegetable Soup

YIELD: 7 SERVINGS

1 3/4 pounds ripe tomatoes (about 4 medium-large),
peeled and diced

2 cups unsalted vegetable broth or water

4 cups chopped cabbage

1 cup fresh or frozen (thawed) whole kernel corn

1 cup fresh or frozen (thawed) cut green beans

1 medium onion, chopped

1 medium carrot, peeled, halved lengthwise,
and sliced

2 tablespoons tomato paste

3/4 teaspoon salt

1/4 teaspoon ground black pepper

1 teaspoon dried thyme or marjoram

1/4 teaspoon celery seed

1. Place the tomatoes and the broth or water in a 4-quart pot, and bring to a boil over high heat. Reduce the heat to low, cover, and simmer for 20 minutes, or until the tomatoes are soft and have broken down.

2. Add all of the remaining ingredients to the pot, and simmer for 15 minutes, or until the vegetables are tender.

3. Ladle the soup into individual serving bowls, and serve hot.

NUTRITIONAL FACTS (PER 1-CUP SERVING)
Cal: 68   Carbs: 12 g   Chol: 0 mg   Fat: 0.8 g
Fiber: 3.7 g   Protein: 2.9 g   Sodium: 256 mg

Cauliflower-Cheese Soup

YIELD: 7 CUPS

1 large head cauliflower (about 2 pounds)
2 cups unsalted chicken or vegetable broth
1 medium yellow onion, chopped
1 teaspoon dry mustard
$1/2$ teaspoon salt
$1/8$ teaspoon ground white pepper
2 cups skim or low-fat milk, divided
3 tablespoons toasted garbanzo flour or unbleached flour
4 ounces nonfat or reduced-fat process Cheddar cheese or reduced-fat Cheddar cheese, shredded or diced (about 1 cup)
$1/4$ cup thinly sliced scallions (garnish)

1. Remove and discard the cauliflower's outer leaves and core. Rinse the cauliflower well, and separate it into small florets.

2. Place the cauliflower florets, broth, onion, dry mustard, salt, and pepper in a 3-quart pot, and bring to a boil over high heat. Reduce the heat to medium-low, cover, and cook, stirring occasionally, for about 10 minutes, or until the cauliflower is tender.

3. Using a slotted spoon, transfer half of the cauliflower to a blender. Add $1^1/2$ cups of the milk and place the lid on the blender, leaving the top slightly ajar to allow steam to escape. Carefully blend at low speed until smooth. Return the puréed mixture to the pot, and stir to mix well.

4. Increase the heat under the pot to medium, and allow the mixture to come to a boil, stirring frequently. Place the remaining $1/2$ cup of milk and the flour in the blender, and process until the flour is dissolved. Slowly stir the flour mixture into the soup. Cook and stir for a minute or 2, or until the mixture thickens slightly. Add the cheese to the pot, and cook, stirring constantly, until the cheese is melted.

5. Ladle the soup into individual serving bowls, and serve hot, topping each serving with a sprinkling of scallions.

NUTRITIONAL FACTS (PER 1-CUP SERVING)
Cal: 86   Carbs: 12 g   Chol: 1 mg   Fat: 0.4 g
Fiber: 2.2 g   Protein: 9.6 g   Sodium: 398 mg

Cream of Cauliflower Soup

YIELD: 4 SERVINGS

1 large head cauliflower (about 2 pounds)
1 cup plus 2 tablespoons water
$1/2$ cup chopped onion
$1^1/4$ teaspoons instant chicken bouillon granules
1 pinch ground white pepper
1 cup skim or low-fat milk
$1/4$ cup grated nonfat Parmesan cheese, or $1/4$ cup regular Parmesan cheese mixed with 2 teaspoons cornstarch
1 pinch ground nutmeg
1 tablespoon finely chopped fresh chives or dill (garnish)

1. Remove and discard the cauliflower's outer leaves and core. Rinse the cauliflower well, and separate it into small florets.

2. Place the cauliflower florets, water, onion, bouillon granules, and pepper in a 2-quart pot, and bring to a boil over high heat. Reduce the heat to medium-low, cover, and cook, stirring occasionally, for about 10 minutes, or until the cauliflower is tender.

3. Using a slotted spoon, transfer half of the cauliflower to a blender. Add the milk, Parmesan, and nutmeg, and place the lid on the blender, leaving the top slightly ajar to allow steam to escape. Carefully blend at low speed until the mixture is smooth. Return the puréed mixture to the pot, and stir to mix well.

4. Place the pot over medium heat, and cook, stirring constantly, just until the soup begins to boil. Add a little more milk if the soup seems too thick.

5. Ladle the soup into individual serving bowls, and serve hot, topping each serving with a sprinkling of chives or dill.

NUTRITIONAL FACTS (PER 1-CUP SERVING)
Cal: 89   Carbs: 11.1 g   Chol: 4 mg   Fat: 0.5 g
Fiber: 2.5 g   Protein: 10 g   Sodium: 372 mg

Fresh Corn Chowder

YIELD: 9 SERVINGS

1 cup water

4 cups diced peeled Yukon Gold potatoes
(about 1½ pounds)

½ cup thinly sliced celery

½ cup chopped onion

2½ teaspoons instant chicken bouillon granules

1½ teaspoons dried savory

⅛ teaspoon ground white pepper

4 cups fresh or frozen (thawed) whole kernel corn
(about 1½ pounds)

3 cups skim or low-fat milk

¼ cup plus 2 tablespoons instant
nonfat dry milk powder

3 tablespoons finely chopped fresh chives
or scallions (garnish)

1. Place the water, potatoes, celery, onion, bouillon granules, savory, and pepper in a 3-quart pot, and bring to a boil over high heat. Reduce the heat to low, cover, and simmer for 15 minutes, or until the potatoes are almost tender.

2. Add the corn to the pot. Cover and simmer for 5 minutes, or until the potatoes and corn are tender.

3. Place the milk in a medium-sized bowl, and stir in the milk powder. Add the mixture to the pot, and cook, stirring constantly, for about 5 minutes, or until the mixture is heated through.

4. Remove 4 cups of soup—including both broth and vegetables—from the pot. Place 2 cups of the removed soup in a blender, and place the lid on the blender, leaving the top slightly ajar to allow steam to escape. Carefully blend the mixture at low speed until smooth. Return the blended mixture to the pot, and repeat this procedure with the remaining 2 cups of soup.

5. Simmer the soup for 5 additional minutes. Ladle the soup into individual serving bowls, and serve hot, topping each serving with a sprinkling of chives or scallions.

NUTRITIONAL FACTS (PER 1-CUP SERVING)
Cal: 164   Carbs: 31 g   Chol: 2 mg   Fat: 1.1 g
Fiber: 3.1 g   Protein: 7.8 g   Sodium: 360 mg

Country Vegetable Soup

YIELD: 8 CUPS

3 cups water, unsalted vegetable broth,
or unsalted beef broth

2 stalks celery, thinly sliced
(include the leaves)

1 cup diced unpeeled potato
(about 1 medium)

1 cup chopped yellow onion

1 medium-large carrot, peeled, halved lengthwise,
and sliced

1 tablespoon instant vegetable or beef bouillon granules

1½ teaspoons dried thyme

¼ teaspoon ground black pepper

2 bay leaves

1 can (14½ ounces) tomatoes, crushed

1 can (15 ounces) red kidney beans, drained

1½ cups coarsely chopped cabbage

1 cup fresh or frozen (unthawed) whole kernel corn

1. Place the water or broth, celery, potato, onion, carrot, bouillon granules, thyme, pepper, and bay leaves in a 4-quart pot, and bring to a boil over high heat. Reduce the heat to low, cover, and simmer, stirring occasionally, for 15 minutes, or until the vegetables are tender.

2. Add all of the remaining ingredients to the pot, and increase the heat to return the mixture to a boil. Reduce the heat to low, cover, and simmer, stirring occasionally, for 15 additional minutes, or until the cabbage is tender and the flavors are well blended.

3. Remove the bay leaves from the soup, and discard. Ladle the soup into individual serving bowls, and serve hot.

NUTRITIONAL FACTS (PER 1-CUP SERVING)
Cal: 126   Carbs: 26 g   Chol: 0 mg   Fat: 0.5 g
Fiber: 7.6 g   Protein: 6 g   Sodium: 373 mg

Barley and Cheese Soup

YIELD: 6 SERVINGS

2 cups water

$^1/_2$ cup plus 1 tablespoon quick-cooking barley

2 tablespoons finely chopped onion

1 teaspoon instant chicken bouillon granules

3 cups skim or low-fat milk, divided

2 tablespoons cornstarch

$^1/_3$ cup instant nonfat dry milk powder

$^1/_8$ teaspoon cayenne pepper or
ground white pepper

4 ounces nonfat or reduced-fat process
Cheddar cheese, or reduced-fat Cheddar cheese,
shredded or diced (about 1 cup)

3 tablespoons thinly sliced scallions (garnish)

1. Place the water, barley, onion, and bouillon granules in a nonstick $2^1/_2$-quart pot, and bring to a boil over high heat. Reduce the heat to low, cover, and simmer for 10 to 12 minutes, or until the barley is tender.

2. Place $^1/_4$ cup of the milk and all of the cornstarch in a small bowl, and stir until the cornstarch dissolves. Set aside.

3. Place the remaining $2^3/_4$ cups of milk, the milk powder, and the pepper in a medium-sized bowl, and mix until smooth. Add the milk mixture to the pot, increase the heat to medium, and cook, stirring constantly, just until the mixture begins to boil.

4. Stir the cornstarch mixture once, and add it to the pot. Cook and stir for 1 minute, or until the mixture thickens slightly.

5. Add the cheese to the pot, and stir until the cheese melts. Remove the pot from the heat.

6. Ladle the soup into individual serving bowls, and serve hot, topping each serving with a sprinkling of scallions.

NUTRITIONAL FACTS (PER 1-CUP SERVING)
Cal: 145   Carbs: 22 g   Chol: 6 mg   Fat: 0.5 g
Fiber: 1.6 g   Protein: 13 g   Sodium: 366 mg

Broccoli-Cheddar Soup

YIELD: 6 SERVINGS

$1^1/_4$ cups unsalted chicken broth

$^1/_3$ cup finely chopped onion

$^1/_2$ teaspoon dried thyme

$^1/_8$ teaspoon ground white pepper

3 cups skim or low-fat milk, divided

$^1/_4$ cup unbleached flour

$^1/_2$ cup instant nonfat dry milk powder

1 package (10 ounces) frozen chopped broccoli,
thawed and squeezed dry

6 ounces nonfat or reduced-fat process
Cheddar cheese, or reduced-fat Cheddar cheese,
shredded or diced (about $1^1/_2$ cups)

1. Place the broth, onion, thyme, and pepper in a 3-quart pot, and bring to a boil over high heat. Reduce the heat to low, cover, and simmer for about 5 minutes, or until the onion is tender.

2. Add $2^1/_2$ cups of the milk to the pot. Increase the heat to medium and cook, stirring constantly, until the mixture begins to boil.

3. Place the flour, the dry milk powder, and the remaining $^1/_2$ cup of milk in a jar with a tight-fitting lid, and shake until smooth. Add the flour mixture to the pot, and cook, stirring constantly, until the mixture begins to boil and thickens slightly.

4. Reduce the heat to medium-low. Add the broccoli and cheese to the pot, and cook, stirring constantly, for about 5 minutes, or until the cheese is melted and the soup is heated through.

5. Ladle the soup into individual serving bowls, and serve hot.

NUTRITIONAL FACTS (PER 1-CUP SERVING)
Cal: 139   Carbs: 16 g   Chol: 6 mg   Fat: 0.3 g
Fiber: 1.5 g   Protein: 17 g   Sodium: 342 mg

Creamy Carrot Soup

YIELD: 6 SERVINGS

4 cups diced carrots (about 6 medium)

1 medium onion, chopped

1 large Yukon Gold potato (about 8 ounces), peeled and diced

3½ cups unsalted chicken broth

½ teaspoon crushed dried marjoram

½ teaspoon salt

⅛ teaspoon ground white pepper

1 can (12 ounces) evaporated skim milk

Minced fresh dill (garnish)

1. Place the carrots, onion, potato, broth, marjoram, salt, and pepper in a 4-quart pot, and bring to a boil over high heat. Reduce the heat to low, cover, and simmer for 25 minutes, or until the carrots are soft.

2. Place 2 cups of the soup—including both vegetables and broth—in a blender, and place the lid on the blender, leaving the top slightly ajar to allow steam to escape. Carefully blend the mixture at low speed until smooth. Repeat this procedure until all of the soup has been blended smooth.

3. Return all of the puréed soup to the pot, and place the pot over medium heat. Add the evaporated milk, and cook, stirring constantly, for several minutes, or until the mixture is heated through.

4. Ladle the soup into individual serving bowls, and serve hot, topping each serving with a sprinkling of fresh dill.

NUTRITIONAL FACTS (PER 1-CUP SERVING)
Cal: 137 Carbs: 24 g Chol: 2 mg Fat: 0.5 g
Fiber: 3.4 g Protein: 8.5 g Sodium: 307 mg

Potato and Leek Soup

YIELD: 9 SERVINGS

2 leeks

4 cups unsalted chicken broth

2½ pounds Yukon Gold potatoes, peeled and diced (6–7 medium)

2 medium stalks celery, thinly sliced (include the leaves)

6 cloves garlic, peeled

1 tablespoon instant chicken bouillon granules

⅛ teaspoon ground white pepper

¾ cup evaporated skim milk

1. Cut the leeks in half lengthwise and rinse well. Thinly slice the white and light green parts, and place in a 4-quart pot. Thinly slice the tender parts of the dark green shoots, and set aside as a garnish.

2. Add the broth, potatoes, celery, garlic cloves, bouillon granules, and pepper to the pot, and bring to a boil over high heat. Reduce heat to low, cover, and simmer, stirring occasionally, for 15 to 20 minutes, or until the potatoes are tender.

3. Transfer half of the vegetables and 1½ cups of the hot broth to a blender. Pick out any garlic cloves that have remained in the pot, and add them to the blender, as well. Place the lid on the blender, leaving the top slightly ajar to allow steam to escape, and carefully blend the mixture at low speed until smooth. Return the puréed mixture to the pot, and stir to mix well.

4. Add the evaporated milk to the pot, and stir to mix. Cook, stirring frequently, for about 2 minutes, or until the mixture is heated through.

5. Ladle the soup into individual serving bowls, and serve hot, topping each serving with a sprinkling of the leek shoots.

NUTRITIONAL FACTS (PER 1-CUP SERVING)
Cal: 143 Carbs: 30.8 g Chol: 1 mg Fat: 0.3 g
Fiber: 2.8 g Protein: 4.2 g Sodium: 308 mg

Lemony Lentil Soup

YIELD: 6 SERVINGS

1 tablespoon extra virgin olive oil
1 teaspoon crushed fresh garlic
1 medium yellow onion, chopped
1 stalk celery, thinly sliced (include the leaves)
4 cups water
1 medium carrot, peeled, halved lengthwise, and sliced
1 medium potato, scrubbed and diced
1 cup dried brown lentils, cleaned (page 302)
1 tablespoon instant chicken or vegetable bouillon granules
$1/2$ teaspoon dried thyme
$1/4$ teaspoon coarsely ground black pepper
2 tablespoons finely chopped fresh parsley, or 2 teaspoons dried
1 tablespoon lemon juice
1 teaspoon freshly grated lemon rind
3 tablespoons grated nonfat or regular Parmesan cheese (garnish)

1. Place the olive oil in a $2^{1}/2$-quart pot, and preheat over medium-high heat. Add the garlic, onion, and celery, and cook, stirring frequently, for about 2 minutes, or until the vegetables are crisp-tender.

2. Add the water, carrot, potato, lentils, bouillon granules, thyme, and pepper to the pot, and bring to a boil. Reduce the heat to low, cover, and simmer, stirring occasionally, for about 45 minutes, or until the lentils are soft and the liquid is thick. Add a little water during cooking if needed.

3. Stir the parsley, lemon juice, and lemon rind into the soup. Cover and simmer for another minute.

4. Ladle the soup into individual serving bowls, and serve hot, topping each serving with a sprinkling of the Parmesan.

NUTRITIONAL FACTS (PER 1-CUP SERVING)
Cal: 179   Carbs: 29 g   Chol: 3 mg   Fat: 2.6 g
Fiber: 8 g   Protein: 11 g   Sodium: 358 mg

Pasta Fagioli

YIELD: 12 SERVINGS

1 pound 95% lean ground beef
1 teaspoon crushed fresh garlic
1 medium Spanish onion, chopped
1 large carrot, peeled, halved lengthwise, and sliced
2 large stalks celery, thinly sliced (include the leaves)
2 cans ($14^{1}/2$ ounces each) unsalted tomatoes, crushed
1 tablespoon instant beef bouillon granules
$2^{1}/2$ teaspoons dried Italian seasoning
$1/4$ teaspoon ground black pepper
4 cups unsalted beef broth or water
1 can (1 pound) red kidney beans or white beans, drained
6 ounces wagon wheel or ziti pasta (about $2^{1}/4$ cups)

1. Coat the bottom of a 4-quart pot with nonstick cooking spray, and preheat over medium heat. Add the ground beef and garlic, and cook, stirring to crumble, until the meat is no longer pink. Drain off and discard any excess fat.

2. Add the onion, carrot, celery, undrained tomatoes, bouillon granules, Italian seasoning, pepper, and broth or water to the pot, and bring to a boil over high heat. Reduce the heat to low, cover, and simmer for 15 minutes, or until the vegetables are tender.

3. Add the beans and pasta to the pot, and bring to a boil over high heat. Reduce the heat to medium-low, cover, and simmer for about 9 minutes, or until the pasta is al dente. (Be careful not to overcook, as the pasta will continue to soften in the hot soup.)

4. Ladle the soup into individual serving bowls, and serve hot.

NUTRITIONAL FACTS (PER 1-CUP SERVING)
Cal: 179   Carbs: 25.7 g   Chol: 24 mg   Fat: 2.1 g
Fiber: 4.9 g   Protein: 14.3 g   Sodium: 287 mg

Lentil Zuppa

YIELD: 8 SERVINGS

2 teaspoons crushed fresh garlic

7 cups unsalted chicken broth or water

1½ cups dried brown lentils, cleaned (page 302)

6 ounces ham, at least 97% lean, diced
(about 1⅛ cups)

1 medium yellow onion, chopped

2 medium stalks celery, chopped
(include the leaves)

1 large carrot, peeled and chopped

2 teaspoons instant chicken bouillon granules

2 bay leaves

1½ teaspoons dried oregano

½ teaspoon ground black pepper

¼ cup grated nonfat or regular
Parmesan cheese (optional)

1. Coat a 4-quart pot with nonstick cooking spray, and preheat over medium heat. Add the garlic, and sauté for about 30 seconds, or just until the garlic begins to turn color.

2. Add all of the remaining ingredients except for the Parmesan to the pot, and bring to a boil over high heat. Reduce the heat to low, cover, and simmer for about 45 minutes, or until the lentils are soft and the liquid is thick. Remove and discard the bay leaves.

3. Transfer 2 cups of the soup—including vegetables and hot broth—to a blender, and place the lid on the blender, leaving the top slightly ajar to allow steam to escape. Carefully blend at low speed until the mixture is smooth. Return the puréed soup to the pot, and stir to mix well.

4. Ladle the soup into individual serving bowls, and serve hot, topping each serving with a rounded teaspoon of the Parmesan, if desired.

NUTRITIONAL FACTS (PER 1-CUP SERVING)
Cal: 186   Carbs: 22.5 g   Chol: 11 mg   Fat: 1.3 g
Fiber: 5.3 g   Protein: 21 g   Sodium: 390 mg

White Bean and Pasta Soup

YIELD: 9 SERVINGS

8 cups water or unsalted chicken broth

1½ cups dried navy beans or Great Northern beans,
cleaned and soaked (page 302)

8 ounces ham, at least 97% lean, diced
(about 1⅔ cups)

1 medium Spanish onion, chopped

2 medium carrots, peeled, halved lengthwise,
and sliced

2 large stalks celery, thinly sliced (include the leaves)

1 tablespoon instant chicken bouillon granules

1 teaspoon crushed fresh garlic

1 teaspoon dried sage

1 bay leaf

½ teaspoon ground black pepper

4 ounces wagon wheel pasta (about 1½ cups)

1. Place all of the ingredients except for the pasta in a 4-quart pot, and bring to a boil over high heat. Reduce the heat to low, cover, and simmer, stirring occasionally, for about 1 hour and 30 minutes, or until the beans are soft. Remove the bay leaf from the soup, and discard.

2. Transfer 3 cups of the soup—including beans, vegetables, and hot broth—to a blender. Place the lid on the blender, leaving the top slightly ajar to allow steam to escape. Carefully blend at low speed until the mixture is smooth. Return the puréed soup to the pot, and stir to mix well.

3. Add the pasta to the pot, and bring to a boil over medium-high heat. Reduce the heat to low, cover, and simmer for about 8 minutes, or until the pasta is al dente. Add a little more water or broth if the soup seems too dry. (Be careful not to overcook, as the pasta will continue to soften in the hot soup.)

4. Ladle the soup into individual serving bowls, and serve hot.

NUTRITIONAL FACTS (PER 1-CUP SERVING)
Cal: 194   Carbs: 32 g   Chol: 13 mg   Fat: 1.3 g
Fiber: 7.1 g   Protein: 13.5 g   Sodium: 411 mg

Dahl (Indian Lentil) Soup

YIELD: 7 CUPS

6 cups water or unsalted chicken broth
1$1/2$ cups dried red lentils, cleaned (page 302)
1$1/4$ cups diced peeled Yukon Gold potato (about 1 large)
1 cup chopped tomato (about 1 medium-large)
1 medium yellow onion, chopped
1 tablespoon instant chicken or vegetable bouillon granules
2–3 teaspoons curry paste
2 teaspoons crushed fresh garlic
$1/8$ teaspoon ground black pepper

1. Place all of the ingredients in a 3-quart pot, and bring to a boil over high heat.

2. Reduce the heat to low, cover, and simmer, stirring occasionally, for about 30 minutes, or until the lentils are soft and the liquid is thick. Add a little water during cooking if needed.

3. Ladle the soup into individual serving bowls, and serve hot.

NUTRITIONAL FACTS (PER 1-CUP SERVING)
Cal: 183   Carbs: 30 g   Chol: 0 mg   Fat: 1.4 g
Fiber: 6.6 g   Protein: 12.5 g   Sodium: 325 mg

Creamy Mushroom Soup

YIELD: 5 SERVINGS

4 cups sliced fresh mushrooms
$1/2$ cup chopped onion
2 tablespoons dry sherry
1 teaspoon dried marjoram or thyme
$1/2$ teaspoon salt
$1/8$ teaspoon ground white pepper
3 cups skim or low-fat milk, divided
1 cup evaporated skim milk
$1/3$ cup toasted garbanzo flour or unbleached flour

1. Place the mushrooms, onion, sherry, marjoram or thyme, salt, and pepper in a nonstick 2$1/2$-quart pot. Place over medium heat, and cook, stirring frequently, until the mushrooms are tender and most of the liquid has evaporated.

2. Add 2$1/2$ cups of the milk and all of the evaporated milk to the pot. Cook and stir until the mixture comes to a simmer.

3. Place the remaining $1/2$ cup of milk and the flour in a jar with a tight-fitting lid, and shake until smooth. Add the flour mixture to the soup, and cook and stir until thickened and bubbly.

4. Ladle the soup into individual serving bowls, and serve hot.

NUTRITIONAL FACTS (PER 1-CUP SERVING)
Cal: 140   Carbs: 21 g   Chol: 0 mg   Fat: 0.9 g
Fiber: 1.9 g   Protein: 12 g   Sodium: 330 mg

Spanish Bean Soup

YIELD: 9 SERVINGS

8 cups unsalted chicken broth or water
1$1/4$ cups dried chickpeas, cleaned and soaked (page 302)
12 ounces unpeeled Yukon Gold potatoes (about 2 medium), diced
1 large Spanish onion, chopped
1 teaspoon crushed fresh garlic
2 cups diced ham, smoked sausage, or kielbasa, at least 97% lean (about 10 ounces)
2 teaspoons instant chicken bouillon granules
$3/8$ teaspoon loosely packed saffron threads
$1/4$ teaspoon ground white pepper
3 tablespoons finely chopped fresh parsley, or 1 tablespoon dried

1. Place the chicken broth or water and the chickpeas in a 4-quart pot, and bring to a boil over high heat. Reduce the heat to low, cover, and simmer, stirring occasionally, for 1$1/2$ to 2 hours, or until the beans are tender.

2. Add all of the remaining ingredients except for the parsley to the pot, cover, and simmer for about 30 minutes, or until the potatoes are tender.

3. Stir the parsley into the soup. Ladle the soup into individual serving bowls, and serve hot.

NUTRITIONAL FACTS (PER 1-CUP SERVING)
Cal: 178   Carbs: 28 g   Chol: 28 mg   Fat: 2.4 g
Fiber: 5.6 g   Protein: 11.3 g   Sodium: 404 mg

Lentil and Sausage Soup

YIELD: 9 CUPS

6 cups water
1 1/2 cups dried brown lentils, cleaned (page 302)
8 ounces smoked sausage or kielbasa, at least 97% lean, sliced 1/4 inch thick (about 1 1/2 cups)
1 cup sliced peeled carrots (about 1 large)
1 cup diced unpeeled potatoes (about 1 medium)
1 medium yellow onion, chopped
1 1/2 teaspoons instant chicken bouillon granules
2 bay leaves
1/4 teaspoon ground black pepper
2 tablespoons tomato paste

1. Place all of the ingredients except for the tomato paste in a 4-quart pot, and bring to a boil over high heat. Reduce the heat to low, cover, and simmer for 45 minutes, or until the lentils are soft and the liquid is thick. Add a little water during cooking if needed.

2. Stir the tomato paste into the soup, and simmer for 5 additional minutes.

3. Remove the bay leaves from the soup, and discard. Ladle the soup into individual serving bowls, and serve hot.

NUTRITIONAL FACTS (PER 1-CUP SERVING)
Cal: 163   Carbs: 25 g   Chol: 11 mg   Fat: 0.9 g
Fiber: 5.1 g   Protein: 13.4 g   Sodium: 399 mg

Country Bean Soup With Ham

YIELD: 9 CUPS

7 cups water or unsalted chicken broth
2 cups dried navy or lima beans, cleaned and soaked (page 302)
2 medium yellow onions, diced
1 stalk celery, finely chopped (include the leaves)
2 teaspoons instant chicken bouillon granules
1/4 teaspoon ground black pepper
2 cups diced ham, at least 97% lean (about 10 ounces)
1 teaspoon dried sage
1 teaspoon dry mustard
2 bay leaves

1. Place the water or broth, beans, onions, celery, bouillon granules, and pepper in a 4-quart pot, and bring to a boil over high heat. Reduce the heat to low, cover, and simmer, stirring occasionally, for 45 minutes.

2. Add all of the remaining ingredients to the pot, increase the heat to medium-high, and allow the mixture to come to a boil. Reduce the heat to low, cover, and simmer, stirring occasionally, for 45 to 60 additional minutes, or until the beans are soft and the liquid is thick. Periodically check the pot during cooking, and add a little more water or broth if needed.

3. Remove the bay leaves from the soup, and discard. Ladle the soup into individual serving bowls, and serve hot.

NUTRITIONAL FACTS (PER 1-CUP SERVING)
Cal: 187   Carbs: 30 g   Chol: 11 mg   Fat: 1.1 g
Fiber: 9 g   Protein: 14.7 g   Sodium: 419 mg

Lightening Up Your Soup Recipes

Almost everyone has a favorite soup recipe or two. Maybe it's a recipe for Mom's Chicken Noodle Soup—the one she always made for you when you were sick. Or maybe it's a recipe for the Vegetable Beef Soup that took the chill off many a winter day. More than likely, though, your favorite soup recipe is a little high in fat—especially if it's a cream soup or if it contains meat. If the recipe uses a commercial broth, it may also be high in salt. Fortunately, it's easy to reduce fat and salt in just about any soup recipe you can think of. Here are some tips.

Reducing Fat

❏ If your recipe contains beef, pork, or poultry, use the leanest cuts available, and trim off any visible fat. (See Chapter 1 for a discussion of lean meats and poultry.) If you have to brown the meat before adding it to the soup, use a nonstick skillet and nonstick cooking spray, and be sure to drain off any fat before transferring the meat in the soup pot.

❏ After preparing a meat stock or soup, refrigerate it for a few hours or overnight to allow the fat to rise to the top and harden. Then lift off the hardened fat for a fat-free broth that has almost no calories.

❏ When there's no time to refrigerate your stock or broth, defat it quickly by placing it in a fat separator cup. This specially designed cup has a spout that pours stock from the *bottom* of the cup. The fat, which floats to the top, stays in the cup.

❏ If you don't have a fat separator cup, quickly defat your soup with ice cubes. Just place a few ice cubes in a pot of warm—not hot—soup, and let the cubes remain in the stock for a few seconds. Then remove the cubes, as well as the fat that clings to them.

❏ If you choose to use a canned broth, keep in mind that most broths are quite low in fat, and that any fat that is present will have floated to the

Split Pea Soup With Ham

YIELD: 6 CUPS

6 cups water or unsalted chicken broth
1½ cups dried green split peas, cleaned (page 302)
1 medium yellow onion, chopped
1 medium carrot, peeled, halved lengthwise, and sliced
1 stalk celery, thinly sliced (include the leaves)
6 ounces ham, at least 97% lean, diced (about 1⅛ cups)
1½ teaspoons instant chicken bouillon granules
1½ teaspoons crushed fresh garlic
1 bay leaf
¼ teaspoon ground black pepper
¼ teaspoon dried thyme

1. Place all of the ingredients in a 3-quart pot, and bring to a boil over high heat. Reduce the heat to low, cover, and simmer, stirring occasionally, for about 1 hour, or until the peas are soft and the liquid is thick.

2. Remove the bay leaf from the soup, and discard. Ladle the soup into individual serving bowls, and serve hot.

NUTRITIONAL FACTS (PER 1-CUP SERVING)
Cal: 211   Carbs: 33 g   Chol: 15 mg   Fat: 0.9 g
Fiber: 4.7 g   Protein: 18 g   Sodium: 483 mg

top. When you open the can, simply spoon out and discard the fat. Now you have a fat-free broth!

❏ If your recipe contains milk, substitute skim or low-fat milk for the whole milk. For a richer taste, add one to two tablespoons of instant nonfat dry milk powder to each cup of skim or low-fat milk.

❏ If your recipe contains cream, substitute evaporated skim milk—or ⅞ cup of skim or low-fat milk mixed with ⅓ cup of instant nonfat dry milk powder—for the high-fat cream.

❏ To add extra richness to low-fat cream soups, remove some of the broth and vegetables from the pot, and purée the mixture in your blender. Then return the mixture to the pot to thicken the soup.

❏ If your recipe contains sour cream, substitute a nonfat or light brand for the full-fat product.

❏ If your recipe contains cheese, use a nonfat or reduced-fat brand. Most reduced-fat cheeses melt well, although they should be finely shredded for best results. When using nonfat cheeses, your best

bet is a process cheese, which is specifically designed to melt during cooking.

Reducing Salt

❏ If your recipe has a stock or bouillon base, either use a commercial sodium-free or reduced-sodium broth, or make your own stock.

❏ To make your soup more flavorful without using salt, reduce your stock or broth by simmering it uncovered until some of the liquid evaporates. This will intensify the flavors.

❏ To prevent your low-salt soup from tasting flat, add a little lemon juice or vinegar to the finished product. These ingredients give the impression of saltiness.

❏ When decreasing the amount of salt or salty bouillon in a recipe, increase the herbs and spices for added flavor.

❏ Add a pinch of white pepper to your pot of low-salt soup. The pungency of the spice will reduce the need for salt.

Golden Split Pea Soup

YIELD: 8 SERVINGS

6 cups unsalted chicken broth or water

1½ cups dried yellow split peas, cleaned (page 302)

1 medium yellow onion, chopped

2 medium sweet potatoes, peeled and diced

1 tablespoon instant chicken bouillon granules

2 teaspoons ground cumin

2 teaspoons ground coriander

½ teaspoon ground ginger

½ teaspoon ground turmeric

⅛ teaspoon ground white pepper

1. Place all of the ingredients in a 3-quart pot, and bring to a boil over high heat. Reduce the heat to low, cover, and simmer, stirring occasionally, for about 1 hour, or until the peas are soft and the liquid is thick.

2. Ladle the soup into individual serving bowls, and serve hot.

NUTRITIONAL FACTS (PER 1-CUP SERVING)
Cal: 177   Carbs: 32 g   Chol: 0 mg   Fat: 0.8 g
Fiber: 7 g   Protein: 10 g   Sodium: 330 mg

Golden Chickpea Soup

YIELD: 9 SERVINGS

6 cloves fresh garlic, crushed

6 cups water or unsalted chicken broth

2 cans (1 pound each) chickpeas, drained

1 large Spanish onion, chopped

2 medium carrots, peeled and diced

2 tablespoons chopped fresh Italian parsley

1 tablespoon instant chicken bouillon granules

2 bay leaves

$1/4$ teaspoon ground black pepper

4 ounces ziti or tube pasta (about $1\frac{1}{2}$ cups)

1. Coat a 4-quart pot with nonstick olive oil cooking spray, and preheat over medium heat. Add the garlic, and sauté for about 30 seconds, or just until the garlic begins to turn color.

2. Add all of the remaining ingredients except for the pasta to the pot, and bring to a boil over high heat. Reduce the heat to low, cover, and simmer for 30 minutes, or until the vegetables are soft. Remove the bay leaves from the soup, and discard.

3. Remove 4 cups of the soup—including vegetables and hot broth—from the pot. Place 2 cups of the removed soup in a blender, and place the lid on the blender, leaving the top slightly ajar to allow steam to escape. Carefully blend at low speed until the mixture is smooth. Return the puréed mixture to the pot, and stir to mix well. Repeat with the remaining 2 cups of removed soup.

4. Add the pasta to the pot, and bring to a boil over medium-high heat. Reduce the heat to medium-low, cover, and simmer for 10 minutes, or until the pasta is al dente. (Be careful not to overcook, as the pasta will continue to soften in the hot soup.)

5. Ladle the soup into individual serving bowls, and serve hot.

NUTRITIONAL FACTS (PER 1-CUP SERVING)
Cal: 172   Carbs: 30.8 g   Chol: 0 mg   Fat: 1.9 g
Fiber: 4.4 g   Protein: 7.9 g   Sodium: 386 mg

French Market Soup

YIELD: 7 SERVINGS

$5\frac{1}{2}$ cups water or unsalted chicken broth

$1\frac{1}{2}$ cups dried 15-bean mixture, cleaned and soaked (page 302)

$1\frac{1}{2}$ teaspoons instant chicken or vegetable bouillon granules

$1\frac{1}{2}$ cups sliced smoked sausage or kielbasa, at least 97% lean (about 8 ounces)

$1\frac{1}{4}$ cups diced unpeeled potato (about 1 medium-large)

$3/4$ cup chopped yellow onion

1 medium carrot, peeled and sliced

1 stalk celery, sliced (include the leaves)

2 teaspoons crushed fresh garlic

2 bay leaves

2 teaspoons ground paprika

$1\frac{1}{2}$ teaspoons dried savory

$1/4$ teaspoon ground black pepper

1. Place the water or broth, beans, and bouillon granules in a 3-quart pot, and bring to a boil over high heat. Reduce the heat to low, cover, and simmer, stirring occasionally, for 45 minutes.

2. Add all of the remaining ingredients to the pot, increase the heat to medium-high, and allow the mixture to come to a boil. Reduce the heat to low, cover, and simmer, stirring occasionally, for 45 to 60 additional minutes, or until the beans are soft and the liquid is thick. Periodically check the pot during cooking, and add a little more water or broth if needed.

3. Remove the bay leaves from the soup, and discard. Ladle the soup into individual serving bowls, and serve hot.

NUTRITIONAL FACTS (PER 1-CUP SERVING)
Cal: 219   Carbs: 37 g   Chol: 14 mg   Fat: 1.5 g
Fiber: 8.7 g   Protein: 16 g   Sodium: 421 mg

Italian White Bean Soup

YIELD: 11 SERVINGS

7 cups water or unsalted chicken broth

2 cups dried navy beans or Great Northern beans,
cleaned and soaked (page 302)

1 large Spanish onion, chopped

6 medium plum tomatoes, peeled and diced

2 medium carrots, peeled,
halved lengthwise, and sliced

2 large stalks celery, thinly sliced
(include the leaves)

1 tablespoon plus 2 teaspoons instant chicken
bouillon granules

2½ teaspoons dried oregano

¼ teaspoon ground black pepper

¼ teaspoon cayenne pepper

1 tablespoon white balsamic or
white wine vinegar

1. Place all of the ingredients except for the vinegar in a 4-quart pot, and bring to a boil over high heat. Reduce the heat to low, cover, and simmer, stirring occasionally, for about 1 hour and 30 minutes, or until the beans are soft.

2. Remove 4 cups of the soup—including vegetables, beans, and hot broth—from the pot. Place 2 cups of the removed soup in a blender, and place the lid on the blender, leaving the top slightly ajar to allow steam to escape. Carefully blend at low speed until the mixture is smooth. Return the puréed soup to the pot, and stir to mix well. Repeat with the remaining 2 cups of removed soup.

3. Add the vinegar to the soup, and stir to mix well. Ladle the soup into individual serving bowls, and serve hot.

NUTRITIONAL FACTS (PER 1-CUP SERVING)
Cal: 134   Carbs: 24.2 g   Chol: 0 mg   Fat: 0.5 g
Fiber: 7.5 g   Protein: 8.2 g   Sodium: 324 mg

Spicy Shrimp Gumbo

YIELD: 6 CUPS

1 medium onion, chopped

1 medium green bell pepper, chopped

½ cup thinly sliced celery (include the leaves)

2 teaspoons crushed fresh garlic

4 ounces smoked sausage or kielbasa,
at least 97% lean, diced (about ⅞ cup)

1 can (15 ounces) unsalted tomato sauce

½ cup chicken broth

2 teaspoons ground paprika

1 teaspoon Cajun seasoning

¾ teaspoon dried thyme

1 bay leaf

1 cup frozen (unthawed) whole kernel corn

1 cup frozen (unthawed) cut okra

12 ounces peeled and deveined raw shrimp

1. Place the onion, green pepper, celery, garlic, sausage, tomato sauce, broth, paprika, Cajun seasoning, thyme, and bay leaf in a 2½-quart pot, and bring to a boil over high heat. Reduce the heat to low, cover, and simmer, stirring occasionally, for 15 minutes, or until the vegetables are tender and the flavors are well blended.

2. Add the corn and okra to the sausage mixture. Increase the heat to high, and bring to a boil. Then reduce the heat to medium-low, cover, and simmer for 5 minutes, or until the okra is barely tender.

3. Add the shrimp to the gumbo, cover, and simmer for 5 additional minutes, or until the shrimp turn pink and are thoroughly cooked.

4. Remove the bay leaf from the gumbo, and discard. Serve hot, spooning the gumbo over brown rice if desired.

NUTRITIONAL FACTS (PER 1-CUP SERVING)
Cal: 137   Carbs: 18 g   Chol: 87 mg   Fat: 1.5 g
Fiber: 3.6 g   Protein: 14 g   Sodium: 406 mg

Old-Fashioned Beef Stew

YIELD: 8 CUPS

1 pound beef top round or lean stew beef, cut into bite-sized pieces
1 can (15 ounces) tomato sauce
2 cups unsalted beef broth
1 tablespoon Worcestershire sauce
2 bay leaves
1 teaspoon dried thyme
1 teaspoon dried marjoram
1/4 teaspoon ground black pepper
2 medium potatoes, scrubbed and diced
2 medium carrots, peeled, halved lengthwise, and sliced
1 medium yellow onion, diced
1 cup sliced fresh mushrooms
1 medium stalk celery, thinly sliced (include the leaves)
1 cup frozen (thawed) green peas

1. Trim any visible fat from the meat. Rinse the meat with cool water, and pat it dry with paper towels

2. Coat a large deep nonstick skillet or Dutch oven with nonstick cooking spray, and preheat over medium-high heat. Add the half of the beef at a time to the skillet, and stir-fry for 2 to 3 minutes, or until nicely browned.

3. Stir the tomato sauce, broth, Worcestershire sauce, herbs, and pepper into the meat, and bring to a boil. Reduce the heat to low, cover, and simmer for 1 hour, or until the meat is tender.

4. Add the potatoes, carrots, onion, mushrooms, and celery to the meat. Cover and simmer for 30 minutes, or until the vegetables are tender. Add the peas, and simmer for 10 additional minutes. Remove and discard the bay leaves, and serve hot.

NUTRITIONAL FACTS (PER 1-CUP SERVING)
Cal: 165   Carbs: 19 g   Chol: 29 mg   Fat: 2.6 g
Fiber: 3.4 g   Protein: 16 g   Sodium: 322 mg

Lentil Chili

YIELD: 8 CUPS

2 cups water
3/4 cup dried brown lentils, cleaned (page 302)
1 can (14 1/2 ounces) tomatoes, crushed
1 medium green bell pepper, chopped
1 medium yellow onion, chopped
1 teaspoon crushed fresh garlic
2 tablespoons chili powder
1/2 teaspoon ground cumin
1/4 teaspoon ground allspice
1 can (15 ounces) tomato sauce
2 cups fresh or frozen (thawed) whole kernel corn

1. Place all of the ingredients except for the tomato sauce and corn in a 2 1/2-quart pot, and bring to a boil over high heat. Reduce the heat to low, cover, and simmer, stirring occasionally, for 30 minutes, or until the lentils are tender.

2. Add the tomato sauce and corn to the lentil mixture. Stir to mix, cover, and simmer for 10 to 15 additional minutes.

3. Ladle the chili into individual serving bowls, and serve hot.

NUTRITIONAL FACTS (PER 1-CUP SERVING)
Cal: 133   Carbs: 27 g   Chol: 0 mg   Fat: 0.8 g
Fiber: 8 g   Protein: 8 g   Sodium: 442 mg

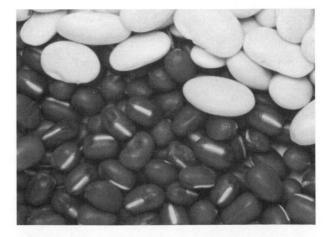

Salsa and Spice Chili

YIELD: 8 SERVINGS

1 pound 95% lean ground beef or
ground turkey

1 can (14$1/2$ ounces) tomatoes, crushed

1 can (8 ounces) unsalted tomato sauce

1 cup bottled salsa, mild or medium

2 cans (15 ounces each)
red kidney beans, drained

1 cup chopped onion

2 tablespoons chili powder

1 teaspoon dried oregano

$1/2$ teaspoon ground cumin

$1/2$ teaspoon ground cinnamon

TOPPINGS

$1/2$ cup shredded nonfat or reduced-fat
Cheddar cheese (optional)

$1/2$ cup nonfat sour cream (optional)

$1/2$ cup chopped scallions (optional)

1. Coat a 3-quart pot with nonstick cooking spray, and preheat over medium heat. Add the beef or turkey, and cook, stirring to crumble, until the meat is no longer pink. Drain off and discard any excess fat.

2. Add the tomatoes, tomato sauce, salsa, beans, onion, chili powder, oregano, cumin, and cinnamon to the pot, and stir to mix. Increase the heat to medium-high, and bring the mixture to a boil. Reduce the heat to low, cover, and simmer, stirring occasionally, for 25 to 30 minutes, or until the onions are soft and the flavors are well blended.

3. Serve hot, topping each serving with some of the cheese, sour cream, and scallions, if desired.

NUTRITIONAL FACTS (PER 1-CUP SERVING)
Cal: 225   Carbs: 29 g   Chol: 30 mg   Fat: 3.4 g
Fiber: 11 g   Protein: 19 g   Sodium: 456 mg

Fiesta Chili

YIELD: 8 SERVINGS

1 pound 95% lean ground beef or ground turkey

1 can (14$1/2$ ounces) unsalted tomatoes, crushed

1 can (15 ounces) tomato sauce

1 can (15 ounces) red kidney beans
or black beans, drained

1 cup chopped onion

2 tablespoons chili powder

$1/2$ teaspoon ground cumin

1$1/2$ cups fresh or frozen (thawed) whole kernel corn

1 can (4 ounces) chopped green chilies, drained

$3/4$ cup shredded nonfat or reduced-fat
Cheddar cheese (optional)

1. Coat a 3-quart pot with nonstick cooking spray, and preheat over medium heat. Add the beef or turkey, and cook, stirring to crumble, until the meat is no longer pink. Drain off and discard any excess fat.

2. Add the tomatoes, tomato sauce, beans, onion, chili powder, and cumin to the pot, and stir to mix. Increase the heat to medium-high, and bring the mixture to a boil. Reduce the heat to low, cover, and simmer, stirring occasionally, for 20 minutes, or until the onions are soft and the flavors are well blended.

3. Add the corn and chilies to the pot. Cover and simmer for 5 minutes, or until the flavors are well blended. Serve hot, topping each serving with a rounded tablespoon of the Cheddar, if desired.

NUTRITIONAL FACTS (PER 1-CUP SERVING)
Cal: 197   Carbs: 26 g   Chol: 30 mg   Fat: 3.4 g
Fiber: 8.2 g   Protein: 17.5 g   Sodium: 489 mg

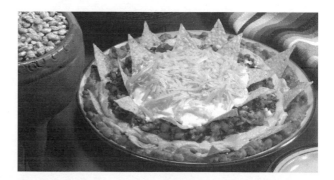

Mexican Bean Soup

YIELD: 7 SERVINGS

4$\frac{1}{2}$ cups water or unsalted chicken broth

1$\frac{1}{2}$ cups dried pinto beans, cleaned and soaked (page 302)

1 medium Spanish onion, chopped

1 medium carrot, peeled, halved lengthwise, and sliced

6 ounces ham, at least 97% lean, diced (about 1$\frac{1}{8}$ cups)

1 tablespoon chopped pickled jalapeño pepper

2$\frac{1}{2}$ teaspoons chili powder

1$\frac{1}{2}$ teaspoons instant chicken bouillon granules

1 teaspoon ground cumin

1. Place all of the ingredients in a 3-quart pot, and bring to a boil over high heat. Reduce the heat to low, cover, and simmer, stirring occasionally, for about 2 hours, or until the beans are soft and the liquid is thick. Add a little more water during cooking if the soup begins to dry out.

2. Ladle the soup into individual serving bowls, and serve hot.

NUTRITIONAL FACTS (PER 1-CUP SERVING)
Cal: 170   Carbs: 25 g   Chol: 11 mg   Fat: 1.5 g
Fiber: 8.6 g   Protein: 14 g   Sodium: 439 mg

7. The Well-Dressed Salad

Salads are among the most versatile of dishes. Depending on their ingredients, they can be light or substantial; sweet or savory; a protein-packed entrée, or a refreshing side dish. Because most salads can be made ahead of time, they are great for entertaining. And because they are portable, they are as much at home at picnics and pot-luck suppers as they are on your own dining room table.

If you're watching your weight, though, beware. Despite the salad's reputation for being a "diet" food, many have no place in a fat- or calorie-controlled menu. Take your typical chef's salad, for instance. A pile of greens topped with strips of full-fat cheese and meat, a hard-boiled egg, and two tablespoons of regular salad dressing can easily deliver 650 calories and 50 grams of fat. And that's if you stop at just two tablespoons of dressing! The truth is that the calories and fat you consume from salads can have a big impact on your overall health. This is especially true when you consider that the average woman gets more fat from salad dressing than from any other food!

Made properly, though, salads are just what the doctor ordered. Ingredients like nonfat and reduced-fat mayonnaise, oil-free and reduced-fat salad dressings, nonfat and light sour cream, nonfat and reduced-fat cheeses, and ultra-lean meats make it possible to create a dazzling array of salads with little or no fat, and with much fewer calories than traditional versions. The recipes in this chapter combine these ingredients with crisp vegetables, ripe fruits, satisfying pastas, and nutritious whole grains to create a variety of fresh salads that will help you get your five-a-day of fruits and veggies in the most healthful and enjoyable way possible.

So whether you're looking for a main-dish grilled chicken salad, a delightful garden side salad, a temptingly sweet fruit salad, or a hearty pasta or bean salad, you need look no further. You'll find that—without sacrificing the flavors you love—you can create a salad that minimizes fat and calories, while maximizing the nutrients that promote a lifetime of good health.

Tuscan Tuna and Pasta Salad

YIELD: 6 SERVINGS

1/2 cup sun-dried tomatoes (not packed in oil)

10 ounces mostaccioli or penne pasta
(about 3 1/3 cups)

2 cups 1-inch pieces young tender green beans
(about 8 ounces)

2 cans (6 ounces each) water-packed
albacore tuna, drained

1/4 cup plus 2 tablespoons sliced black olives

DRESSING

1/2 cup bottled nonfat or reduced-fat
red wine vinaigrette salad dressing

1 tablespoon lemon juice

1 teaspoon crushed fresh garlic

1 teaspoon dried thyme

1/8 teaspoon ground black pepper

1. Place the tomatoes in a heatproof bowl, and add boiling water just to cover. Set aside for 10 minutes, or until the tomatoes have plumped. Drain well, and slice the tomatoes into thin strips. Set aside.

2. Cook the pasta al dente according to package directions. About 4 minutes before the pasta is done, add the green beans, and cook until the pasta is al dente and the beans are crisp-tender. Drain, rinse with cold water, and drain again.

3. Place the pasta mixture in a large bowl. Add the tuna, olives, and tomatoes, and toss to mix well.

4. Place the dressing ingredients in a small bowl, and stir to mix. Pour the dressing over the pasta mixture, and toss to mix well.

5. Cover the salad, and chill for at least 2 hours before serving. Toss in a little more dressing just before serving if the salad seems too dry.

NUTRITIONAL FACTS (PER 1 3/4-CUP SERVING)
Cal: 284   Carbs: 44 g   Chol: 16 mg   Fat: 2.4 g
Fiber: 3.4 g   Protein: 21 g   Sodium: 571 mg

Broccoli and Basil Pasta Salad

YIELD: 10 SERVINGS

8 ounces rotini pasta (about 3 cups)
or radiatore pasta (about 2 2/3 cups)

2 cups fresh broccoli florets

2/3 cup diagonally sliced carrots (about 1 large)

1/2 cup matchstick-sized pieces red bell pepper
(about 1/2 medium)

DRESSING

1/2 cup nonfat or reduced-fat mayonnaise

1/3 cup nonfat or light sour cream

2 tablespoons orange juice

2 teaspoons Dijon mustard

1 tablespoon finely chopped fresh basil,
or 1 teaspoon dried

1/8 teaspoon ground white pepper

1. Cook the pasta al dente according to package directions. About 1 minute before the pasta is done, add the broccoli and carrots, and cook until the pasta is al dente and the broccoli turns bright green and is crisp-tender. Drain, rinse with cold water, and drain again.

2. Place the pasta mixture in a large bowl, and toss in the red pepper.

3. Place the dressing ingredients in a small bowl, and stir to mix. Pour the dressing over the pasta and vegetables, and toss gently to mix well.

4. Cover the salad, and chill for at least 2 hours or overnight before serving. Stir in a little more mayonnaise just before serving if the salad seems too dry.

NUTRITIONAL FACTS (PER 3/4-CUP SERVING)
Cal: 111   Carbs: 22 g   Chol: 0 mg   Fat: 0.5 g
Fiber: 1.5 g   Protein: 4 g   Sodium: 111 mg

Sesame Shrimp and Noodle Salad

For variety, substitute thin strips of cooked chicken breast for the shrimp.

YIELD: 6 SERVINGS

8 ounces fettuccine pasta

2 cups cooked shrimp (about 10 ounces)

1 medium red bell pepper, cut into thin strips

1 medium cucumber, peeled, seeded, and diced

4 scallions, thinly sliced

DRESSING

1/3 cup seasoned rice wine vinegar

2 tablespoons reduced-sodium soy sauce

1 tablespoon sesame oil

1 teaspoon crushed fresh garlic

1/4 teaspoon ground ginger

1/8 teaspoon ground white pepper

1. Cook the fettuccine al dente according to package directions. Drain, rinse with cold water, and drain again.

2. Place the fettuccine in a large bowl. Add the shrimp and vegetables, and toss to mix.

3. Place the dressing ingredients in a small bowl, and stir to mix. Pour the dressing over the pasta mixture, and toss to mix well.

4. Cover the salad, and chill for several hours before serving.

NUTRITIONAL FACTS (PER 1⅓-CUP SERVING)

Cal: 226   Carbs: 32 g   Chol: 92 mg   Fat: 3.4 g
Fiber: 1.6 g   Protein: 15 g   Sodium: 571 mg

Italian Pasta Salad

This is a basic salad that can be varied in many ways.

YIELD: 8 SERVINGS

8 ounces rotini pasta (about 3 cups) or penne pasta (about 2⅔ cups)

1 medium tomato, chopped

1/4 cup sliced scallions

1/4 cup sliced black olives

1/3 cup bottled nonfat or reduced-fat Italian salad dressing

1/4 cup grated nonfat or regular Parmesan cheese

1. Cook the pasta al dente according to package directions. Drain, rinse with cold water, and drain again.

2. Place the pasta in a large bowl. Add the tomato, scallions, and olives, and toss to mix well. Add the Italian dressing and cheese, and toss to mix well.

3. Cover the salad, and chill for at least 2 hours or overnight before serving. Toss in a little more dressing just before serving if the salad seems too dry.

NUTRITIONAL FACTS (PER ¾-CUP SERVING)

Cal: 130   Carbs: 25 g   Chol: 2 mg   Fat: 0.9 g
Fiber: 1.1 g   Protein: 4.9 g   Sodium: 226 mg

VARIATIONS

For variety, add any of the following ingredients:

- 1/2 cup chopped seeded cucumber and 1/2 cup chopped red bell pepper
- 1 cup lightly steamed broccoli florets
- 12 ounces cooked shrimp
- 1 cup chopped artichoke hearts
- 1/2 cup zucchini cut into matchstick-sized pieces and 1/2 cup grated carrot
- 1 cup cooked or canned kidney beans, chickpeas, or white beans

Minestrone Salad

YIELD: 9 CUPS

8 ounces rotini pasta (about 3 cups)

1 cup 1-inch pieces young tender green beans (about ⅓ pound), or 1 cup frozen (unthawed) green beans

1 can (15 ounces) red kidney beans, rinsed and drained

1 small zucchini, quartered lengthwise and thinly sliced (about 1 cup)

1 cup coarsely shredded cabbage

1 cup chopped seeded plum tomatoes (about 3 medium)

½ cup bottled nonfat or reduced-fat Italian salad dressing

¼ cup grated nonfat or regular Parmesan cheese

1 teaspoon dried basil

⅛ teaspoon ground black pepper

1. Cook the pasta al dente according to package directions. About 4 minutes before the pasta is done, add the green beans, and cook until the pasta is al dente and the beans are crisp-tender. Drain, rinse with cold water, and drain again.

2. Place the pasta mixture in a large bowl. Add the kidney beans, zucchini, cabbage, and tomatoes, and toss to mix well. Add the salad dressing, Parmesan, basil, and pepper, and toss to mix well.

3. Cover the salad, and chill for at least 2 hours before serving. Toss in a little more dressing just before serving if the salad seems too dry.

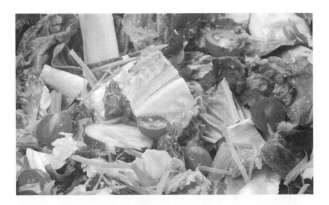

NUTRITIONAL FACTS (PER 1-CUP SERVING)
Cal: 163   Carbs: 31 g   Chol: 1 mg   Fat: 0.7 g
Fiber: 3.9 g   Protein: 7.9 g   Sodium: 213 mg

Antipasto Pasta Salad

YIELD: 10 CUPS

8 ounces penne pasta (about 2⅔ cups) or rotini pasta (about 3 cups)

1 cup sliced fresh mushrooms

4 ounces ham, at least 97% lean, thinly sliced and cut into thin strips

1 cup diced nonfat or reduced-fat mozzarella cheese

1 cup chopped frozen (thawed) or canned (drained) artichoke hearts

½ cup thin strips commercial roasted red pepper (half of a 7-ounce jar)

½ cup thinly sliced scallions or leeks

½ cup sliced black olives

½ cup bottled nonfat or reduced-fat red wine vinaigrette salad dressing

½ teaspoon dried oregano

1. Cook the pasta al dente according to package directions. About 2 minutes before the pasta is done, add the mushrooms, and cook until the pasta is al dente and the mushrooms are lightly cooked. Drain, rinse with cold water, and drain again.

2. Place the pasta mixture in a large bowl. Add the ham, cheese, artichoke hearts, roasted pepper, scallions or leeks, and olives, and toss to mix. Add the dressing and oregano, and toss to mix well.

3. Cover the salad, and chill for at least 2 hours before serving. Toss in a little more salad dressing just before serving if the salad seems too dry.

NUTRITIONAL FACTS (PER 1-CUP SERVING)
Cal: 133   Carbs: 20 g   Chol: 8 mg   Fat: 1.4 g
Fiber: 1 g   Protein: 8 g   Sodium: 311 mg

Orzo and Broccoli Salad

YIELD: 6 SERVINGS

1/3 cup chopped sun-dried tomatoes
(not packed in oil)

1 cup orzo pasta

2 cups chopped fresh broccoli

2 tablespoons pine nuts (optional)

DRESSING

1/4 cup plus 2 tablespoons bottled nonfat
or reduced-fat Italian salad dressing

1/2 teaspoon crushed fresh garlic

1/2 teaspoon dried basil

1/8 teaspoon ground black pepper

1. Place the tomatoes in a heatproof bowl, and add boiling water just to cover. Set aside for 10 minutes, or until the tomatoes have plumped. Drain well, and set aside.

2. Cook the orzo al dente according to package directions. About 1 minute before the pasta is done, add the broccoli, and cook until the pasta is al dente and the broccoli turns bright green and is crisp-tender. Drain, rinse with cold water, and drain again.

3. Place the pasta mixture in a large bowl. Toss in the tomatoes and, if desired, the pine nuts.

4. Place the dressing ingredients in a small bowl, and stir to mix. Pour the dressing over the pasta mixture, and toss to mix well.

5. Cover the salad, and chill for at least 4 hours before serving. Toss in a little more dressing just before serving if the salad seems too dry.

NUTRITIONAL FACTS (PER 2/3-CUP SERVING)		
Cal: 131 Carbs: 26 g Chol: 0 mg Fat: 0.6 g		
Fiber: 1.9 g Protein: 4.9 g Sodium: 192 mg		

Shrimp and Pasta Salad

YIELD: 5 SERVINGS

10 ounces small seashell pasta (about 3 1/2 cups)

1 1/2 cups (about 8 ounces) cooked shrimp
or crab meat

3/4 cup chopped frozen (thawed) artichoke hearts,
canned (drained) artichoke hearts,
or frozen (thawed) green peas

1/2 cup finely chopped celery

1/2 cup diced red bell pepper

1/4 cup chopped onion

DRESSING

1/2 cup nonfat or reduced-fat mayonnaise

3 tablespoons grated nonfat or regular
Parmesan cheese

1 tablespoon lemon juice

1/2 teaspoon dried Italian seasoning

1/8 teaspoon ground white pepper

1. Cook the pasta al dente according to package directions. Drain, rinse with cold water, and drain again.

2. Place the pasta in a large bowl. Add the seafood and vegetables, and toss to mix well.

3. Place the dressing ingredients in a small bowl, and stir to mix. Pour the dressing over the pasta mixture, and toss to mix well.

4. Cover the salad, and chill for at least 2 hours before serving. Toss in a little more mayonnaise just before serving if the salad seems too dry.

NUTRITIONAL FACTS (PER 1 3/4-CUP SERVING)		
Cal: 302 Carbs: 52 g Chol: 90 mg Fat: 1.5 g		
Fiber: 2.9 g Protein: 19 g Sodium: 353 mg		

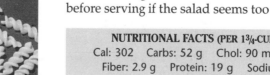

Slim Caesar Salad

YIELD: 6 SERVINGS

12 cups torn romaine lettuce

3 tablespoons grated nonfat or regular
Parmesan cheese

GARLIC CROUTONS

1 tablespoon crushed fresh garlic

2½ cups Italian or French bread cubes

1 tablespoon grated nonfat or regular
Parmesan cheese

¼ teaspoon dried Italian seasoning

Nonstick olive oil cooking spray

DRESSING

½ cup nonfat or reduced-fat mayonnaise

¼ cup fat-free egg substitute

¼ cup grated nonfat or regular Parmesan cheese

1 tablespoon white wine vinegar

1 tablespoon lemon juice

2 teaspoons chopped anchovy fillets,
or 1 teaspoon anchovy paste

1 teaspoon crushed fresh garlic

1. To make the croutons, rub the garlic over the inside of a medium-sized bowl. Place the bread cubes in the bowl, add the Parmesan and Italian seasoning, and toss gently to mix well and to coat the cubes with the garlic and other seasonings.

2. Coat a baking sheet with nonstick cooking spray, and arrange the cubes in a single layer on the sheet. Spray the cubes lightly with the cooking spray, and bake at 350°F for 8 minutes. Turn the cubes with a spatula, spray again, and bake for 4 additional minutes, or until the croutons are lightly browned and crisp.

3. Turn the oven off, and allow the croutons to cool in the oven with the door ajar for 15 minutes. Store in an airtight container until ready to use.

4. Place all of the dressing ingredients in a blender, and blend for about 1 minute, or until smooth.

5. Place the lettuce in a large salad bowl. Pour the dressing over the lettuce, and toss to mix well. Add the croutons and Parmesan, and toss to mix well. Serve immediately.

NUTRITIONAL FACTS (PER 2-CUP SERVING)
Cal: 95   Carbs: 15 g   Chol: 5 mg   Fat: 0.9 g
Fiber: 2.3 g   Protein: 7 g   Sodium: 336 mg

TIME-SAVING TIP
To prepare Slim Caesar Salad in no time flat, substitute 2 cups of ready-made fat-free or low-fat garlic or Caesar croutons for the homemade croutons.

Seashell Seafood Salad

YIELD: 6 SERVINGS

12 ounces small seashell pasta (about 3½ cups)

2 cups (about 10 ounces) cooked lump crab meat,
lobster, or shrimp

1 cup frozen (thawed) green peas

½ cup chopped red bell pepper

⅓ cup chopped onion

DRESSING

⅔ cup nonfat or reduced-fat mayonnaise

⅓ cup nonfat or light sour cream

1 tablespoon plus 1 teaspoon lemon juice

1 tablespoon minced fresh dill, or 1 teaspoon dried

1. Cook the pasta al dente according to package directions. Drain, rinse with cold water, and drain again.

2. Place the pasta in a large bowl. Add the seafood and vegetables, and toss to mix.

3. Place the dressing ingredients in a small bowl, and stir to mix. Pour the dressing over the pasta mixture, and toss to mix well.

4. Cover the salad, and chill for several hours before serving.

NUTRITIONAL FACTS (PER 1½-CUP SERVING)
Cal: 310   Carbs: 57 g   Chol: 30 mg   Fat: 1.5 g
Fiber: 2.8 g   Protein: 17 g   Sodium: 382 mg

Gorgonzola Garden Salad

YIELD: 4 SERVINGS

8 cups mixed salad greens or torn butter crunch or romaine lettuce

1 can (10 ounces) mandarin orange sections, well drained

1/2 cup diagonally sliced celery

4 thin slices red or sweet white onion, separated into rings

1/4 cup crumbled Gorgonzola or blue cheese

1/4 cup dark raisins

1/4 cup chopped walnuts (optional)

1/2 cup bottled nonfat or low-fat raspberry or balsamic vinaigrette salad dressing

1. Arrange 2 cups of the salad greens on each of 4 salad plates. Top the lettuce on each plate with a quarter of the mandarin oranges, 2 tablespoons of celery, and a quarter of the onion rings. Sprinkle with 1 tablespoon each of cheese, raisins, and if desired, walnuts.

2. Drizzle 2 tablespoons of the dressing over each salad, and serve immediately.

> **NUTRITIONAL FACTS (PER 2½-CUP SERVING)**
> Cal: 141   Carbs: 26.5 g   Chol: 6 mg   Fat: 2.7 g
> Fiber: 4.3 g   Protein: 4.7 g   Sodium: 222 mg

Primavera Pasta Salad

YIELD: 8 SERVINGS

8 ounces rotini or wagon wheel pasta (about 3 cups)

2 cups fresh broccoli florets, fresh snow peas, or fresh asparagus spears, cut into 1-inch pieces

1 cup sliced carrots

1/2 cup sliced fresh mushrooms

1/2 cup matchstick-sized pieces red bell pepper

1/3 cup thinly sliced scallions

1/2 cup bottled nonfat or reduced-fat Italian salad dressing

1/4 cup grated nonfat or regular Parmesan cheese

1/2 teaspoon dried Italian seasoning

1. Cook the pasta al dente according to package directions. About 2 minutes before the pasta is done, add the broccoli, snow peas, or asparagus; carrots; and mushrooms. Cook until the pasta is al dente and the vegetables are crisp-tender. Drain well, rinse with cold water, and drain again.

2. Place the pasta mixture in a large bowl. Add the red pepper and scallions, and toss to mix well. Add the dressing, Parmesan, and Italian seasoning, and toss to mix well.

3. Cover the salad, and chill for at least 2 hours before serving. Add a little more dressing just before serving if the salad seems too dry.

> **NUTRITIONAL FACTS (PER 1-CUP SERVING)**
> Cal: 141   Carbs: 28 g   Chol: 1 mg   Fat: 0.6 g
> Fiber: 1.8 g   Protein: 6 g   Sodium: 181 mg

Berry Delicious Spinach Salad

YIELD: 4 SERVINGS

4 cups fresh spinach

1½ cups sliced fresh strawberries

1/2 cup diced nonfat or low-fat mozzarella cheese

1/4 cup diagonally sliced celery

4 thin slices red onion, separated into rings

1/2 cup bottled nonfat or low-fat raspberry vinaigrette salad dressing

1/4 cup golden raisins

1/4 cup toasted chopped pecans or almonds (page 348) (optional)

1. Place the spinach, strawberries, cheese, celery, and onion rings in a large bowl, and toss to mix well. Pour the dressing over the salad, and toss to mix well.

2. Divide the salad among 4 salad bowls. Top each serving with a tablespoon of the raisins and, if desired, a tablespoon of the pecans or almonds. Serve immediately.

> **NUTRITIONAL FACTS (PER 1¾-CUP SERVING)**
> Cal: 124   Carbs: 28 g   Chol: 1 mg   Fat: 0.5 g
> Fiber: 3.3 g   Protein: 7 g   Sodium: 183 mg

Italian Ham and Cheese Salad

YIELD: 5 SERVINGS
8 ounces penne pasta (about 2²/₃ cups)
1 cup diced ham, at least 97% lean (about 5 ounces)
1 cup diced nonfat or reduced-fat mozzarella cheese
1 cup frozen (thawed) green peas
²/₃ cup matchstick-sized pieces red bell pepper
¹/₃ cup sliced black olives
3 scallions, thinly sliced

DRESSING

¹/₄ cup nonfat or light sour cream
¹/₄ cup plus 2 tablespoons nonfat or reduced-fat mayonnaise
1 tablespoon Dijon mustard
³/₄ teaspoon dried Italian seasoning

1. Cook the pasta al dente according to package directions. Drain, rinse with cold water, and drain again.

2. Place the pasta in a large bowl. Add the ham, mozzarella, peas, red pepper, olives, and scallions, and toss to mix.

3. Place the dressing ingredients in a small bowl, and stir to mix. Pour the dressing over the pasta mixture, and toss to mix well.

4. Cover the salad, and chill for at least 2 hours before serving. Toss in a little more mayonnaise just before serving if the salad seems too dry.

NUTRITIONAL FACTS (PER 1²/₃-CUP SERVING)
Cal: 300 Carbs: 47 g Chol: 10 mg Fat: 2.8 g
Fiber: 3.4 g Protein: 21 g Sodium: 778 mg

Neptune Pasta Salad

For variety, substitute fresh asparagus pieces for the broccoli.

YIELD: 5 SERVINGS
8 ounces tricolor rotini pasta (about 3 cups)
1¹/₃ cups fresh broccoli florets
2 cups cooked crab meat or shrimp (about 10 ounces)
²/₃ cup matchstick-sized pieces red bell pepper
3 scallions, thinly sliced

DRESSING

¹/₂ cup nonfat or reduced-fat mayonnaise
¹/₄ cup bottled nonfat or reduced-fat Italian salad dressing
2¹/₄ teaspoons finely chopped fresh oregano, or ³/₄ teaspoon dried

1. Cook the pasta al dente according to package directions. About 1 minute before the pasta is done, add the broccoli, and cook until the pasta is al dente and the broccoli is bright green and crisp-tender. Drain, rinse with cold water, and drain again.

2. Place the pasta mixture in a large bowl. Add the crab meat or shrimp, red pepper, and scallions, and toss to mix.

3. Place the dressing ingredients in a small bowl, and stir to mix. Pour the dressing over the pasta, and toss to mix well.

4. Cover the salad, and chill for at least 2 hours before serving. Toss in a little more mayonnaise just before serving if the salad seems too dry.

NUTRITIONAL FACTS (PER 1²/₃-CUP SERVING)
Cal: 252 Carbs: 41 g Chol: 36 mg Fat: 1.4 g
Fiber: 2.4 g Protein: 17 g Sodium: 537 mg

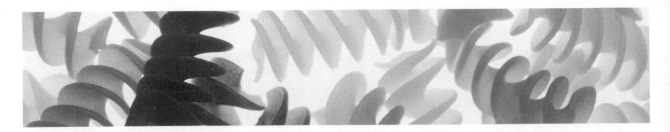

Pasta Salad Niçoise

YIELD: 5 SERVINGS

8 ounces penne pasta (about $2^2/_3$ cups)

$1^1/_2$ cups young tender fresh green beans

1 can (9 ounces) water-packed albacore tuna, drained

$3/_4$ cup chopped frozen (thawed) or canned (drained) artichoke hearts

$3/_4$ cup matchstick-sized pieces red bell pepper

$1/_2$ cup diced red onion

$1/_3$ cup sliced black olives

$1^1/_2$ tablespoons finely chopped fresh lemon thyme, or $1^1/_2$ teaspoons dried thyme

DRESSING

$1/_2$ cup bottled nonfat or reduced-fat Italian salad dressing

2 teaspoons Dijon mustard

$3/_4$ teaspoon crushed fresh garlic

1. Cook the pasta al dente according to package directions. About 4 minutes before the pasta is done, add the green beans, and cook until the beans are crisp-tender and the pasta is al dente. Drain, rinse with cold water, and drain again.

2. Place the pasta mixture in a large bowl. Add the tuna, artichoke hearts, red pepper, onion, olives, and thyme, and toss gently to mix well.

3. Place the dressing ingredients in a small bowl, and stir to mix well. Pour the dressing over the pasta mixture, and toss gently to mix.

4. Cover the salad, and chill for at least 2 hours before serving. Toss in a little more dressing just before serving if the salad seems too dry.

> **NUTRITIONAL FACTS** (PER $1^3/_4$-CUP SERVING)
> Cal: 284   Carbs: 45 g   Chol: 14 mg   Fat: 2.5 g
> Fiber: 4.5 g   Protein: 19.6 g   Sodium: 543 mg

Old-Fashioned Macaroni Salad

YIELD: 8 SERVINGS

8 ounces elbow macaroni (about $1^3/_4$ cups)

$1/_4$ cup sliced black olives

$1/_4$ cup thinly sliced celery

$1/_4$ cup finely chopped red bell pepper, or $1/_4$ cup shredded carrot

$1/_4$ cup chopped onion

1 tablespoon minced fresh chives or dill, or 1 teaspoon dried

DRESSING

$1/_2$ cup nonfat or reduced-fat mayonnaise

$1/_4$ cup nonfat or light sour cream

1 tablespoon spicy mustard

$1/_8$ teaspoon ground black pepper

1. Cook the macaroni al dente according to package directions. Drain, rinse with cold water, and drain again.

2. Place the macaroni in a large bowl. Add the olives, celery, red pepper or carrots, onion, and chives or dill, and toss to mix.

3. Place the dressing ingredients in a small bowl, and stir to mix. Pour the dressing over the macaroni mixture, and toss to mix well.

4. Cover the salad, and chill for several hours before serving. Toss in a little more mayonnaise just before serving if the salad seems too dry.

> **NUTRITIONAL FACTS** (PER $2/_3$-CUP SERVING)
> Cal: 130   Carbs: 26.6 g   Chol: 0 mg   Fat: 0.8 g
> Fiber: 1 g   Protein: 4.1 g   Sodium: 177 mg

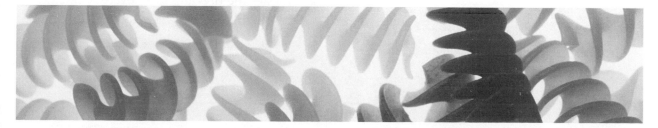

The Crowning Touch

Salads are among the most healthful dishes you can add to your diet. But if you top your fresh salad with an oily dressing, you're probably taking a big bite out of your fat budget. And while supermarkets now stock a wide range of low-fat and nonfat dressings, it's important to keep in mind that many commercial dressings still contain far too much sodium. What's the alternative? The following dressings—which are a snap to prepare—will be not only low in sodium and fat, but also full of the fresh-made flavor that only homemade dressings can offer.

Tangy Tomato Dressing

YIELD: 2 CUPS

1 can (10¾ ounces) condensed tomato soup, undiluted

½ cup chopped onion

¼ cup plus 2 tablespoons white wine vinegar

2 tablespoons sugar or honey

2 tablespoons extra virgin olive oil

2 teaspoons ground paprika

1 teaspoon dry mustard

1 teaspoon dried thyme

¼ teaspoon ground black pepper

4 cloves garlic

1. Place all of the ingredients in a blender, and process for 1 minute, or until smooth.

2. Transfer the dressing to a covered container, and chill for several hours before serving.

NUTRITIONAL FACTS (PER TABLESPOON)
Cal: 19   Carbs: 2.9 g   Chol: 0 mg   Fat: 1 g
Fiber: 0.1 g   Protein 0.2 g   Sodium: 53 mg

Roasted Red Pepper Dressing

YIELD: 1 CUP

½ cup chopped commercial roasted red pepper

¼ cup balsamic vinegar

¼ cup water

¼ cup grated nonfat or regular Parmesan cheese

2 tablespoons extra virgin olive oil

2 teaspoons crushed fresh garlic

½ teaspoon dried Italian seasoning

¼ teaspoon salt

⅛ teaspoon ground black pepper

1. Place all of the ingredients in a blender, and process for about 1 minute, or until smooth.

2. Transfer the mixture to a covered container, and chill for several hours before serving.

NUTRITIONAL FACTS (PER TABLESPOON)
Cal: 22   Carbs: 1 g   Chol: 1 mg   Fat: 1.7 g
Fiber: 0 g   Protein: 0.6 g   Sodium: 70 mg

Honey Mustard Dressing

YIELD: 1¼ CUPS

¾ cup nonfat or reduced-fat mayonnaise

3 tablespoons honey

3 tablespoons Dijon mustard

2 tablespoons water

1. Place all of the ingredients in a small bowl, and stir to mix well.

2. Transfer the dressing to a covered container, and chill for several hours before serving

NUTRITIONAL FACTS (PER TABLESPOON)
Cal: 17   Carbs: 4 g   Chol: 0 mg   Fat: 0.1 g
Fiber: 0.1 g   Protein: 0.1 g   Sodium: 92 mg

Creamy Italian Dressing

YIELD: 1²/₃ CUPS

1¹/₄ cups nonfat or reduced-fat mayonnaise

¹/₄ cup skim or low-fat milk

¹/₄ cup grated nonfat or regular Parmesan cheese

2 tablespoons white wine vinegar

2 teaspoons crushed fresh garlic

¹/₂ teaspoon dried Italian seasoning

¹/₈ teaspoon ground white pepper

1. Place all of the ingredients in small bowl, and stir to mix well.

2. Transfer the dressing to a covered container, and chill for several hours before serving.

NUTRITIONAL FACTS (PER TABLESPOON)
Cal: 11   Carbs: 2.3 g   Chol: 1 mg   Fat: 0 g
Fiber: 0 g   Protein: 0.4 g   Sodium: 72 mg

Thick and Creamy Thousand Island Dressing

YIELD: 1¹/₂ CUPS

³/₄ cup nonfat or reduced-fat mayonnaise

¹/₃ cup nonfat or light sour cream

¹/₄ cup chili sauce

2 tablespoons sweet pickle relish

2 teaspoons finely chopped onion

¹/₄ teaspoon garlic powder

¹/₈ teaspoon ground white pepper

1. Place the mayonnaise and sour cream in a small bowl, and stir to mix well. Add the remaining ingredients, and stir to mix well.

2. Transfer the dressing to a covered container, and chill for several hours before serving.

NUTRITIONAL FACTS (PER TABLESPOON)
Cal: 13   Carbs: 3 g   Chol: 0 mg   Fat 0 g
Fiber: 0 g   Protein: 0.3 g   Sodium: 102 mg

Sour Cream-Blue Cheese Dressing

YIELD: 1¹/₂ CUPS

³/₄ cup nonfat or reduced-fat mayonnaise

¹/₂ cup nonfat or light sour cream

1 teaspoon crushed fresh garlic

¹/₈ teaspoon ground white pepper

¹/₂ cup plus 2 tablespoons crumbled
blue cheese, divided

1. Place all of the ingredients except for half of the blue cheese in a blender or food processor, and process to mix well. Stir in the remaining blue cheese. Add a little milk if the mixture is too thick.

2. Serve immediately or transfer the dressing to a covered container, and chill for several hours before serving. This dressing is best used within 12 hours. After that, it will start to develop a thinner consistency.

NUTRITIONAL FACTS (PER TABLESPOON)
Cal: 21   Carbs: 2 g   Chol: 2 mg   Fat: 1 g
Fiber: 0 g   Protein: 1 g   Sodium: 105 mg

Tex-Mex Salad Dressing

YIELD: 1¹/₈ CUPS

¹/₃ cup nonfat or light sour cream

¹/₃ cup nonfat or reduced-fat
mayonnaise

¹/₂ cup bottled chunky salsa

1. Place the sour cream and mayonnaise in a small bowl, and stir to mix well. Stir in the salsa.

2. Transfer the dressing to a covered container, and chill for several hours before serving.

NUTRITIONAL FACTS (PER TABLESPOON)
Cal: 10   Carbs: 2.4 g   Chol: 0 mg   Fat: 0 g
Fiber: 0 g   Protein: 0.1 g   Sodium: 68 mg

Spruced-Up Spinach Salad

YIELD: 6 SERVINGS

9 cups fresh spinach leaves

2 cups sliced fresh mushrooms

1 small red bell pepper, sliced into thin strips

3 thin slices sweet or red onion, separated into rings

3/4 cup shredded nonfat or reduced-fat
Cheddar cheese

6 slices extra-lean turkey bacon, cooked,
drained, and crumbled

2 hard boiled eggs. chopped

3/4 cup Tangy Tomato Dressing (page 188)
or bottled nonfat or reduced-fat French,
honey mustard, or ranch salad dressing

1. Place the spinach, mushrooms, red pepper, and onion in a large salad bowl, and toss to mix well.

2. Divide the salad among 4 salad bowls. Top each serving with some of the cheese, bacon, and eggs, and a few spoonsful of the dressing. Serve immediately.

NUTRITIONAL FACTS (PER 2-CUP SERVING)
Cal: 132   Carbs: 11.3 g   Chol: 91 mg   Fat: 4.5 g
Fiber: 2.3 g   Protein: 12 g   Sodium: 395 mg

Italian Garden Salad

YIELD: 6 SERVINGS

6 cups torn romaine or iceberg lettuce

1 1/2 cups coarsely chopped radicchio lettuce
or coarsely shredded purple cabbage

2 thin slices red onion, separated into rings

1 cup sliced fresh mushrooms

2 plum tomatoes, sliced

3/4 cup canned chickpeas, rinsed and drained

1 medium carrot, peeled

1/4 cup grated nonfat or regular Parmesan cheese

1 teaspoon dried oregano

1/2 cup bottled nonfat or reduced-fat red wine
vinaigrette or Italian salad dressing

1. Place the lettuce, radicchio or cabbage, onion, mushrooms, tomatoes, and chickpeas in a large salad bowl. Using a potato peeler, shred the carrot into thin strips and add it to the bowl. Add the Parmesan and oregano, and toss to mix well.

2. Drizzle the dressing over the salad, and toss to mix well. Serve immediately.

NUTRITIONAL FACTS (PER 2-CUP SERVING)
Cal: 101   Carbs: 18.3 g   Chol: 0 mg   Fat: 0.9 g
Fiber: 3.2 g   Protein: 6.2 g   Sodium: 241 mg

Fiesta Layered Salad

YIELD: 8 SERVINGS

3/4 cup nonfat or light sour cream

3/4 cup nonfat or reduced-fat mayonnaise

8 cups torn romaine lettuce

1 can (1 pound) red kidney beans, rinsed and drained

1 cup shredded nonfat or reduced-fat Cheddar cheese

1 cup chopped green bell pepper

1/2 medium sweet onion, thinly sliced

1 cup diced plum tomato

1 cup diced avocado

GARNISH

1/4 cup shredded nonfat or reduced-fat
Cheddar cheese

1/4 cup sliced black olives

1. Place the sour cream and mayonnaise in a small bowl. Stir to mix well, and set aside.

2. Place the lettuce in a 3-quart glass serving bowl. Arrange the kidney beans in a layer over the lettuce, followed by layers of cheese, green pepper, onion, tomato, and avocado. Spread the sour cream mixture over the avocado layer, and garnish with a sprinkling of cheese and olives.

3. Cover the salad, and chill for 3 to 5 hours. Toss to mix well just before serving.

NUTRITIONAL FACTS (PER 1 1/2-CUP SERVING)
Cal: 166   Carbs: 22.6 g   Chol: 4 mg   Fat: 3.5 g
Fiber: 5.2 g   Protein: 11 g   Sodium: 413 mg

Rocket Salad

YIELD: 4 SERVINGS
6 cups arugula
12 cherry tomatoes, halved
3/4 cup shredded nonfat or reduced-fat mozzarella cheese
3/4 cup ready-made herb-flavored fat-free or low-fat croutons
1/2 cup bottled nonfat or reduced-fat balsamic vinaigrette salad dressing

1. Arrange $1^1/_2$ cups of arugula over the bottom of each of 4 salad plates. Top the arugula with 6 cherry tomato halves, 3 tablespoons of mozzarella, and 3 tablespoons of croutons.

2. Drizzle 2 tablespoons of the dressing over each salad, and serve immediately.

NUTRITIONAL FACTS (PER SERVING)
Cal: 116   Carbs: 16 g   Chol: 2 mg   Fat: 0.7 g
Fiber: 2.4 g   Protein: 8.8 g   Sodium: 450 mg

Antipasto Salad

YIELD: 6 SERVINGS
6 cups torn romaine lettuce
2 medium plum tomatoes, thinly sliced
6 thin slices red onion, separated into rings
3 ounces nonfat or reduced-fat mozzarella cheese or reduced-fat provolone cheese, thinly sliced and cut into thin strips
3 ounces ham, at least 97% lean, thinly shaved and cut into thin strips
1 cup canned kidney beans or chickpeas, rinsed and drained
6 small canned (drained) or frozen (thawed) artichoke hearts, halved
6 cherry peppers or Greek salad peppers
6 large pitted black olives
3/4 cup Creamy Italian Dressing (page 189) or bottled nonfat or reduced-fat Italian salad dressing

1. Arrange the lettuce over the bottom of a large serving platter. Lay first the tomato and then the onion rings over the lettuce. Arrange the mozzarella or provolone and the ham strips over the onions. Arrange the kidney beans or chickpeas, artichoke hearts, peppers, and olives around the outer edges of the lettuce.

2. Serve immediately, topping each serving with 2 tablespoons of the dressing.

NUTRITIONAL FACTS (PER 1³⁄₄-CUP SERVING)
Cal: 134   Carbs: 19 g   Chol: 10 mg   Fat: 1.5 g
Fiber: 4.3 g   Protein: 13 g   Sodium: 382 mg

Fresh Tomato Salad

To keep the tomatoes bright and firm, make this salad no more than 2 to 4 hours before serving.

YIELD: 6 SERVINGS
4 medium ripe tomatoes, cut into wedges (about 3 cups)
1 medium sweet onion, cut into thin wedges (about 1 cup)
1 medium green bell pepper, cut into thin strips (about 1 cup)

DRESSING
3 tablespoons red wine vinegar
1 tablespoon extra virgin olive oil
1 tablespoon sugar
1 tablespoon finely chopped fresh basil, or 1 teaspoon dried
1/4 teaspoon salt

1. Place all of the vegetables in a shallow dish, and toss to mix.

2. Place the dressing ingredients in a small bowl, and stir to mix. Pour the dressing over the salad, and toss to mix well.

3. Cover the salad, and chill for 2 to 4 hours, stirring occasionally, before serving.

NUTRITIONAL FACTS (PER ³⁄₄-CUP SERVING)
Cal: 60   Carbs: 9.4 g   Chol: 0 mg   Fat: 2.6 g
Fiber: 1.7 g   Protein: 1.2 g   Sodium: 106 mg

Chinese Cucumber Salad

YIELD: 8 SERVINGS

3 cups peeled, sliced cucumber (about 3 medium)

1 medium onion, thinly sliced

DRESSING

¼ cup seasoned rice wine vinegar

1 tablespoon reduced-sodium soy sauce

1 teaspoon sesame oil

⅛ teaspoon ground white pepper

1. Place the cucumber and onion in a shallow dish, and toss to mix.

2. Place the dressing ingredients in a small bowl, and stir to mix. Pour the dressing over the vegetables, and toss to mix well.

3. Cover the salad, and chill for several hours or overnight before serving.

NUTRITIONAL FACTS (PER ½-CUP SERVING)
Cal: 29   Carbs: 5 g   Chol: 0 mg   Fat: 0.7 g
Fiber: 1.1 g   Protein: 1.1 g   Sodium: 174 mg

Oriental Asparagus Salad

YIELD: 8 SERVINGS

1¼ pounds fresh asparagus spears

1 medium red bell pepper,
cut into matchstick-sized pieces

1 can sliced water chestnuts, drained

DRESSING

¼ cup seasoned rice wine vinegar

1 tablespoon reduced-sodium soy sauce

2 teaspoons sesame oil

½ teaspoon crushed fresh garlic

⅛ teaspoon ground ginger

1. Rinse the asparagus under cool running water, and snap off the tough stem ends. Cut the spears into 1-inch pieces. Fill a 2-quart pot half-full with water, and bring to a boil over high heat. Add the asparagus to the boiling water, and boil for about 30 seconds, or just until the asparagus pieces turn bright green and are crisp-tender.

2. Drain the asparagus, and plunge them into a large bowl of ice water to stop the cooking process. Drain once more, and transfer to a shallow dish.

3. Add the red pepper and water chestnuts to the asparagus, and toss to mix.

4. Place the dressing ingredients in a small bowl, and stir to mix. Pour the dressing over the vegetable mixture, and toss to mix well.

5. Cover the salad, and chill for 8 hours or overnight, stirring every few hours, before serving.

NUTRITIONAL FACTS (PER ¾-CUP SERVING)
Cal: 42   Carbs: 6 g   Chol: 0 mg   Fat: 1.3 g
Fiber: 2 g   Protein: 1.8 g   Sodium: 150 mg

Company Carrot-Raisin Salad

YIELD: 7 SERVINGS

4 cups grated carrot (about 8 medium)

⅔ cup thinly sliced celery

¾ cup dark raisins

DRESSING

⅓ cup nonfat or reduced-fat mayonnaise

⅓ cup nonfat or light sour cream

2 tablespoons frozen (thawed)
apple juice concentrate

1. Place the carrot, celery, and raisins in a large bowl, and toss to mix well.

2. Place the dressing ingredients in a small bowl, and stir to mix. Pour the dressing over the carrot mixture, and toss to mix well.

3. Cover the salad, and chill for several hours or overnight before serving.

NUTRITIONAL FACTS (PER ⅔-CUP SERVING)
Cal: 102   Carbs: 24 g   Chol: 0 mg   Fat: 0.2 g
Fiber: 3.2 g   Protein: 1.8 g   Sodium: 126 g

California Carrot Salad

YIELD: 8 SERVINGS

6 cups grated carrots (about 12 medium)

1 cup golden raisins

1/3 cup toasted slivered almonds
(page 348) (optional)

DRESSING

3 tablespoons frozen (thawed)
orange juice concentrate

1/2 cup nonfat or reduced-fat mayonnaise

1/3 cup nonfat or light sour cream

1. Place the carrots, raisins, and almonds, if desired, in a large bowl, and toss to mix well.

2. Place the dressing ingredients in a small bowl, and stir to mix. Pour the dressing over the carrot mixture, and toss to mix well.

3. Cover the salad, and chill for several hours or overnight before serving.

> **NUTRITIONAL FACTS (PER 2/3-CUP SERVING)**
> Cal: 118   Carbs: 28 g   Chol: 0 mg   Fat: 0.2 g
> Fiber: 3.2 g   Protein: 2.2 g   Sodium: 109 mg

Sunshine Carrot Salad

YIELD: 6 SERVINGS

2 cups grated carrot (about 4 medium)

1 can (8 ounces) crushed pineapple in juice,
drained well

1 can (11 ounces) mandarin
orange sections, drained

1/2 cup golden raisins

DRESSING

1/4 cup plus 2 tablespoons nonfat or
light sour cream

1/4 cup nonfat or reduced-fat mayonnaise

1 tablespoon sugar

1. Place the carrot, pineapple, mandarin oranges, and raisins in a large bowl, and toss gently to mix.

2. Place the dressing ingredients in a small bowl, and stir to mix. Spread the dressing over the carrot mixture, and toss gently to mix well.

3. Cover the salad, and chill for several hours or overnight before serving.

> **NUTRITIONAL FACTS (PER 1/2-CUP SERVING)**
> Cal: 110   Carbs: 26 g   Chol: 0 mg   Fat: 0.3 g
> Fiber: 2.2 g   Protein: 2 g   Sodium: 98 mg

Fresh Broccoli Salad

YIELD: 10 SERVINGS

1 head fresh broccoli (about 1 1/4 pounds)

1/2 cup chopped red onion

1/2 cup dark raisins

1/2 cup salted roasted sunflower seeds

DRESSING

1 cup nonfat or reduced-fat mayonnaise

2 tablespoons sugar

1 tablespoon apple cider vinegar

1. Peel the tough outer skin from the broccoli stalk. Chop the stalks into 1/2-inch pieces, and separate the top into small florets. Measure the broccoli. There should be about 6 cups of florets and stems. Adjust the amount if necessary.

2. Place the broccoli, onion, raisins, and sunflower seeds in a large bowl, and toss to mix well.

3. Place the dressing ingredients in a small bowl, and stir to mix. Add the dressing to the broccoli mixture, and toss to mix well.

4. Cover the salad, and chill for several hours or overnight before serving.

> **NUTRITIONAL FACTS (PER 2/3-CUP SERVING)**
> Cal: 107   Carbs: 16 g   Chol: 0 mg   Fat: 3.9 g
> Fiber: 2.5 g   Protein: 3.4 g   Sodium: 224 mg

Zesty German Potato Salad

YIELD: 8 SERVINGS

1/4 cup plus 2 tablespoons chicken broth, divided
1 tablespoon plus 1 teaspoon unbleached flour
3/4 teaspoon dry mustard
1/8 teaspoon ground black pepper
1 2/3 pounds unpeeled potatoes (about 5 medium)
1/4 teaspoon salt
4 slices extra-lean turkey bacon
1/2 cup sliced celery
1/2 cup chopped onion
1/3 cup apple cider vinegar
2 tablespoons sugar
1 tablespoon minced fresh parsley

1. Place 1/4 cup of the broth and all of the flour, mustard, and pepper in a small jar with a tight-fitting lid. Shake until smooth, and set aside.

2. Halve the potatoes lengthwise. Then slice them 1/4-inch thick. Measure the potatoes. There should be 5 cups. Adjust the amount if necessary.

3. Place the potatoes in a 4-quart pot. Cover with water, add the salt, and bring to a boil over high heat. Reduce the heat to medium-low, cover, and cook for 8 to 10 minutes, or just until tender. Drain well, and return the potatoes to the pot. Set aside.

4. While the potatoes are cooking, arrange the bacon on a large plate lined with a paper towel. Cover the bacon with another paper towel, and microwave on high power for about 4 minutes, or until crisp and browned. Alternatively, cook the bacon until crisp according to package directions. Set aside.

5. Coat a large nonstick skillet with nonstick cooking spray, and preheat over medium-high heat. Add the celery and onion, and cook, stirring frequently, for about 2 minutes, or until crisp-tender.

6. Add the vinegar, sugar, and remaining 2 tablespoons of chicken broth to the skillet, and bring to a boil, stirring frequently to dissolve the sugar. Reduce the heat to low.

7. Shake the flour mixture, and add it to the skillet. Cook, stirring constantly, until the mixture starts to boil and thickens slightly.

8. Add the potatoes to the skillet, and toss gently to coat with the dressing. Remove the skillet from the heat.

9. Crumble the bacon, and add it to the skillet. Then toss in the parsley. Serve warm or at room temperature.

> **NUTRITIONAL FACTS (PER 2/3-CUP SERVING)**
> Cal: 116   Carbs: 25 g   Chol: 10 mg   Fat: 0.4 g
> Fiber: 2.2 g   Protein: 3.6 g   Sodium: 191 mg

Sweet Potato Salad

YIELD: 6 SERVINGS

1 pound sweet potatoes (about 2 medium)
1 can (8 ounces) crushed pineapple in juice, well drained
1/4 cup diced celery
1/4 cup plus 2 tablespoons golden raisins
1/4 cup toasted chopped pecans (page 348)
3 tablespoons shredded sweetened coconut

DRESSING

1/4 cup nonfat or light sour cream
1/4 cup nonfat or reduced-fat mayonnaise
1/8 teaspoon ground ginger

1. Peel the potatoes, and cut into 5/8-inch cubes. Measure the potatoes. There should be 3 cups. Adjust the amount if necessary.

2. Place the potatoes in a 2-quart pot. Add enough water to barely cover, and bring to a boil over high heat. Reduce the heat to medium, cover, and cook for 5 minutes, or just until tender. Drain, rinse with cold water, and drain again.

3. Place the potatoes in a large bowl. Add the drained pineapple, celery, raisins, pecans, and coconut, and toss to mix well.

4. Place the dressing ingredients in a small bowl, and stir to mix. Add the dressing to the salad, and toss to mix well.

5. Cover the salad, and chill for at least 3 hours before serving.

NUTRITIONAL FACTS (PER ⅔-CUP SERVING)
Cal: 137   Carbs: 24 g   Chol: 8 mg   Fat: 4.6 g
Fiber: 2.5 g   Protein: 1.7 g   Sodium: 19 mg

Dillicious Potato Salad

YIELD: 9 SERVINGS

2 pounds unpeeled potatoes (about 6 medium)
¼ teaspoon salt
1 cup (about 6 ounces) frozen (thawed) green peas
⅓ cup grated carrot
⅓ cup chopped onion

DRESSING

¼ cup plus 2 tablespoons nonfat or light sour cream
¼ cup plus 2 tablespoons nonfat or reduced-fat mayonnaise
2 tablespoons Dijon mustard
1 tablespoon finely chopped fresh dill, or 1 teaspoon dried
⅛ teaspoon ground white pepper

1. Cut the potatoes in ¾-inch pieces, and place in a 3-quart pot. Cover with water, add the salt, and bring to a boil over high heat. Reduce the heat to medium-low, cover, and cook for about 10 minutes, or just until tender. Drain, rinse with cold water, and drain again.

2. Place the potatoes in a large bowl. Add the peas, carrot, and onion, and toss gently to mix.

3. Place the dressing ingredients in a small bowl, and stir to mix. Pour the dressing over the potato mixture, and toss gently to mix well.

4. Cover the salad, and chill for at least 2 hours before serving.

NUTRITIONAL FACTS (PER ¾-CUP SERVING)
Cal: 145   Carbs: 32 g   Chol: 0 mg   Fat: 0.2 g
Fiber: 3.4 g   Protein: 3.7 g   Sodium: 177 mg

All-American Potato Salad

YIELD: 8 SERVINGS

2 pounds unpeeled medium-sized red potatoes
¼ teaspoon salt
⅓ cup thinly sliced celery
⅓ cup finely chopped onion
⅓ cup grated carrot
2 tablespoons sweet pickle relish

DRESSING

⅓ cup nonfat or reduced-fat mayonnaise
⅓ cup nonfat or light sour cream
2 tablespoons spicy mustard
⅛ teaspoon ground black pepper

1. Cut the potatoes into ¾-inch pieces, and place in a 3-quart pot. Cover with water, add the salt, and bring to a boil over high heat. Reduce the heat to medium-low, cover, and cook for about 10 minutes, or just until tender. Drain, rinse with cold water, and drain again.

2. Place the potatoes in a large bowl. Add the celery, onion, carrot, and relish, and toss gently to mix.

3. Place the dressing ingredients in a small bowl, and stir to mix. Pour the dressing over the potato mixture, and toss gently to mix.

4. Cover the salad, and chill for at least 2 hours before serving.

NUTRITIONAL FACTS (PER ¾-CUP SERVING)
Cal: 139   Carbs: 31 g   Chol: 0 mg   Fat: 0.2 g
Fiber: 2.9 g   Protein: 3.5 g   Sodium: 220 mg

Terrific Taco Salad

YIELD: 6 SERVINGS

6 flour tortillas (8- to 10-inch rounds),
warmed to room temperature

9 cups shredded romaine lettuce

TACO FILLING

1 pound 95% lean ground beef

1 can (1 pound) black beans or pinto beans,
drained and coarsely mashed

1 cup bottled salsa

$\frac{1}{2}$ cup chopped onion

1 tablespoon chili powder

GARNISH

2 medium tomatoes, diced

1 cup nonfat or reduced-fat shredded
Cheddar cheese

$\frac{3}{4}$ cup nonfat or light sour cream

1. To make the shells, invert six 6-ounce custard cups on a large baking sheet, and coat the bottom of each cup with nonstick cooking spray. Place each tortilla over a cup, allowing the sides of the tortilla to drape down over the sides of the inverted cup. (Note that the tortilla will not drape enough to touch the sides of the cup, but will bend just enough to form a basket for the salad.) Bake at 350°F for 10 to 12 minutes, or until the tortillas are crisp and the edges are lightly browned.

2. Remove the pan from the oven, and allow the shells to cool to room temperature. Remove the shells from the custard cups, and transfer each one to an individual serving plate.

3. To make the taco filling, coat a large nonstick skillet with nonstick cooking spray, and preheat over medium-high heat. Add the ground beef, and cook, stirring to crumble, until the meat is no longer pink. Drain off and discard any excess fat.

4. Add the beans, salsa, onion, and chili powder to the skillet, and stir to mix well. Reduce the heat to

low, cover the skillet, and cook for 5 minutes, or until the onions are tender and the flavors are blended. Add a little water or extra salsa if the mixture seems too dry. Remove the skillet from the heat.

5. To assemble the salads, arrange $1\frac{1}{2}$ cups of the lettuce over the bottom of each tortilla shell, and top with a sixth of the meat mixture. Garnish with the tomatoes, cheese, and sour cream, and serve immediately, accompanying the salad with Tex-Mex Salad Dressing (page 189), if desired.

NUTRITIONAL FACTS (PER SERVING)
Cal: 385   Carbs: 48 g   Chol: 42 mg   Fat: 6.1 g
Fiber: 8.8 g   Protein: 32 g   Sodium: 728 mg

Seven-Layer Slaw

YIELD: 10 SERVINGS

2 teaspoons lemon juice

2 teaspoons sugar

$1\frac{1}{2}$ cups chopped peeled apples
(about $1\frac{1}{2}$ medium)

1 cup nonfat or light sour cream

1 cup nonfat or reduced-fat mayonnaise

6 cups shredded cabbage
(about $\frac{1}{2}$ medium head)

1 can (8 ounces) sliced water chestnuts,
drained

1 cup (about 6 ounces) frozen (thawed)
green peas

$\frac{3}{4}$ cup shredded nonfat or reduced-fat
Cheddar cheese

$\frac{1}{4}$ cup chopped toasted pecans (page 348)

1. Place the lemon juice and sugar in a small bowl. Add the apples, and toss to mix. Set aside.

2. Place the sour cream and mayonnaise in a small bowl, and stir to mix well. Set aside.

3. Place the cabbage in a $2\frac{1}{2}$-quart glass serving bowl. Arrange the apple mixture in a layer over the cabbage, followed by a layer of water chestnuts and a layer of peas. Spread the sour cream mixture over the peas, and sprinkle the cheese over the sour cream. Top with a sprinkling of nuts.

4. Cover the salad, and chill for several hours or overnight. Toss to mix well just before serving.

NUTRITIONAL FACTS (PER ¾-CUP SERVING)
Cal: 121   Carbs: 19 g   Chol: 1 mg   Fat: 2.3 g
Fiber: 3.2 g   Protein: 5.6 g   Sodium: 292 mg

Creamy Coleslaw

YIELD: 8 SERVINGS

6 cups coarsely shredded cabbage
(about ½ medium head)

1 cup shredded carrot (about 2 medium)

1 medium green bell pepper,
cut into very thin strips

DRESSING

¾ cup nonfat or reduced-fat mayonnaise

3 tablespoons distilled white vinegar

2 tablespoons sugar

1 tablespoon Dijon mustard

¼ teaspoon celery seed

⅛ teaspoon ground white pepper

1. Place the cabbage, carrot, and green pepper in a large bowl, and toss to mix well.

2. Place the dressing ingredients in a small bowl, and stir to mix. Pour the dressing over the cabbage mixture, and toss to mix well.

3. Cover the salad, and chill for 8 hours or overnight before serving.

NUTRITIONAL FACTS (PER ⅔-CUP SERVING)
Cal: 56   Carbs: 10 g   Chol: 0 mg   Fat: 1.4 g
Fiber: 1.2 g   Protein: 0.8 g   Sodium: 199 mg

Crunchy Chicken and Rice Salad

YIELD: 5 SERVINGS

2½ cups water

1 cup wild rice

2 cups diced cooked chicken or turkey breast
(about 10 ounces)

1½ cups halved seedless green grapes
or diced peeled apples

1 can (8 ounces) water chestnuts, drained and
coarsely chopped

½ cup chopped celery

½ cup toasted slivered almonds, cashews,
or pecans (page 348) (optional)

DRESSING

½ cup nonfat or reduced-fat mayonnaise

½ cup nonfat or light sour cream

⅛ teaspoon ground ginger

1. Place the water and rice in a 2-quart pot, and bring to a boil over high heat. Reduce the heat to low, cover, and simmer without stirring for 50 to 60 minutes, or until the water is absorbed and the rice is tender. Remove the pot from the heat, and let sit covered for 5 minutes. Then uncover the pot and allow the rice to cool to room temperature, or transfer to a covered container and chill until ready to assemble the salad.

2. Place the cooled rice, chicken or turkey, grapes or apples, water chestnuts, celery, and nuts, if desired, in a large bowl, and toss to mix well.

3. Place the dressing ingredients in a small bowl, and stir to mix. Add the dressing to the salad, and toss to mix well.

4. Cover the salad, and chill for at least 2 hours before serving.

NUTRITIONAL FACTS (PER 1⅔-CUP SERVING)
Cal: 283   Carbs: 40 g   Chol: 48 mg   Fat: 2.6 g
Fiber: 2.4 g   Protein: 23 g   Sodium: 254 mg

Greek Grilled Chicken Salad

YIELD: 4 SERVINGS

4 boneless skinless chicken breast halves (about 5 ounces each)

2–3 tablespoons Lemon-Herb Rub (page 137)

Nonstick olive oil cooking spray

10 cups torn romaine lettuce or mixed salad greens

1 medium cucumber, peeled, quartered lengthwise, and sliced

12 cherry tomatoes, halved

1/4 cup sliced black olives

4 thin slices red onion, separated into rings

1/2 cup crumbled nonfat or reduced-fat feta cheese

8 Greek salad peppers (optional)

3/4 cup bottled nonfat or reduced-fat red wine vinaigrette, Caesar, or balsamic vinaigrette salad dressing

1. Rinse the chicken with cool water, and pat it dry with paper towels. Using your fingers, rub both sides of each piece of chicken with some of the rub. If you have time, set the chicken aside for 15 to 30 minutes to allow the flavors to better penetrate the meat.

2. Coat a broiler pan with nonstick cooking spray, and arrange the chicken on the pan. Spray the tops of the chicken breasts lightly with the cooking spray, and, turning occasionally, cook over medium coals or broil 6 inches under a preheated broiler for 12 to 15 minutes, or until the meat is nicely browned and no longer pink inside. Set the chicken aside to cool.

3. Slice the chicken thinly across the grain. Set aside. (Note that the chicken can be cooked the day before, refrigerated, and sliced just before assembling the salads.)

4. To serve, arrange 2 1/2 cups of lettuce or other greens over the bottom of each of 4 plates. Arrange some of the cucumber, tomatoes, and olives around the outer edges of the lettuce on each plate. Top the

lettuce with some of the onion rings. Arrange a sliced chicken breast over the lettuce, sprinkle with some of the feta, and garnish with 2 Greek salad peppers, if desired. Serve immediately, accompanied by some of the dressing and, if desired, wedges of warm pita bread.

NUTRITIONAL FACTS (PER SERVING)

Cal: 302　Carbs: 28 g　Chol: 82 mg　Fat: 3.2 g
Fiber: 3.9 g　Protein: 39 g　Sodium: 988 mg

Pacific Chicken Salad

YIELD: 6 SERVINGS

3 cups cooked brown rice

2 cups diced cooked chicken or turkey breast (about 10 ounces)

2 cups diced fresh pineapple, or 1 can (20 ounces) unsweetened pineapple chunks, drained

1 can (8 ounces) sliced water chestnuts, drained

3/4 cup matchstick-sized pieces celery

DRESSING

1/2 cup nonfat or reduced-fat mayonnaise

2 tablespoons mango chutney

1 teaspoon curry paste

1/4 teaspoon ground ginger

1/8 teaspoon ground white pepper

1. Place the rice, chicken or turkey, pineapple, water chestnuts, and celery in a large bowl, and toss to mix well.

2. Place the dressing ingredients in a small bowl, and stir to mix. Pour the dressing over the rice mixture, and toss to mix well.

3. Cover the salad, and chill for several hours before serving.

NUTRITIONAL FACTS (PER 1 1/3-CUP SERVING)

Cal: 244　Carbs: 38 g　Chol: 36 mg　Fat: 2.3 g
Fiber: 3.5 g　Protein: 17.4 g　Sodium: 238 mg

Greek Couscous Salad

YIELD: 7 SERVINGS
1½ cups water
1 cup whole wheat couscous
1¼ cups peeled, seeded, chopped cucumber (about 1 large)
1 cup chopped seeded plum tomato (3–4 medium)
½ cup chopped red onion
½ cup chopped black olives
½ cup crumbled nonfat or reduced-fat feta cheese
2 tablespoons finely chopped fresh mint

DRESSING

3 tablespoons lemon juice
1 tablespoon extra virgin olive oil
2 teaspoons Dijon mustard
2 teaspoons sugar
¼ teaspoon salt
¼ teaspoon ground black pepper

1. Place the water and couscous in a medium-sized pot, and bring to a boil over high heat. Cover the pot, remove from the heat, and allow to stand for 5 minutes, or until all of the water is absorbed. Uncover the pot and allow the couscous to cool to room temperature, or transfer to a covered container and chill until ready to assemble the salad.

2. Place the cooled couscous, cucumber, tomato, onion, olives, feta cheese, and mint in a large bowl, and toss to mix well.

3. Place the dressing ingredients in a small bowl, and stir to mix. Pour the dressing over the salad, and toss to mix well.

4. Cover the salad, and chill for at least 2 hours before serving.

NUTRITIONAL FACTS (PER ¾-CUP SERVING)
Cal: 145   Carbs: 24 g   Chol: 1 mg   Fat: 3.3 g
Fiber: 4.8 g   Protein: 5.7 g   Sodium: 332 mg

Southwestern Grilled Chicken Salad

YIELD: 4 SERVINGS
4 boneless skinless chicken breast halves (about 5 ounces each)
2–3 tablespoons Spicy Tex-Mex Rub (page 137)
Nonstick olive oil cooking spray
10 cups torn romaine lettuce or mixed salad greens
¾ cup chopped tomato
4 thin slices red onion, separated into rings
½ cup shredded nonfat or reduced-fat Cheddar cheese
¼ cup sliced black olives
60 baked tortilla chips (about 3 ounces)
¾ cup bottled nonfat or low-fat Ranch salad dressing

1. Rinse the chicken with cool water, and pat it dry with paper towels. Using your fingers, rub both sides of each piece of chicken with some of the rub. If you have time, set the chicken aside for 15 to 30 minutes to allow the flavors to better penetrate the meat.

2. Coat a broiler pan with nonstick cooking spray, and arrange the chicken on the pan. Spray the tops of the chicken breasts lightly with the cooking spray, and, turning occasionally, cook over medium coals or broil 6 inches under a preheated broiler for 12 to 15 minutes, or until the meat is nicely browned and no longer pink inside. Set the chicken aside for 15 minutes.

3. Slice the chicken thinly across the grain. Set aside. (Note that the chicken can be cooked the day before, refrigerated, and sliced just before assembling the salads.)

4. To serve, arrange 2½ cups of lettuce over the bottom of each of 4 plates. Sprinkle some of the tomato over the lettuce on each plate, and top with some of the onion rings. Arrange a sliced chicken breast over the lettuce, and sprinkle with 2 tablespoons of cheese and a tablespoon of olives. Arrange 15 chips around the outer edge of each plate, and serve immediately, accompanied by some of the dressing.

NUTRITIONAL FACTS (PER SERVING)
Cal: 386   Carbs: 43 g   Chol: 83 mg   Fat: 3.8 g
Fiber: 5.8 g   Protein: 42 g   Sodium: 881 mg

Brown Rice and Lentil Salad

YIELD: 6 SERVINGS

2 cups cooked brown rice

1 cup cooked brown lentils

¾ cup chopped seeded plum tomato
(about 3 medium)

¼ cup thinly sliced scallions

DRESSING

1 tablespoon balsamic vinegar

1 tablespoon extra virgin olive oil

1 teaspoon Dijon mustard

½ teaspoon dried oregano

¼ teaspoon salt

1. Place the rice, lentils, tomato, and scallions in a medium-sized bowl, and toss to mix well.

2. Place the dressing ingredients in a small bowl, and stir to mix. Pour the dressing over the salad, and toss to mix well.

3. Cover the salad, and chill for 2 to 5 hours before serving.

NUTRITIONAL FACTS (PER ⅔-CUP SERVING)
Cal: 141   Carbs: 23 g   Chol: 0 mg   Fat: 3.2 g
Fiber: 4.6 g   Protein: 5 g   Sodium: 126 mg

Rice-Almond Salad

YIELD: 6 SERVINGS

2½ cups cooked brown rice

½ cup finely chopped celery

½ cup finely chopped carrot

¼ cup toasted slivered almonds (page 348)

¼ cup golden raisins

DRESSING

¼ cup plus 2 tablespoons nonfat or
reduced-fat mayonnaise

1 tablespoon mango chutney

½ teaspoon ground ginger

½ teaspoon curry paste

1. Place the rice, celery, carrot, almonds, and raisins in a large bowl, and toss to mix well.

2. Place the dressing ingredients in a small bowl, and stir to mix. Add the dressing to the rice mixture, and toss to mix well, adding a little more mayonnaise if the mixture seems too dry.

3. Cover the salad, and chill for at least 2 hours before serving.

NUTRITIONAL FACTS (PER ⅔-CUP SERVING)
Cal: 142   Carbs: 25 g   Chol: 0 mg   Fat: 3.7 g
Fiber: 2.3 g   Protein: 3.1 g   Sodium: 139 mg

Mediterranean Chef's Salad

YIELD: 4 SERVINGS

10 cups torn romaine lettuce or
mixed salad greens

1 medium cucumber, peeled and sliced

8 cherry tomatoes, halved

1 can (12 ounces) water-packed
albacore tuna, drained

1 can (15 ounces) white beans, rinsed and drained

½ cup crumbled nonfat or reduced-fat feta cheese

¼ cup sliced black olives

4 slices red onion, separated into rings

½ cup bottled nonfat or reduced-fat Italian or
Caesar salad dressing

1. Arrange a quarter of the lettuce over the bottom of each of 4 large plates. Arrange a quarter of the cucumber slices and 4 cherry tomato halves around the edges of each plate.

2. Top the greens on each plate with ⅓ cup of the tuna; then scatter ⅓ cup of the beans over the tuna. Sprinkle with 2 tablespoons of feta and a tablespoon of olives. Top with some of the onion rings.

3. Drizzle 2 tablespoons of the dressing over each salad, and serve immediately.

NUTRITIONAL FACTS (PER SERVING)
Cal: 224   Carbs: 27 g   Chol: 28 mg   Fat: 1.9 g
Fiber: 4.2 g   Protein: 25 g   Sodium: 676 mg

Terrific Tabbouleh

YIELD: 8 SERVINGS

1 cup bulgur wheat

2 cups boiling water

1 cup chopped tomatoes
(about 2 medium)

1 cup peeled, seeded, chopped cucumber
(about 1 large)

½ cup (packed) chopped fresh parsley

½ cup thinly sliced scallions

1–2 tablespoons finely chopped fresh mint

DRESSING

¼ cup lemon juice

1–2 tablespoons extra virgin olive oil

1 teaspoon crushed fresh garlic

¼ teaspoon salt

⅛ teaspoon ground black pepper

1. Place the bulgur wheat in a large heatproof bowl, and pour the boiling water over the wheat. Stir to mix, cover, and set aside for 30 to 45 minutes, or until most of the liquid is absorbed. Drain off any excess liquid. (Alternatively, prepare according to package directions.)

2. Add the tomatoes, cucumber, parsley, scallions, and mint to the bulgur, and toss to mix well.

3. Place the dressing ingredients in a small bowl, and stir to mix. Pour the dressing over the salad, and toss to mix well.

4. Cover the salad, and chill for at least 3 hours before serving.

NUTRITIONAL FACTS (PER ⅔-CUP SERVING)
Cal: 86   Carbs: 16 g   Chol: 0 mg   Fat: 2 g
Fiber: 3.9 g   Protein: 2.7 g   Sodium: 75 mg

Mediterranean White Bean Salad

YIELD: 6 SERVINGS

⅔ cup bulgur wheat

1⅓ cups boiling water

1 can white beans (15 ounces),
rinsed and drained

½ cup thinly sliced celery

½ cup chopped red onion

¼ cup finely chopped fresh parsley

DRESSING

3 tablespoons lemon juice

1 tablespoon extra virgin olive oil

2 teaspoons Dijon mustard

1 teaspoon sugar

1 teaspoon crushed fresh garlic

¼ teaspoon ground cumin

1 pinch ground black pepper

1. Place the bulgur wheat in a large heatproof bowl, and pour the boiling water over the wheat. Stir to mix, cover, and set aside for 30 to 45 minutes, or until most of the liquid is absorbed. Drain off any excess liquid. (Alternatively, prepare according to package directions.)

2. Add the beans, celery, onion, and parsley to the bulgur, and toss to mix well.

3. Place the dressing ingredients in a small bowl, and stir to mix. Pour the dressing over the salad, and toss to mix well.

4. Cover the salad, and chill for at least 2 hours before serving.

NUTRITIONAL FACTS (PER ⅔-CUP SERVING)
Cal: 172   Carbs: 30 g   Chol: 0 mg   Fat: 2.8 g
Fiber: 7.4 g   Protein: 8 g   Sodium: 212 mg

White Bean, Basil, and Tomato Salad

YIELD: 8 SERVINGS

2 cans (15 ounces each) white beans or navy beans, rinsed and drained

1 pound fresh plum tomatoes, seeded and chopped (6–8 medium)

¼ cup plus 2 tablespoons coarsely chopped fresh basil

DRESSING

3 tablespoons white wine vinegar

1 tablespoon extra virgin olive oil

2 teaspoons Dijon mustard

2 teaspoons sugar

1 teaspoon crushed fresh garlic

⅛ teaspoon ground black pepper

¼ teaspoon salt

1. Place the beans, tomatoes, and basil in a large shallow bowl, and toss to mix well.

2. Place the dressing ingredients in a small bowl, and stir to mix well. Pour the dressing over the bean mixture, and toss to mix well.

3. Cover the salad, and chill for 2 to 5 hours, stirring occasionally, before serving.

NUTRITIONAL FACTS (PER ⅔-CUP SERVING)
Cal: 121   Carbs: 20 g   Chol: 0 mg   Fat: 2.1 g
Fiber: 6.1 g   Protein: 6.2 g   Sodium: 167 mg

Rosemary Rice Salad

YIELD: 8 SERVINGS

3 cups cooked brown rice

1 cup finely chopped peeled fresh broccoli stems

½ cup grated carrot (about 1 medium)

⅓ cup finely chopped celery

¼ cup dark or golden raisins

DRESSING

¼ cup orange juice

2 tablespoons white wine vinegar

1 tablespoon extra virgin olive oil

1 teaspoon crushed fresh garlic

1 tablespoon chopped fresh rosemary, or 1 teaspoon dried

1 teaspoon sugar

¼ teaspoon ground ginger

¼ teaspoon salt

1. Place the rice, broccoli, carrot, celery, and raisins in a large bowl, and toss to mix well.

2. Place the dressing ingredients in a small bowl, and stir to mix. Pour the dressing over the rice mixture, and toss to mix well.

3. Cover the salad, and chill for at least 2 hours or overnight before serving.

NUTRITIONAL FACTS (PER ⅔-CUP SERVING)
Cal: 122   Carbs: 23 g   Chol: 0 mg   Fat: 2.2 g
Fiber: 2.1 g   Protein: 2.5 g   Sodium: 81 mg

Curried Rice and Bean Salad

YIELD: 8 SERVINGS

3 cups cooked brown rice

1 can (1 pound) red kidney beans, rinsed and drained

½ cup chopped green bell pepper

½ cup thinly sliced celery

⅓ cup thinly sliced scallions

¼ cup dark raisins

DRESSING

⅓ cup nonfat or reduced-fat mayonnaise

⅓ cup plain nonfat yogurt

1–2 teaspoons curry paste

⅛ teaspoon ground black pepper

1. Place the rice, beans, green pepper, celery, scallions, and raisins in a large bowl, and toss to mix well.

2. Place the dressing ingredients in a small bowl, and stir to mix. Pour the dressing over the rice mixture, and toss to mix well.

3. Cover the salad, and chill for at least 2 hours or overnight before serving.

NUTRITIONAL FACTS (PER ¾-CUP SERVING)
Cal: 166   Carbs: 33 g   Chol: 0 mg   Fat: 1.2 g
Fiber: 4.9 g   Protein: 6.2 g   Sodium: 227 mg

Tuscan Lentil Salad

YIELD: 8 SERVINGS
¾ cup dried brown lentils, cleaned (page 302)
2 cups water
¼ teaspoon salt
2 cups frozen (thawed) whole kernel corn, or 1 can (15 ounces) whole kernel corn, drained
1 cup chopped frozen (thawed) or canned (drained) whole artichoke hearts
½ cup diced commercial roasted red bell pepper
¼ cup chopped onion

DRESSING

⅓ cup bottled nonfat or reduced-fat Italian salad dressing
1 teaspoon Dijon mustard
½ teaspoon dried oregano

1. Place the lentils, water, and salt in a 1½-quart pot, and bring to a boil over high heat. Reduce the heat to low, cover, and simmer for about 20 minutes, or until the lentils are tender but not mushy. Remove the pot from the heat, and set aside to cool to room temperature.

2. Drain any excess water from the cooled lentils, and place them in a large bowl. Add the corn, artichoke hearts, roasted pepper, and onion, and toss to mix.

3. Place the dressing ingredients in a small bowl, and stir to mix. Pour the dressing over the lentil mixture, and toss to mix well.

4. Cover the salad, and chill for several hours or overnight before serving.

NUTRITIONAL FACTS (PER ¾-CUP SERVING)
Cal: 114   Carbs: 20 g   Chol: 0 mg   Fat: 0.4 g
Fiber: 4.5 g   Protein: 7.1 g   Sodium: 182 mg

Cuban Black Bean Salad

YIELD: 8 SERVINGS
1 can (1 pound) black beans, rinsed and drained
2½ cups cooked brown rice, chilled
1 medium tomato, seeded and chopped
½ cup thinly sliced celery
½ cup chopped green bell pepper
½ cup chopped sweet onion

DRESSING

3 tablespoons white wine vinegar
1 tablespoon extra virgin olive oil
1 teaspoon dried oregano
1 teaspoon crushed fresh garlic
1 teaspoon sugar
¼ teaspoon salt

1. Place the beans, rice, tomato, celery, green pepper, and onion in a large bowl, and toss to mix well.

2. Place the dressing ingredients in a small bowl, and stir to mix. Pour the dressing over the bean mixture, and toss to mix well.

3. Cover the salad, and chill for at least 2 hours before serving.

NUTRITIONAL FACTS (PER ¾-CUP SERVING)
Cal: 130   Carbs: 27 g   Chol: 0 mg   Fat: 2.3 g
Fiber: 4.3 g   Protein: 4.6 g   Sodium 153 mg

Refreshing Fruit Salad

YIELD: 10 SERVINGS

2 cups sliced bananas (about 2 large)

2 cups diced fresh pineapple (about 1/2 large)

2 cups sliced fresh strawberries

3 kiwis, peeled and cut into chunks

DRESSING

1 block (8 ounces) nonfat or reduced-fat cream cheese, softened to room temperature

3 tablespoons honey

2 tablespoons orange juice

1 tablespoon poppy seeds

1. Place the cream cheese and honey in the bowl of an electric mixer, and beat until smooth. Beat in the orange juice, and stir in the poppy seeds. Set aside.

2. Place the fruits in a large bowl, and toss to mix well.

3. To assemble the salads, place $3/4$ cup of fruit in each of 10 serving bowls, and top with 2 tablespoons of the dressing. Serve immediately.

> **NUTRITIONAL FACTS (PER 3/4-CUP SERVING)**
> Cal: 112   Carbs: 22 g   Chol: 1 mg   Fat: 0.9 g
> Fiber: 2.3 g   Protein: 4.2 g   Sodium: 112 mg

Waldorf Salad

YIELD: 8 SERVINGS

4 cups diced unpeeled red Delicious apples (about 5 1/2 medium)

1 1/2 cups thinly sliced celery

1/2 cup dark raisins

1/2 cup chopped toasted walnuts or pecans (page 348)

DRESSING

1/3 cup nonfat or reduced-fat mayonnaise

1/3 cup nonfat or light sour cream

1. Place the apples, celery, raisins, and walnuts or pecans in a large bowl, and toss to mix well.

2. Place the dressing ingredients in a small bowl. and stir to mix. Add the dressing to the apple mixture, and toss to mix well.

3. Cover the salad, and chill for 1 to 3 hours before serving.

> **NUTRITIONAL FACTS (PER 3/4-CUP SERVING)**
> Cal: 128   Carbs: 19 g   Chol: 0 mg   Fat: 4.9 g
> Fiber: 2.6 g   Protein: 2 g   Sodium: 94 mg

Spiked Fruit Salad

YIELD: 8 SERVINGS

4 plums or apricots, sliced

2 apples, peeled and sliced

2 pears, peeled and sliced

2 peaches or nectarines, peeled and sliced

1 1/2 cups seedless red grapes

DRESSING

1 teaspoon cornstarch

1/2 cup orange juice

1/2 cup dry white wine

1/4 cup honey

1 tablespoon freshly grated orange rind, or 1 teaspoon dried orange rind

1. Place the cornstarch and juice in a small saucepan, and stir to dissolve the cornstarch. Add the wine, honey, and orange rind, and stir to mix well. Cook over medium heat, stirring constantly, for several minutes, or until the mixture begins to boil and thickens slightly. Remove the pot from the heat, and allow to cool to room temperature.

2. Pour the dressing into a large bowl. Add the fruits, and toss to mix well. Cover and chill for 3 to 6 hours before serving.

> **NUTRITIONAL FACTS (PER 7/8-CUP SERVING)**
> Cal: 132   Carbs: 31 g   Chol: 0 mg   Fat: 0.6 g
> Fiber: 2.5 g   Protein: 0.8 g   Sodium: 2 mg

Winter Fruit Salad

YIELD: 8 SERVINGS

3 cups diced unpeeled golden Delicious apples (about 4 medium)
1 cup sliced celery
1 cup seedless red grapes, halved
1/2 cup dark raisins
1/2 cup chopped toasted almonds or pecans (page 348)

DRESSING

1/3 cup nonfat or reduced-fat mayonnaise
1/3 cup nonfat or light sour cream

1. Place the apples, celery, grapes, raisins, and nuts in a large bowl, and toss to mix well.

2. Place the dressing ingredients in a small bowl, and stir to mix. Pour the dressing over the apple mixture, and toss to mix well.

3. Cover the salad, and chill for 1 to 3 hours before serving.

NUTRITIONAL FACTS (PER 3/4-CUP SERVING)
Cal: 132   Carbs: 21 g   Chol: 0 mg   Fat: 4.5 g
Fiber: 2.7 g   Protein: 2.8 g   Sodium: 94 mg

Rainbow Fruit Salad

YIELD: 5 SERVINGS

1 cup sliced fresh strawberries
1 cup cubed cantaloupe
1 cup diced kiwi fruit (about 3 medium)
1 cup sliced bananas (about 1 large)
1 cup fresh blueberries

DRESSING

2 tablespoons frozen (thawed) orange juice concentrate
1 tablespoon honey
3/4 teaspoon poppy seeds

1. Place the fruit in a large bowl, and toss to mix.

2. Place the dressing ingredients in a small bowl, and stir to mix. Pour the dressing over the fruit, and toss to mix well.

3. Cover the salad, and chill for 1 to 3 hours before serving.

NUTRITIONAL FACTS (PER 1-CUP SERVING)
Cal: 121   Carbs: 26 g   Chol: 0 mg   Fat: 0.8 g
Fiber: 4 g   Protein: 1.7 g   Sodium: 7 mg

Festive Fruit Salad

This light and delicious fruit salad has a dressing of yogurt cheese, which you make yourself using nonfat yogurt. In a hurry? Use nonfat or light sour cream instead of the homemade cheese.

YIELD: 6 SERVINGS

1 can (8 ounces) pineapple chunks i n juice, drained
1 can (10 ounces) mandarin orange sections, drained
2 large bananas, sliced
1/2 cup miniature marshmallows
1/4 cup shredded sweetened coconut
1/3 cup toasted almonds or pecans (page 348) (optional)
1/2 cup vanilla yogurt cheese (page 12)

1. Place the fruit, marshmallows, coconut, and, if desired, the nuts in a large bowl, and toss to mix. Add the yogurt cheese to the fruit mixture, and toss to mix.

2. Cover the salad, and chill for 1 to 3 hours before serving.

NUTRITIONAL FACTS (PER 2/3-CUP SERVING)
Cal: 123   Carbs: 26 g   Chol: 0 mg   Fat: 1.8 g
Fiber: 2.3 g   Protein: 2.5 g   Sodium: 27 mg

Shamrock Fruit Salad

YIELD: 9 SERVINGS

2 cans (8 ounces each) unsweetened
crushed pineapple in juice, undrained

½ cup boiling water

1 package (4-serving size) sugar-free
or regular lime gelatin

1 block (8 ounces) nonfat or reduced-fat
cream cheese, softened to room temperature

1½ cups nonfat or light whipped topping

1 can (10 ounces) mandarin orange sections, drained

⅓ cup chopped pecans (optional)

1. Drain the pineapple, pouring the juice into a 1-cup measure. If necessary, add water to bring the volume up to ½ cup. Set aside.

2. Pour the boiling water into a blender, and add the gelatin. Cover the blender, and carefully blend at low speed for about 30 seconds, or until the gelatin is completely dissolved. Add the pineapple juice, and blend again. Allow the mixture to sit in the blender for about 20 minutes, or until it reaches room temperature. Add the cream cheese, and blend until smooth.

3. Pour the cream cheese mixture into a large bowl, and chill for 40 minutes. Stir the mixture; it should be the consistency of pudding. If it is too thin, return it to the refrigerator for a few minutes, or until it reaches the proper consistency.

4. When the gelatin reaches the proper consistency, stir with a wire whisk until smooth. Gently fold in first the whipped topping, and then the drained pineapple, mandarin oranges, and, if desired, the pecans.

5. Pour the mixture into an 8-inch square pan, and chill for 8 hours, or until firm. Cut into squares to serve.

NUTRITIONAL FACTS (PER ¾-CUP SERVING)
Cal: 71   Carbs: 12 g   Chol: 2 mg   Fat: 0.5 g
Fiber: 0.7 g   Protein: 4.6 g   Sodium: 153 mg

Blueberry-Banana Salad

YIELD: 6 SERVINGS

2 cups sliced bananas (about 2 large)

1 cup fresh blueberries

½ cup miniature marshmallows

¼ cup shredded sweetened coconut

½ cup nonfat or light sour cream

1 can (10 ounces) mandarin orange sections,
well drained

1. Place the bananas, blueberries, marshmallows, and coconut in a medium-sized bowl, and toss to mix. Add the sour cream to the fruit mixture, and toss to mix. Add the oranges, and toss gently.

2. Cover the salad, and chill for 1 to 3 hours before serving.

NUTRITIONAL FACTS (PER ¾-CUP SERVING)
Cal: 128   Carbs: 27 g   Chol: 0 mg   Fat: 1.8 g
Fiber: 2.9 g   Protein: 2.3 g   Sodium: 29 mg

8. Smart Side Dishes

Side dishes often pose a dilemma when people first adopt a light and healthy lifestyle. Noodles swimming in creamy sauces, rice dishes made with butter, and casseroles laden with cheese are side dish specialties in many households. It may come as no surprise that many of these dishes have as much or more fat and calories than the entreé they're accompanying!

So what can you serve alongside your favorite entrée? Fresh vegetables and whole grains are the best choices by far. Busy cooks will be happy to know that the less you do to vegetables in the way of cooking, the better off your side dish will be nutritionally. Simple methods like steaming and stir-frying are superb techniques for preserving nutrients, flavor, and color. Or cook your vegetables in a covered skillet with a few tablespoons of broth or wine.

It is equally easy to base your side dishes on whole grains like brown rice, barley, bulgur wheat, and whole wheat couscous. Your grocery store has many flavorful, nutrient-rich brands of quick-cooking brown rice and barley. And bulgur wheat and couscous have always been a snap to fix. Serve these grains alone, or combine them with vegetables for super-delicious side dishes that are special enough for any occasion.

The recipes in this chapter use garden-fresh vegetables, whole grains, zesty herbs and spices, and a variety of terrific no- and low-fat products to give side dishes flavor without fat—and without an unhealthy dose of sodium, too. Thanks to products like nonfat and reduced-fat cheeses and nonfat and light sour cream, you will find that even vegetable casseroles and creamy cheese toppings can be prepared with little or no fat. As a bonus, the recipes that follow often replace boiling with steaming and other cooking techniques that minimize nutrient loss while keeping veggies bright in color and flavorful.

So take out a selection of grains and the freshest vegetables available, and treat your family to smart and savory side dishes. You'll be delighted to learn that even crisp-coated onion rings can take their place at your table—once you know the secrets of healthy cooking.

Glorious Green Bean Casserole

YIELD: 6 SERVINGS

½ cup evaporated skim milk

3 tablespoons unbleached flour

⅛ teaspoon ground white pepper

1 pound frozen (unthawed) French-cut or regular-cut green beans

½ cup chicken or vegetable broth

1 can (4 ounces) sliced mushrooms, drained

3 tablespoons toasted sliced almonds (page 348)

1 medium-small yellow onion, very thinly sliced and separated into rings

TOPPING

2 tablespoons grated Parmesan cheese*

2 tablespoons Italian-style seasoned dried bread crumbs

Nonstick butter-flavored cooking spray

* In this recipe, use regular Parmesan cheese, not a fat-free brand.

1. To make the topping, place the Parmesan cheese and bread crumbs in a small dish, and stir to mix well. Set aside.

2. Place the evaporated milk, flour, and pepper in a jar with a tight-fitting lid, and shake until smooth. Set aside.

3. Place the green beans and broth in a 2½-quart pot, and bring to a boil over high heat. Reduce the heat to medium, cover, and cook for about 1 minute, or just until the beans are completely thawed and heated through.

4. Shake the milk mixture, and, stirring constantly, add it to the pot. Continue to cook and stir for a minute or 2, or until the mixture is thickened and bubbly. Remove the pot from the heat, and stir in the mushrooms and almonds.

5. Coat a shallow 1-quart casserole dish or a 9-inch deep dish pie pan with nonstick cooking spray, and spread the green bean mixture evenly in the dish. Spread the onion rings over the top, and sprinkle with the topping. Spray lightly with the cooking spray.

6. Bake uncovered at 350°F for 30 minutes, or until bubbly and nicely browned. Remove the dish from the oven, and let sit for 5 minutes before serving.

NUTRITIONAL FACTS (PER ½-CUP SERVING)
Cal: 92   Carbs: 12 g   Chol: 2 mg   Fat: 2.6 g
Fiber: 3 g   Protein: 5.2 g   Sodium: 244 mg

Asparagus With Honey Mustard Sauce

YIELD: 5 SERVINGS

1½ pounds fresh asparagus spears

SAUCE

¼ cup plus 2 tablespoons nonfat or reduced-fat mayonnaise

1 tablespoon plus 1 teaspoon Dijon mustard

1 tablespoon plus 1 teaspoon lemon juice

1 tablespoon plus 1 teaspoon honey

1. Rinse the asparagus under cool running water, and snap off the tough stem ends. Arrange the asparagus spears in a microwave or conventional steamer. Cover and cook on high power or over medium-high heat for about 4 minutes, or just until the spears are crisp-tender. Transfer to a serving dish.

2. While the asparagus are cooking, place all of the sauce ingredients in a 1-quart saucepan, and stir to mix well. Cook over medium-low heat, stirring constantly, just until the sauce is heated through. Alternatively, place the sauce in a microwave-safe bowl, and microwave uncovered on high power for 1 to 2 minutes, or just until heated through. Add a few teaspoons of water if the sauce seems too thick.

3. Drizzle the sauce over the asparagus, and serve hot.

NUTRITIONAL FACTS (PER SERVING)
Cal: 61   Carbs: 12 g   Chol: 0 mg   Fat: 0.6 g
Fiber: 2.5 g   Protein: 2.9 g   Sodium: 221 mg

Cooking Country Style

Southern-style vegetables are typically seasoned with bacon, lard, or ham hocks. Delicious? Absolutely! Healthy? As you might expect, these dishes are loaded with fat and salt. Fortunately, a variety of ingredients can be substituted for the usual Southern flavorings, resulting in mouthwatering dishes that are untraditionally low in fat. Here are some ideas:

❑ *Bouillon granules.* Ham bouillon granules can be added to a pot of beans or cabbage as a fat-free alternative to ham or bacon. Look for a brand like Goya, which is usually located in the ethnic foods section of grocery stores. Chicken- and vegetable-flavored bouillons are still another option. What about sodium? A teaspoon of the granules typically contains 1,000 milligrams of sodium—about half the amount in a teaspoon of salt. You can eliminate salt worries, though, by choosing a brand like Vogue Vege Base, a vegetable bouillon made mostly of powdered vegetables. Do keep in mind that most bouillons contain monosodium glutamate (MSG), and read labels carefully if you want to avoid this ingredient.

❑ *Lean ham.* Many hams—both turkey and pork—are very low in fat. Look for brands that are at least 97-percent lean. Then dice the ham and add small amounts to bean soups, greens, or other vegetable dishes.

❑ *Smoked turkey sausage.* Like lean ham, this product will add a smoky flavor to a variety of dishes. Look for brands like Healthy Choice, which is 97-percent lean, and use the sausage as you would lean ham.

❑ *Smoked turkey parts.* This is a great alternative to ham hocks. Add chunks of skinless smoked turkey to bean soups, green beans, and other vegetables.

❑ *Herbs and spices.* Because sage, fennel, and thyme are traditionally used to flavor sausage, these spices can be used instead of meat to add a country-style taste to bean soups and many vegetable dishes. Dry mustard also enhances the flavors of cabbage, greens, and green beans, reducing the need for fat and salt.

❑ *Vinegar.* A splash of vinegar or lemon juice tossed into vegetables just before serving adds zip, reducing the need for salty seasonings. Experiment with different types of vinegar, such as cider, white wine, red wine, rice wine, malt, and balsamic.

Country-Style Green Beans

YIELD: 6 SERVINGS

1½ pounds fresh green beans, trimmed and cut into 1-inch pieces (about 6 cups)

¾ cup water

1½ teaspoons instant ham bouillon granules, or 3 ounces ham, at least 97% lean, diced

1 teaspoon dry mustard

⅛ teaspoon ground black pepper

1. Place all of the ingredients in a 2½-quart pot, and stir to mix. Bring to a boil over high heat.

2. Reduce the heat to medium-low, and simmer uncovered, stirring occasionally, for 2 to 3 minutes, or until the beans turn bright green.

3. Cover the pot, and simmer, stirring occasionally, for 12 to 15 minutes, or until the beans are just tender. Serve hot.

NUTRITIONAL FACTS (PER ¾-CUP SERVING)
Cal: 37   Carbs: 7 g   Chol: 0 mg   Fat: 0.2 g
Fiber: 3.9 g   Protein: 2.2 g   Sodium: 176 mg

Green Beans Pomodoro

YIELD: 6 SERVINGS

1 teaspoon crushed fresh garlic

1 pound fresh green beans, trimmed and snapped into 2-inch pieces (about 4 cups)

1 can (14½ ounces) Italian-style stewed tomatoes

1 tablespoon extra virgin olive oil

1. Coat a large nonstick skillet with nonstick cooking spray, and preheat over medium-high heat. Add the garlic, and stir-fry for about 30 seconds, or just until the garlic begins to turn color.

2. Add the green beans, the tomatoes with their juice, and the olive oil to the skillet, and stir to mix. Bring the mixture to a boil, reduce the heat to low, and cover. Simmer, stirring occasionally, for about 15 minutes.

3. Place the skillet cover slightly ajar to allow steam to escape, and cook for 10 additional minutes, or until the beans are tender. Serve hot.

> **NUTRITIONAL FACTS (PER ¾-CUP SERVING)**
> Cal: 64   Carbs: 8 g   Chol: 0 mg   Fat: 2.6 g
> Fiber: 3.3 g   Protein: 2 g   Sodium: 176 mg

Green Beans and Mushrooms

YIELD: 5 SERVINGS

1 pound fresh green beans, trimmed and cut into 1-inch pieces (about 4 cups)

1 cup sliced fresh mushrooms

½ cup water

1 teaspoon instant chicken bouillon granules

1 teaspoon crushed fresh garlic

½ teaspoon dried thyme

1. Place all of the ingredients in a 2½-quart pot, and stir to mix well. Bring to a boil over high heat.

2. Reduce the heat to medium-low, cover, and simmer, stirring occasionally, for 12 to 15 minutes, or until the beans are just tender. Serve hot.

> **NUTRITIONAL FACTS (PER ¾-CUP SERVING)**
> Cal: 32   Carbs: 7 g   Chol: 0 mg   Fat: 0.2 g
> Fiber: 3.2 g   Protein: 1.9 g   Sodium: 119 mg

Green Beans With Glazed Onions

YIELD: 6 SERVINGS

1 cup chicken or vegetable broth

1 pound fresh green beans, trimmed and snapped into 1½-inch pieces (about 4 cups)

2–3 teaspoons extra virgin olive oil

½ large Spanish onion, sliced into very thin wedges

¾ teaspoon dried thyme

¼ teaspoon salt

⅛ teaspoon ground black pepper

1 teaspoon sugar

1 tablespoon balsamic vinegar

1. Place the broth in the bottom of a stove top or microwave steamer, and add the beans. Cover and cook over high heat or on high power for 10 minutes, or until tender.

2. While the beans are cooking, coat a large nonstick skillet with the olive oil, and preheat over medium heat. Add the onion, thyme, salt, and pepper, and sauté for about 5 minutes, or until the onions are wilted and just starting to brown. (Cover the skillet periodically if it becomes too dry, or add a few teaspoons of broth as needed.) Add the sugar, and sauté for another minute. Add the vinegar, and stir to mix well.

3. Add the beans, along with 2 tablespoons of the broth used for steaming, to the skillet. Toss the beans and onions together for a minute or 2 over medium heat, and serve hot.

> **NUTRITIONAL FACTS (PER ¾-CUP SERVING)**
> Cal: 48   Carbs: 7 g   Chol: 0 mg   Fat: 1.6 g
> Fiber: 2.8 g   Protein: 1.6 g   Sodium: 94 mg

Cabbage and Potato Curry

YIELD: 6 SERVINGS

2 medium unpeeled potatoes, sliced 1/4 inch thick

1/2 cup chicken or vegetable broth

1/2 medium head cabbage, halved and cut into 1-inch pieces (about 1 pound)

2–3 teaspoons curry paste

1. Place the potatoes and broth in a large nonstick skillet. Place the skillet over medium-low heat, cover, and cook, stirring occasionally, for about 5 minutes, or until the potatoes start to soften.

2. Add the cabbage and curry paste to the skillet, and stir to mix. Cover and cook, stirring occasionally, for 7 to 9 minutes, or until the cabbage and potatoes are tender. Add more broth during cooking if the skillet becomes too dry. Serve hot.

NUTRITIONAL FACTS (PER 3/4-CUP SERVING)		
Cal: 93 Carbs: 17 g Chol: 0 mg Fat: 1.2 g		
Fiber: 2.9 g Protein: 2.8 g Sodium: 133 mg		

Braised Cabbage With Bacon and Onions

YIELD: 4 SERVINGS

3 strips extra-lean turkey bacon, diced, or 1 1/2 ounces diced Canadian bacon (about 1/3 cup)

1/2 medium-large head cabbage, halved and cut into 1/2-inch slices (about 1 pound)

1/2 medium onion, thinly sliced

1/4 cup chicken or vegetable broth

1/8 teaspoon ground black pepper

1. Coat a large nonstick skillet with nonstick cooking spray, and preheat over medium heat. Add the bacon, and cook, stirring frequently, for about 3 minutes, or until nicely browned.

2. Add the cabbage, onion, broth, and pepper to the skillet. Cover and cook over medium heat, stirring occasionally, for about 5 minutes, or until the cabbage begins to wilt. Add a few more tablespoons of broth if the skillet seems too dry, but only enough to keep the cabbage from scorching.

3. Reduce the heat to medium-low, cover, and cook for 10 additional minutes, or until the cabbage is wilted and tender. Serve hot.

NUTRITIONAL FACTS (PER 3/4-CUP SERVING)		
Cal: 44 Carbs: 6 g Chol: 11 mg Fat: 0.7 g		
Fiber: 3.2 g Protein: 3.9 g Sodium: 153 mg		

Carrots Marsala

YIELD: 5 SERVINGS

1 pound carrots (about 6 medium), peeled and cut into matchstick-sized pieces (about 4 cups)

1/2 cup chicken broth

1/4 cup dry Marsala

1 tablespoon sugar

1/8 teaspoon ground black pepper

1 tablespoon plus 1 teaspoon reduced-fat margarine or light butter

1 tablespoon finely chopped fresh parsley (garnish)

1. Place the carrots, broth, Marsala, sugar, and pepper in a large nonstick skillet, and stir to mix well. Bring the mixture to a boil over high heat. Reduce the heat to medium-low, cover, and cook, stirring occasionally, for about 6 minutes, or until the carrots are tender. Add a little more broth if the skillet becomes too dry.

2. Stir the margarine or butter into the carrot mixture. Increase the heat to medium-high, and cook uncovered for about 3 minutes, or until most of the liquid has evaporated. Sprinkle the parsley over the top, and serve hot.

NUTRITIONAL FACTS (PER 2/3-CUP SERVING)		
Cal: 75 Carbs: 12 g Chol: 0 mg Fat: 1.6 g		
Fiber: 2.7 g Protein: 0.8 g Sodium: 111 mg		

Celery Crunch Casserole

YIELD: 8 SERVINGS

¾ cup evaporated skim milk

3 tablespoons plus 1 teaspoon unbleached flour

3 cups thinly sliced celery (about 6 medium stalks)

1 tablespoon water

1 cup chicken broth

1 can (8 ounces) sliced water chestnuts, drained

1 can (4 ounces) sliced mushrooms, drained

2 tablespoons toasted sliced almonds
(page 348) (optional)

TOPPING

2 tablespoons grated Parmesan cheese*

2 tablespoons plain dried bread crumbs

Nonstick butter-flavored cooking spray

* In this recipe, use regular Parmesan cheese, not a fat-free product.

1. To make the topping, place the Parmesan cheese and bread crumbs in a small dish, and stir to mix well. Set aside.

2. Place the evaporated milk and flour in a jar with a tight-fitting lid, and shake until smooth. Set aside.

3. Place the celery and water in a large nonstick skillet. Cover and cook over medium heat, stirring frequently, for about 3 minutes, or until the celery is crisp-tender. (Add a little more water if the skillet becomes too dry.) Carefully drain off any excess liquid.

4. Add the broth to the skillet, and allow the mixture to come to a boil. Shake the milk mixture, and, stirring constantly, add it to the celery mixture. Reduce the heat to medium, and continue to cook and stir for another minute or 2, or until the mixture is thickened and bubbly.

5. Remove the skillet from the heat, and stir in the water chestnuts, mushrooms, and if desired, the almonds. Set aside.

6. Coat a shallow 1½-quart casserole dish or a 9-inch deep dish pie pan with nonstick cooking spray,

and spread the vegetable mixture evenly in the dish. Sprinkle the topping over the vegetables, and spray the top lightly with the cooking spray.

7. Bake uncovered at 350°F for about 23 minutes, or until the mixture is bubbly around the edges and the top is nicely browned. Remove the dish from the oven, and let sit for 5 minutes before serving.

NUTRITIONAL FACTS (PER ½-CUP SERVING)			
Cal: 67	Carbs: 12 g	Chol: 2 mg	Fat: 0.8 g
Fiber: 2.5 g	Protein: 3.7 g	Sodium: 235 mg	

Cauliflower au Gratin

*For variety, substitute broccoli
for the cauliflower.*

YIELD: 5 SERVINGS

1 recipe Cheddar Cheese Sauce (page 219)

1 package (1 pound) frozen cauliflower florets,
thawed and drained

2 tablespoons finely ground cracker crumbs
(onion or herb flavor) or seasoned
dried bread crumbs

Nonstick butter-flavored cooking spray

1. Prepare the cheese sauce in a 2-quart pot. Add the cauliflower and cook uncovered, stirring frequently, for about 2 minutes, or just until heated through.

2. Coat a shallow 1½-quart casserole dish or a 9-inch deep dish pie pan with nonstick cooking spray, and spread the mixture evenly in the dish. Sprinkle the crumbs over the top of the mixture, and spray the crumbs lightly with the cooking spray.

2. Bake uncovered at 350°F for about 20 minutes, or until the top is browned and the edges are bubbly. Remove the dish from the oven, and let sit for 5 minutes before serving.

NUTRITIONAL FACTS (PER ¾-CUP SERVING)			
Cal: 80	Carbs: 10 g	Chol: 4 mg	Fat: 0.3 g
Fiber: 1.8 g	Protein: 9 g	Sodium: 221 mg	

Glazed Rosemary Carrots

YIELD: 5 SERVINGS

1 pound carrots (about 6 medium), peeled and
cut into matchstick-sized pieces (about 4 cups)

1/2 cup plus 2 tablespoons apple juice

1/2 teaspoon dried rosemary, finely crumbled

1/8 teaspoon salt

1 tablespoon light brown sugar or honey

1 tablespoon plus 1 teaspoon reduced-fat
margarine or light butter

1. Place the carrots, apple juice, rosemary, and salt in
a large nonstick skillet, and stir to mix well. Bring the
mixture to a boil over high heat. Reduce the heat to
medium-low, cover, and cook, stirring occasionally,
for about 6 minutes, or until the carrots are tender.
Add a little more juice if the skillet becomes too dry.

2. Stir the brown sugar or honey and the margarine
or butter into the carrot mixture. Increase the heat to
medium-high, and cook uncovered for a few additional minutes, or until most of the liquid has evaporated. Serve hot.

NUTRITIONAL FACTS (PER 2/3-CUP SERVING)		
Cal: 75 Carbs: 15 g Chol: 0 mg Fat: 1.7 g		
Fiber: 2.6 g Protein: 0.9 g Sodium: 109 mg		

Country-Style Collards

YIELD: 5 SERVINGS

1 pound frozen (unthawed) chopped
collard or turnip greens

3/4 cup water

1/2 cup diced ham, at least 97% lean

3/4 teaspoon dry mustard

1/2 teaspoon instant ham or chicken bouillon granules

1. Place all of the ingredients in a 2-quart pot, and
bring to a boil over high heat. Stir to mix well, reduce
the heat to medium-low, and cover.

2. Simmer the greens, stirring occasionally, for about
20 minutes, or until tender. Serve hot.

NUTRITIONAL FACTS (PER 2/3-CUP SERVING)		
Cal: 48 Carbs: 5 g Chol: 5 mg Fat: 0.8 g		
Fiber: 2.6 g Protein: 5.3 g Sodium: 260 mg		

Country Corn Pudding

YIELD: 7 SERVINGS

2 cups skim or low-fat milk

1/2 cup quick-cooking yellow corn grits*

1/4 cup finely chopped onion

1 tablespoon sugar

1/8 teaspoon ground white pepper

1 can (8 ounces) creamed corn

1 can (8 ounces) whole kernel corn, drained

1/4 cup plus 2 tablespoons evaporated skim milk

3/4 cup fat-free egg substitute

1/2 teaspoon baking powder

* Look for grits that cook in 3 to 5 minutes.

1. Place the milk, grits, onion, sugar, and pepper in a
2 1/2-quart nonstick pot, and stir to mix. Cook over
medium heat, stirring frequently, until the mixture
begins to boil. Reduce the heat to low, cover, and simmer, stirring frequently, for about 5 minutes, or until
thick and bubbly.

2. Remove the pot from the heat, and stir in first the
creamed and whole kernel corn, then the evaporated
milk, and, finally, the egg substitute. Sprinkle the
baking powder over the top, and stir to mix well.

3. Coat a 2-quart casserole dish with nonstick cooking spray, and pour the pudding mixture into the
dish. Place the dish in a large roasting pan, and add
hot tap water to the pan until it reaches halfway up
the sides of the dish.

4. Bake uncovered at 350°F for 50 minutes, or until a
sharp knife inserted in the center of the dish comes
out clean. Remove the dish from the oven, and let sit
for 10 minutes before serving.

NUTRITIONAL FACTS (PER 2/3-CUP SERVING)		
Cal: 136 Carbs: 25 g Chol: 2 mg Fat: 0.6 g		
Fiber: 1.3 g Protein: 8 g Sodium: 259 mg		

Stuffed Eggplant Extraordinaire

YIELD: 4 SERVINGS

2 slices whole wheat bread

2 small eggplants (about 8 ounces each)

1 medium tomato, finely chopped

1/3 cup finely chopped green bell pepper

1/3 cup finely chopped onion

1/3 cup finely chopped celery

1/8 teaspoon salt

1/4 teaspoon ground black pepper

2 tablespoons minced fresh parsley,
or 2 teaspoons dried

2 tablespoons plus 2 teaspoons grated
Parmesan cheese*

Nonstick olive oil cooking spray

* In this recipe, use regular Parmesan cheese, not a fat-free product.

1. Tear the bread into pieces, and place the pieces in a blender or food processor. Process into fine crumbs, and set aside.

2. Cut each eggplant in half lengthwise, and scoop out and reserve the flesh, leaving a 3/8-inch-thick shell. Trim a small piece off the bottom of each shell, if necessary, to allow the half to sit upright. Set aside.

3. Coat a large skillet with nonstick cooking spray. Finely chop the removed eggplant, and transfer it to the skillet. Add the tomato, green pepper, onion, celery, salt, and black pepper to the skillet, and place over medium heat. Cover and cook, stirring occasionally, for about 5 minutes, or until the vegetables are almost tender.

4. Remove the skillet from the heat, and stir in the bread crumbs and parsley. Divide the eggplant mixture among the 4 hollowed-out eggplant shells.

5. Coat a shallow baking dish with nonstick cooking spray, and arrange the stuffed shells in the dish. Sprinkle 2 teaspoons of cheese over the top of each stuffed shell, and spray the tops lightly with the

cooking spray. Bake uncovered at 350ºF for 25 minutes, or until the filling is heated through and the tops are golden brown. Serve hot.

NUTRITIONAL FACTS (PER SERVING)		
Cal: 87 Carbs: 12 g Chol: 1 mg Fat: 1.8 g		
Fiber: 4.5 g Protein: 5.1 g Sodium: 182 mg		

Italian Oven-Fried Eggplant

YIELD: 4 SERVINGS

1 large eggplant (about 1 pound)

1/4 cup fat-free egg substitute

1/3 cup Italian-style seasoned dried bread crumbs

3 tablespoons grated Parmesan cheese*

1 tablespoon plus 1 teaspoon unbleached flour

Nonstick olive oil cooking spray

* In this recipe, use regular Parmesan cheese, not a fat-free product.

1. Trim a couple of inches off each end of the eggplant, and discard. Slice the eggplant crosswise into eight rounds, each 1/2-inch thick. Set aside.

2. Coat a large baking sheet with nonstick olive oil cooking spray, and set aside.

3. Place the egg substitute in a shallow bowl. Place the bread crumbs, Parmesan cheese, and flour in another shallow bowl, and stir to mix well. Dip the eggplant slices first in the egg substitute, and then in the crumb mixture, turning to coat both sides well. Arrange the slices in a single layer on the prepared sheet, and spray the tops lightly with the cooking spray.

4. Bake uncovered at 400°F for 10 minutes. Turn the slices, and bake for 10 additional minutes, or until golden brown and tender. Serve hot.

NUTRITIONAL FACTS (PER SERVING)		
Cal: 87 Carbs: 13 g Chol: 3 mg Fat: 1.7 g		
Fiber: 2.5 g Protein: 5.4 g Sodium: 229 mg		

Spiced Sweet Potato Soufflé

YIELD: 8 SERVINGS

2 pounds unpeeled sweet potatoes
(about 4 medium)

1/2 cup apple or orange juice

3 tablespoons maple syrup or honey

1/2 teaspoon ground cinnamon

1/2 teaspoon ground nutmeg

1/4 cup plus 2 tablespoons golden raisins
or chopped dates

3 egg whites, brought to room temperature

1/2 teaspoon cream of tartar

TOPPING

1/4 cup light brown sugar

1/4 cup honey crunch wheat germ or finely
chopped pecans

3 tablespoons shredded sweetened coconut

1. To cook the sweet potatoes in a conventional oven, bake them at 400°F for about 45 minutes, or until tender. To cook in a microwave oven, prick each potato in several places with a fork, and microwave on high power for about 15 minutes, or until tender. Set aside to cool.

2. To make the topping, place all of the topping ingredients in a small bowl, and stir to mix well. Set aside.

3. When the potatoes have cooled, peel them and cut them into chunks. Place the potatoes, fruit juice, maple syrup or honey, cinnamon, and nutmeg in a large bowl, and, using an electric mixer or a potato masher, beat or mash the potatoes until smooth. Stir in the raisins or dates, and set the mixture aside.

4. Place the egg whites in a large glass bowl, and sprinkle the cream of tartar over the top. Using an electric mixer, beat for several minutes, or until stiff peaks form when the beaters are lifted. Gently fold the egg whites into the potato mixture.

5. Coat a 2-quart casserole dish with nonstick cooking spray, and spread the sweet potato mixture evenly in the dish. Sprinkle the topping over the potatoes.

6. Bake uncovered at 350°F for about 45 minutes, or until the topping is golden brown and a sharp knife inserted near the center of the casserole comes out clean. Cover the casserole loosely with aluminum foil during the last few minutes of baking if the top starts to brown too quickly. Serve hot.

NUTRITIONAL FACTS (PER 2/3-CUP SERVING)
Cal: 168   Carbs: 37 g   Chol: 0 mg   Fat: 1.2 g
Fiber: 2.6 g   Protein: 3.5 g   Sodium: 35 mg

Southwestern Roasted Sweet Potatoes

YIELD: 6 SERVINGS

1 3/4 pounds unpeeled sweet potatoes
(about 3 medium-large)

3–4 teaspoons chili powder

1/4 teaspoon salt

1 tablespoon extra virgin olive oil

1. Peel the potatoes, and cut into 1/4-inch-thick slices. Measure the potatoes; there should be 5 cups. Adjust the amount if necessary.

2. Place the potatoes in a large bowl. Sprinkle with the chili powder and salt, and drizzle with the olive oil. Toss well to coat.

3. Coat a nonstick 9-x-13-inch pan with nonstick cooking spray, and spread the potatoes evenly in the pan. Cover the pan with aluminum foil, and bake at 400°F for 15 minutes. Remove the foil, and bake for 10 additional minutes. Turn the potatoes, and bake for 10 minutes more, or until tender. Serve hot.

NUTRITIONAL FACTS (PER 2/3-CUP SERVING)
Cal: 106   Carbs: 20 g   Chol: 0 mg   Fat: 2.5 g
Fiber: 2.8 g   Protein: 1.6 g   Sodium: 109 mg

Sweet Potato-Apple Casserole

YIELD: 8 SERVINGS

1¾ pounds unpeeled sweet potatoes
(about 3 medium-large)

4 medium Granny Smith or golden Delicious apples

¼ cup plus 2 tablespoons dark raisins

3 tablespoons orange juice

2 tablespoons honey

2 tablespoons light brown sugar

1½ teaspoons cornstarch

1 teaspoon dried grated orange rind

1. Peel the potatoes, halve lengthwise, and cut into ⅛-inch-thick slices. Measure the potatoes; there should be 5 cups. Adjust the amount if necessary.

2. Peel the apples, and cut into ¼-inch-thick slices. Measure the apples; there should be 3 cups. Adjust the amount if necessary.

Buttery-Tasting Potatoes Without the Fat

Naturally fat-free and rich in potassium, potatoes star in many of our favorite side dishes, in addition to making a hearty addition to soups and stews. Unfortunately, most of us add far too much fat to our potatoes, turning a nutritious food into one that has no place in a light and healthy lifestyle.

If you love buttery-tasting potatoes but not the fat or calories, you will be happy to know that several varieties of "golden" potatoes are now widely available in grocery stores. These all-purpose potatoes have a light butter-colored flesh and a smooth buttery flavor that needs no added fat, making them perfect for all your lighter recipes. Look for brands like Yukon Gold and Yellow Finn.

---

3. Coat a 2-quart casserole dish with nonstick butter-flavored cooking spray, and spread half of the potatoes over the bottom of the dish. Top with half of the apples and half of the raisins. Repeat the layers.

4. Place all of the remaining ingredients in a small bowl, and stir until the cornstarch is dissolved. Pour the juice mixture over the casserole. Cover the dish with aluminum foil, and, using a sharp knife, cut four 1-inch slits in the foil to allow steam to escape.

5. Bake at 350°F for 1 hour, or until all of the layers are tender. Serve hot.

NUTRITIONAL FACTS (PER ⅔-CUP SERVING)
Cal: 131   Carbs: 33 g   Chol: 0 mg   Fat: 0.2 g
Fiber: 2.7 g   Protein: 1.3 g   Sodium: 8 mg

Pineapple-Sweet Potato Casserole

YIELD: 6 SERVINGS

2 cans (15 ounces each) cut sweet potatoes
in light syrup, drained

1 can (8 ounces) crushed pineapple
in juice, undrained

¼ teaspoon ground cinnamon

¼ cup golden raisins or chopped dates

¼ cup chopped toasted pecans
(page 348) (optional)

1½ cups miniature marshmallows

1. Cut the potatoes into bite-sized pieces, and place in a large bowl. Add all of the remaining ingredients except the marshmallows, and toss to mix.

2. Coat a 9-inch deep dish pie pan with nonstick cooking spray, and place the sweet potato mixture in the pan. Top with the marshmallows.

3. Bake uncovered at 350°F for about 35 minutes, or until the sweet potato mixture is bubbly around the edges and the top is lightly browned. If the top starts to brown too quickly, loosely cover the dish with aluminum foil during the last 10 minutes of baking. Serve hot.

NUTRITIONAL FACTS (PER ⅔-CUP SERVING)
Cal: 184   Carbs: 44 g   Chol: 0 mg   Fat: 0.2 g
Fiber: 2.5 g   Protein: 1.8 g   Sodium: 33 mg

Cheddar-Stuffed Potatoes

YIELD: 4 SERVINGS

4 medium Yukon Gold or russet baking potatoes (about 6 ounces each)
1/4 cup skim milk
1/4 cup nonfat or light sour cream
1/8 teaspoon salt
1/2 cup shredded nonfat or reduced-fat Cheddar cheese
3 tablespoons finely chopped onion
1 tablespoon finely chopped fresh parsley, chives, or dill
Nonstick butter-flavored cooking spray
Ground paprika (garnish)

1. To cook the potatoes in a conventional oven, wrap each potato in aluminum foil, and bake at 400°F for about 40 minutes, or until tender. To cook in a microwave oven, prick each potato in several places with a fork, and microwave on high power for about 12 minutes, or until tender. Allow the potatoes to cool until they can be handled easily.

2. Cut a 1/2-inch-deep lengthwise slice from the top of each potato, and carefully scoop out the pulp, leaving a 1/4-inch-thick shell. Place the scooped-out potato flesh and the milk, sour cream, and salt in a medium-sized bowl, and mash with a potato masher. Add the cheese, onion, and parsley, and stir to mix well.

3. Spoon the filling back into the potato skins. Arrange the potatoes in an 8-x-8-inch baking dish, spray the tops lightly with the cooking spray, and sprinkle some paprika over each. Bake at 350°F for 25 to 30 minutes, or until the filling is heated through and the tops are lightly browned. Serve hot.

NUTRITIONAL FACTS (PER SERVING)
Cal: 199   Carbs: 39 g   Chol: 2 mg   Fat: 0.5 g
Fiber: 3.6 g   Protein: 9.2 g   Sodium: 152 mg

Cheddar Scalloped Potatoes

YIELD: 6 SERVINGS

1 1/4 pounds unpeeled Yukon Gold or russet potatoes (3–4 medium)
1 recipe Cheddar Cheese Sauce (page 219)
2 tablespoons plain dried bread crumbs
Nonstick butter-flavored cooking spray

1. To cook the potatoes in a microwave oven, prick each potato in several places with a fork, and microwave on high power for about 12 minutes, or until tender. To cook the potatoes in a conventional oven, wrap each potato in aluminum foil, and bake at 400°F for about 40 minutes, or until tender. Set aside to cool.

2. When the potatoes have cooled, slice them into 1/4-inch-thick slices. There should be about 3 1/2 cups of cooked potatoes. Set aside.

3. Prepare the Cheddar Cheese Sauce in a 2-quart pot, increasing the amount of milk called for in the recipe to 1 1/4 cups. Remove the sauce from the heat, add the potatoes, and toss to mix well.

4. Coat a shallow 1 1/2-quart casserole dish or a 9-inch deep dish pie pan with nonstick cooking spray, and spread the mixture evenly in the dish. Sprinkle the crumbs over the top of the mixture, and spray the top lightly with the cooking spray.

5. Bake uncovered at 350°F for about 25 minutes, or until the edges are bubbly and the top is lightly browned. Remove the dish from the oven, and let sit for 5 minutes before serving.

NUTRITIONAL FACTS (PER 2/3-CUP SERVING)
Cal: 149   Carbs: 26 g   Chol: 2 mg   Fat: 0.5 g
Fiber: 2 g   Protein: 9 g   Sodium: 181 mg

Sauce It Up!

Butter- and cheese-based sauces can do so much to enhance the flavor of vegetables. Unfortunately, these same sauces can also add an unhealthy amount of fat and calories. But take heart. Made properly, creamy, rich-tasting sauces can still adorn your favorite veggies. Here are some ideas for light and luscious toppings.

Creamy Lemon Sauce

This sauce can beautifully replace hollandaise in any of your favorite recipes.

YIELD: 1½ CUPS
3 tablespoons instant nonfat dry milk powder
2 tablespoons cornstarch
Pinch ground white pepper
Pinch dry mustard
Pinch ground nutmeg
1 cup skim or low-fat milk
¼ cup fat-free egg substitute
1 tablespoon reduced-fat margarine or light butter
3 tablespoons lemon juice
1 teaspoon freshly grated lemon rind
¼ teaspoon salt

1. Place the milk powder, cornstarch, pepper, mustard, and nutmeg in a 1-quart glass bowl, and stir to mix well. Add ¼ cup of the milk, and stir with a wire whisk until smooth. Whisk in the remaining milk and the egg substitute. Add the margarine or butter to the milk mixture. (There is no need to melt the margarine or butter.)

2. Place the bowl containing the milk mixture in a microwave oven, and microwave uncovered on high power for 1½ minutes. Then whisk to mix well. Microwave for an additional 1½ to 2 minutes, whisking every 30 seconds, until the mixture is thickened. (Note that the mixture may seem curdled when you first stir it, but will become smooth as you keep whisking.)

3. Remove the mixture from the microwave oven, and whisk in the lemon juice, lemon rind, and salt. Serve hot over steamed asparagus, green beans, cauliflower, or other vegetables.

NUTRITIONAL FACTS (PER TABLESPOON)
Cal: 12   Carbs: 1.6 g   Chol: 0 mg   Fat: 0.3 g   Fiber: 0 g   Protein: 0.8 g   Sodium: 39 mg

Sour Cream-Dill Sauce

YIELD: 1⅛ CUPS
½ cup plus 1 tablespoon nonfat or light mayonnaise
½ cup plus 1 tablespoon nonfat or light sour cream
1 tablespoon plus 1½ teaspoons water
1 tablespoon lemon juice
Pinch ground white pepper
2 tablespoons finely chopped fresh dill

1. Place the mayonnaise, sour cream, water, lemon juice, and pepper in a small saucepan, and stir with a wire whisk to mix well. Place the pan over medium heat, and cook, stirring constantly, until the sauce is heated through.

2. Stir the dill into the sauce, and remove the pot from the heat. Serve hot over steamed cauliflower, asparagus, green beans, potatoes, or other vegetables.

NUTRITIONAL FACTS (PER TABLESPOON)
Cal: 12   Carbs: 2.4 g   Chol: 0 mg   Fat: 0 g   Fiber: 0 g   Protein: 0.2 g   Sodium: 56 mg

Cheddar Cheese Sauce

YIELD: 1¼ CUPS

1 cup skim or low-fat milk, divided

2 tablespoons plus 1½ teaspoons unbleached flour

2 tablespoons instant nonfat dry milk powder

⅛ teaspoon ground white pepper

¾ cup diced or shredded nonfat or reduced-fat process Cheddar cheese

1. Place ⅓ cup of the milk and all of the flour, milk powder, and pepper in a small jar with a tight-fitting lid. Shake to mix well, and set aside.

2. Place the remaining ⅔ cup of milk in a 1-quart saucepan. Place over medium heat, and cook, stirring constantly, until the milk starts to boil. Stir in the flour mixture, and continue to cook and stir for a few seconds, or until the sauce is thickened and bubbly.

3. Reduce the heat to medium-low, add the cheese, and continue to stir until the cheese melts. Serve hot over steamed broccoli, cauliflower, asparagus, potatoes, or other vegetables.

NUTRITIONAL FACTS (PER TABLESPOON)
Cal: 15   Carbs: 1.6 g   Chol: 1 mg   Fat: 0 g
Fiber: 0 g   Protein: 2 g   Sodium: 45 mg

Honey Mustard Sauce

YIELD: 1¼ CUPS

¾ cup nonfat or light mayonnaise

¼ cup Dijon mustard

2–3 tablespoons honey

1 tablespoon water

1. Place all of the ingredients in a 1-quart saucepan, and stir to mix well. Place over medium-low heat, and cook, stirring constantly, just until the sauce is heated through.

2. Serve hot over steamed broccoli, cauliflower, asparagus, or other vegetables.

NUTRITIONAL FACTS (PER TABLESPOON)
Cal: 16   Carbs: 3.3 g   Chol: 0 mg   Fat: 0.3 g
Fiber: 0 g   Protein: 0.2 g   Sodium: 130 mg

Golden Mashed Potatoes

YIELD: 8 SERVINGS

1 medium rutabaga (about 1½ pounds)

1½ pounds baking potatoes (4–5 medium)

¼ teaspoon salt

⅛ teaspoon ground white pepper

⅓ cup nonfat or light sour cream or plain nonfat yogurt

1. Peel the rutabaga, and dice it into ½-inch cubes. Place the rutabaga in a 3-quart pot, add enough water to barely cover, and bring to a boil over high heat. Reduce the heat to medium-low, cover, and simmer, stirring occasionally, for about 20 minutes, or until the rutabaga is almost tender.

2. Peel the potatoes, and cut them into 1-inch pieces. Add the potatoes to the cooking rutabaga, adding water if needed to barely cover the vegetables. Increase the heat to high, and bring to a second boil. Reduce the heat to medium-low, cover, and simmer for about 15 minutes, or until the vegetables are very tender.

3. Remove the pot from the heat, and drain off and reserve the cooking liquid. Add the salt and pepper to the vegetables, and mash with a potato masher or beat with an electric mixer until smooth.

4. Stir the sour cream or yogurt into the mashed vegetables, adding a little of the reserved cooking liquid if the mixture is too stiff. Serve hot.

NUTRITIONAL FACTS (PER ⅔-CUP SERVING)
Cal: 96   Carbs: 21 g   Chol: 0 mg   Fat: 0.2 g
Fiber: 3 g   Protein: 2.5 g   Sodium: 97 mg

Garlic Mashed Potatoes

YIELD: 6 SERVINGS

2 pounds Yukon Gold or russet potatoes
(about 6 medium)

5–6 cloves garlic, peeled

1/2 cup plain nonfat yogurt or nonfat or light sour cream

1/4 teaspoon salt

Pinch ground white pepper

1. Peel the potatoes, and cut them into chunks. Place the potatoes and the garlic in a 3-quart pot, add water just to cover, and bring to a boil over high heat. Reduce the heat to medium, cover, and cook for about 12 minutes, or until soft.

2. Drain the potatoes and garlic, reserving 1/2 cup of the cooking liquid. Return the vegetables to the pot, and stir in the yogurt or sour cream, salt, pepper, and 1/4 cup of the reserved cooking liquid.

3. Beat the potatoes with an electric mixer or mash with a potato masher until smooth. If the potatoes are too stiff, add enough of the reserved cooking liquid to achieve the desired consistency. Serve hot.

NUTRITIONAL FACTS (PER 3/4-CUP SERVING)
Cal: 130   Carbs: 29 g   Chol: 0 mg   Fat: 0.2 g
Fiber: 2 g   Protein: 3.6 g   Sodium: 111 mg

Greek Cottage Fries

*For variety, substitute peeled sweet potatoes
for the baking potatoes.*

YIELD: 4 SERVINGS

1 1/2 pounds unpeeled baking potatoes
(about 3 extra large)

2–3 teaspoons extra virgin olive oil

1 teaspoon crushed fresh garlic

3/4 teaspoon dried rosemary, finely crumbled

1/4 teaspoon salt

1. Scrub the potatoes, dry well, and cut lengthwise into strips that are 3/8-inch thick and 3/4-inch wide. Place the strips in a large bowl.

2. Drizzle the olive oil over the potatoes. Add the garlic, rosemary, and salt, and toss to mix well.

3. Coat a large nonstick baking sheet with nonstick olive oil cooking spray, and arrange the potatoes in a single layer on the sheet. Make sure that the strips aren't touching one another.

4. Bake uncovered at 400°F for 20 minutes. Turn the potatoes, and bake for 10 additional minutes, or until nicely browned and tender. Serve hot.

NUTRITIONAL FACTS (PER SERVING)
Cal: 167   Carbs: 34 g   Chol: 0 mg   Fat: 2.4 g
Fiber: 3.1 g   Protein: 3.2 g   Sodium: 152 mg

Herb-Roasted Onions

YIELD: 6 SERVINGS

2 pounds Spanish or sweet onions (about 4 large)

1 tablespoon balsamic vinegar

1 1/2 teaspoons dried thyme or rosemary,
or 1 1/2 tablespoons chopped fresh

1/4 teaspoon salt

1/4 teaspoon ground black pepper

1 tablespoon extra virgin olive oil (optional)

Nonstick olive oil cooking spray

1. Peel the onions, trim the ends off, and cut into 3/4-inch-thick wedges. Measure the onions; there should be about 6 cups. Adjust the amount if necessary.

2. Place the onions in a large bowl, and add the vinegar, thyme or rosemary, salt, pepper, and, if desired, the olive oil. Toss to mix well.

3. Coat a 9-x-13-inch pan with the cooking spray, and spread the onions over the bottom of the pan. If you did not use the olive oil, spray the tops of the onions with the cooking spray.

4. Bake uncovered at 450°F for 20 minutes. Stir well, and bake for 15 additional minutes, or until tender and nicely browned. Serve hot.

NUTRITIONAL FACTS (PER 3/4-CUP SERVING)
Cal: 52   Carbs: 12 g   Chol: 0 mg   Fat: 0.2 g
Fiber: 2.2 g   Protein: 1.6 g   Sodium: 93 mg

Hearty Oven Fries

YIELD: 5 SERVINGS

1½ pounds unpeeled baking potatoes
(about 3 extra large)

1 egg white, lightly beaten, or 2 tablespoons
fat-free egg substitute

Nonstick cooking spray

COATING

2 teaspoons ground paprika

1 teaspoon garlic powder

¼ teaspoon salt

⅛ teaspoon ground black pepper

1. To make the coating, place all of the coating ingredients in a small dish, and stir to mix well. Set aside.

2. Scrub the potatoes, dry well, and cut lengthwise into ½-inch-thick strips. Place the potatoes in a large bowl. Pour the egg white or egg substitute over the potatoes, and toss to coat evenly. Sprinkle the coating over the potatoes, and toss again to coat.

3. Coat a large baking sheet with nonstick cooking spray, and arrange the potatoes in a single layer on the sheet. Make sure that the potato strips aren't touching one another.

4. Spray the tops lightly with cooking spray, and bake uncovered at 400°F for 15 minutes. Turn the potatoes, and bake for 15 additional minutes, or until nicely browned and tender. Serve hot.

NUTRITIONAL FACTS (PER SERVING)
Cal: 123   Carbs: 28 g   Chol: 0 mg   Fat: 0.3 g
Fiber: 2.7 g   Protein: 2.7 g   Sodium: 125 mg

VARIATION
To make Crispy Cajun Fries, substitute 1½ teaspoons of Cajun seasoning mixed with 1½ teaspoons of ground paprika for the coating mixture.

NUTRITIONAL FACTS (PER SERVING)
Cal: 124   Carbs: 28 g   Chol: 0 mg   Fat: 0.3 g
Fiber: 2.7 g   Protein: 2.7 g   Sodium: 151 mg

Crispy Onion Rings

YIELD: 5 SERVINGS

2 medium-large sweet onions (about 8 ounces each)

Nonstick cooking spray

EGG COATING

¼ cup plus 2 tablespoons unbleached flour

¼ cup plus 2 tablespoons fat-free egg substitute

¼ cup skim or low-fat milk

CORN FLAKE COATING

3½ cups corn flakes

¼ cup grated Parmesan cheese*

¼ teaspoon dried thyme

¼ teaspoon ground black pepper

* In this recipe, use regular Parmesan cheese, not a fat-free product.

1. Peel the onions, and cut into ½-inch-thick slices. Separate the slices into rings, and set aside.

2. Place all of the egg coating ingredients in a shallow bowl, and stir with a wire whisk until smooth. Set aside.

3. Place all of the corn flake coating ingredients in a food processor or blender, and process into fine crumbs. Transfer the corn flake mixture to a shallow dish.

4. Coat a large baking sheet with nonstick cooking spray. Dip the onion rings first in the egg mixture, turning to coat well, and then in the corn flake mixture. Arrange the rings in a single layer on the prepared sheet, and spray them lightly with the cooking spray.

5. Bake uncovered at 400°F for 10 to 12 minutes, or until the onion rings are crisp and nicely browned. Serve hot.

NUTRITIONAL FACTS (PER SERVING)
Cal: 169   Carbs: 30 g   Chol: 2 mg   Fat: 1.8 g
Fiber: 2.7 g   Protein: 8 g   Sodium: 156 mg

Spinach-Stuffed Tomatoes

YIELD: 8 SERVINGS

4 large tomatoes (about 8 ounces each)

1 cup whole wheat couscous

1½ cups vegetable or chicken broth

1½ teaspoons crushed fresh garlic

3 cups (packed) chopped fresh spinach

¼ cup finely chopped fresh basil

¼ cup grated Parmesan cheese*

Nonstick butter-flavored cooking spray

½ cup shredded reduced-fat mozzarella cheese

* In this recipe, use regular Parmesan cheese, not a fat-free product.

1. Cut each tomato in half crosswise, and scoop out the pulp, leaving just the shell. Discard the pulp or reserve it for another use, and set the tomato shells aside.

2. Place the couscous and broth in a 1-quart pot, and bring to a boil over high heat. Stir the mixture, reduce the heat to low, and cover. Simmer for about 3 minutes, or until the liquid is absorbed and the couscous is tender. Remove the pot from the heat, and set aside to cool slightly.

3. Coat a large nonstick skillet with nonstick cooking spray, and preheat over medium heat. Add the garlic, and stir-fry for about 30 seconds, or just until the garlic begins to turn color. Add the spinach, and stir-fry for another minute or 2, or until the spinach is wilted.

4. Remove the skillet from the heat, and add the couscous, basil, and Parmesan. Toss to mix well.

5. Coat a 7-x-11-inch pan with nonstick cooking spray. Spoon the spinach mixture into the tomato shells, mounding the tops slightly, and arrange the tomatoes in the prepared pan. Spray the tops lightly with the cooking spray.

6. Bake uncovered at 350°F for 20 minutes. Sprinkle 1 tablespoon of mozzarella over the top of each tomato, and bake for 5 additional minutes, or until the tomatoes are tender, the filling is heated through, and the cheese is melted. Serve hot.

NUTRITIONAL FACTS (PER SERVING)
Cal: 149   Carbs: 23 g   Chol: 3 mg   Fat: 2.6 g
Fiber: 4.3 g   Protein: 8 g   Sodium: 216 mg

Rosemary Roasted Vegetables

YIELD: 4 SERVINGS

2 medium carrots, peeled and sliced ¾-inch thick

2 medium yellow onions, cut into ¾-inch-thick wedges

2 medium potatoes (unpeeled), cut into 1-inch cubes

8 ounces whole fresh mushrooms, cut in half

6 cloves garlic, peeled

1 tablespoon balsamic vinegar

1 tablespoon broth or water

1 tablespoon fresh rosemary, or 1 teaspoon dried

¼ teaspoon coarsely ground black pepper

¼ teaspoon salt

1 tablespoon extra virgin olive oil (optional)

Nonstick olive oil cooking spray

1. Place the vegetables and garlic cloves in a large bowl, and toss to mix well. Add the vinegar, broth or water, rosemary, pepper, salt, and, if desired, the olive oil, and stir to mix well.

2. Coat a 9-x-13-inch nonstick pan with the cooking spray, and spread the vegetables in an even layer in the pan. If you did not use the olive oil, spray the tops of the vegetables with the cooking spray.

3. Cover the pan with aluminum foil, and bake at 450°F for 20 minutes. Remove the foil, and bake for 15 additional minutes. Turn the vegetables, and bake for 15 minutes more, or until the vegetables are tender and nicely browned. Serve hot.

NUTRITIONAL FACTS (PER ¾-CUP SERVING)
Cal: 136   Carbs: 30 g   Chol: 0 mg   Fat: 1 g
Fiber: 3.7 g   Protein: 4 g   Sodium: 154 mg

Summary Squash Casserole

YIELD: 6 SERVINGS

1½ pounds fresh yellow squash (8–10 medium)

½ cup chopped onion

2 tablespoons water

⅛ teaspoon ground black pepper

1 tablespoon unbleached flour

¾ cup nonfat or low-fat cottage cheese

¾ cup fat-free egg substitute

¾ cup shredded nonfat or reduced-fat
Cheddar cheese

2 tablespoons Italian-style seasoned
dried bread crumbs

Nonstick butter-flavored cooking spray

1. Cut each squash in half lengthwise. Then cut into slices slightly less than ¼-inch thick. Measure the squash; there should be 5 cups. Adjust the amount if necessary.

2. Place the squash, onion, water, and pepper in a large nonstick skillet, and stir to mix. Cover and cook over medium heat for about 4 minutes, or until the squash starts to soften. Reduce the heat to medium-low, and cook, stirring occasionally, for 7 additional minutes, or until the squash is tender. Add a little water during cooking if needed, but only enough to prevent sticking and burning.

3. If any excess water remains in the skillet, cook uncovered until the liquid evaporates, or carefully drain the liquid off. Remove the skillet from the heat, and set aside for about 10 minutes to cool slightly.

4. Stir the flour into the cottage cheese. Then add the cottage cheese to the squash, stirring to mix well. Stir in first the egg substitute and then the cheese.

5. Coat an 8-inch square (2-quart) baking dish with nonstick cooking spray, and spread the squash mixture evenly in the pan. Sprinkle the bread crumbs over the top, and spray the top lightly with the cooking spray.

6. Bake uncovered at 375°F for about 45 minutes, or until the mixture is bubbly around the edges, the top is lightly browned, and a sharp knife inserted in the center of the casserole comes out clean. Remove the dish from the oven, and let sit for 10 minutes before serving.

> **NUTRITIONAL FACTS (PER ¾-CUP SERVING)**
> Cal: 96   Carbs: 10 g   Chol: 4 mg   Fat: 0.4 g
> Fiber: 2.4 g   Protein: 13.4 g   Sodium: 321 mg

Cranapple Acorn Squash

YIELD: 4 SERVINGS

2 medium acorn squash (about 1 pound each)

¼ teaspoon ground nutmeg

Nonstick butter-flavored cooking spray

FILLING

2 cups finely chopped peeled apple
(about 3 medium)

¼ cup dried sweetened cranberries

¼ cup golden raisins

3 tablespoons light brown sugar

2 tablespoons chopped toasted pecans
(page 348) (optional)

1. Cut each squash in half crosswise, and scoop out and discard the seeds. If necessary, trim a small piece off the bottom of each half to allow it to sit upright. Set aside.

2. To make the filling, place all of the filling ingredients in a medium-sized bowl, and stir to mix well. Spoon a quarter of the mixture into the cavity of each squash half, and sprinkle a pinch of nutmeg over each stuffed shell.

3. Coat a 9-x-13-inch pan with nonstick cooking spray, and arrange the filled squash halves in the pan. Spray the tops lightly with the cooking spray, cover the dish with aluminum foil, and bake at 350°F for about 1 hour, or until tender. Serve hot.

> **NUTRITIONAL FACTS (PER SERVING)**
> Cal: 202   Carbs: 51 g   Chol: 0 mg   Fat: 0.8 g
> Fiber: 8.5 g   Protein: 2 g   Sodium: 11 mg

Baked Butternut Pudding

YIELD: 8 SERVINGS

3 pounds butternut squash (about 2 medium)

2 cups apple juice

2 tablespoons light brown sugar

1 tablespoon plus 1 teaspoon
butter-flavored sprinkles

1/2 teaspoon ground cinnamon

1/4 teaspoon ground nutmeg

1/2 cup fat-free egg substitute

TOPPING

3 tablespoons light brown sugar

3 tablespoons honey crunch wheat germ or
finely chopped toasted pecans (page 348)

1. Peel and seed the squash, and cut the remaining flesh into cubes. Place the squash and the apple juice in a 4-quart pot, and bring to a boil over high heat. Reduce the heat to low, cover, and simmer, stirring occasionally, for 25 minutes, or until the squash is very tender.

2. Remove the pot from the heat, and drain off and discard the juice. Add the brown sugar, butter-flavored sprinkles, cinnamon, and nutmeg to the squash, and mash the mixture with a potato masher until smooth.

3. Place the egg substitute in a small bowl, and stir in 1/2 cup of the hot mashed squash. Return the mixture to the pot, and stir to mix. Set aside.

4. To make the topping, place the topping ingredients in a small bowl, and stir to mix well. Set aside.

5. Coat a 2-quart casserole dish with nonstick cooking spray, and spread the squash mixture evenly in the dish. Sprinkle the topping over the squash, and bake uncovered at 350°F for 45 to 50 minutes, or until a sharp knife inserted in the center of the dish comes out clean. Remove the dish from the oven, and let sit for 5 minutes before serving.

NUTRITIONAL FACTS (PER 2/3-CUP SERVING)
Cal: 115   Carbs: 23 g   Chol: 0 mg   Fat: 0.6 g
Fiber: 4.5 g   Protein: 3.8 g   Sodium: 43 mg

Skillet Squash and Onions

YIELD: 6 SERVINGS

1 1/2 pounds zucchini or yellow squash (about
4–5 medium zucchini or 8–10 medium squash)

1 medium yellow onion, sliced 1/4-inch thick

2 tablespoons water

1 tablespoon minced fresh dill, or 1 teaspoon dried

2 teaspoons butter-flavored sprinkles,
or 1/4 teaspoon salt

1/8 teaspoon ground black pepper

1. Cut each squash in half lengthwise. Then cut into 1/4-inch-thick slices. Measure the squash; there should be 6 cups. Adjust the amount if necessary.

2. Place the squash and onion in a large nonstick skillet, and stir to mix. Sprinkle the water, dill, butter-flavored sprinkles or salt, and pepper over the top, and place the skillet over medium heat. Cover and cook, stirring occasionally, for 7 to 9 minutes, or just until the vegetables are tender. Serve hot.

NUTRITIONAL FACTS (PER 2/3-CUP SERVING)
Cal: 25   Carbs: 4 g   Chol: 0 mg   Fat: 0.2 g
Fiber: 1.6 g   Protein: 1.5 g   Sodium: 30 mg

Stuffed Acorn Squash

YIELD: 4 SERVINGS

2 medium acorn squash (about 1 pound each)

FILLING

1/2 cup quick-cooking brown rice

1 can (8 ounces) crushed pineapple in juice,
undrained

1/4 cup finely chopped onion

1/4 cup finely chopped celery

1/4 cup golden raisins

1/4 cup vegetable or chicken broth

1 teaspoon curry paste

1. Cut each squash in half crosswise, and scoop out and discard the seeds. If necessary, trim a small piece off the bottom of each half to allow it to sit upright. Set aside.

2. To make the filling, place all of the filling ingredients in a 1-quart pot, and stir to mix well. Bring to a boil over medium-high heat. Reduce the heat to low, cover, and simmer without stirring for about 10 minutes, or until the rice is tender and the liquid has been absorbed. Spoon a quarter of the mixture into the cavity of each squash half.

3. Coat a 9-x-13-inch pan with nonstick cooking spray, and arrange the filled squash halves in the pan. Cover the pan with aluminum foil, and bake at 350°F for 50 to 60 minutes, or until tender. Serve hot.

NUTRITIONAL FACTS (PER SERVING)			
Cal: 201	Carbs: 44 g	Chol: 0 mg	Fat: 1.3 g
Fiber: 7.5 g	Protein: 3.3 g	Sodium: 92 mg	

Italian Squash and Onions

YIELD: 6 SERVINGS
4 ounces Turkey Italian Sausage (page 251)
4 medium pattypan or zucchini squash, sliced ¼-inch thick (about 5 cups)
1 medium yellow onion, sliced ¼-inch thick and separated into rings

1. Coat a large nonstick skillet with nonstick cooking spray, and preheat over medium heat. Add the sausage, and cook, stirring to crumble, until the meat is no longer pink. Drain off and discard any excess fat.

2. Add the squash and onions to the skillet. Cover and cook, stirring occasionally, for about 7 minutes, or until the vegetables are tender. Add a few tablespoons of water or chicken broth if the skillet becomes too dry. Serve hot.

NUTRITIONAL FACTS (PER ¾-CUP SERVING)			
Cal: 50	Carbs: 5 g	Chol: 12 mg	Fat: 0.9 g
Fiber: 1.8 g	Protein: 6 g	Sodium: 82 mg	

Spinach-Noodle Casserole

For variety, substitute frozen chopped broccoli for the spinach.

YIELD: 8 SERVINGS
4 ounces extra-broad no-yolk noodles
1 package (10 ounces) frozen chopped spinach, thawed and squeezed dry
1 cup nonfat or low-fat cottage cheese
1 cup shredded nonfat or reduced-fat mozzarella cheese
½ cup evaporated skim milk
½ cup fat-free egg substitute

TOPPING
3 tablespoons grated Parmesan cheese*
1 tablespoon plus 1½ teaspoons Italian-style seasoned dried bread crumbs
Nonstick butter-flavored cooking spray

* In this recipe, use regular Parmesan cheese, not a fat-free product.

1. Cook the noodles al dente according to package directions. Drain well, and return to the pot.

2. Add the spinach, cottage cheese, mozzarella, milk, and egg substitute to the noodles, and toss to mix well. Set aside.

3. To make the topping, place the Parmesan cheese and bread crumbs in a small dish, and stir to mix well. Set aside.

4. Coat an 8-inch square (2-quart) baking dish with nonstick cooking spray. Spread the spinach mixture evenly in the dish, and sprinkle with the topping. Spray the top lightly with the cooking spray.

5. Cover the dish with aluminum foil, and bake at 350°F for 35 minutes. Remove the foil and bake for 10 additional minutes, or until the mixture is bubbly around the edges and the top is lightly browned.

6. Remove the dish from the oven, and let sit for 10 minutes before cutting into squares and serving.

NUTRITIONAL FACTS (PER ¾-CUP SERVING)			
Cal: 138	Carbs: 16 g	Chol: 6 mg	Fat: 1.1 g
Fiber: 1.2 g	Protein: 15 g	Sodium: 335 mg	

Down-Home Lima Beans

YIELD: 9 SERVINGS

4 cups unsalted chicken broth or water

2 cups dried large lima beans,
cleaned and soaked (page 302)

1 medium-large onion, chopped

2½ teaspoons instant ham or
chicken bouillon granules

2 teaspoons dried sage

1 bay leaf

¼ teaspoon ground black pepper

1. Place all of the ingredients in a 3-quart pot, and bring to a boil over high heat. Reduce the heat to low, cover, and simmer, stirring occasionally, for 1 hour and 30 minutes, or until the beans are soft and the liquid is thick. Periodically check the pot during cooking, and add a little more broth or water if needed.

2. Remove the pot from the heat, and discard the bay leaf. Serve hot.

NUTRITIONAL FACTS (PER ⅔-CUP SERVING)
Cal: 140   Carbs: 26 g   Chol: 0 mg   Fat: 0.2 g
Fiber: 8 g   Protein: 8.5 g   Sodium: 222 mg

Savory Baked Tomatoes

*For variety, substitute sweet onions
for the tomatoes.*

YIELD: 4 SERVINGS

2 large tomatoes, halved crosswise

3 tablespoons grated Parmesan cheese*

½ teaspoon dried Italian seasoning or dried basil

* In this recipe, use regular Parmesan cheese, not a fat-free product.

1. Coat an 8-inch square baking dish with nonstick cooking spray, and arrange the tomatoes, cut side up, in the pan.

2. Place the Parmesan cheese and Italian seasoning or basil in a small bowl, and stir to mix well. Sprinkle some of the mixture over the top of each tomato half.

3. Bake uncovered at 350°F for 30 to 35 minutes, or until the tomatoes are tender and the topping is lightly browned. Serve hot.

NUTRITIONAL FACTS (PER SERVING)
Cal: 45   Carbs: 6 g   Chol: 3 mg   Fat: 1.7 g
Fiber: 1.8 g   Protein: 2.9 g   Sodium: 97 mg

Sautéing Vegetables Without Fat

Sautéed or stir-fried vegetables add savory flavor to many recipes, and make a delicious and nutritious side dish, as well. However, the traditional method of sautéing often calls for unhealthful—and unnecessary—amounts of oil, butter, or margarine. Indeed, some recipes call for several tablespoons of oil! But as the recipes in this chapter show, all that extra oil is simply not necessary.

To make flavorful sautéed vegetables with a minimum of added fat and calories, spray a thin film of nonstick cooking spray over the bottom of a nonstick skillet, or coat the bottom of the skillet with just a few teaspoons of extra virgin olive oil. Then preheat the skillet over medium to medium-high heat, and cook the vegetables, stirring frequently, until they reach the desired degree of doneness. If the skillet becomes too dry, periodically cover it so that the steam released from the cooking vegetables can moisten the mixture and prevent scorching. Add a few teaspoons of water or broth to the skillet if necessary, but keep only enough moisture in the skillet to prevent sticking and burning. Too much liquid will steam the vegetables instead of giving them the lovely browned finish and savory caramelized flavor that is characteristic of sautéed foods.

Zucchini With Red Peppers and Onions

YIELD: 5 SERVINGS

2–3 teaspoons extra virgin olive oil

1 pound zucchini (about 3 medium), cut into 2-x-$\frac{1}{2}$-inch strips

1 small yellow onion, cut into thin wedges

1 medium red bell pepper, cut into thin strips

$\frac{1}{2}$ teaspoon dried Italian seasoning

$\frac{1}{4}$ teaspoon salt

$\frac{1}{8}$ teaspoon ground black pepper

1. Coat a large nonstick skillet with the olive oil, and preheat over medium-high heat.

2. Add all of the remaining ingredients to the skillet, and stir-fry for about 4 minutes, or until the vegetables start to brown and become crisp-tender. Cover the skillet periodically or add a little wine or chicken broth if the skillet becomes too dry. Serve hot.

NUTRITIONAL FACTS (PER $\frac{3}{4}$-CUP SERVING)
Cal: 40   Carbs: 4.1 g   Chol: 0 mg   Fat: 2 g
Fiber: 1.7 g   Protein: 1.4 g   Sodium: 110 mg

Oven-Fried Zucchini

YIELD: 6 SERVINGS

$\frac{1}{2}$ cup plus 2 tablespoons fat-free egg substitute

$\frac{1}{2}$ cup plain dried bread crumbs

$\frac{1}{2}$ cup grated nonfat or regular Parmesan cheese

1 teaspoon dried Italian seasoning

4 medium-large zucchini (about 1$\frac{3}{4}$ pounds)

Nonstick olive oil cooking spray

1. Place the egg substitute in a shallow bowl, and set aside. Place the bread crumbs, Parmesan, and Italian seasoning in another shallow dish. Stir to mix well, and set aside.

2. Diagonally slice the zucchini into $\frac{3}{8}$-inch-thick slices. Dip each slice first in the egg substitute, and then in the crumb mixture, turning to coat each side.

3. Coat a large baking sheet with olive oil cooking spray, and arrange the zucchini slices in a single layer on the sheet. Spray the tops lightly with the cooking spray.

4. Bake at 400°F for 8 minutes. Turn the slices, and bake for 7 additional minutes, or until golden brown. Serve hot.

NUTRITIONAL FACTS (PER SERVING)
Cal: 79   Carbs: 13 g   Chol: 6 mg   Fat: 0.7 g
Fiber: 2 g   Protein: 7.3 g   Sodium: 167 mg

Dilled Zucchini and Carrots

YIELD: 5 SERVINGS

2 medium-large zucchini

3 medium-large carrots

2–3 teaspoons extra virgin olive oil

1 teaspoon crushed fresh garlic

1$\frac{1}{2}$ teaspoons finely chopped fresh dill, or $\frac{1}{2}$ teaspoon dried

$\frac{1}{4}$ teaspoon salt

1. Diagonally cut the zucchini into $\frac{1}{4}$-inch-thick slices. Measure the zucchini; there should be 3 cups. Adjust the amount if necessary.

2. Peel the carrots, and diagonally cut into $\frac{1}{8}$-inch-thick slices. Measure the carrots; there should be 3 cups. Adjust the amount if necessary.

3. Coat a large, deep nonstick skillet with the olive oil, and preheat over medium-high heat. Add the zucchini, the carrots, and all of the remaining ingredients, and cook, stirring frequently, for about 4 minutes, or until the vegetables are crisp-tender. Cover the skillet periodically if it begins to dry out. (The steam released from the cooking vegetables will moisten the skillet.) Serve hot.

NUTRITIONAL FACTS (PER $\frac{3}{4}$-CUP SERVING)
Cal: 61   Carbs: 10 g   Chol: 0 mg   Fat: 2 g
Fiber: 3.3 g   Protein: 1.7 g   Sodium: 146 mg

Garden Rice

*For variety, substitute whole wheat couscous
or bulgur wheat for the rice.*

YIELD: 4 SERVINGS

1 tablespoon plus 1 teaspoon reduced-fat margarine or light butter
2/3 cup chopped fresh broccoli
2/3 cup fresh or frozen (unthawed) whole kernel corn
1/3 cup chopped red bell pepper
1/3 cup chopped fresh mushrooms
3 tablespoons sliced scallions
2 cups cooked brown rice
2 tablespoons vegetable or chicken broth
1/8 teaspoon salt

1. Place the margarine or butter in a large nonstick skillet, and melt over medium-high heat. Add the broccoli, corn, red pepper, mushrooms, and scallions; cover; and cook, stirring frequently, for about 3 minutes, or until the vegetables are crisp-tender.

2. Add the rice, broth, and salt to the skillet, and cook uncovered for another minute or 2, or until the mixture is heated through. Add a little more broth if the mixture seems too dry. Serve hot.

NUTRITIONAL FACTS (PER 7/8-CUP SERVING)
Cal: 155   Carbs: 30 g   Chol: 0 mg   Fat: 2.8 g
Fiber: 3.2 g   Protein: 4 g   Sodium: 95 mg

Spinach and Mushroom Sauté

YIELD: 4 SERVINGS

2 teaspoons extra virgin olive oil
1 1/2 teaspoons crushed fresh garlic
2 cups sliced fresh mushrooms (about 8 ounces)
10 cups (packed) fresh spinach leaves (about 10 ounces)
1/4 teaspoon salt
1/8 teaspoon ground black pepper

1. Coat a large nonstick skillet with the olive oil, and preheat over medium-high heat. Add the garlic and mushrooms, and stir-fry for about 2 minutes, or just until the mushrooms start to brown and begin to release their juices.

2. Add the spinach, salt, and pepper to the skillet, and stir-fry for another 2 minutes, or just until the spinach is wilted. Add a little water or broth if the skillet becomes too dry. Serve hot.

NUTRITIONAL FACTS (PER 3/4-CUP SERVING)
Cal: 45   Carbs: 4 g   Chol: 0 mg   Fat: 2.7 g
Fiber: 2.4 g   Protein: 2.8 g   Sodium: 189 mg

Savory Sautéed Mushrooms

YIELD: 6 SERVINGS

1 teaspoon crushed fresh garlic
1 pound fresh mushrooms, sliced
1/4 teaspoon dried thyme
1/4 teaspoon ground black pepper
1/4 teaspoon salt
1/4 cup dry white wine
2 tablespoons finely chopped fresh Italian parsley (garnish)

1. Coat a large nonstick skillet with olive oil cooking spray, and preheat over medium-high heat. Add the garlic, mushrooms, thyme, pepper, and salt, and stir-fry for several minutes, or just until the mushrooms start to brown and begin to release their juices. Cover the skillet periodically if it begins to dry out. (The steam from the cooking vegetables will moisten the skillet.)

2. Add the wine to the skillet, and reduce the heat to medium. Cook and stir for several minutes, or until all but a few tablespoons of the wine have evaporated.

3. Transfer the mushrooms to a serving dish, and sprinkle the parsley over the top. Serve hot.

NUTRITIONAL FACTS (PER 1/2-CUP SERVING)
Cal: 22   Carbs: 3.2 g   Chol: 0 mg   Fat: 0.3 g
Fiber: 1 g   Protein: 1.6 g   Sodium: 92 mg

Spiced Spinach and Potatoes

YIELD: 6 SERVINGS
1/3 cup finely chopped onion
2 teaspoons crushed fresh garlic
1 teaspoon whole cumin seeds
1/2 teaspoon ground ginger
1/4 teaspoon coarsely ground black pepper
1 pound white or sweet potatoes, peeled and cut into 3/4-inch chunks (about 3 1/2 cups)
2 cups chicken or vegetable broth
5 cups (moderately packed) coarsely chopped fresh spinach (about 8 ounces), or 1 package (10 ounces) frozen chopped spinach, thawed and drained

1. Coat a large nonstick skillet with nonstick cooking spray, and preheat over medium-high heat. Add the onion, garlic, cumin seeds, ginger, and pepper, and stir to mix. Cover and cook, stirring frequently, for about 2 minutes, or until the onion begins to soften and the mixture is fragrant. Add a little broth or water to the skillet if it becomes too dry.

2. Add the potatoes and broth to the skillet, and allow the mixture to come to a boil. Reduce the heat to medium-low, cover, and cook, stirring occasionally, for about 10 minutes, or until the potatoes are tender.

3. Remove the lid from the skillet, increase the heat to medium-high, and cook uncovered for several minutes, or until all but about 1/2 cup of the cooking liquid has evaporated.

4. Add the spinach to the skillet, and stir-fry for about 2 minutes, or just until the spinach has wilted. (If you are using frozen spinach, cook just until the spinach is heated through.) Serve hot.

NUTRITIONAL FACTS (PER 3/4-CUP SERVING)
Cal: 71   Carbs: 16 g   Chol: 0 mg   Fat: 0.2 g
Fiber: 2.6 g   Protein: 2.7 g   Sodium: 229 mg

Barley, Spinach, and Mushroom Pilaf

YIELD: 5 SERVINGS
1 cup quick-cooking barley
2 cups vegetable or chicken broth
2–3 teaspoons extra virgin olive oil
1 1/2 teaspoons crushed fresh garlic
1 1/2 cups sliced fresh mushrooms
1/2 teaspoon dried thyme
1/8 teaspoon ground black pepper
1 1/2 cups (packed) chopped fresh spinach

1. Place the barley and broth in a 1-quart pot, and bring to a boil over high heat. Reduce the heat to low, cover, and simmer for 10 to 12 minutes, or until the liquid is absorbed and the barley is tender. Remove the pot from the heat, and set aside.

2. Coat a large nonstick skillet with the olive oil, and preheat over medium-high heat. Add the garlic, and stir-fry for about 30 seconds, or just until the garlic begins to turn color. Add the mushrooms, thyme, and pepper, and stir-fry for about 2 minutes, or until the mushrooms are tender. Add the spinach, and stir-fry for about 1 additional minute, or just until the spinach is wilted. Add a little water or broth if the skillet becomes too dry.

3. Add the barley to the skillet, and stir-fry for another minute, or until well mixed and heated through. Serve hot.

NUTRITIONAL FACTS (PER 3/4-CUP SERVING)
Cal: 141   Carbs: 26 g   Chol: 0 mg   Fat: 2.5 g
Fiber: 3.8 g   Protein: 4.3 g   Sodium: 258 mg

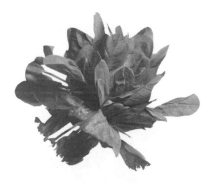

9. *Main Dish Pastabilities*

Featured prominently in some of the world's most healthful cuisines, pasta is the perfect solution when you need a low-fat meal in a matter of minutes. And contrary to popular belief, pasta is not fattening. One cup of cooked pasta—about two ounces dry—has only about two hundred calories and one gram of fat. Pasta is also loaded with energizing complex carbohydrates. And when your pasta contains whole grain flour rather than refined flour, it is also a rich source of fiber, B vitamins, and minerals, making it a truly valuable addition to your diet.

Considering pasta's healthful profile, it may seem odd that this food is so often thought of as being fattening. The problem is not with the pasta—it's with what so often goes on top. Cream-enriched sauces, pools of olive oil, greasy sausage, and gobs of high-fat cheese are just a few of the toppings that can turn a lean plate of pasta into a fat and calorie budget-busting nightmare. But can these fatty ingredients be eliminated without sacrificing flavor? Absolutely. This chapter first presents a selection of light but luscious sauces that you can use to top your favorite pasta dishes. Following this, you'll find a wide range of recipes that combine pasta with nonfat and low-fat dairy products, ultra-lean meats, seafood, beans, vegetables, savory herbs and spices, and other wholesome ingredients. The result? Healthy pasta creations that are every bit as tempting as their calorie-laden counterparts. And you may be surprised to find that pasta is also a snap to prepare. In fact, many of the dishes in this chapter can be whipped up in less than thirty minutes, making pasta a real boon to the busy cook.

Whether you enjoy pasta only occasionally or are a true lover of this culinary pleasure, this chapter is sure to delight you with a wealth of "pastabilities" for preparing one of the most satisfying of comfort foods. So take out your pasta pot, and get ready to create pasta dishes that are as guilt-free as they are delectable. It's easy—once you know the secrets of healthy cooking.

PASTA SAUCES

Red Clam Sauce

YIELD: 4 SERVINGS

1 tablespoon extra virgin olive oil (optional)

1½ teaspoons crushed fresh garlic

2 cans (6½ ounces each)
chopped clams, undrained

1¼ pounds fresh plum tomatoes
(7–8 medium), peeled and finely chopped

½ teaspoon dried Italian seasoning

¼ teaspoon ground black pepper

¼ teaspoon crushed red pepper

¼ cup finely chopped fresh parsley

1. Coat a large nonstick skillet with nonstick olive oil cooking spray or with the olive oil, and preheat over medium heat. Add the garlic, and stir-fry for about 30 seconds, or just until the garlic begins to turn color.

2. Drain the juice from the clams, reserving the juice, and set the clams aside. Add the clam juice, tomatoes, Italian seasoning, and black and red pepper to the skillet. Increase the heat to medium-high, and allow the mixture to come to a boil. Then cook over medium heat, stirring frequently, for about 5 minutes, or until the liquid is reduced by about half, the tomatoes are soft, and mixture has cooked down into a sauce.

3. Add the clams and parsley to the skillet, and cook for another minute or 2, or until the mixture is heated through. Serve hot over your choice of pasta.

NUTRITIONAL FACTS (PER ½-CUP SERVING)
Cal: 104   Carbs: 9.4 g   Chol: 33 mg   Fat: 1.4 g
Fiber: 1.6 g   Protein: 14 g   Sodium: 162 mg

Roasted Tomato Sauce

YIELD: 3 CUPS

1¾ pounds fresh plum tomatoes
(about 8 medium-large), quartered lengthwise

1 medium-large yellow onion, cut into thin wedges

2 cups sliced fresh mushrooms

1 large red bell pepper, cut into ¼-inch-thick strips

10 cloves garlic, peeled

1 tablespoon balsamic vinegar

1 teaspoon dried oregano

¼ teaspoon salt

¼ teaspoon coarsely ground black pepper

1 tablespoon extra virgin olive oil (optional)

Nonstick olive oil cooking spray

1. Place the vegetables and garlic cloves in a large bowl, and toss to mix well. Add the vinegar, oregano, salt, pepper, and, if desired, the olive oil, and stir to mix well.

2. Coat a 9-x-13-inch nonstick pan with nonstick olive oil cooking spray, and spread the vegetables in a single layer in the pan. If you did not use the olive oil, spray the tops of the vegetables with the cooking spray.

3. Cover the pan with aluminum foil, and bake at 450°F for 20 minutes. Remove the foil, and bake for 30 additional minutes, or until the vegetables are tender and nicely browned. Serve hot over your choice of pasta.

NUTRITIONAL FACTS (PER ¾-CUP SERVING)
Cal: 57   Carbs: 12.8 g   Chol: 0 mg   Fat: 0.6 g
Fiber: 3 g   Protein: 2.4 g   Sodium: 145 mg

Arrabbiata Sauce

A simple spicy sauce.

YIELD: 3½ CUPS

1 tablespoon extra virgin olive oil
1½ teaspoons crushed fresh garlic
1 can (28 ounces) crushed tomatoes
½ cup chicken, beef, or vegetable broth
3 tablespoons finely chopped fresh parsley
1 teaspoon crushed red pepper

1. Coat a 2-quart pot with the olive oil, and preheat over medium heat. Add the garlic, and stir-fry for about 30 seconds, or just until the garlic begins to turn color. Add all of the remaining ingredients, increase the heat to medium-high, and bring the mixture to a boil.

2. Reduce the heat to low, cover, and simmer, stirring occasionally, for 20 minutes, or until the sauce is thick and the flavors are well blended. Serve hot over your choice of pasta.

> **NUTRITIONAL FACTS (PER ½-CUP SERVING)**
> Cal: 55   Carbs: 8 g   Chol: 0 mg   Fat: 1.9 g
> Fiber: 2 g   Protein: 2 g   Sodium: 223 mg

Broiled Tomato-Basil Sauce

YIELD: 4 SERVINGS

1 pound fresh plum tomatoes (about 6 medium), coarsely chopped
1 medium-large yellow onion, cut into very thin wedges
½ cup coarsely chopped fresh basil
2 teaspoons crushed fresh garlic
¼ teaspoon salt
¼ teaspoon ground black pepper
1 tablespoon extra virgin olive oil (optional)
Nonstick olive oil cooking spray

1. Place all of the ingredients in a large bowl, and toss to mix well.

2. Coat a large baking sheet with nonstick olive oil cooking spray, and spread the mixture in a single layer on the sheet. If you did not use the olive oil, spray the top of the tomato mixture lightly with the cooking spray.

3. Place the tomato mixture 6 inches below a preheated broiler, and broil for about 5 minutes, or until the tomatoes are soft and the onions begin to brown. Serve hot over your choice of pasta.

> **NUTRITIONAL FACTS (PER ⅔-CUP SERVING)**
> Cal: 35   Carbs: 8 g   Chol: 0 mg   Fat: 0.4 g
> Fiber: 1.8 g   Protein: 1.4 g   Sodium: 144 mg

Puttanesca Sauce

YIELD: 4 CUPS

1 tablespoon extra virgin olive oil (optional)
2 teaspoons crushed fresh garlic
½ cup chopped onion
⅓ cup sliced black olives
¼ cup finely chopped fresh parsley
1 can (28 ounces) crushed tomatoes
½ cup chicken broth
3 tablespoons chopped capers
1 tablespoon dark brown sugar
2–3 teaspoons mashed anchovy fillets (optional)
¼ teaspoon crushed red pepper

1. Coat a 2-quart pot with nonstick olive oil cooking spray or with the olive oil, and preheat over medium heat. Add the garlic, and stir-fry for about 30 seconds, or just until the garlic begins to turn color. Add all of the remaining ingredients, increase the heat to medium-high, and bring the mixture to a boil.

2. Reduce the heat to low, cover, and simmer, stirring occasionally, for 20 minutes, or until the onions are soft, the sauce is thick, and the flavors are well blended. Serve hot over your choice of pasta.

> **NUTRITIONAL FACTS (PER ½-CUP SERVING)**
> Cal: 50   Carbs: 10 g   Chol: 0 mg   Fat: 0.7 g
> Fiber: 2.3 g   Protein: 2.1. g   Sodium: 363 mg

Almost Alfredo Sauce

YIELD: 3 CUPS

3/4 cup grated nonfat Parmesan cheese, or 1/2 cup regular Parmesan cheese mixed with 2 1/2 tablespoons cornstarch
1/2 cup evaporated skim milk
1/8 teaspoon ground white pepper
Pinch ground nutmeg
2 1/2 cups skim or low-fat milk

1. Place the Parmesan cheese, evaporated milk, pepper, and nutmeg in a small bowl, and stir to mix well. Set aside.

2. Place the milk in a 1 1/2-quart pot, and bring to a boil over medium heat, stirring constantly. Add the evaporated milk mixture to the pot, and cook, still stirring, for about 2 minutes, or until the mixture is thickened and bubbly. Add a little more milk if the sauce seems too thick. Serve hot over pasta or vegetables, or use in casseroles as you would condensed cream soups.

NUTRITIONAL FACTS (PER 1/2-CUP SERVING)
Cal: 82   Carbs: 11 g   Chol: 12 mg   Fat: 0.2 g
Fiber: 0 g   Protein: 9 g   Sodium: 167 mg

Broiled Mushroom and Plum Tomato Sauce

YIELD: 4 SERVINGS

2 cups sliced fresh mushrooms (about 4 ounces)
2 cups chopped fresh plum tomatoes (about 6 medium)
2 teaspoons crushed fresh garlic
1 teaspoon dried oregano
1/4 teaspoon salt
1/4 teaspoon coarsely ground black pepper
1 tablespoon extra virgin olive oil (optional)
Nonstick olive oil cooking spray

Creamy Sauces Without the Cream

Cream is a key ingredient in many deliciously rich pasta dishes. But with over 800 calories and 88 grams of fat per cup, this is one ingredient you would be better off without. Does this mean giving up creamy, satisfying sauces? Fortunately, there are a variety of ways to create rich and creamy sauces without using high-fat cream.

One of the simplest ways to eliminate the cream from your pasta sauce is to replace it with evaporated skim milk. For a slightly thicker consistency, dissolve a little cornstarch into the milk—1 to 1 1/2 teaspoons per cup—before cooking the sauce. Or stir a little grated nonfat Parmesan cheese into the sauce before cooking. (1 to 2 tablespoons per cup should do it.) When you bring the sauce to a boil, it will thicken slightly.

Nonfat or reduced-fat ricotta cheese, cream cheese, and soft curd farmer cheese blended until smooth with an equal amount of skim or low-fat milk are still other delicious options for creating creamy, rich-tasting sauces. Just be sure to cook these sauces only until they are heated through. Do *not* let them boil, as they may separate.

So don't be afraid to experiment with different ingredients to create lighter, healthier versions of your treasured pasta recipes. And keep in mind that when you use these ingredients in your slimmed-down recipes, not only do you eliminate lots of calories and artery-clogging saturated fat, but you also add nutrients like protein, calcium, and potassium to your dishes, making them as nutritious as they are delicious.

1. Place all of the ingredients in a large bowl, and toss to mix well.

2. Coat a large baking sheet with olive oil cooking spray, and spread the mixture in a single layer over the sheet. If you did not use the olive oil, spray the top of the tomato mixture lightly with the cooking spray.

3. Place the tomato mixture 6 inches below a preheated broiler, and broil for about 5 minutes, or until the tomatoes are soft and the mushrooms begin to brown. Serve hot over your choice of pasta.

> **NUTRITIONAL FACTS** (PER ⅔-CUP SERVING)
> Cal: 31   Carbs: 5.3 g   Chol: 0 mg   Fat: 0.8 g
> Fiber: 1.8 g   Protein: 1.3 g   Sodium: 142 mg

Chunky Garden Marinara Sauce

YIELD: 3½ CUPS

| 1 tablespoon extra virgin olive oil (optional) |
| 2 teaspoons crushed fresh garlic |
| 1 cup chopped fresh mushrooms |
| ¾ cup chopped red or green bell pepper |
| ½ cup chopped onion |
| 1 can (28 ounces) crushed tomatoes |
| 2 teaspoons instant vegetable or beef bouillon granules |
| 1½ teaspoons dried Italian seasoning |
| 1½ teaspoons sugar (optional) |
| ¼ teaspoon crushed red pepper |

1. Coat a large nonstick skillet with nonstick cooking spray or with the olive oil, and preheat over medium heat. Add the garlic, mushrooms, bell pepper, and onion. Cover, and cook, stirring occasionally, for about 5 minutes, or until the vegetables start to soften and release their juices.

2. Add all of the remaining ingredients to the skillet, and stir to mix. Increase the heat to medium-high, and bring the mixture to a boil. Reduce the heat to low, cover, and simmer, stirring occasionally, for about 20 minutes, or until the sauce is thick and the

flavors are well blended. Serve hot over your choice of pasta.

> **NUTRITIONAL FACTS** (PER ½-CUP SERVING)
> Cal: 48   Carbs: 10 g   Chol: 0 mg   Fat: 0.1 g
> Fiber: 2.7 g   Protein: 2.5 g   Sodium: 228 mg

Savory Meat Sauce

YIELD: 5⅓ CUPS

| 12 ounces 95% lean ground beef |
| 1 medium yellow onion, chopped |
| 1½ cups sliced fresh mushrooms |
| ½ cup chopped green bell pepper |
| ½ cup finely chopped celery (include the leaves) |
| 2 teaspoons crushed fresh garlic |
| 2½ teaspoons dried Italian seasoning |
| 2 teaspoons instant beef bouillon granules |
| 2 teaspoons sugar (optional) |
| 1 can (28 ounces) crushed tomatoes |

1. Coat a large nonstick skillet with nonstick cooking spray, and preheat over medium heat. Add the ground beef, and cook, stirring to crumble, until the meat is no longer pink. Drain off and discard any excess fat.

2. Add all of the remaining ingredients except for the tomatoes to the skillet, and stir to mix. Cover and cook, stirring occasionally, for about 5 minutes, or until the vegetables start to soften and release their juices.

3. Add the tomatoes to the skillet, and stir to mix. Increase the heat to medium-high, and bring the mixture to a boil. Reduce the heat to low, cover, and simmer, stirring occasionally, for 20 to 25 minutes, or until the sauce is thick and the flavors are well blended. Serve hot over your choice of pasta.

> **NUTRITIONAL FACTS** (PER ⅔-CUP SERVING)
> Cal: 97   Carbs: 9.2 g   Chol: 26 mg   Fat: 2 g
> Fiber: 2.2 g   Protein: 10.5 g   Sodium: 225 mg

White Clam Sauce

YIELD: 4 SERVINGS

1–2 tablespoons extra virgin olive oil

2 teaspoons crushed fresh garlic

2 cups sliced fresh mushrooms

2 cans (6$\frac{1}{2}$ ounces each)
chopped clams, undrained

$\frac{1}{4}$ cup dry white wine

1$\frac{1}{2}$ teaspoons lemon juice

$\frac{1}{4}$ teaspoon coarsely ground black pepper

$\frac{1}{2}$ cup thinly sliced scallions

$\frac{1}{4}$ cup plus 2 tablespoons chopped fresh parsley

1. Coat a large nonstick skillet with the olive oil, and preheat over medium-high heat. Add the garlic and mushrooms, and sauté for about 3 minutes, or until the mushrooms begin to brown and start to release their juices.

2. Add the clams with their juice and the wine, lemon juice, and pepper to the skillet. Reduce the heat to medium and cook, stirring frequently, for several minutes, or until the liquid is reduced by about a fourth.

3. Remove the skillet from the heat, stir in the scallions and parsley, and serve hot over your choice of pasta.

NUTRITIONAL FACTS (PER $\frac{1}{2}$-CUP SERVING)
Cal: 129　Carbs: 6 g　Chol: 33 mg　Fat: 4.6 g
Fiber: 1 g　Protein: 14 g　Sodium: 155 mg

PASTA DISHES

Slim Spaghetti Carbonara

YIELD: 4 SERVINGS

8 ounces thin spaghetti

1$\frac{1}{4}$ cups evaporated skim milk

$\frac{1}{4}$ cup fat-free egg substitute

$\frac{1}{4}$ teaspoon coarsely ground black pepper

1$\frac{1}{2}$ teaspoons crushed fresh garlic

4 slices extra-lean turkey bacon, cooked,
drained, and crumbled

$\frac{1}{4}$ cup thinly sliced scallions

2 tablespoons finely chopped fresh parsley

$\frac{1}{3}$ cup grated nonfat or regular Parmesan cheese

1. Cook the pasta al dente according to package directions. Drain well, return to the pot, and cover to keep warm.

2. Place the evaporated milk, egg substitute, and pepper in a small bowl. Stir to mix well, and set aside.

3. Coat a large nonstick skillet with nonstick butter-flavored cooking spray, and preheat over medium-high heat. Add the garlic, and stir-fry for 30 seconds, or just until the garlic begins to turn color.

4. Reduce the heat under the skillet to medium-low, and add the spaghetti. Slowly pour the milk mixture over the spaghetti, and toss gently for a minute or 2, or until the sauce thickens slightly. Add a little more evaporated milk if the sauce seems too dry.

5. Add the bacon, scallions, and parsley to the skillet mixture, and toss to mix well. Remove the skillet from the heat, toss in the Parmesan, and serve hot.

NUTRITIONAL FACTS (PER 1$\frac{1}{3}$-CUP SERVING)
Cal: 322　Carbs: 55 g　Chol: 29 mg　Fat: 1.6 g
Fiber: 1.6 g　Protein: 20 g　Sodium: 312 mg

Rigatoni and Sausage Primavera

YIELD: 4 SERVINGS

8 ounces rigatoni pasta (about 3¼ cups) or rotini pasta (about 3 cups)
8 ounces sliced smoked sausage or kielbasa (about 1¼ cups), at least 97% lean
1 medium zucchini, halved lengthwise and sliced ¼-inch thick
1 cup sliced fresh mushrooms
¾ cup matchstick-sized pieces red bell pepper
1 teaspoon crushed fresh garlic
1 cup chicken or vegetable broth
¾ teaspoon dried oregano
1 cup chopped fresh plum tomatoes (about 3 medium)
¼ cup grated nonfat or regular Parmesan cheese (optional)

1. Cook the pasta al dente according to package directions. Drain well, return to the pot, and cover to keep warm.

2. While the pasta is cooking, coat a large nonstick skillet with nonstick olive oil cooking spray, and preheat over medium-high heat. Add the sausage or kielbasa, zucchini, mushrooms, red pepper, and garlic, and stir-fry for about 3 minutes, or until the sausage is browned and the vegetables are crisp-tender. Cover the skillet periodically if it begins to dry out. (The steam from the cooking vegetables will moisten the skillet.) Add a few teaspoons of water to the skillet if needed.

3. Transfer the sausage and vegetables to a large bowl, and cover to keep warm. Add the broth and oregano to the skillet, and cook uncovered over medium-high heat, stirring frequently, for a couple of minutes, or until the broth is reduced by half.

4. Add the tomatoes to the skillet, cover, and cook over medium-high heat for about 1 minute, or until the tomatoes are heated through and beginning to soften.

5. Reduce the heat to medium, and add the pasta and the sausage-vegetable mixture to the skillet. Toss

for a minute or 2 to blend the flavors, adding a little more broth if the mixture seems too dry. Serve hot, topping each serving with a tablespoon of Parmesan, if desired.

NUTRITIONAL FACTS (PER 2-CUP SERVING)			
Cal: 306	Carbs: 52 g	Chol: 25 mg	Fat: 2.7 g
Fiber: 2.8 g	Protein: 17.7 g	Sodium: 638 mg	

Penne With Sausage, Peppers, and Onions

YIELD: 5 SERVINGS

8 ounces penne or ziti pasta (about 2⅔ cups)
12 ounces Turkey Italian Sausage (page 251)
1 can (14½ ounces) stewed tomatoes, crushed
1 medium yellow onion, cut into thin wedges
1 medium green bell pepper, cut into strips
1 medium red bell pepper, cut into strips
3 tablespoons tomato paste
1 teaspoon dried Italian seasoning

1. Cook the pasta al dente according to package directions. Drain well, return to the pot, and cover to keep warm.

2. While the pasta is cooking, coat a large nonstick skillet with nonstick cooking spray, and preheat over medium heat. Add the sausage to the skillet, and cook, stirring to crumble, until the meat is no longer pink. Drain off and discard any excess fat.

3. Add all of the remaining ingredients to the skillet, and stir to mix. Cover and cook over medium heat, stirring occasionally, for 7 to 10 minutes, or until the vegetables are tender and the flavors are well blended.

4. Pour the skillet mixture over the pasta, and toss to mix well. Serve hot.

NUTRITIONAL FACTS (PER 1¾-CUP SERVING)			
Cal: 318	Carbs: 48 g	Chol: 43 mg	Fat: 3.6 g
Fiber: 3.8 g	Protein: 23 g	Sodium: 393 mg	

Spaghetti With Garlic, Chicken, and Sun-Dried Tomatoes

YIELD: 4 SERVINGS

1/4 cup diced sun-dried tomatoes (not packed in oil)
1 cup chicken broth, divided
1 teaspoon cornstarch
1/8 teaspoon ground white pepper
8 ounces thin spaghetti
12 ounces boneless skinless chicken breasts
1/4 teaspoon salt
1 tablespoon extra virgin olive oil (optional)
1 tablespoon crushed fresh garlic
1/4 cup plus 2 tablespoons sliced scallions
1/4 cup grated nonfat or regular Parmesan cheese

1. Place the tomatoes and 1/4 cup of the broth in a small saucepan, and bring to a boil over medium heat. Reduce the heat to low, cover, and simmer for about 2 minutes, or until the tomatoes are plumped and the liquid is absorbed. Remove the pot from the heat, and cover to keep warm.

2. Place the remaining 3/4 cup of broth in a small dish. Add the cornstarch and pepper, and stir to dissolve the cornstarch. Set aside.

3. Cook the pasta al dente according to package directions. Drain well, return to the pot, and cover to keep warm.

4. While the pasta is cooking, rinse the chicken with cool water, and pat it dry with paper towels. Cut the chicken into bite-sized pieces, sprinkle with the salt, and set aside.

5. Coat a large skillet with nonstick olive oil cooking spray or with the olive oil, and preheat over medium-high heat. Add the garlic and chicken, and stir-fry for about 4 minutes, or until the chicken is nicely browned and no longer pink inside.

6. Reduce the heat under the skillet to medium, and add the sun-dried tomatoes and pasta to the skillet mixture. Stir the cornstarch mixture, and pour it over the pasta. Toss gently for a minute or 2, or until the sauce thickens slightly.

7. Add the scallions to the pasta mixture, and toss to mix well. Remove the skillet from the heat, and serve hot, topping each serving with a tablespoon of the Parmesan.

NUTRITIONAL FACTS (PER 1²/₃-CUP SERVING)
Cal: 346   Carbs: 50 g   Chol: 52 mg   Fat: 2.1 g
Fiber: 2 g   Protein: 31 g   Sodium: 482 mg

Italian Country Linguine

YIELD: 4 SERVINGS

8 ounces linguine pasta
4 ounces ham, at least 97% lean, thinly sliced and cut into thin strips
1 teaspoon crushed fresh garlic
2 cups thinly sliced fresh mushrooms
3 tablespoons dry white wine or chicken broth
2 cups coarsely chopped fresh plum tomatoes (about 4 medium)
1 teaspoon dried oregano
1/4 cup sliced scallions
1/4 cup grated nonfat or regular Parmesan cheese

1. Cook the pasta al dente according to package directions. Drain well, return to the pot, and cover to keep warm.

2. While the pasta is cooking, coat a large nonstick skillet with nonstick cooking spray, and preheat over medium-high heat. Add the ham and garlic, and stir-fry for about 2 minutes, or until the ham begins to brown.

3. Add the mushrooms and wine or broth to the skillet, and stir-fry for about 2 minutes, or until the mushrooms begin to release their juices. Add a little more broth or wine if the skillet becomes too dry.

4. Add the tomatoes and oregano to the skillet, and reduce the heat to medium. Cover and cook for about 3 minutes, or just until the tomatoes are heated through and are beginning to soften.

5. Add the pasta and scallions to the skillet, and toss to mix well. Serve hot, topping each serving with a tablespoon of Parmesan.

NUTRITIONAL FACTS (PER 1²⁄₃-CUP SERVING)
Cal: 290   Carbs: 51 g   Chol: 18 mg   Fat: 2 g
Fiber: 2.6 g   Protein: 17 g   Sodium: 307 mg

Pasta Piselli

YIELD: 4 SERVINGS

8 ounces thin spaghetti

³⁄₄ cup frozen (unthawed) green peas

1¹⁄₄ cups evaporated skim milk

¹⁄₄ cup fat-free egg substitute

1 cup sliced fresh mushrooms

5 ounces ham, at least 97% lean,
cut into thin strips (about 1 cup)

1 teaspoon crushed fresh garlic

3 tablespoons grated nonfat or
regular Parmesan cheese

1. Cook the pasta al dente according to package directions. About 2 minutes before the pasta is done, add the peas to the pot, and cook until the peas are thawed and the pasta is al dente. Drain well, return the pasta and peas to the pot, and cover to keep warm.

2. Place the evaporated milk and egg substitute in a small bowl. Stir to mix well, and set aside.

3. Coat a large nonstick skillet with nonstick cooking spray, and preheat over medium-high heat. Add the mushrooms, ham, and garlic, and stir-fry for about 4 minutes, or until the mushrooms are tender and the ham is nicely browned. Cover the skillet periodically if it begins to dry out. (The steam from the cooking vegetables will moisten the skillet.)

4. Reduce the heat under the skillet to medium-low, and add the pasta to the skillet mixture. Slowly pour the evaporated milk mixture over the pasta, and toss gently for a minute or 2, or until the sauce thickens slightly. Add a little more evaporated milk if the sauce seems too dry. Remove the skillet from the heat, toss in the Parmesan, and serve hot.

NUTRITIONAL FACTS (PER 1²⁄₃-CUP SERVING)
Cal: 360   Carbs: 58 g   Chol: 22 mg   Fat: 2.2 g
Fiber: 3.2 g   Protein: 26 g   Sodium: 533 mg

Angel Hair With Ham and Artichoke Hearts

YIELD: 4 SERVINGS

8 ounces capellini (angel hair) pasta

5 ounces ham, at least 97% lean, thinly sliced
and cut into thin strips

1 teaspoon crushed fresh garlic

1 cup coarsely chopped frozen (thawed)
or canned (drained) artichoke hearts

¹⁄₄ cup chicken broth or dry white wine

³⁄₄ teaspoon dried Italian seasoning

SAUCE

1 cup nonfat or low-fat ricotta cheese

1 cup skim or low-fat milk

2 tablespoons grated nonfat or regular
Parmesan cheese

¹⁄₄ teaspoon ground white pepper

1. To make the sauce, place all of the sauce ingredients in a blender or food processor, and blend until smooth. Set aside.

2. Cook the pasta al dente according to package directions. Drain well, return to the pot, and cover to keep warm.

3. While the pasta is cooking, coat a large nonstick skillet with nonstick cooking spray, and preheat over medium-high heat. Add the ham and garlic, and stir-fry for about 2 minutes, or until the ham is lightly browned.

4. Add the artichoke hearts, broth or wine, and Italian seasoning to the skillet, and cook uncovered for about 2 minutes, or until the artichoke hearts are heated through and the liquid is reduced by half.

5. Reduce the heat to medium, add the pasta to the skillet, and toss to mix well. Pour the sauce over the pasta mixture, and toss gently for a minute or 2, or until the sauce is heated through. (Do not allow the sauce to boil.) Add a little more milk if the sauce seems too dry. Serve hot.

NUTRITIONAL FACTS (PER 1¹⁄₂-CUP SERVING)
Cal: 352   Carbs: 55 g   Chol: 24 mg   Fat: 2.2 g
Fiber: 3.6 g   Protein: 27.6 g   Sodium: 463 mg

Lemon Chicken Linguine

*For variety, substitute scallops or shrimp
for the chicken.*

YIELD: 4 SERVINGS
8 ounces linguine pasta
12 ounces boneless skinless chicken breasts
1/4 teaspoon salt
1/8 teaspoon ground black pepper
1/4 cup chicken broth
3 tablespoons lemon juice
1 tablespoon freshly grated lemon rind
1 cup evaporated skim milk
1 1/2 teaspoons cornstarch
2 teaspoons crushed fresh garlic
1/4 cup sliced scallions
1/4 cup finely chopped fresh parsley
3 tablespoons grated nonfat or regular Parmesan cheese

1. Cook the pasta al dente according to package directions. Drain well, return to the pot, and cover to keep warm.

2. While the pasta is cooking, rinse the chicken with cool water, and pat it dry with paper towels. Cut the chicken into 3/4-inch cubes, sprinkle with the salt and pepper, and set aside.

3. Place the broth, lemon juice, and lemon rind in a small bowl, stir to mix, and set aside.

4. Place 1 tablespoon of the evaporated milk and all of the cornstarch in another bowl, and stir to dissolve the cornstarch. Stir in the remaining evaporated milk, and set aside.

5. Coat a large nonstick skillet with nonstick olive oil cooking spray, and preheat over medium-high heat. Add the garlic and chicken, and stir-fry for about 4 minutes, or until the chicken is nicely browned and no longer pink inside.

6. Reduce the heat under the skillet to medium, and add the pasta. Pour the broth mixture over the pasta and chicken, and toss to mix well. Slowly pour the milk mixture over the pasta, and toss gently for a minute or 2, or until the sauce just begins to boil and thickens slightly. Add a little more evaporated milk if the mixture seems too dry.

7. Add the scallions and parsley to the skillet, and toss to mix well. Remove the skillet from the heat, toss in the Parmesan, and serve hot.

NUTRITIONAL FACTS (PER 1 2/3-CUP SERVING)
Cal: 381   Carbs: 56 g   Chol: 54 mg   Fat: 2.2 g
Fiber: 1.7 g   Protein: 34 g   Sodium: 392 mg

Bow Ties With Tuna and Tomatoes

YIELD: 4 SERVINGS
1 1/2 cups chopped fresh plum tomatoes (about 5 medium)
1 can (9 ounces) water-packed albacore tuna, drained
5 thin slices red onion
1/3 cup chopped fresh basil
1/4 cup chopped black olives
1/4 cup bottled nonfat or reduced-fat Italian salad dressing
1 1/2 teaspoons crushed fresh garlic
1/8 teaspoon coarsely ground black pepper
10 ounces bow tie pasta (about 3 3/4 cups) or rigatoni pasta (about 4 cups)
1/4 cup grated nonfat or regular Parmesan cheese (optional)

1. Place the tomatoes, tuna, onion, basil, olives, salad dressing, garlic, and pepper in a large bowl, and toss gently to mix well. Set aside for 30 minutes.

2. Cook the pasta al dente according to package directions. Drain well, and return to the pot.

3. Add the tomato-tuna mixture to the pasta, and toss gently to mix well. Serve hot, topping each serving with a tablespoon of Parmesan, if desired.

NUTRITIONAL FACTS (PER 2-CUP SERVING)
Cal: 375   Carbs: 61 g   Chol: 17 mg   Fat: 2.8 g
Fiber: 3 g   Protein: 25 g   Sodium: 462 mg

Spaghetti and Shrimp Florentine

YIELD: 4 SERVINGS

12 ounces peeled and deveined raw shrimp
1/4 teaspoon salt
1/4 teaspoon ground black pepper
8 ounces thin spaghetti
1 tablespoon extra virgin olive oil (optional)
1 1/2 teaspoons crushed fresh garlic
1/2 cup dry white wine
1 tablespoon lemon juice
3/4 teaspoon dried oregano
4 cups (packed) chopped fresh spinach
1/3 cup thin strips commercial roasted red pepper
3/4 cup reduced-sodium chicken broth
1 teaspoon cornstarch
1/4 cup grated nonfat or regular Parmesan cheese

1. Rinse the shrimp with cool water, and pat them dry with paper towels. Sprinkle with the salt and pepper, and set aside.

2. Cook the pasta al dente according to package directions. Drain well, return to the pot, and toss with the olive oil if desired. Cover to keep warm.

3. While the pasta is cooking, coat a large nonstick skillet with nonstick olive oil cooking spray, and preheat over medium-high heat. Add the garlic, and stir-fry for 30 seconds, or just until the garlic begins to turn color. Add the shrimp, and stir-fry for about 4 minutes, or until the shrimp turn pink.

4. Add the wine, lemon juice, and oregano to the skillet, and cook for about 2 minutes, or until the volume is reduced by half. Reduce the heat to medium, add the spinach, and stir-fry for a minute or 2, or just until the spinach is wilted. Stir in the roasted peppers.

5. Add the pasta to the skillet. Place the chicken broth in a small bowl, and stir in the cornstarch. Pour the mixture over the pasta and toss gently for about 1 minute, or until the sauce thickens slightly. Add a little more broth if the mixture seems too dry.

6. Remove the skillet from the heat, and serve hot, topping each serving with a tablespoon of the Parmesan.

NUTRITIONAL FACTS (PER 1 1/2-CUP SERVING)
Cal: 320   Carbs: 50 g   Chol: 141 mg   Fat: 1.8 g
Fiber: 2.1 g   Protein: 26 g   Sodium: 512 mg

Ragin' Cajun Pasta

YIELD: 6 SERVINGS

12 ounces fettuccine pasta
8 ounces peeled and deveined raw shrimp
2 teaspoons crushed fresh garlic
5 ounces smoked sausage or kielbasa, at least 97% lean, thinly sliced (about 1 cup)
1/2 cup chopped onion
1/2 cup chopped green bell pepper
1 can (14 1/2 ounces) stewed tomatoes, crushed
1 1/2 teaspoons Cajun seasoning

1. Cook the pasta al dente according to package directions. Drain well, return to the pot, and cover to keep warm.

2. While the pasta is cooking, rinse the shrimp with cool water, and pat them dry with paper towels.

3. Coat a large deep nonstick skillet with nonstick olive oil cooking spray, and preheat over medium-high heat. Add the garlic, sausage or kielbasa, onion, and green pepper, and cook, stirring frequently, for about 4 minutes, or until the sausage is nicely browned and the vegetables start to soften. Cover the skillet periodically if it begins to dry out. (The steam from the cooking vegetables will moisten the skillet.)

4. Stir the tomatoes, including their juice, the shrimp, and the Cajun seasoning into the skillet mixture. Allow the mixture to come to a boil. Then reduce the heat to low, cover, and simmer for 10 minutes, or until the shrimp turn pink and the onions and peppers are tender.

5. Add the pasta to the sauce, and toss gently to mix well. Serve hot.

NUTRITIONAL FACTS (PER 1 2/3-CUP SERVING)
Cal: 313   Carbs: 52 g   Chol: 62 mg   Fat: 2.3 g
Fiber: 2.8 g   Protein: 19 g   Sodium: 522 mg

Spicy Spaghetti and Shrimp

YIELD: 4 SERVINGS

8 ounces thin spaghetti

12 ounces peeled and deveined raw shrimp

2 teaspoons extra virgin olive oil (optional)

1 1/2 teaspoons crushed fresh garlic

1 can (14 1/2 ounces) stewed tomatoes, crushed

1/4 cup coarsely chopped black olives

1 tablespoon plus 1 teaspoon small capers*

3/4 teaspoon dried oregano or basil

1/4 teaspoon crushed red pepper

1/4 cup grated nonfat or regular Parmesan cheese

* If only large capers are available, coarsely chop them before using.

1. Cook the pasta al dente according to package directions. Drain well, return to the pot, and cover to keep warm.

2. While the pasta is cooking, rinse the shrimp with cool water, and pat them dry with paper towels. Set aside.

3. Coat a large nonstick skillet with the olive oil or with nonstick olive oil cooking spray, and preheat over medium-high heat. Add the garlic and stir-fry for about 30 seconds, or just until the garlic begins to turn color.

4. Add the shrimp, undrained tomatoes, olives, capers, oregano or basil, and crushed red pepper to the skillet, and bring to a boil over medium-high heat. Reduce the heat to low, cover, and simmer, stirring occasionally, for about 5 minutes, or until the flavors are well blended and the shrimp turn pink.

5. Add the pasta to the skillet, and toss to mix well. Serve hot, topping each serving with a tablespoon of the Parmesan.

NUTRITIONAL FACTS (PER 1 1/2-CUP SERVING)
Cal: 361   Carbs: 53 g   Chol: 126 mg   Fat: 3.3 g
Fiber: 3.2 g   Protein: 27 g   Sodium: 564 mg

Linguine With Creamy Clam Sauce

YIELD: 4 SERVINGS

2 cans (6 1/2 ounces each) chopped clams, undrained

8 ounces linguine pasta

1 cup evaporated skim milk

1 1/2 teaspoons cornstarch

1/8 teaspoon ground white pepper

2 teaspoons crushed fresh garlic

1/3 cup grated nonfat or regular Parmesan cheese

1/4 cup finely chopped fresh scallions

1/4 cup finely chopped fresh parsley

1. Drain the clams, reserving the juice. Set aside.

2. Cook the pasta al dente according to package directions. Drain well, return to the pot, and cover to keep warm.

3. Place 1 tablespoon of the evaporated milk and all of the cornstarch and pepper in a small bowl, and stir to dissolve the cornstarch. Stir in the remaining evaporated milk, and set aside.

4. Coat a large nonstick skillet with nonstick olive oil cooking spray, and preheat over medium-high heat. Add the garlic, and stir-fry for about 30 seconds, or just until the garlic begins to turn color.

5. Reduce the heat under the skillet to medium, and add the pasta, clams, and 1/4 cup of the reserved clam juice. Toss gently to mix well.

6. Stir the evaporated milk mixture. Pour the mixture over the pasta, and toss gently for a minute or 2, or until the mixture thickens slightly. Add a little more evaporated milk if the mixture seems too dry.

7. Remove the skillet from the heat, and toss in the Parmesan, scallions, and parsley. Serve hot.

NUTRITIONAL FACTS (PER 1 1/3-CUP SERVING)
Cal: 374   Carbs: 58 g   Chol: 43 mg   Fat: 2.2 g
Fiber: 1.7 g   Protein: 30 g   Sodium: 270 mg

Linguine With Clam Sauce

YIELD: 4 SERVINGS

2 cans (6 ounces each) chopped clams, undrained

8 ounces linguine pasta

1 tablespoon olive oil (optional)

1 medium yellow onion, diced

1 cup sliced fresh mushrooms

1/2 cup thinly sliced celery (include the leaves)

2 teaspoons crushed fresh garlic

1 1/2 teaspoons butter-flavored sprinkles

3/4 teaspoon dried basil

3/4 teaspoon dried oregano

1/8 teaspoon ground white pepper

1/4 cup minced fresh parsley

1/3 cup grated nonfat or regular Parmesan cheese

1. Drain the clams, reserving 1/2 cup of the juice, and set aside.

2. Cook the pasta al dente according to package directions. Drain well, return to the pot, and toss with the olive oil if desired. Cover to keep warm.

3. While the linguine is cooking, place the onion, mushrooms, celery, garlic, butter-flavored sprinkles, basil, oregano, and pepper in a large skillet. Add the clams and the reserved juice, and bring to a boil over high heat. Reduce the heat to low, cover, and simmer, stirring occasionally, for 10 minutes, or until the vegetables are tender.

4. Add the cooked linguine and the parsley to the clam mixture, and toss gently until well mixed. Serve hot, topping each serving with a rounded tablespoon of the Parmesan.

NUTRITIONAL FACTS (PER 1 1/2-CUP SERVING)
Cal: 318   Carbs: 53 g   Chol: 36 mg   Fat: 1.9 g
Fiber: 2.4 g   Protein: 22 g   Sodium: 308 mg

Sonoma Spaghetti

YIELD: 4 SERVINGS

1/2 cup chopped sun-dried tomatoes (not packed in oil)

1/2 cup water

8 ounces spaghetti or fettuccine pasta

1 block (8 ounces) nonfat or reduced-fat cream cheese

1 cup skim or low-fat milk

1/8 teaspoon ground white pepper

4 scallions, thinly sliced

2 tablespoons minced fresh basil

1/4 cup grated nonfat or regular Parmesan cheese

1. Place the sun-dried tomatoes and water in a 1-quart saucepan, and bring to a boil over high heat. Reduce the heat to low, cover, and simmer for 2 minutes, or until the tomatoes are plumped. Remove the pot from the heat, and set aside.

2. Cook the pasta al dente according to package directions. Drain well, return to the pot, and cover to keep warm.

3. While the pasta is cooking, place the cream cheese, milk, and pepper in a blender or food processor, and process until smooth. Pour the mixture into a 1-quart saucepan, and place over low heat. Cook and stir for about 2 minutes, or just until the sauce is heated through. Do not allow the sauce to boil. The sauce should be the consistency of heavy cream. Add a few tablespoons of skim milk, if necessary, to thin it to the desired consistency.

4. Drain any remaining liquid from the sun-dried tomatoes, and add the tomatoes to the pasta. Add the sauce, scallions, and basil, and toss gently to mix. Serve hot, topping each serving with a tablespoon of the Parmesan.

NUTRITIONAL FACTS (PER 1 1/2-CUP SERVING)
Cal: 317   Carbs: 56 g   Chol: 10 mg   Fat: 1.2 g
Fiber: 2.4 g   Protein: 20.4 g   Sodium: 493 mg

Spaghetti With Scallops and Tomato Cream Sauce

YIELD: 4 SERVINGS
8 ounces thin spaghetti
12 ounces large raw scallops
1½ teaspoons crushed fresh garlic
¼ cup thinly sliced scallions
¼ cup grated nonfat or regular Parmesan cheese

SAUCE
½ cup chopped sun-dried tomatoes (not packed in oil)
¾ cup chicken broth
1¼ cups evaporated skim milk
1½ teaspoons cornstarch
1 teaspoon dried oregano or basil
⅛ teaspoon ground black pepper

1. To make the sauce, place the tomatoes and broth in a small saucepan, and bring to a boil over medium heat. Reduce the heat to low, cover, and simmer for 2 minutes, or until the tomatoes are plumped. Remove the pot from the heat, and set aside to cool slightly. (Do not drain.)

2. Place 2 tablespoons of the evaporated milk and all of the cornstarch, oregano or basil, and pepper in a small bowl, and stir to dissolve the cornstarch. Add the remaining evaporated milk, and stir to mix well. Add the evaporated milk mixture to the tomato mixture, stir to mix well, and set aside.

3. Cook the pasta al dente according to package directions. Drain well, return to the pot, and cover to keep warm.

4. While the pasta is cooking, rinse the scallops with cool water, and pat them dry with paper towels. Set aside.

5. Coat a large nonstick skillet with nonstick cooking spray, and preheat over medium-high heat. Add the garlic, and stir-fry for 30 seconds, or just until the garlic begins to turn color. Add the scallops, and stir-fry for about 4 minutes, or just until the scallops turn opaque and are thoroughly cooked.

6. Reduce the heat under the skillet to medium-low. Add the pasta to the skillet, and pour the sauce over the pasta. Toss gently over low heat for about 2 minutes, or until the sauce thickens slightly. Add the scallions, and toss to mix well. Remove the skillet from the heat, toss in the Parmesan, and serve hot.

NUTRITIONAL FACTS (PER 1⅔-CUP SERVING)
Cal: 380   Carbs: 60 g   Chol: 34 mg   Fat: 1.7 g
Fiber: 1.5 g   Protein: 31 g   Sodium: 421 mg

Rigatoni With Spicy Olive Sauce

YIELD: 4 SERVINGS
8 ounces rigatoni pasta (about 3¼ cups)
2 teaspoons crushed fresh garlic
1¼ pounds fresh plum tomatoes (about 8 medium), chopped
⅓ cup sliced black olives
¼ cup olive brine (from the can of olives)
2 teaspoons dried Italian seasoning
¼–½ teaspoon crushed red pepper
¼ cup grated nonfat or regular Parmesan cheese
1 cup diced nonfat or reduced-fat mozzarella cheese

1. Cook the pasta al dente according to package directions. Drain well, return to the pot, and cover to keep warm.

2. While the pasta is cooking, coat a large skillet with nonstick cooking spray, and preheat over medium-high heat. Add the garlic, and stir-fry for about 30 seconds, or just until the garlic begins to turn color.

3. Add the tomatoes, olives, brine, Italian seasoning, and red pepper to the skillet, and stir to mix. Reduce the heat to medium, cover, and cook, stirring constantly, for 8 to 10 minutes, or until the tomatoes are soft.

4. Add the pasta to the skillet, and toss to mix well. Remove the skillet from the heat, and toss in first the Parmesan and then the mozzarella. Serve hot.

NUTRITIONAL FACTS (PER 1½-CUP SERVING)
Cal: 321   Carbs: 54 g   Chol: 8 mg   Fat: 2.7 g
Fiber: 3.4 g   Protein: 20 g   Sodium: 523 mg

Penne California

YIELD: 4 SERVINGS

10 ounces penne pasta (about 3$\frac{1}{3}$ cups)
1 can (15 ounces) white beans, rinsed and drained, divided
1 tablespoon extra virgin olive oil (optional)
2–3 teaspoons crushed fresh garlic
2 cups unsalted chicken or vegetable broth
$\frac{3}{4}$ cup chopped sun-dried tomatoes (not packed in oil)
1 teaspoon dried Italian seasoning
$\frac{1}{4}$ teaspoon coarsely ground black pepper
$\frac{1}{2}$ cup sliced scallions
$\frac{1}{4}$ cup sliced black olives
$\frac{1}{4}$ cup grated nonfat or regular Parmesan cheese (optional)

1. Cook the pasta al dente according to package directions. Drain well, return to the pot, and cover to keep warm.

2. While the pasta is cooking, place $\frac{1}{4}$ cup of the beans in a small bowl. Mash with a fork until smooth, and set aside.

3. Coat a large nonstick skillet with nonstick olive oil cooking spray or with the olive oil, and preheat over medium-heat. Add the garlic, and stir-fry for about 30 seconds, or just until the garlic begins to turn color.

4. Add the broth, sun-dried tomatoes, Italian seasoning, and pepper to the skillet, and bring to a boil over medium-high heat. Reduce the heat to low, cover, and simmer for about 5 minutes, or until the tomatoes are soft. Add the mashed white beans to the skillet, and stir to mix well. (This will thicken the sauce slightly.)

5. Add the pasta, the remaining white beans, the scallions, and the olives to the skillet, and toss gently over low heat for a minute or 2, or until the beans are heated through and the flavors are well blended. Add a little more broth if the mixture seems too dry. Serve hot, topping each serving with a tablespoon of the Parmesan, if desired.

NUTRITIONAL FACTS (PER 2-CUP SERVING)
Cal: 408   Carbs: 78 g   Chol: 0 mg   Fat: 2.6 g
Fiber: 8 g   Protein: 18 g   Sodium: 472 mg

Penne With Spinach Cream Sauce

YIELD: 5 SERVINGS

12 ounces penne or tube pasta (about 4 cups)
1$\frac{1}{2}$ teaspoons crushed fresh garlic
4 cups (packed) chopped fresh spinach
$\frac{1}{2}$ teaspoon dried Italian seasoning
$\frac{1}{4}$ cup plus 2 tablespoons grated nonfat or regular Parmesan cheese

SAUCE

1 cup nonfat or low-fat ricotta cheese
1 cup skim or low-fat milk
1 teaspoon butter-flavored sprinkles
$\frac{1}{8}$ teaspoon ground white pepper

1. Cook the pasta al dente according to package directions. Drain well, return to the pot, and cover to keep warm.

2. While the pasta is cooking, place all of the sauce ingredients in a blender or food processor, and process until smooth. Set aside.

3. Coat a large nonstick skillet with nonstick butter-flavored cooking spray, and preheat over medium heat. Add the garlic, and stir-fry for about 30 seconds, or just until the garlic begins to turn color. Add the spinach and Italian seasoning, and stir-fry for about 1 minute, or just until the spinach is wilted.

4. Add the pasta to the skillet. Reduce the heat to low, and pour the sauce over the pasta mixture. Toss gently over low heat for a minute or 2, or just until the sauce is heated through. Do not allow the sauce to boil. Add a little more milk if the sauce seems too dry.

5. Remove the skillet from the heat, and toss in the Parmesan. Serve hot.

NUTRITIONAL FACTS (PER 1$\frac{1}{2}$-CUP SERVING)
Cal: 346   Carbs: 62 g   Chol: 6 mg   Fat: 1.2 g
Fiber: 2.2 g   Protein: 22 g   Sodium: 245 mg

Fabulous Fettuccine Alfredo

YIELD: 4 SERVINGS

10 ounces fettuccine pasta

1/2 cup grated nonfat or regular Parmesan cheese

1/4 cup thinly sliced scallions (garnish)

2 tablespoons chopped fresh parsley (garnish)

SAUCE

1 can (12 ounces) evaporated skim milk

1 1/2 teaspoons cornstarch

1/8 teaspoon ground white pepper

1. Cook the pasta al dente according to package directions. Drain well, return to the pot, and cover to keep warm.

2. While the pasta is cooking, place 1 tablespoon of the evaporated milk and all of the cornstarch and pepper in a small bowl, and stir to dissolve the cornstarch. Stir in the remaining evaporated milk.

3. Place the pot containing the pasta over medium heat, and pour the sauce over the pasta. Toss gently for a minute or 2, or until the sauce is heated through, is just beginning to boil, and has thickened slightly. Add a little more milk if the sauce seems too dry.

4. Remove the pot from the heat, and toss in the Parmesan. Serve hot, topping each serving with some of the scallions and parsley.

NUTRITIONAL FACTS (PER 1 1/2-CUP SERVING)
Cal: 390   Carbs: 71 g   Chol: 9 mg   Fat: 1.3 g
Fiber: 1.9 g   Protein: 22 g   Sodium: 352 mg

VARIATION

To make Fettuccine Alfredo With Sun-Dried Tomatoes, place 1/3 cup of sun-dried tomatoes and 1/3 cup of water in a small pot, and bring to a boil over high heat. Reduce the heat to low, cover, and simmer for 2 minutes, or until the tomatoes are plumped. Remove the pot from the heat and drain off any excess liquid. Add the plumped tomatoes to the pasta after tossing the pasta in the sauce in Step 3.

NUTRITIONAL FACTS (PER 1 1/2-CUP SERVING)
Cal: 401   Carbs: 74 g   Chol: 9 mg   Fat: 1.5 g
Fiber: 2.5 g   Protein: 23 g   Sodium: 445 mg

Bow Ties With Spicy Artichoke Sauce

YIELD: 4 SERVINGS

8 ounces bow tie pasta (about 3 cups) or rigatoni pasta (about 3 1/4 cups)

1 pound fresh tomatoes (about 3 medium), diced

1 medium yellow onion, diced

1 cup sliced fresh mushrooms

1/4 cup vegetable or chicken broth

1 tablespoon crushed fresh garlic

1 teaspoon dried basil

1 teaspoon dried oregano

1/4 teaspoon salt

1/8 teaspoon cayenne pepper

1/8 teaspoon ground black pepper

1 can (14 ounces) artichoke hearts, drained and quartered

1/2 red bell pepper, cut into thin strips

1 tablespoon lemon juice

1/4 cup plus 2 tablespoons grated nonfat or regular Parmesan cheese

1. Cook the pasta al dente according to package directions. Drain well, return to the pot, and cover to keep warm.

2. While the pasta is cooking, place the tomatoes, onion, mushrooms, broth, garlic, basil, oregano, salt, cayenne pepper, and black pepper in a large skillet. Place over medium-low heat, cover, and cook, stirring occasionally, for about 10 minutes, or until the tomatoes are soft.

3. Add the artichoke hearts, red pepper, and lemon juice to the skillet mixture. Cover and cook for 3 additional minutes, or until the peppers are crisp-tender. Reduce the heat to low.

4. Add the pasta to the skillet mixture, and toss gently to mix. Serve hot, topping each serving with some of the Parmesan cheese.

NUTRITIONAL FACTS (PER 1 3/4-CUP SERVING)
Cal: 325   Carbs: 66 g   Chol: 7 mg   Fat: 1.6 g
Fiber: 9.7 g   Protein: 14.5 g   Sodium: 294 mg

Pasta Primavera

YIELD: 5 SERVINGS

1 1/2 cups evaporated skim milk

2 teaspoons cornstarch

1/8 teaspoon ground white pepper

8 ounces spaghetti or fettuccine pasta

2 teaspoons crushed fresh garlic

1/2 cup thinly sliced carrots

1/2 cup sliced fresh mushrooms

2 cups fresh broccoli florets

1/2 small red bell pepper, cut into thin strips

1 medium onion, cut into thin wedges

1 tablespoon water

1/2 cup plus 2 tablespoons grated nonfat or regular Parmesan cheese

1. Place 1 tablespoon of the evaporated milk and all of the cornstarch and pepper in a small bowl, and stir to dissolve the cornstarch. Stir in the remaining milk, and set aside.

2. Cook the pasta al dente according to package directions. Drain well, return to the pot, and cover to keep warm.

3. Coat a large skillet with nonstick cooking spray, and preheat over medium-high heat. Add the garlic, and stir-fry for 30 seconds, or just until the garlic begins to turn color.

4. Add the vegetables and water to the skillet, cover, and cook, stirring occasionally, for 3 to 5 minutes, or until the vegetables are crisp-tender. Add a little more water if the skillet becomes too dry.

5. Reduce the heat to medium, and add the pasta to the skillet mixture. Stir the milk mixture, and add it to the skillet. Toss gently over medium heat for about 2 minutes, or just until the sauce begins to boil and thickens slightly. Add a little more evaporated milk if the mixture seems too dry.

6. Remove the skillet from the heat, and add the Parmesan cheese. Toss gently to mix, and serve hot.

NUTRITIONAL FACTS (PER 1 1/2-CUP SERVING)
Cal: 291   Carbs: 53 g   Chol: 10 mg   Fat: 1.1 g
Fiber: 3.2 g   Protein: 17 g   Sodium: 194 mg

Capellini With Pesto Cheese Sauce

YIELD: 4 SERVINGS

10 ounces capellini (angel hair) pasta

1 block (8 ounces) nonfat or reduced-fat cream cheese, or 8 ounces soft curd farmer cheese

3/4 cup skim or low-fat milk

1 cup chopped fresh plum tomatoes (about 3 medium)

1/4 cup pine nuts

PESTO

1/2 cup (packed) fresh basil

1/2 cup (packed) fresh parsley

1/4 cup plus 2 tablespoons grated nonfat or regular Parmesan cheese

2 teaspoons crushed fresh garlic

1. Cook the pasta al dente according to package directions. Drain well, return to the pot, and cover to keep warm.

2. While the pasta is cooking, place all of the pesto ingredients in a food processor, and process until the herbs are finely chopped. Transfer the mixture to a small bowl, and set aside.

3. Place the cream cheese or farmer cheese and the milk in the food processor, and process until smooth. Set aside.

4. Add the cheese mixture to the pasta, and toss over low heat for a minute or two, or just until the sauce is warmed through. Do not allow the sauce to boil. Add a little more milk if the sauce seems too thick. Remove the pot from the heat, add the pesto, and toss to mix well.

5. Serve hot, topping each serving with 1/4 cup of the chopped tomatoes and a tablespoon of the pine nuts.

NUTRITIONAL FACTS (PER 1 3/4-CUP SERVING)
Cal: 398   Carbs: 65 g   Chol: 12 mg   Fat: 5 g
Fiber: 2.8 g   Protein: 24.7 g   Sodium: 378 mg

Penne With Roasted Red Pepper Sauce

YIELD: 4 SERVINGS

12 ounces penne pasta (about 4 cups)

1/4 cup grated nonfat or regular Parmesan cheese

3/4 teaspoon dried basil, or 2 1/4 teaspoons
finely chopped fresh basil

SAUCE

1 jar (7 ounces) roasted red peppers,
drained and chopped

1 cup evaporated skim milk

1/3 cup grated nonfat or regular Parmesan cheese

1 tablespoon finely chopped fresh basil,
or 1 teaspoon dried

1 teaspoon crushed fresh garlic

1/4 teaspoon ground black pepper

1. Cook the pasta al dente according to package directions. Drain well, return to the pot, and cover to keep warm.

2. While the pasta is cooking, place all of the sauce ingredients in a blender or food processor, and process until smooth.

3. Place the pot containing the pasta over low heat, and pour the sauce over the pasta. Cook and stir for a minute or 2, or until the sauce is heated through. Do not allow the sauce to boil. Add a little more evaporated milk if the mixture seems too dry.

4. Serve hot, topping each serving with a tablespoon of the Parmesan and a sprinkling of basil.

NUTRITIONAL FACTS (PER 1 1/2-CUP SERVING)
Cal: 416   Carbs: 78 g   Chol: 14 mg   Fat: 1.8 g
Fiber: 2.4 g   Protein: 21 g   Sodium: 364 mg

Pasta With Crab and Asparagus

YIELD: 4 SERVINGS

8 ounces penne or small sea shell pasta
(about 2 3/4 cups)

8 ounces fresh asparagus spears, cut into
1-inch pieces (about 1 3/4 cups)

6 ounces (about 1 cup) flaked cooked crab meat
or drained canned crab meat

1/4 cup grated nonfat or regular Parmesan cheese

SAUCE

1 cup nonfat or low-fat ricotta cheese

2 scallions, chopped

2 tablespoons dry sherry

2 tablespoons lemon juice

1/4 teaspoon dried oregano

1/8 teaspoon ground white pepper

1. To make the sauce, place all of the sauce ingredients in a blender or food processor, and process until smooth. Set aside.

2. Cook the pasta al dente according to package directions. About 1 minute before the pasta is done, add the asparagus, and cook until the asparagus are crisp-tender and the pasta is al dente. Drain the pasta and asparagus, and return the mixture to the pot.

3. Add the crab meat to the pasta mixture, and top with the sauce. Place the pot over low heat, and, tossing gently, cook just until the sauce is heated through. Do not allow the sauce to boil. If the sauce is too thick, add a little skim milk.

4. Serve hot, topping each serving with a tablespoon of the Parmesan.

NUTRITIONAL FACTS (PER 1 1/2-CUP SERVING)
Cal: 337   Carbs: 51 g   Chol: 47 mg   Fat: 1.6 g
Fiber: 2.7 g   Protein: 29 g   Sodium: 332 mg

Bow Ties With Broccoli and Tomatoes

YIELD: 4 SERVINGS
8 ounces bow tie pasta (about 3 cups)
3 cups fresh broccoli florets
2 teaspoons crushed fresh garlic
1 pound fresh plum tomatoes (6–7 medium), diced
1/4 cup chicken or vegetable broth
1 1/2 teaspoons dried Italian seasoning
1/4–1/2 teaspoon crushed red pepper
1/4 cup grated nonfat or regular Parmesan cheese
1 cup nonfat or low-fat ricotta cheese

1. Cook the pasta al dente according to package directions. About 2 minutes before the pasta is done, add the broccoli to the pot. Cook until the broccoli turns bright green and is crisp-tender and the pasta is al dente. Drain well, return to the pot, and cover to keep warm.

2. While the pasta is cooking, coat a large nonstick skillet with nonstick olive oil cooking spray, and pre-heat over medium-high heat. Add the garlic, and stir-fry for about 30 seconds, or just until the garlic begins to turn color.

3. Add the tomatoes, broth, Italian seasoning, and red pepper to the skillet, and reduce the heat to medium-low. Cover and cook, stirring occasionally, for 4 to 5 minutes, or just until the tomatoes are heated through and just beginning to soften.

4. Add the pasta mixture to the skillet, and toss to mix well. Remove the skillet from the heat, and toss in the Parmesan. Serve hot, topping each serving with 1/4 cup of the ricotta.

NUTRITIONAL FACTS (PER 2-CUP SERVING)
Cal: 326   Carbs: 56 g   Chol: 5 mg   Fat: 1.5 g
Fiber: 4.5 g   Protein: 22 g   Sodium: 264 mg

Spaghetti With Shrimp and Sun-Dried Tomatoes

YIELD: 4 SERVINGS
8 ounces thin spaghetti
1 tablespoon extra virgin olive oil (optional)
1 pound peeled and deveined raw shrimp
1/2 cup diced sun-dried tomatoes (not packed in oil)
1/2 cup chicken broth
2 tablespoons dry white wine
2 teaspoons crushed fresh garlic
1 teaspoon dried rosemary
1/4 teaspoon coarsely ground black pepper
1/4 cup minced fresh parsley
1/3 cup crumbled nonfat or reduced-fat feta cheese

1. Cook the pasta al dente according to package directions. Drain well, return to the pot, and toss with the olive oil if desired. Cover to keep warm.

2. While the pasta is cooking, rinse the shrimp with cool water, and pat them dry with paper towels.

3. Coat a large nonstick skillet with nonstick olive oil cooking spray. Add the shrimp, sun-dried tomatoes, broth, wine, garlic, rosemary, and pepper, and stir to mix. Cover and cook over medium heat for 4 minutes, or until the shrimp turn pink and the tomatoes have plumped. Reduce the heat to low.

4. Add the pasta to the shrimp mixture. Tossing gently, cook for a minute or 2, or until the mixture is heated through. Toss in the parsley, and serve hot, topping each serving with some of the feta cheese.

NUTRITIONAL FACTS (PER 1 1/2-CUP SERVING)
Cal: 328   Carbs: 47 g   Chol: 162 mg   Fat: 2.2 g
Fiber: 2.3 g   Protein: 28 g   Sodium: 584 mg

Garden Vegetable Linguine

YIELD: 4 SERVINGS

1/4 cup diced sun-dried tomatoes
(not packed in oil)

1 cup plus 2 tablespoons vegetable broth, divided

8 ounces linguine or spinach fettuccine pasta

2 teaspoons crushed fresh garlic

1 1/2 cups fresh broccoli florets

2 medium-small yellow squash,
halved lengthwise and sliced (about 1 cup)

1 cup sliced fresh mushrooms

1/2 cup diagonally sliced carrots

1 tablespoon finely chopped fresh oregano,
or 1 teaspoon dried

1/4 cup chopped toasted pecans
(page 348) (optional)

1 teaspoon cornstarch

1/4 cup grated nonfat or regular Parmesan cheese

1. Place the sun-dried tomatoes and 1/4 cup of the broth in a small saucepan, and bring to a boil over high heat. Reduce the heat to low, cover, and simmer for about 2 minutes, or until the tomatoes are plumped. Remove the pot from the heat, and cover to keep warm.

2. Cook the pasta al dente according to package directions. Drain well, return to the pot, and cover to keep warm.

3. While the pasta is cooking, coat a large nonstick skillet with nonstick cooking spray, and preheat over medium-high heat. Add the garlic, and stir-fry for about 30 seconds, or just until the garlic begins to turn color. Add the vegetables, oregano, and 1/4 cup of the remaining broth. Cover and cook for 1 to 2 minutes, or until the vegetables are crisp-tender.

4. Reduce the heat under the skillet to medium-low, and add the pasta, the undrained sun-dried tomatoes, and, if desired, the pecans to the skillet mixture. Stir the cornstarch into the remaining 1/2 cup plus 2 tablespoons of broth, and pour over the pasta and vegetables. Toss gently for about 1 minute, or until the sauce thickens slightly. Add a little more broth if the mixture seems too dry.

5. Remove the skillet from the heat, and toss in the Parmesan. Serve hot.

NUTRITIONAL FACTS (PER 1¾-CUP SERVING)
Cal: 274   Carbs: 52 g   Chol: 3 mg   Fat: 1.5 g
Fiber: 3.8 g   Protein: 12.5 g   Sodium: 467 mg

Pasta Pesto Primavera

YIELD: 4 SERVINGS

8 ounces thin spaghetti

3/4 cup thinly sliced cauliflower florets

3/4 cup yellow squash, halved lengthwise
and sliced 1/4-inch thick

3/4 cup thin strips red bell pepper

3/4 cup sliced fresh mushrooms

1/2 cup warm chicken or vegetable broth

PESTO SAUCE

2/3 cup (tightly packed) fresh basil

2/3 cup (tightly packed) fresh spinach

1/2 cup plus 2 tablespoons grated nonfat or
regular Parmesan cheese

1/3 cup chopped walnuts or pine nuts (optional)

1 tablespoon plus 1 teaspoon extra virgin olive oil

3–4 cloves garlic, peeled

1/4 teaspoon ground white pepper

1. Cook the pasta al dente according to package directions. About 1 minute before the pasta is done, add the vegetables, and cook until the vegetables are crisp-tender and the pasta is al dente. Drain well, return the pasta and vegetables to the pot, and cover to keep warm.

2. While the pasta is cooking, place all of the pesto ingredients in a blender or food processor, and process until finely ground.

3. Add the pesto to the pasta and vegetables, and toss to mix well. Add the broth, and toss to mix well. Add a little more broth if the sauce seems too dry, and serve hot.

NUTRITIONAL FACTS (PER 1⅔-CUP SERVING)
Cal: 318   Carbs: 52 g   Chol: 8 mg   Fat: 4.6 g
Fiber: 3.7 g   Protein: 16 g   Sodium: 323 mg

Baked Rigatoni With Sausage, Tomatoes, and Cheese

YIELD: 8 SERVINGS

12 ounces rigatoni pasta (about 4⁷⁄₈ cups)

1 pound Turkey Italian Sausage (below)

1 can (28 ounces) crushed tomatoes

½ cup chopped onion

1 teaspoon dried oregano

¼–½ teaspoon crushed red pepper (optional)

¼ cup grated nonfat or regular Parmesan cheese

1 cup shredded nonfat or reduced-fat mozzarella cheese

½ cup shredded reduced-fat provolone cheese

1. Cook the pasta al dente according to package directions. Drain well, return to the pot, and cover to keep warm.

2. While the pasta is cooking, coat a large nonstick skillet with nonstick cooking spray, and preheat over medium heat. Add the sausage, and cook, stirring to crumble, until the meat is no longer pink. Drain off and discard any excess fat.

3. Add the tomatoes, onion, oregano, and red pepper to the skillet, and bring to a boil over medium-high heat. Reduce the heat to low, cover, and cook, stirring occasionally, for 10 minutes, or until the onions are tender and the flavors are blended.

4. Pour the tomato mixture over the pasta, and toss to mix well. Add the Parmesan cheese, and toss to mix well.

5. Coat a 9-x-13-inch baking pan with nonstick cooking spray, and spread the pasta mixture evenly in the dish. Sprinkle first with the mozzarella and then with the provolone.

6. Cover the dish with aluminum foil, and bake at 350°F for 25 minutes. Remove the foil, and bake uncovered for 10 additional minutes, or until the cheese is lightly browned. Serve hot.

NUTRITIONAL FACTS (PER 1⅔-CUP SERVING)
Cal: 317   Carbs: 40 g   Chol: 43 mg   Fat: 3.7 g
Fiber: 2.9 g   Protein: 28 g   Sodium: 363 mg

Making Your Own Italian Sausage

Italian sausage is used to add richness and a distinctive flavor to a variety of pasta creations, and to many other dishes as well. Fortunately, it's easy to make a sausage mixture that is just as flavorful as a traditional one, but contains a fraction of the fat and calories. Stir Turkey Italian Sausage into sauces or use it to top your favorite pizza, and enjoy an authentic taste of Italy.

Turkey Italian Sausage

YIELD: 1 POUND

1 pound 96–93% lean ground turkey or ground pork sirloin

2 teaspoons crushed fresh garlic

2 teaspoons ground paprika

1½ teaspoons whole fennel seeds

1 teaspoon dried Italian seasoning

¼ teaspoon crushed red pepper

½ teaspoon salt

1. Place all of the ingredients in a medium-sized bowl, and mix thoroughly. Cover and refrigerate for several hours to allow the flavors to blend.

2. To precook for use in recipes, coat a large skillet with nonstick cooking spray, and preheat over medium heat. Add the sausage, and cook, stirring to crumble, until the meat is no longer pink. Use as directed in your recipe.

NUTRITIONAL FACTS (PER 2-OUNCE COOKED SERVING)
Cal: 105   Carbs: 0 g   Chol: 46 mg   Fat: 3 g
Fiber: 0 g   Protein: 18 g   Sodium: 235 mg

Sicilian Baked Ziti

YIELD: 8 SERVINGS

12 ounces ziti pasta (about 4½ cups)

¼ cup plus 2 tablespoons grated nonfat or regular Parmesan cheese

2 cups shredded nonfat or reduced-fat mozzarella cheese

SAUCE

1 can (28 ounces) crushed tomatoes

2 cups diced peeled eggplant (about 1 medium-small)

2 cups sliced fresh mushrooms

1 medium onion, chopped

1½ teaspoons crushed fresh garlic

2 teaspoons dried Italian seasoning

½ teaspoon crushed red pepper

1 jar (12 ounces) roasted red peppers, drained and coarsely chopped

1. To make the sauce, place all of the sauce ingredients except for the roasted peppers in a 3-quart pot, and bring to a boil over medium-high heat. Reduce the heat to low, cover, and simmer for 25 minutes, or until the vegetables are tender. Add the peppers, and simmer for 5 additional minutes. Remove the pot from the heat, and set 1½ cups of the sauce aside in a medium-sized bowl.

2. Cook the ziti al dente according to package directions. Drain the pasta, and return it to the pot. Add the sauce (except for the reserved sauce) and the Parmesan, and toss to mix.

3. Coat a 9-x-13-inch baking pan with cooking spray, and spread the ziti mixture evenly in the pan. Top first with the reserved sauce, and then with the mozzarella.

4. Cover the pan with aluminum foil, and bake at 350°F for 25 minutes. Remove the foil, and bake uncovered for 15 additional minutes, or until the cheese is bubbly and lightly browned. Serve hot.

NUTRITIONAL FACTS (PER 1⅔-CUP SERVING)
Cal: 277   Carbs: 46 g   Chol: 6 mg   Fat: 1.2 g
Fiber: 4 g   Protein: 19 g   Sodium: 591 mg

Savory Baked Ziti

YIELD: 10 SERVINGS

1 pound ziti pasta (about 6 cups)

5 cups Savory Meat Sauce (page 235)

¼ cup grated nonfat or regular Parmesan cheese

1 cup shredded nonfat or reduced-fat mozzarella cheese

CHEESE FILLING

3 cups nonfat or low-fat ricotta cheese

½ cup grated nonfat or regular Parmesan cheese

¼ cup plus 2 tablespoons fat-free egg substitute

3 tablespoons finely chopped fresh parsley

1. Cook the ziti until barely al dente according to package directions. Drain well, and return to the pot. Add 3 cups of the sauce, and toss to mix well. Set aside.

2. To make the cheese filling, place all of the filling ingredients in a medium-sized bowl, and stir to mix well. Set aside.

3. To assemble the casserole, coat a 9-x-13-inch baking pan with nonstick cooking spray, and spread half of the ziti in the pan. Spread all of the filling over the ziti. Then cover the filling with the remaining ziti. Spread the remaining 2 cups of sauce over the top, and sprinkle with the ¼ cup of Parmesan.

4. Cover the pan with aluminum foil, and bake at 350°F for 40 minutes, or until hot and bubbly. Remove the foil, spread the mozzarella over the top, and bake uncovered for 10 additional minutes, or until the cheese is melted.

5. Remove the dish from the oven, and let sit for 10 minutes before cutting into squares and serving.

NUTRITIONAL FACTS (PER SERVING)
Cal: 362   Carbs: 51 g   Chol: 27 mg   Fat: 2.3 g
Fiber: 3.1 g   Protein: 33 g   Sodium: 522 mg

Pesto Pasta With Sun-Dried Tomatoes

YIELD: 4 SERVINGS

$\frac{1}{2}$ cup chopped sun-dried tomatoes (not packed in oil)

$\frac{1}{2}$ cup unsalted chicken broth

8 ounces fettuccine or linguine pasta

$\frac{1}{4}$ cup pine nuts (optional)

PESTO SAUCE

$\frac{3}{4}$ cup (packed) chopped fresh spinach

$\frac{1}{2}$ cup plus 2 tablespoons grated nonfat or regular Parmesan cheese

$\frac{1}{2}$ cup (packed) chopped fresh basil

$\frac{1}{2}$ cup unsalted chicken broth

1 tablespoon plus 1 teaspoon extra virgin olive oil

4 cloves garlic, peeled

$\frac{1}{4}$ teaspoon coarsely ground black pepper

1. Place the sun-dried tomatoes and the broth in a small pot, and bring to a boil over high heat. Reduce the heat to low, cover, and simmer for 2 minutes, or until the tomatoes have plumped. Remove the pot from the heat, and drain off any excess liquid. Cover the pot and set aside.

2. Cook the pasta al dente according to package directions. Drain well, return to the pot, and cover to keep warm.

3. While the pasta is cooking, place all of the pesto ingredients in a blender or food processor, and process until the herbs are finely chopped.

4. Add the pesto to the pasta, and toss to mix well. Add the sun-dried tomatoes and, if desired, the pine nuts, and toss to mix well. Add a little more broth if the sauce seems too dry, and serve hot.

NUTRITIONAL FACTS (PER 1$\frac{1}{3}$-CUP SERVING)		
Cal: 334 Carbs: 54 g Chol: 7 mg Fat: 5.6 g		
Fiber: 2.7 g Protein: 17 g Sodium: 419 mg		

Vegetable Manicotti Alfredo

YIELD: 7 SERVINGS

14 manicotti tubes (about 8 ounces)

1 recipe Almost Alfredo Sauce (page 234)

1 cup shredded nonfat or reduced-fat mozzarella cheese

FILLING

15 ounces nonfat or low-fat ricotta cheese

1 cup nonfat or low-fat cottage cheese

1 cup shredded nonfat or reduced-fat mozzarella cheese

1 package (10 ounces) frozen chopped spinach or broccoli, thawed and squeezed dry

1 can (4 ounces) chopped mushrooms, drained

$\frac{1}{4}$ cup fat-free egg substitute

$\frac{1}{4}$ cup grated nonfat or regular Parmesan cheese

1. Cook the manicotti al dente according to package directions. Drain well, and set aside.

2. To make the filling, place all of the filling ingredients in a large bowl, and stir to mix well.

3. Coat a 9-x-13-inch baking pan with nonstick cooking spray, and spoon a thin layer of sauce over the bottom of the pan. Using a small spoon, stuff about $\frac{1}{3}$ cup of the filling mixture into each of the tubes, and arrange the filled tubes in the pan. Pour the remaining sauce evenly over the manicotti.

4. Bake uncovered at 350°F for about 30 minutes, or until heated through. Sprinkle the cup of mozzarella over the top, and bake for 5 additional minutes, or just until the cheese is melted.

5. Remove the dish from the oven, and let sit for 10 minutes before serving.

NUTRITIONAL FACTS (PER SERVING)		
Cal: 347 Carbs: 45 g Chol: 19 mg Fat: 0.9 g		
Fiber: 2.1 g Protein: 38 g Sodium: 694 mg		

Lasagna Roll-Ups

YIELD: 4 SERVINGS

8 lasagna noodles (about 6$\frac{1}{2}$ ounces)

1 cup shredded nonfat or reduced-fat mozzarella cheese

FILLING

15 ounces nonfat or low-fat ricotta cheese

1 package (10 ounces) frozen chopped spinach, thawed and squeezed dry

$\frac{1}{2}$ cup grated carrot

2 tablespoons minced fresh parsley

SAUCE

1 can (14$\frac{1}{2}$ ounces) unsalted tomatoes, crushed

1 can (6 ounces) tomato paste

$\frac{1}{4}$ cup unsalted vegetable broth or water

1 medium yellow onion, chopped

1 teaspoon dried Italian seasoning

1 teaspoon crushed fresh garlic

1. To make the sauce, place all of the sauce ingredients in a 1$\frac{1}{2}$-quart pot, and bring to a boil over medium-high heat. Reduce the heat to low, cover, and simmer for 20 minutes.

2. To make the filling, place all of the filling ingredients in a medium-sized bowl, and stir to mix well. Set aside.

3. Cook the noodles al dente according to package directions. Drain, rinse with cool water, and drain again.

4. Coat a 2$\frac{1}{2}$-quart casserole dish with nonstick cooking spray. To assemble the roll-ups, arrange the noodles on a flat surface, and spread an eighth of the filling mixture along the length of each noodle. Roll each noodle up jelly-roll style, and place in the prepared dish, seam side down. Pour the sauce over the roll-ups.

5. Cover the dish with aluminum foil, and bake at 350°F for 30 minutes. Remove the foil, top with the mozzarella, and bake uncovered for 10 additional minutes, or until the cheese is melted. Serve hot.

NUTRITIONAL FACTS (PER SERVING)
Cal: 384   Carbs: 57 g   Chol: 22 mg   Fat: 1.4 g
Fiber: 6 g   Protein: 35 g   Sodium: 437 mg

TIME-SAVING TIP
In a hurry? Instead of preparing homemade sauce for your Lasagna Roll-Ups, use 3 cups of bottled marinara sauce.

Manicotti Florentine

YIELD: 7 SERVINGS

14 manicotti tubes (about 8 ounces)

1 recipe Chunky Garden Marinara Sauce (page 235), or 3$\frac{1}{2}$ cups bottled marinara sauce

1 cup shredded nonfat or reduced-fat mozzarella cheese

FILLING

3$\frac{1}{2}$ cups nonfat or low-fat ricotta cheese

1 package (10 ounces) frozen chopped spinach, thawed and squeezed dry

$\frac{1}{4}$ cup fat-free egg substitute

$\frac{1}{2}$ cup grated nonfat or regular Parmesan cheese

1. Cook the manicotti al dente according to package directions. Drain well, and set aside.

2. To make the filling, place all of the filling ingredients in a large bowl, and stir to mix well.

3. Coat a 9-x-13-inch baking pan with nonstick cooking spray, and spoon a thin layer of sauce over the bottom of the pan. Using a small spoon, stuff about $\frac{1}{3}$ cup of the filling mixture into each of the tubes, and arrange the filled tubes in the pan. Pour the remaining sauce evenly over the manicotti.

4. Bake uncovered at 350°F for about 30 minutes, or until heated through. Sprinkle the mozzarella over the top, and bake for 5 additional minutes, or just until the cheese is melted.

5. Remove the dish from the oven, and let sit for 10 minutes before serving.

NUTRITIONAL FACTS (PER SERVING)
Cal: 327   Carbs: 47 g   Chol: 10 mg   Fat: 0.7 g
Fiber: 4.4 g   Protein: 33.5 g   Sodium: 547 mg

Florentine Stuffed Shells

YIELD: 8 SERVINGS

24 jumbo pasta shells

1 cup shredded nonfat or reduced-fat mozzarella cheese

FILLING

15 ounces nonfat or low-fat ricotta cheese

$1/2$ cup shredded nonfat or reduced-fat mozzarella cheese

$1/4$ cup grated nonfat or regular Parmesan cheese

1 package (10 ounces) frozen chopped spinach or broccoli, thawed and squeezed dry

$1/4$ cup finely chopped onion

$1/2$ teaspoon dried Italian seasoning

SAUCE

1 can ($14 1/2$ ounces) unsalted tomatoes, crushed

1 can (6 ounces) tomato paste

$1/2$ cup finely chopped onion

1 teaspoon crushed fresh garlic

$1/4$ cup dry red wine, beef broth, or vegetable broth

2 tablespoons grated nonfat or regular Parmesan cheese

2 teaspoons dried Italian seasoning

$1/4$ teaspoon ground black pepper

1. To make the sauce, place all of the sauce ingredients in a $1 1/2$-quart pot, and bring to a boil over medium-high heat. Reduce the heat to low, cover, and simmer for 20 minutes.

2. To make the filling, place all of the filling ingredients in a medium-sized bowl, and stir to mix well. Set aside.

3. Cook the pasta al dente according to package directions. Drain, rinse with cool water, and drain again. Set aside.

4. To assemble the dish, coat a 9-x-13-inch baking pan with nonstick cooking spray. Spoon 1 rounded tablespoon of the filling into each shell, and arrange the stuffed shells in a single layer in the prepared pan. Pour the sauce over the shells.

5. Bake uncovered at 350°F for 25 to 30 minutes, or until heated through. Top with the cup of mozzarella, and bake for 5 additional minutes, or until the cheese is melted. Serve hot.

NUTRITIONAL FACTS (PER SERVING)
Cal: 279   Carbs: 44 g   Chol: 10 mg   Fat: 1.1 g
Fiber: 3.6 g   Protein: 22 g   Sodium: 482 mg

TIME-SAVING TIP
To speed preparation, make Florentine Stuffed Shells with 3 cups of bottled marinara sauce instead of the homemade sauce.

Rigatoni Cannellini

YIELD: 6 SERVINGS

12 ounces rigatoni pasta (about $4 7/8$ cups)

1 pound fresh plum tomatoes (about 8 medium), cut into $3/4$-inch pieces

1 can (15 ounces) cannellini or navy beans, rinsed and drained

$1/2$ cup sliced scallions

$1/4$ cup plus 2 tablespoons sliced black olives

2 teaspoons crushed fresh garlic

$1/2$ teaspoon crushed red pepper

$1/4$ cup grated nonfat or regular Parmesan cheese

$1/4$ cup finely chopped fresh basil

1 cup diced nonfat or reduced-fat mozzarella cheese

1. Cook the pasta al dente according to package directions. Drain well, return to the pot, and cover to keep warm.

2. While the pasta is cooking, place the tomatoes, beans, scallions, olives, garlic, and pepper in a large deep skillet. Place the skillet over medium heat, cover, and cook for about 5 minutes, or until the mixture is heated through and the tomatoes are just beginning to soften.

3. Add the pasta to the skillet mixture, and toss to mix well.

4. Remove the skillet from the heat, add the Parmesan and basil, and toss to mix. Add the diced mozzarella, toss to mix, and serve hot.

NUTRITIONAL FACTS (PER $1 3/4$-CUP SERVING)
Cal: 357   Carbs: 63 g   Chol: 4 mg   Fat: 2.4 g
Fiber: 6.1 g   Protein: 20 g   Sodium: 538 mg

Three-Cheese Manicotti

YIELD: 7 SERVINGS

14 manicotti tubes (about 8 ounces)

1 recipe Chunky Garden Marinara Sauce (page 235),
1 recipe Arrabbiata Sauce (page 233),
or 3½ cups Savory Meat Sauce (page 235)

1 cup shredded nonfat or reduced-fat
mozzarella cheese

CHEESE FILLING

3 cups nonfat or low-fat ricotta cheese

1½ cups shredded nonfat or reduced-fat
mozzarella cheese

¼ cup fat-free egg substitute

⅓ cup grated nonfat or regular Parmesan cheese

3 tablespoons finely chopped fresh parsley

1. Cook the manicotti al dente according to package directions. Drain well, and set aside.

2. To make the filling, place all of the filling ingredients in a large bowl, and stir to mix well.

3. Coat a 9-x-13-inch baking pan with nonstick cooking spray, and spoon a thin layer of sauce over the bottom of the pan. Using a small spoon, stuff about ⅓ cup of the filling mixture into each of the tubes, and arrange the filled tubes in the pan. Pour the remaining sauce evenly over the manicotti.

4. Bake uncovered at 350°F for about 30 minutes, or until heated through. Sprinkle the cup of mozzarella over the top, and bake for 5 additional minutes, or just until the cheese is melted. Remove the dish from the oven, and let sit for 10 minutes before serving.

NUTRITIONAL FACTS (PER SERVING)
Cal: 343　　Carbs: 46 g　　Chol: 12 mg　　Fat: 0.7 g
Fiber: 4.4 g　　Protein: 38 g　　Sodium: 539 mg

Chinese Chicken and Noodles

YIELD: 4 SERVINGS

8 ounces linguine or fettuccine pasta

12 ounces boneless skinless chicken breasts

2 teaspoons peanut or vegetable oil (optional)

1½ teaspoons crushed fresh garlic

1½ teaspoons freshly grated ginger root,
or ½ teaspoon ground ginger

1 small red bell pepper, cut into thin strips

1 cup sliced fresh mushrooms

2 cups (packed) chopped bok choy
or napa cabbage

SAUCE

½ cup chicken broth

2 teaspoons cornstarch

¼ cup seasoned rice wine vinegar

2 tablespoons reduced-sodium soy sauce

2 teaspoons dark brown sugar

1½ teaspoons sesame oil

¼–½ teaspoon crushed red pepper

1. Cook the pasta al dente according to package directions. Drain well, return to the pot, and cover to keep warm.

2. While the pasta is cooking, place 1 tablespoon of the chicken broth and all of the cornstarch in a small dish, and stir to dissolve the cornstarch. Add the remaining broth and sauce ingredients, and stir to mix well. Set aside.

3. Rinse the chicken with cool water, and pat it dry with paper towels. Cut the chicken into bite-sized pieces.

4. Coat a large nonstick skillet with nonstick cooking spray or with the oil, and preheat over medium-high heat. Add the garlic, ginger, and chicken, and stir-fry for about 4 minutes, or until the chicken is nicely browned and no longer pink inside.

5. Add the red pepper and mushrooms to the skillet mixture, and stir-fry for 1 to 2 minutes, or until the vegetables are almost crisp-tender. Periodically place a lid over the skillet if it begins to dry out. (The steam released from the cooking vegetables will moisten the skillet.) Add a few teaspoons of water or broth if needed.

6. Add the bok choy or cabbage to the skillet, and stir-fry for another minute, or until the bok choy starts to wilt and the vegetables are crisp-tender. Again, add a little water or broth if the skillet becomes too dry.

7. Reduce the heat under the skillet to medium, and add the pasta. Stir the sauce, and pour it over the skillet mixture. Gently toss the mixture for a minute or 2, or until the sauce thickens. Serve hot.

NUTRITIONAL FACTS (PER 1⅔-CUP SERVING)
Cal: 357   Carbs: 52 g   Chol: 49 mg   Fat: 3.8 g
Fiber: 2.3 g   Protein: 29 g   Sodium: 503 mg

Tofu Lo Mein

YIELD: 5 SERVINGS

1 pound reduced-fat firm or extra-firm tofu, frozen, thawed, and squeezed dry (page 313)
Nonstick cooking spray
10 ounces linguine pasta
1½ teaspoons crushed fresh garlic
2 cups small fresh broccoli florets
1 cup sliced fresh mushrooms
1 medium red bell pepper, cut into thin strips
½ cup sliced scallions

SAUCE

1 cup vegetable or chicken broth
¼ cup reduced-sodium soy sauce
¼ cup dry sherry
2 tablespoons dark brown sugar
2–3 teaspoons sesame oil
1 teaspoon ground ginger
2 teaspoons cornstarch

1. To make the sauce, place all of the sauce ingredients except for the cornstarch in a small bowl, and stir to mix well. Cut the tofu into ½-inch cubes and place the cubes in a shallow nonmetal container. Pour ¼ cup of the sauce mixture over the tofu, toss to mix, and set aside for 10 minutes. Add the cornstarch to the remaining sauce, stir to dissolve the cornstarch, and set aside.

2. Coat a large nonstick baking sheet with nonstick cooking spray. Drain off any sauce that the tofu has not soaked up, and spread the tofu cubes in a single layer on the sheet. Spray the tops of the cubes lightly with the cooking spray, and bake at 375ºF for 10 minutes. Turn the cubes with a spatula, and bake for 10 additional minutes, or until the cubes are nicely browned, crisp on the outside, and chewy on the inside. Remove the tofu cubes from the oven, and set aside.

3. While the tofu is cooking, cook the pasta al dente according to package directions. Drain well, return to the pot, and cover to keep warm.

4. Coat a large nonstick skillet with nonstick cooking spray. Place the skillet over medium-high heat, and add the garlic, broccoli, mushrooms, red pepper, and scallions. Stir-fry the vegetables for about 4 minutes, or until crisp-tender, covering the skillet periodically if it begins to dry out (the steam from the cooking vegetables will moisten the skillet). Add a few teaspoons of water or broth to the skillet only if necessary. Add the tofu, and toss to mix well. Add the pasta, and toss to mix well.

5. Stir the reserved sauce, and add it to the skillet. Toss the mixture for a minute or 2, or until the sauce thickens slightly. Serve hot.

NUTRITIONAL FACTS (PER 2-CUP SERVING)
Cal: 356   Carbs: 55 g   Chol: 0 mg   Fat: 5.9 g
Fiber: 3.2 g   Protein: 18 g   Sodium: 546 mg

Tempting Turkey Tetrazzini

YIELD: 6 SERVINGS

| 8 ounces spaghetti |
| 2¼ cups chicken broth, divided |
| ¼ cup unbleached flour |
| 2 tablespoons dry sherry or white wine |
| 1½ cups sliced fresh mushrooms |
| 1 can (12 ounces) evaporated skim milk |
| ½ teaspoon dried thyme |
| ⅛ teaspoon ground nutmeg |
| ⅛ teaspoon ground white pepper |
| 2 cups diced cooked turkey or chicken breast |
| ¼ cup grated Parmesan cheese* |

* In this recipe, use regular Parmesan cheese, not a fat-free product.

1. Cook the pasta al dente according to package directions. Drain well, return to the pot, and cover to keep warm.

2. While the pasta is cooking, place ½ cup of the broth and all of the flour in a jar with a tight-fitting lid, and shake until smooth. Set aside.

3. Coat a large deep skillet with nonstick cooking spray, and preheat over medium-high heat. Add the sherry or wine and the mushrooms, and sauté for several minutes, or until the mushrooms begin to soften and release their juices.

4. Add the remaining 1¾ cups of broth and the evaporated milk, thyme, nutmeg, and pepper to the skillet. Reduce the heat to medium, and cook, stirring frequently, until the mixture begins to boil. Add the flour mixture, and cook, stirring constantly, for about 2 minutes, or until the mixture is bubbly and slightly thickened.

5. Remove the skillet from the heat. Add the pasta and the turkey or chicken, and toss to mix well.

6. Coat an 8-x-12-inch baking pan with nonstick cooking spray. Spread the pasta mixture evenly in the dish, and sprinkle with the Parmesan.

7. Bake uncovered at 350°F for 35 minutes, or until the pasta mixture is hot and bubbly. Remove the dish from the oven, and let sit for 5 to 10 minutes before serving.

NUTRITIONAL FACTS (PER 1½-CUP SERVING)
Cal: 297   Carbs: 40 g   Chol: 45 mg   Fat: 2.6 g
Fiber: 1.3 g   Protein: 26 g   Sodium: 399 mg

Seafood Lasagna Roll-Ups

YIELD: 4 SERVINGS

| 8 lasagna noodles (about 6½ ounces) |
| 2 cups Almost Alfredo Sauce (page 234) |
| ½ cup shredded nonfat or reduced-fat mozzarella cheese |

FILLING

| 15 ounces nonfat or low-fat ricotta cheese |
| ¼ cup grated nonfat or regular Parmesan cheese |
| 3 tablespoons fat-free egg substitute |
| 2 tablespoons finely chopped fresh parsley |
| 1 cup cooked crab meat or diced cooked shrimp (or ½ cup each) |

1. To make the filling, place the ricotta, Parmesan, egg substitute, and parsley in a medium-sized bowl, and stir to mix well. Add the crab meat or shrimp, and stir to mix. Set aside.

2. Cook the noodles al dente according to package directions. Drain, rinse with cool water, and drain again.

3. Coat a 2½-quart casserole dish with nonstick cooking spray. To assemble the roll-ups, arrange the noodles on a flat surface, and spread an eighth of the filling mixture along the length of each noodle. Roll each noodle up jelly-roll style, and place in the prepared dish, seam side down. Pour the sauce over the roll-ups.

4. Cover the dish with aluminum foil, and bake at 350°F for 30 minutes. Remove the foil, top with the mozzarella, and bake uncovered for 10 additional minutes, or until the cheese is melted. Serve hot.

NUTRITIONAL FACTS (PER SERVING)
Cal: 430   Carbs: 56 g   Chol: 45 mg   Fat: 1.4 g
Fiber: 1.1 g   Protein: 46 g   Sodium: 569 mg

Linguine With Roasted Vegetables

YIELD: 4 SERVINGS

1 cup fresh halved mushrooms

1 cup ¾-inch cubes eggplant

1 medium zucchini, halved lengthwise and sliced ½-inch thick

1 medium yellow onion, cut into thin wedges

¼ teaspoon salt

1 tablespoon balsamic vinegar

Nonstick olive oil cooking spray

8 ounces linguine pasta

1 tablespoon extra virgin olive oil (optional)

2 teaspoons crushed fresh garlic

1 pound fresh plum tomatoes (6–7 medium), chopped

¼ cup chicken or vegetable broth

1½ teaspoons dried oregano, or 1½ tablespoons fresh

¼–½ teaspoon crushed red pepper

¼ cup plus 2 tablespoons nonfat or regular Parmesan cheese or crumbled nonfat or reduced-fat feta cheese

1. Place the mushrooms, eggplant, zucchini, and onion in a large bowl. Sprinkle with the salt and vinegar, and toss to mix well.

2. Coat a large baking sheet with nonstick olive oil cooking spray, and arrange the vegetables on the sheet in a single layer. Spray the vegetables lightly with the cooking spray, and bake uncovered at 475°F for 10 minutes. Turn the vegetables, and bake for 10 additional minutes, or until nicely browned. Remove the vegetables from the oven, and set aside.

3. Cook the pasta al dente according to package directions. Drain well, return to the pot, and toss with the olive oil if desired. Cover to keep warm.

4. Coat a large nonstick skillet with the cooking spray, and preheat over medium-high heat. Add the garlic, and stir-fry for about 30 seconds, or just until the garlic begins to turn color.

5. Reduce the heat to medium, and add the tomatoes, broth, oregano, and red pepper to the skillet.

Cover and cook for about 8 minutes, or until the tomatoes soften and begin to break down.

6. Add the roasted vegetables and pasta to the skillet, and toss to mix well. Add a little more broth if the sauce seems too dry. Serve hot, topping each serving with a rounded tablespoon of the Parmesan or feta cheese.

> **NUTRITIONAL FACTS (PER 1½-CUP SERVING)**
> Cal: 297   Carbs: 55 g   Chol: 5 mg   Fat: 1.9 g
> Fiber: 4 g   Protein: 16 g   Sodium: 339 mg

Light and Lazy Lasagna

This lasagna is "lazy" because you don't cook the noodles before layering them in the pan. You can also prepare this entrée to the point of baking several hours—or even a day—in advance, and then refrigerate it until it's time to pop the dish into the oven.

YIELD: 10 SERVINGS

12 lasagna noodles (about 9 ounces)

2 cups shredded nonfat or reduced-fat mozzarella cheese

¼ cup grated nonfat or regular Parmesan cheese

FILLING

15 ounces nonfat or low-fat ricotta cheese

1 cup nonfat or low-fat cottage cheese

¼ cup grated nonfat or regular Parmesan cheese

2 tablespoons finely chopped fresh parsley, or 2 teaspoons dried

SAUCE

1 pound 95% lean ground beef or Turkey Italian Sausage (page 251)

2 cans (8 ounces each) unsalted tomato sauce

1 can (28 ounces) crushed tomatoes

2 tablespoons tomato paste

2 cups sliced fresh mushrooms

1 medium onion, chopped

1½ teaspoons crushed fresh garlic

2½ teaspoons dried Italian seasoning

1. To make the sauce, coat a 4-quart pot with non-stick cooking spray, and preheat over medium heat. Add the beef or sausage, and cook, stirring to crumble, until the meat is no longer pink. Drain off and discard any excess fat.

2. Add all of the remaining sauce ingredients to the browned meat, increase the heat to high, and bring to a boil. Reduce the heat to low, cover, and simmer for 25 minutes, or until the vegetables are tender. Set aside.

3. To make the filling, place all of the filling ingredients in a large bowl, and stir to mix well. Set aside.

4. To assemble the lasagna, coat a 9-x-13-inch baking pan with nonstick cooking spray. Spoon 1 cup of the sauce over the bottom of the pan. Lay 4 of the uncooked noodles over the bottom of the pan, arranging 3 of the noodles lengthwise and 1 noodle crosswise. Allow a little space between the noodles

for expansion. (You will have to break 1 inch off the crosswise noodle to make it fit in the pan.)

5. Top the noodles with half of the filling mixture, $3/4$ cup of the mozzarella, and $13/4$ cups of the sauce. Repeat the noodles, filling, mozzarella, and sauce layers. Finally, top with the remaining noodles, sauce, Parmesan, and mozzarella.

6. Spray a large sheet of aluminum foil with non-stick cooking spray, and cover the pan with the foil, placing the sprayed side down. Bake at 350°F for 45 minutes. Remove the foil, and bake uncovered for 15 additional minutes, or until the edges are bubbly and the top is browned. Remove the dish from the oven, and let sit for 15 minutes before cutting and serving.

NUTRITIONAL FACTS (PER SERVING)		
Cal: 307 Carbs: 36 g Chol: 34 mg Fat: 2.9 g		
Fiber: 3 g Protein: 33 g Sodium: 510 mg		

10. *Hearty Home-Style Entrées*

Many people believe that adopting a healthy diet means waving good-bye to the hearty home-style dishes they love so much. But the truth is that you don't have to give up crispy fried chicken, savory meat loaf, saucy skillet dinners, or any of your other favorites just because you've opted for a healthier way of eating. Nor do you have to spend hours in specialty stores searching for exotic ingredients, or added time in the kitchen learning complicated cooking methods. By replacing high-fat ingredients with lighter foods, and by using a few simple cooking techniques, you can still enjoy all of your favorite foods—and many new ones, too. This chapter will show you how.

The entrées in this chapter begin with the freshest seafood or the leanest cuts of poultry, beef, or pork. Then fat and calories are kept to a minimum by using nonstick skillets and nonstick cooking sprays, and by replacing full-fat dairy products with their healthful lower-fat counterparts. Of course, fresh vegetables, hearty grains, and savory seasonings play an important role in these dishes by adding their own great flavors and textures, and by boosting nutrition, too. The result? Satisfying home-style entrées that will fill you up, but not out!

As you glance through the pages of this chapter, remember that these are just *some* of the light and healthy main dishes that are within your reach. Delicious pasta entrées are presented in Chapter 9, crowd-pleasing meatless main dishes can be found in Chapter 11, and a variety of main dish salads can be found in Chapter 7. And, of course, many of your own family favorites can be easily "slimmed down" and given a nutritional boost with the techniques and ingredients used within this chapter.

The following pages present a wide range of hearty home-style entrées guaranteed to provide a delicious answer to that age-old question, "What's for dinner?" And every dish—from Chicken Breasts With Sourdough Stuffing, to Skillet Stroganoff, to Pot Roast With Sour Cream Gravy, to Jiffy Jambalaya—will prove to family and friends that healthy food can be great food, as well.

Chicken Breasts With Sourdough Stuffing

YIELD: 4 SERVINGS

4 bone-in skinless chicken breast halves
(about 6 ounces each)

1/4 teaspoon salt

1/4 teaspoon ground black pepper

Nonstick butter-flavored cooking spray

STUFFING

5 slices sourdough bread

1 cup coarsely chopped fresh mushrooms

1/4 cup finely chopped onion

1/4 cup finely chopped celery
(include the leaves)

1/2 teaspoon poultry seasoning

1/2 cup chicken broth

1. Rinse the chicken with cool water, and pat it dry with paper towels. Lightly sprinkle both sides with the salt and pepper, and set aside.

2. Place 2 1/2 of the bread slices in a blender or food processor, and process into coarse crumbs. There should be 2 cups. Cut the remaining bread slices into 1/2-inch cubes. There should be 2 1/4 cups. Set the bread crumbs and cubes aside.

3. Coat a large nonstick skillet with nonstick cooking spray, and preheat over medium-high heat. Add the mushrooms, onion, and celery, and cook, stirring frequently, until the vegetables start to soften. Add a little broth if the skillet becomes too dry.

4. Remove the skillet from the heat, and stir in the poultry seasoning. Then toss in the bread crumbs and cubes. Tossing gently, slowly add just enough broth to make a moist, but not wet, stuffing that holds together. Set aside.

5. Coat a 9-x-13-inch baking pan with nonstick cooking spray, and lay the chicken in the pan with the bone side up. Mound a quarter of the stuffing into the depression of the breast bone of each piece of chicken. Spray the stuffing lightly with the cooking spray.

6. Cover the pan with aluminum foil, and bake at 350°F for 40 minutes. Remove the foil, and bake uncovered for 20 additional minutes, or until the chicken is tender and no longer pink inside, and the stuffing is lightly browned. Serve hot.

NUTRITIONAL FACTS (PER SERVING)

Cal: 256   Carbs: 18 g   Chol: 82 mg   Fat: 3.4 g
Fiber: 1.5 g   Protein: 36 g   Sodium: 515 mg

Making Savory Fat-Free Stuffings

Savory stuffings add a down-home touch that makes any meal special. However, these flavorful mixtures of bread, seasonings, and vegetables are typically moistened with a liberal amount of butter or margarine, which can raise both fat and calorie counts to unhealthful levels. The good news is that you can make moist and delicious stuffings with absolutely no fat. Simply substitute half as much broth or a liquid butter substitute such as Butter Buds for the butter or margarine called for in the recipe. For instance, if the recipe calls for one stick (1/2 cup) of butter, use 1/4 cup of broth instead. Slowly pour the broth over the stuffing, tossing gently to mix until all of the liquid has been incorporated. Then add a little more broth if the stuffing seems too dry. It should be moist, but not wet, and should hold together nicely.

Eggs are frequently added to stuffings to bind the mixture together. You can save more fat and cholesterol by replacing any eggs in the recipe with an equal amount of egg whites or fat-free egg substitute. And while you're modifying your stuffing recipe, boost its fiber and nutrition by substituting whole grain bread for refined white bread. With these modifications, you will turn a high-fat, nutrient-poor food into a healthful and delicious dish.

Crusty Chicken Pot Pie

YIELD: 5 SERVINGS

FILLING

1 can (10¾ ounces) low-fat condensed cream of celery soup, undiluted

¾ cup skim or low-fat milk

2 cups cooked diced chicken or turkey breast (about 10 ounces), or 3 cans (5 ounces each) chunk white chicken or turkey breast in water, drained

1 package (10 ounces) frozen (thawed) mixed vegetables, drained

CRUST

1 cup unbleached flour

¼ cup oat bran or quick-cooking oats

1½ teaspoons baking powder

3 tablespoons reduced-fat margarine or light butter, cut into pieces

⅓ cup nonfat or low-fat buttermilk

1. To make the filling, place the soup and milk in a 2-quart pot, and stir to mix well. Place the pot over medium heat and cook, stirring frequently, until the mixture comes to a boil. Add the chicken or turkey and the vegetables, and heat until the mixture is warmed through.

2. Coat a 9-inch deep dish pie pan with cooking spray, and spread the warm chicken mixture evenly in the pan. Set aside.

3. To make the crust, place the flour, oat bran or oats, and baking powder in a medium-sized bowl, and stir to mix well. Using a pastry cutter or 2 knives, cut in the margarine or butter until the mixture resembles coarse meal. Add enough of the buttermilk to form a stiff dough that leaves the sides of the bowl and forms a ball. Turn the dough onto a floured surface, and pat it into a 5-inch circle. Then, using a rolling pin, roll the dough into a 10-inch circle.

4. Using a sharp knife or a pizza wheel, cut the dough into ¾-inch-wide strips. Lay half of the crust strips over the filling, spacing them ½ inch apart. Lay the remaining strips over the filling in the oppo-

site direction to form a lattice top. Trim the edges to make the dough conform to the shape of the pan.

5. Bake uncovered at 375°F for 25 to 30 minutes, or until the filling is bubbly and the crust is lightly browned. Remove the dish from the oven, and let sit for 5 minutes before serving.

NUTRITIONAL FACTS (PER SERVING)			
Cal: 296	Carbs: 34 g	Chol: 46 mg	Fat: 6.4 g
Fiber: 3.6 g	Protein: 25 g	Sodium: 516 mg	

Tex-Mex Chicken and Rice

YIELD: 5 SERVINGS

1 pound boneless skinless chicken breasts

¼ teaspoon salt

1 teaspoon crushed fresh garlic

2 cups quick-cooking brown rice

1 can (1 pound) red kidney beans, drained

1¾ cups unsalted chicken broth

½ cup bottled salsa

⅓ cup finely chopped green bell pepper

⅓ cup finely chopped onion

1 tablespoon chili powder

1. Rinse the chicken with cool water, and pat it dry with paper towels. Cut the chicken into bite-sized pieces, and sprinkle with the salt.

2. Coat a large nonstick skillet with nonstick cooking spray, and preheat over medium-high heat. Add the chicken and garlic, and stir-fry for about 5 minutes, or until the chicken is browned and no longer pink inside.

3. Add all of the remaining ingredients to the skillet. Stir to mix well, and bring to a boil. Reduce the heat to low, cover, and simmer for about 8 minutes, or until the rice is tender and the liquid is absorbed.

4. Remove the skillet from the heat, cover, and let stand for 5 minutes. Serve hot.

NUTRITIONAL FACTS (PER 1½-CUP SERVING)			
Cal: 359	Carbs: 51 g	Chol: 53 mg	Fat: 2.8 g
Fiber: 8 g	Protein: 32 g	Sodium: 371 mg	

Chicken Dijon

YIELD: 4 SERVINGS

1/3 cup chicken broth, divided

1 1/2 teaspoons cornstarch

4 boneless skinless chicken breast halves
(about 4 ounces each)

1 1/2 teaspoons crushed fresh garlic,
or 3/8 teaspoon garlic powder

1/4 teaspoon ground black pepper

2 cups sliced fresh mushrooms

2 tablespoons Dijon mustard

1 teaspoon sugar

3/4 cup nonfat or light sour cream

1. Place 1 tablespoon of the broth and all of the cornstarch in a small bowl, and stir to dissolve the cornstarch. Set aside.

2. Rinse the chicken with cool water, and pat it dry with paper towels. Spread the garlic over the chicken, and sprinkle with the pepper.

3. Coat a large nonstick skillet with nonstick cooking spray, and preheat over medium-high heat. Place the chicken in the skillet, and cook for 2 minutes on each side, or until nicely browned.

4. Reduce the heat to low, and pour the remaining broth into the bottom of the skillet. Arrange the mushrooms around the chicken, cover, and cook for 15 minutes, or until the chicken is tender and no longer pink inside.

5. Transfer the chicken to a warm serving platter. Remove the mushrooms from the skillet with a slotted spoon, and place on top of the chicken. Cover the platter to keep it warm.

6. Stir the cornstarch mixture, and add it to the skillet. Cook over medium heat, whisking constantly, until the mixture comes to a boil and thickens slightly.

7. Add the mustard and sugar to the liquid in the skillet, and whisk over low heat to mix well. Add the sour cream, and whisk until the sauce is smooth and heated through. Spoon the sauce over the chicken and mushrooms, and serve hot with wild rice, brown rice, or noodles, if desired.

NUTRITIONAL FACTS (PER SERVING)
Cal: 197   Carbs: 12 g   Chol: 67 mg   Fat: 2.2 g
Fiber: 0.6 g   Protein: 30 g   Sodium: 350 mg

Crispy Cajun Chicken

Finely crushed corn flakes give this ultra-lean oven-fried chicken its crispy coating.

YIELD: 8 SERVINGS

8 bone-in skinless chicken breast halves
(about 6 ounces each), or 3 pounds bone-in
skinless chicken breast halves, legs, and thighs

1 1/4 cups nonfat or low-fat buttermilk or yogurt

Nonstick cooking spray

COATING

5 cups corn flakes

1 tablespoon ground paprika

2–3 teaspoons Cajun seasoning

1. Rinse the chicken with cool water, and pat it dry with paper towels. Place the chicken in a shallow nonmetal dish, and pour the buttermilk or yogurt over the chicken. Turn the pieces to coat, cover, and refrigerate for 6 to 24 hours.

2. To make the coating, place the corn flakes in a blender or food processor, and process into crumbs. You should have about 1 1/4 cups of crumbs. Adjust the amount if necessary.

3. Place the corn flake crumbs and all of the remaining coating ingredients in a gallon-sized plastic bag. Close the bag, and shake well to mix.

4. Remove 2 pieces of chicken from the buttermilk, place in the coating bag, and shake to coat evenly. Repeat with the remaining chicken.

5. Coat a large baking sheet with nonstick cooking spray, and arrange the chicken on the pan. Lightly spray each piece of chicken with cooking spray, and bake uncovered at 400°F for 50 minutes, or until the meat is tender and the chicken is no longer pink inside. Serve hot.

NUTRITIONAL FACTS (PER SERVING)
Cal: 207   Carbs: 16 g   Chol: 72 mg   Fat: 3.2 g
Fiber: 0.4 g   Protein: 28 g   Sodium: 285 mg

Southern-Style Smothered Chicken

YIELD: 4 SERVINGS

4 boneless skinless chicken breast halves
(about 4 ounces each)

1/2 cup plus 2 tablespoons unbleached flour

1/2 teaspoon poultry seasoning

1/4 teaspoon salt

1/4 teaspoon ground black pepper

1/4 cup evaporated skim milk

1/4 cup fat-free egg substitute

Nonstick cooking spray

1 cup chicken broth

1. Rinse the chicken with cool water, and pat it dry with paper towels. Place the chicken on a flat surface, and use a meat mallet to pound each half to 1/4-inch thickness.

2. Place the flour, poultry seasoning, salt, and pepper in a shallow dish, and stir to mix well. Remove 2 tablespoons of the mixture, and place it and the evaporated milk in a small jar with a tight-fitting lid. Shake to mix well, and set aside.

3. Place the egg substitute in a shallow dish. Dip the chicken pieces first in the egg substitute and then in the flour mixture, turning to coat both sides.

4. Coat a large nonstick skillet with nonstick cooking spray, and preheat over medium-high heat. Place the chicken in the skillet, and cook for 2 to 3 minutes, or until nicely browned. Spray the tops of the chicken breasts lightly with the cooking spray, turn, and cook for 2 to 3 additional minutes, or until nicely browned on both sides.

5. Pour the broth around the chicken. Reduce the heat to low, and stir the evaporated milk mixture into the broth. Cover the skillet and simmer for about 10 minutes, scraping the bottom of the pan occasionally, until the chicken is tender and the gravy is thick. Serve hot with potatoes or brown rice, if desired.

NUTRITIONAL FACTS (PER SERVING)
Cal: 180   Carbs: 12 g   Chol: 67 mg   Fat: 1.9 g
Fiber: 0.3 g   Protein: 29 g   Sodium: 345 mg

Italian Baked Chicken

YIELD: 4 SERVINGS

4 boneless skinless chicken breast halves
(about 5 ounces each)

3/4 teaspoon dried Italian seasoning

1/2 teaspoon garlic powder, or 2 teaspoons
crushed fresh garlic

1/4 teaspoon coarsely ground black pepper

1/4 teaspoon salt

1 can (14 1/2 ounces) Italian-style stewed
tomatoes, undrained

2 tablespoons tomato paste

1 medium zucchini, halved lengthwise and
sliced 3/4-inch thick

2 cups halved fresh mushrooms

1 medium yellow onion, cut into 1/2-inch-thick wedges

1. Rinse the chicken with cool water, and pat it dry with paper towels. Place the Italian seasoning, garlic powder or garlic, pepper, and salt in a small bowl, and stir to mix well. Rub both sides of the chicken with the spice mixture.

2. Coat a large oven-proof nonstick skillet with non-stick olive oil cooking spray, and preheat over medium-high heat. Add the chicken to the skillet, and cook for 2 to 3 minutes on each side, or until nicely browned. Remove the skillet from the heat, and set aside.

3. Place the tomatoes and tomato paste in a large bowl, and stir to mix well. Add the zucchini, mushrooms, and onion, and stir to mix well. Spread the vegetable mixture over and around the chicken in the skillet.

4. Cover the skillet with aluminum foil, and bake at 350°F for about 35 minutes, or until the vegetables are tender and the chicken is no longer pink inside. Serve hot with brown rice or pasta, if desired.

NUTRITIONAL FACTS (PER SERVING)
Cal: 220   Carbs: 13 g   Chol: 82 mg   Fat: 2 g
Fiber: 3.4 g   Protein: 35 g   Sodium: 484 mg

Baked Chicken With Garlic and Sun-Dried Tomatoes

As the garlic cloves cook, they become sweet and mild. For a real treat, spread the cloves on hot French bread instead of using butter.

YIELD: 4 SERVINGS

4 boneless skinless chicken breast halves (about 4 ounces each)

20 cloves garlic, peeled (about 2 heads)

1/4 teaspoon salt

1 tablespoon extra virgin olive oil (optional)

1 medium onion, sliced 1/4-inch thick and separated into rings

1/2 cup chopped sun-dried tomatoes (not packed in oil)

1/2 cup chicken broth

1/4 cup dry white wine

1 teaspoon dried oregano

1/4 teaspoon coarsely ground black pepper

1. Rinse the chicken with cool water, and pat it dry with paper towels. Crush 2 of the garlic cloves, and spread them over the chicken. Sprinkle the chicken with the salt, and set aside.

2. Coat a large oven-proof skillet with nonstick olive oil cooking spray or with the olive oil, and preheat over medium-high heat. Place the chicken in the skillet, and arrange the remaining garlic cloves around the chicken.

3. Cook the chicken for about 2 minutes on each side, or until the chicken and garlic cloves are nicely browned. If necessary, remove the garlic cloves from the skillet before the chicken is browned to prevent the cloves from burning. Remove the chicken from the skillet, and set aside. Remove the skillet from the heat.

4. Scatter the garlic cloves over the bottom of the skillet, and arrange the onions and dried tomatoes over the garlic cloves. Arrange the chicken in a single layer over the vegetables. Pour the broth and wine

over the chicken, and sprinkle with the oregano and pepper.

5. Cover and bake at 350°F for 30 minutes, or until the chicken is tender and no longer pink inside.

6. Serve hot, accompanying each chicken breast with some of the vegetables and pan juices. Serve over brown rice or noodles, if desired.

NUTRITIONAL FACTS (PER SERVING)
Cal: 209   Carbs: 15 g   Chol: 72 mg   Fat: 3.3 g
Fiber: 1.7 g   Protein: 30 g   Sodium: 448 mg

Chicken Rollatini

YIELD: 4 SERVINGS

4 boneless skinless chicken breast halves (about 4 ounces each)

1/4 teaspoon ground black pepper

1 teaspoon crushed fresh garlic

3 tablespoons chicken broth

STUFFING

1/4 cup finely chopped celery (include the leaves)

1/4 cup finely chopped shallots or onions

1/4 cup chopped golden raisins

1 cup soft whole wheat bread crumbs*

1/4 cup grated nonfat or regular Parmesan cheese

1/2 teaspoon poultry seasoning

1/4 cup chicken broth

SAUCE

1/2 cup dry white wine

1/4 cup plus 2 tablespoons chicken broth

1 teaspoon cornstarch

* To make soft bread crumbs, tear about 1 1/3 slices of bread into chunks, place the chunks in a food processor or blender, and process into crumbs.

1. To make the stuffing, coat a large nonstick skillet with butter-flavored cooking spray, and preheat over medium-high heat. Add the celery and the shallots or onions, and stir-fry for about 3 minutes, or until the vegetables start to soften. Add a little chicken broth to the skillet if it becomes too dry. Remove the skillet from the heat, and set aside for a few minutes to cool slightly.

2. Add the raisins, bread crumbs, Parmesan, and poultry seasoning to the skillet, and toss to mix well. Tossing gently, slowly add just enough broth to make a moist, but not wet, stuffing that holds together. Set aside.

3. Rinse the chicken with cool water, and pat it dry with paper towels. Place the chicken pieces on a flat surface, and use a meat mallet to pound each piece to $1/4$-inch thickness.

4. Spread each piece of chicken with a fourth of the stuffing, extending the stuffing to within $1/2$ inch of each edge. Starting at the short end, roll each piece of chicken up jelly roll-style, and tie in 3 places with string. Sprinkle each roll with some of the pepper.

5. Coat a large nonstick skillet with nonstick butter-flavored cooking spray, and preheat over medium-high heat. Arrange the chicken rolls in the skillet and cook for about 7 minutes, turning every few minutes, until nicely browned on all sides.

6. Add the garlic and the 3 tablespoons of broth to the skillet. Reduce the heat to low, cover, and simmer for 5 minutes. Turn the rolls over, and simmer for 5 additional minutes, or until the chicken is no longer pink inside. Add a little more broth if the skillet becomes dry. Transfer the rolls to a serving platter, and cover to keep warm.

7. To make the sauce, increase the heat under the skillet to medium, and add the wine. Cook, stirring frequently, until the wine is reduced by half.

8. Place the chicken broth in a small bowl, and stir in the cornstarch. Add the cornstarch mixture to the skillet, and cook, stirring constantly, for about 2 minutes, or until the mixture begins to boil and thickens slightly.

9. Pour the sauce over the chicken rolls, and serve hot.

NUTRITIONAL FACTS (PER SERVING)
Cal: 226   Carbs: 19 g   Chol: 69 mg   Fat: 2 g
Fiber: 2.2 g   Protein: 32 g   Sodium: 328 mg

Honey Crunch Chicken

For variety, substitute coarsely ground toasted pecans for half of the wheat germ.

YIELD: 8 SERVINGS
8 bone-in skinless chicken breast halves (about 6 ounces each), or 3 pounds bone-in skinless chicken breast halves, legs, and thighs
$1\frac{1}{2}$ cups nonfat or low-fat buttermilk
Nonstick cooking spray

COATING
4 cups corn flakes
$1/2$ cup honey crunch wheat germ
1 teaspoon poultry seasoning
$1/4$ teaspoon ground black pepper
$1/4$ teaspoon salt

1. Rinse the chicken with cool water, and pat it dry with paper towels. Place the chicken in a shallow nonmetal dish, and pour the buttermilk over the chicken. Turn the pieces to coat, cover, and refrigerate for 6 to 24 hours.

2. To make the coating, place the corn flakes in a blender or food processor, and process into crumbs. You should have about 1 cup plus 2 tablespoons of crumbs. Adjust the amount if necessary.

3. Place the corn flake crumbs and all of the remaining coating ingredients in a gallon-sized plastic bag. Close the bag, and shake well to mix.

4. Remove 2 pieces of chicken from the buttermilk, place in the coating bag, and shake to coat evenly. Repeat with the remaining chicken.

5. Coat a large baking sheet with nonstick cooking spray, and arrange the chicken on the pan. Lightly spray each piece of chicken with the cooking spray, and bake uncovered at 400°F for 50 minutes, or until the meat is tender and the chicken is no longer pink inside. Serve hot.

NUTRITIONAL FACTS (PER SERVING)
Cal: 224   Carbs: 13 g   Chol: 83 mg   Fat: 2.5 g
Fiber: 1.1 g   Protein: 36 g   Sodium: 283 mg

Down-Home Chicken and Dumplings

YIELD: 6 SERVINGS

½ cup skim or low-fat milk

¼ cup plus 2 tablespoons unbleached flour

3 cups chicken broth

1 medium carrot, peeled,
halved lengthwise, and sliced

1 stalk celery, thinly sliced (include the leaves)

½ cup chopped onion

¼ teaspoon poultry seasoning

⅛ teaspoon ground white pepper

2 cups diced cooked chicken breast
(about 10 ounces)

1 cup frozen (unthawed) green peas

DUMPLINGS

1½ cups unbleached flour

2 teaspoons baking powder

1 teaspoon sugar

¾ cup nonfat or low-fat buttermilk

1. Place the milk and flour in a jar with a tight-fitting lid, and shake until smooth. Set aside.

2. Place the broth, carrot, celery, onion, poultry seasoning, and pepper in a 4-quart pot or a large, deep nonstick skillet (at least 3-quart capacity), and bring to a boil over high heat. Reduce the heat to low, cover, and simmer for 5 minutes, or until the vegetables are almost tender.

3. Add the chicken and peas to the pot, and increase the heat to return the mixture to a boil. Reduce the heat to medium, shake the milk mixture, and slowly pour it into the pot while stirring constantly. Cook and stir for a minute or 2, or until the mixture is thickened and bubbly. Reduce the heat to low.

4. To make the dumplings, place the flour, baking powder, and sugar in a medium-sized bowl, and stir to mix well. Add the buttermilk, and stir just until moistened. Add a little more buttermilk if needed to make a thick batter.

5. Drop heaping teaspoonfuls of the batter onto the simmering stew. Cover and simmer over low heat for 10 to 12 minutes, or until the dumplings are fluffy and cooked through. Serve hot.

NUTRITIONAL FACTS (PER 1½-CUP SERVING)
Cal: 241   Carbs: 36 g   Chol: 34 mg   Fat: 1.2 g
Fiber: 2.7 g   Protein: 20 g   Sodium: 591 mg

Chicken With White Wine and Mushroom Sauce

YIELD: 4 SERVINGS

4 boneless skinless chicken breast halves
(about 4 ounces each)

¼ cup fat-free egg substitute

¼ cup plus 2 tablespoons unbleached flour

½ teaspoon salt

¼ teaspoon ground black pepper

Nonstick butter-flavored cooking spray

SAUCE

½ cup plus 2 tablespoons evaporated skim milk

1 teaspoon cornstarch

½ cup dry white wine, divided

2 teaspoons crushed fresh garlic

2 cups sliced fresh mushrooms

1. Rinse the chicken with cool water, and pat it dry with paper towels. Place the chicken pieces on a flat surface, and use a meat mallet to pound each piece to ¼-inch thickness.

2. Place the egg substitute in a shallow dish. Place the flour, salt, and pepper in another shallow dish, and stir to mix well. Dip each chicken piece first in the egg, and then in the flour mixture, turning to coat each side. Set aside.

3. Coat a large nonstick skillet with nonstick butter-flavored cooking spray, and preheat over medium-high heat. Add the chicken and cook for about 3 minutes, or until nicely browned. Spray the top of the chicken lightly with the cooking spray, turn, and cook for 3 additional minutes, or until nicely browned and no longer pink inside. Transfer the chicken to a serving platter, and cover to keep warm.

4. To make the sauce, place the evaporated milk and cornstarch in a jar with a tight-fitting lid, and shake to mix well. Set aside.

5. Place 1/4 cup of the wine in the skillet, and cook over medium-high heat, stirring frequently, until most of the wine has evaporated. Add the garlic and mushrooms, and stir-fry for about 3 minutes, or until the mushrooms begin to brown and release their juices. Add the remaining 1/4 cup of wine, and cook, stirring frequently, until the wine is reduced by half.

6. Reduce the heat under the skillet to medium, shake the evaporated milk mixture, and add it to the skillet. Cook, stirring constantly, until the mixture boils and thickens slightly. Pour the sauce over the chicken, and serve hot.

> **NUTRITIONAL FACTS (PER SERVING)**
> Cal: 220   Carbs: 14.5 g   Chol: 67 mg   Fat: 2 g
> Fiber: 0.8 g   Protein: 32 g   Sodium: 407 mg

Baked Chicken Paprika

YIELD: 4 SERVINGS

4 bone-in skinless chicken breast halves (about 8 ounces each)

1/2 teaspoon garlic powder

1/4 teaspoon salt

1/4 teaspoon ground black pepper

1 medium-large Spanish onion, sliced and separated into rings

1 tablespoon ground paprika

1/4 cup plus 2 tablespoons tomato juice

SAUCE

2 teaspoons cornstarch

2 teaspoons chicken broth

1/2 cup nonfat or light sour cream

1. Rinse the chicken with cool water, and pat it dry with paper towels. Place the garlic powder, salt, and pepper in a small bowl, and stir to mix well. Rub both sides of the chicken with the spice mixture.

2. Coat a large nonstick oven-proof skillet with nonstick cooking spray, and preheat over medium-high heat. Place the chicken in the skillet, and cook for about 2 minutes on each side, or until nicely browned. Transfer the chicken to a plate, and set aside.

3. Arrange half of the onion rings over the bottom of the skillet, and sprinkle with 1 teaspoon of the paprika. Pour the tomato juice over the onions, and arrange the chicken over the onions. Sprinkle 1 teaspoon of the remaining paprika over the chicken, top with the remaining onion rings, and sprinkle with the remaining paprika.

4. Cover the skillet tightly with aluminum foil, and bake at 350°F for 40 minutes. Remove the foil, and bake uncovered for 20 additional minutes, or until the chicken is tender and no longer pink inside. Transfer the chicken and onions to a serving platter, and cover to keep warm.

5. Measure the pan juices; there should be 1 cup. Adjust the amount if necessary by adding chicken broth, and return the juices to the skillet.

6. Place the cornstarch and chicken broth in a small bowl, and stir to mix well. Add the mixture to the skillet. Stir the sour cream, and add it to the skillet mixture, whisking until smooth.

7. Place the skillet over medium heat, and cook, stirring constantly, for about 2 minutes, or until the mixture is thickened and bubbly. Transfer the sauce to a warmed gravy boat or pitcher, and serve hot with the chicken. Serve with noodles or brown rice, if desired.

> **NUTRITIONAL FACTS (PER SERVING)**
> Cal: 216   Carbs: 12 g   Chol: 82 mg   Fat: 2.1 g
> Fiber: 1.4 g   Protein: 35 g   Sodium: 316 mg

Chicken and Mushroom Risotto

YIELD: 4 SERVINGS

8 ounces boneless skinless chicken breasts

1/8 teaspoon salt

1/8 teaspoon ground black pepper

3/4 cup sliced fresh mushrooms

1 teaspoon crushed fresh garlic

3 3/4 cups unsalted chicken broth

1 1/2 cups arborio rice

3/4 cup frozen green peas

1/4 cup plus 2 tablespoons evaporated skim milk

3 tablespoons grated nonfat or regular
Parmesan cheese

1. Rinse the chicken with cool water, and pat it dry with paper towels. Cut the chicken into 1/2-inch pieces, and sprinkle with the salt and pepper.

2. Coat a large nonstick skillet with nonstick butter-flavored cooking spray, and preheat over medium-high heat. Add the chicken, and stir-fry for 3 to 4 minutes, or until nicely browned. Add the mushrooms and garlic, and stir-fry for another minute or 2, or until the mushrooms begin to brown and start to release their juices. (Add a little white wine or chicken broth if the skillet becomes too dry.)

3. Stir the broth and rice into the skillet mixture, and bring to a boil. Reduce the heat to low, cover, and simmer without stirring for about 12 minutes, or until about three-fourths of the liquid has been absorbed. Stir in the peas, and cook covered for another 3 minutes, or until most of the liquid has been absorbed.

4. Add the evaporated milk to the skillet, and, if necessary, increase the heat slightly to return the mixture to a simmer. Cook uncovered, stirring frequently, for about 5 minutes, or until the rice is tender but still a little firm to the bite, and most of the liquid has been absorbed. Add a little more broth during cooking if needed, leaving just enough liquid to make the mixture moist and creamy.

5. Stir the Parmesan cheese into the risotto. If the mixture seems too dry at this point, add a little more evaporated milk or broth. Serve hot, topping each serving with a rounded teaspoon of additional Parmesan, if desired.

NUTRITIONAL FACTS (PER 1 1/2-CUP SERVING)
Cal: 411   Carbs: 65 g   Chol: 36 mg   Fat: 1.7 g
Fiber: 2.7 g   Protein: 31.5 g   Sodium: 302 mg

Chicken With Black Bean Salsa

YIELD: 6 SERVINGS

6 boneless skinless chicken breast halves
(about 4 ounces each)

1 tablespoon crushed fresh garlic,
or 3/4 teaspoon garlic powder

1/4 teaspoon coarsely ground black pepper

3 tablespoons chicken broth

1 can (15 ounces) black beans, undrained

1/2 cup bottled salsa

3 tablespoons thinly sliced scallions

1. Rinse the chicken with cool water, and pat it dry with paper towels. Spread each piece with some of the garlic, and sprinkle with the pepper.

2. Coat a large skillet with nonstick cooking spray, and preheat over medium-high heat. Arrange the chicken in the skillet, and cook for about 2 minutes on each side, or until nicely browned. Reduce the heat to low, and add the broth. Cover and simmer for 10 to 12 minutes, or until the chicken is tender and no longer pink inside. Add a little more broth during cooking if necessary, but only enough to keep the skillet barely moist. Transfer the chicken to a serving platter, and cover to keep warm.

3. Drain any liquid from the skillet, and add the undrained black beans and the salsa. Cook and stir over medium heat until heated through. Spoon the bean mixture over the chicken, sprinkle with the scallions, and serve hot, accompanying the dish with brown rice, if desired.

NUTRITIONAL FACTS (PER SERVING)
Cal: 212   Carbs: 15 g   Chol: 72 mg   Fat: 3.4 g
Fiber: 4.9 g   Protein: 30 g   Sodium: 436 mg

Chicken Cacciatore

YIELD: 4 SERVINGS

1 can (14$^1/_2$ ounces) unsalted tomatoes, crushed
2 tablespoons tomato paste
1 teaspoon dried Italian seasoning
$^1/_4$ teaspoon crushed red pepper
4 boneless skinless chicken breast halves (about 4 ounces each)
$^1/_2$ teaspoon salt
$^1/_2$ teaspoon coarsely ground black pepper
$^1/_4$ cup dry white wine or chicken broth
1$^1/_2$ teaspoons crushed fresh garlic
1 medium yellow onion, cut into thin wedges
1 medium green pepper, cut into thin strips
1$^1/_2$ cups sliced fresh mushrooms
$^1/_4$ cup grated nonfat or regular Parmesan cheese (optional)

1. Place the tomatoes, tomato paste, Italian seasoning, and red pepper in a medium-sized bowl, and stir to mix well. Set aside.

2. Rinse the chicken with cool water, and pat it dry with paper towels. Place the chicken pieces on a flat surface, and use a meat mallet to pound each piece to $^1/_4$-inch thickness. Sprinkle both sides of the chicken pieces with the salt and pepper.

3. Coat a large nonstick skillet with nonstick olive oil cooking spray, and preheat over medium-high heat. Place the chicken in the skillet, and cook for 3 to 4 minutes on each side, or until nicely browned and no longer pink inside. Transfer the chicken to a platter, and cover to keep warm.

4. Add the wine or broth to the skillet, and cook over medium-high heat for a minute or 2, or until most of the liquid has evaporated. Add the garlic, onion, green pepper, and mushrooms, and stir-fry for about 4 minutes, or until the vegetables are crisp-tender. Add a little more wine or broth if the skillet becomes too dry.

5. Move the vegetables to one side of the skillet, and return the chicken to the skillet. Arrange the vegetables over and around the chicken.

6. Pour the tomato mixture over the chicken and vegetables, and bring to a boil over medium-high heat. Reduce the heat to low, cover, and simmer for about 10 minutes, or until the flavors are well blended and the vegetables are tender. Serve hot with your choice of pasta, topping each serving with a tablespoon of Parmesan, if desired.

> **NUTRITIONAL FACTS (PER SERVING)**
> Cal: 199   Carbs: 9.2 g   Chol: 82 mg   Fat: 2.2 g
> Fiber: 2.5 g   Protein: 35 g   Sodium: 358 mg

Lemon-Herb Chicken With Vegetables

YIELD: 4 SERVINGS

4 boneless skinless chicken breast halves (about 4 ounces each)
$^1/_4$ cup chicken broth
16 medium whole fresh mushrooms (about 8 ounces)
2 medium carrots, peeled, halved lengthwise, and cut into 2-inch pieces
2 medium zucchini, halved lengthwise and cut into $^1/_2$-inch slices

MARINADE

2 tablespoons lemon juice
1 tablespoon brown sugar
1 teaspoon crushed fresh garlic
$^1/_2$ teaspoon coarsely ground black pepper
$^1/_4$ teaspoon salt
1 teaspoon dried thyme, oregano, or rosemary

1. Rinse the chicken with cool water, and pat it dry with paper towels. Place the chicken in a shallow nonmetal container.

2. Place the marinade ingredients in a small bowl, and stir to mix. Pour the mixture over the chicken pieces. Turn the chicken to coat, cover, and refrigerate for several hours or overnight.

3. Coat a large skillet with nonstick cooking spray, and preheat over medium-high heat. Arrange the chicken in the skillet, reserving the marinade, and cook for about 2 minutes on each side, or until nicely browned.

4. Reduce the heat to low, and add the reserved marinade and the broth, mushrooms, and carrots to the skillet. Cover and simmer for 10 minutes. Add the zucchini, and simmer for an additional 5 minutes, or until the chicken is no longer pink inside and the vegetables are tender.

5. Serve hot, accompanying each chicken breast with some of the vegetables and pan juices. Serve over brown rice, if desired.

NUTRITIONAL FACTS (PER SERVING)
Cal: 192   Carbs: 11 g   Chol: 72 mg   Fat: 3.4 g
Fiber: 2.7 g   Protein: 29 g   Sodium: 263 mg

Almost Veal Parmesan

Turkey breast has a taste and texture similar to that of veal, and substitutes nicely for the fattier meat in dishes like Veal Parmesan and Veal Marsala.

YIELD: 4 SERVINGS
4 turkey breast cutlets (about 4 ounces each)
¼ cup fat-free egg substitute
3 tablespoons unbleached flour
3 tablespoons grated nonfat or regular Parmesan cheese
¼ teaspoon ground black pepper
2 cups Chunky Garden Marinara Sauce (page 235) or bottled marinara sauce
2 tablespoons chicken broth or water
Nonstick olive oil cooking spray
¾ cup shredded nonfat or reduced-fat mozzarella cheese

1. Rinse the turkey with cool water, and pat it dry with paper towels. Place the turkey pieces on a flat surface, and use a meat mallet to pound each piece to ³/₈-inch thickness.

2. Place the egg substitute in a shallow dish. Place the flour, Parmesan, and pepper in another shallow dish, and stir to mix well. Dip each turkey piece first in the egg substitute and then in the flour mixture, turning to coat both sides. Set aside.

3. Place the marinara sauce and the broth or water in a medium-sized bowl, and stir to mix well. Set aside.

4. Coat a large oven-proof skillet with nonstick olive oil cooking spray, and preheat over medium-high heat. Add the turkey pieces, and cook for about 3 minutes, or until nicely browned. Spray the top of the turkey lightly with the cooking spray, turn, and cook for 3 additional minutes, or until nicely browned and no longer pink inside.

5. Remove the skillet from the heat, and carefully pour the marinara sauce over and around the turkey pieces. (Be aware that the sauce may splatter a little when it hits the hot skillet.) Lift the turkey pieces to allow the sauce to cover the bottom of the skillet.

6. Place the skillet in a 400°F oven, and bake uncovered for 10 minutes, or until the sauce is hot and bubbly. Sprinkle the mozzarella over the top, and bake for 5 additional minutes, or until the cheese is melted. Serve hot with your choice of pasta.

NUTRITIONAL FACTS (PER SERVING)
Cal: 257   Carbs: 21 g   Chol: 79 mg   Fat: 1.3 g
Fiber: 3.9 g   Protein: 39 g   Sodium: 471 mg

Almost Veal Marsala

YIELD: 4 SERVINGS
1 pound turkey breast tenderloin, sliced crosswise into 8 equal pieces
¼ cup fat-free egg substitute
¼ cup plus 2 tablespoons unbleached flour
½ teaspoon salt
½ teaspoon ground black pepper
½ cup chicken broth
¾ teaspoon cornstarch
Nonstick butter-flavored cooking spray
2 cups sliced fresh mushrooms
¾ cup dry Marsala
2 tablespoons chopped fresh Italian parsley (garnish)

1. Rinse the turkey with cool water, and pat it dry with paper towels. Place the turkey pieces on a flat surface, and use a meat mallet to pound each piece to $3/8$-inch thickness.

2. Place the egg substitute in a shallow dish. Place the flour, salt, and pepper in another shallow dish, and stir to mix well. Dip each turkey piece first in the egg substitute and then in the flour mixture, turning to coat both sides. Set aside.

3. Place 1 teaspoon of the chicken broth in a small bowl. Add all of the cornstarch, and stir to dissolve. Stir in the remaining broth, and set aside.

4. Coat a large nonstick skillet with nonstick butter-flavored cooking spray, and preheat over medium-high heat. Add the turkey pieces, and cook for about 3 minutes, or until nicely browned. Spray the top of the turkey lightly with the cooking spray, turn, and cook for 3 additional minutes, or until nicely browned and no longer pink inside. Transfer the turkey to a platter, and cover to keep warm.

5. Add the mushrooms to the skillet, and stir-fry for about 2 minutes, or until the mushrooms begin to brown and start to release their juices. (Add a little broth if the skillet becomes too dry.) Return the turkey to the skillet, and arrange the mushrooms over and around the turkey pieces.

6. Add the Marsala to the skillet, and bring to a boil. Reduce the heat to medium and cook uncovered for 2 minutes, or until the Marsala is reduced by half.

7. Stir the cornstarch mixture and add it to the skillet. Increase the heat if necessary to bring the broth to a boil. Reduce the heat to medium-low, cover, and simmer for about 3 minutes, or until the sauce is slightly thickened and the flavors are well blended.

8. Transfer the turkey and sauce to a serving platter, sprinkle with the parsley, and serve hot.

NUTRITIONAL FACTS (PER SERVING)
Cal: 205   Carbs: 12 g   Chol: 73 mg   Fat: 1.3 g
Fiber: 0.9 g   Protein: 29 g   Sodium: 429 mg

Savory Turkey and Rice

YIELD: 6 SERVINGS
1 pound turkey breast tenderloins
5¼ cups unsalted chicken broth, divided
2 cups brown rice
2 teaspoons instant chicken bouillon granules
1¼ cups sliced fresh mushrooms
1 medium yellow onion, chopped
2 tablespoons dry sherry
1 teaspoon crushed fresh garlic
¾ teaspoon poultry seasoning
¼ teaspoon ground black pepper
1 cup frozen (thawed) green peas

1. Rinse the turkey with cool water, and pat it dry with paper towels. Coat a 9-inch square pan with cooking spray, and arrange the turkey in a single layer in the pan. Add 2 tablespoons of the broth, cover with aluminum foil, and bake at 350°F for 20 minutes. Remove the foil, and bake uncovered for 10 additional minutes, or until the meat is tender and the turkey is no longer pink inside.

2. Remove the turkey from the pan, and allow to cool to room temperature. Tear the meat into bite-sized pieces, and set aside.

3. Place the rice, 5 cups of the broth, and the bouillon granules in a 2½-quart pot. Bring the mixture to a boil over high heat, stir, and reduce the heat to low. Cover and simmer without stirring for 45 to 50 minutes, or until the liquid has been absorbed and the rice is tender. Remove the pot from the heat, and allow to sit, covered, for 5 minutes.

4. Place the mushrooms, onion, sherry, garlic, poultry seasoning, and pepper in a large nonstick skillet. Sauté over medium heat until the mushrooms are tender and most of the liquid has evaporated. Add the peas, rice, turkey, and remaining 2 tablespoons of broth, and toss until heated through. Serve hot.

NUTRITIONAL FACTS (PER 1½-CUP SERVING)
Cal: 341   Carbs: 54 g   Chol: 49 mg   Fat: 2.8 g
Fiber: 3.8 g   Protein: 24 g   Sodium: 403 mg

Glazed Turkey Tenderloins

For variety, substitute pork tenderloin
for the turkey tenderloins.

YIELD: 4 SERVINGS

1 pound turkey breast tenderloin, sliced crosswise into 8 equal pieces
¼ teaspoon garlic powder
¼ teaspoon salt
¼ teaspoon coarsely ground black pepper
1 teaspoon dried fines herbes* or dried rosemary

GLAZE

¼ cup orange marmalade
¼ cup chicken broth
1 tablespoon balsamic vinegar
1½ teaspoons Dijon mustard

* A blend of thyme, oregano, sage, rosemary, marjoram, and basil, fines herbes can be found in the dried spice section of most grocery stores.

1. To make the glaze, place all of the glaze ingredients in a small bowl, and stir to mix well. Set aside.

2. Rinse the turkey with cool water, and pat it dry with paper towels. Place the turkey pieces on a flat surface, and use a meat mallet to pound each piece to ¼-inch thickness.

3. Place the garlic powder, salt, pepper, and fines herbes or rosemary in a small bowl, and stir to mix well. Rub some of the herb mixture over both sides of each piece.

4. Coat a large nonstick skillet with nonstick cooking spray, and preheat over medium-high heat. Add the turkey, and cook for about 2 minutes on each side, or until nicely browned and no longer pink inside. Transfer the turkey to a plate, and cover to keep warm.

5. Reduce the heat under the skillet to medium. Stir the glaze mixture, and pour it into the skillet. Cook, stirring constantly, for about 1 minute, or until the glaze is reduced by about a third and is thickened and bubbly.

6. Return the turkey to the skillet, and turn it in the glaze to coat well. Serve hot, accompanied by brown rice or whole wheat couscous, if desired.

NUTRITIONAL FACTS (PER SERVING)			
Cal: 181	Carbs: 14 g	Chol: 70 mg	Fat: 1 g
Fiber: 0.1 g	Protein: 28 g	Sodium: 296 mg	

Turkey Piccata

YIELD: 4 SERVINGS

1 pound turkey breast tenderloin, sliced crosswise into 8 equal pieces
⅓ cup fat-free egg substitute
½ cup unbleached flour
½ teaspoon dried tarragon
¼ teaspoon salt
¼ teaspoon ground black pepper
1 tablespoon extra virgin olive oil
1½ cups sliced fresh mushrooms
1 cup chicken broth
1 tablespoon plus 1½ teaspoons lemon juice
¼ cup thinly sliced scallions
1 teaspoon crushed fresh garlic
1 tablespoon freshly grated lemon rind
2 tablespoons finely chopped fresh parsley

1. Rinse the turkey with cool water, and pat it dry with paper towels. Place the turkey pieces on a flat surface, and use a meat mallet to pound each piece to ⅜-inch thickness.

2. Place the egg substitute in a shallow dish. Place the flour, tarragon, salt, and pepper in another shallow dish, and stir to mix. Dip each turkey piece first in the egg substitute and then in the flour mixture, turning to coat both sides.

3. Coat a large nonstick skillet with the olive oil, and preheat over medium heat. Add the turkey, and cook for about 2 minutes on each side, or until golden brown and no longer pink inside. Transfer the turkey to a warm serving platter, and cover to keep warm.

4. Add the mushrooms to the skillet, and stir-fry for about 1 minute, or until the mushrooms begin to soften. (Add a little water or broth if the skillet becomes too dry.) Add the broth, lemon juice, scallions, and garlic to the skillet. Cook, stirring occasionally, for 4 to 6 minutes, or just until the mushrooms are tender and the liquid is reduced by half.

5. Remove the skillet from the heat, and stir in the lemon rind and parsley. Spoon the sauce over the turkey and serve hot, accompanied by angel hair pasta, if desired.

> **NUTRITIONAL FACTS (PER SERVING)**
> Cal: 235   Carbs: 16 g   Chol: 73 mg   Fat: 5 g
> Fiber: 2.2 g   Protein: 31 g   Sodium: 398 mg

Breast of Turkey Provençal

YIELD: 4 SERVINGS
1 pound turkey breast tenderloin, sliced crosswise into 8 equal pieces
1/3 cup unbleached flour
1/4 teaspoon salt
1/4 teaspoon ground black pepper
1/2 cup dry white wine
2 teaspoons crushed fresh garlic
1 teaspoon dried rosemary
1 teaspoon dried oregano
1 tablespoon extra virgin olive oil
1 bay leaf
1/2 cup chicken broth
1 medium tomato, cut into 8 wedges
1/4 cup minced fresh parsley (garnish)

1. Rinse the turkey with cool water, and pat it dry with paper towels. Place the turkey pieces on a flat surface, and use a meat mallet to pound each piece to $3/8$-inch thickness.

2. Place the flour, salt, and pepper in a plastic bag. Close the bag, and shake well to mix. Place the turkey, 2 pieces at a time, in the coating bag, and shake well until evenly coated. Set aside.

3. Place the wine, garlic, rosemary, and oregano in a small bowl, and stir to mix. Set aside.

4. Coat a large nonstick skillet with the olive oil, and preheat over medium-high heat. Add the turkey, and cook for about 2 minutes on each side, or until nicely browned and no longer pink inside.

5. Pour the wine mixture over the turkey, and add the bay leaf. Reduce the heat to medium-low, and cook until the wine is reduced by half, periodically scraping the bottom of the skillet. Add the chicken broth, and arrange the tomato wedges around the meat. Cover and simmer for 5 to 7 minutes, or until the turkey and tomatoes are tender. Remove and discard the bay leaf.

6. Transfer the turkey, tomatoes, and sauce to a serving platter, and sprinkle with the parsley. Serve over noodles or pasta, if desired.

> **NUTRITIONAL FACTS (PER SERVING)**
> Cal: 207   Carbs: 13 g   Chol: 73 mg   Fat: 4.8 g
> Fiber: 0.8 g   Protein: 28 g   Sodium: 283 mg

Mexican Skillet Dinner

YIELD: 6 SERVINGS
1 pound 95% lean ground beef
1 can (14 1/2 ounces) Mexican-style stewed tomatoes, crushed
2 1/2 cups fresh or frozen (thawed) whole kernel corn
8 ounces elbow macaroni (about 1 3/4 cups)
1 2/3 cups beef broth
1 teaspoon crushed fresh garlic
1 tablespoon chili powder
1/2 teaspoon dried oregano
1/4 teaspoon ground black pepper

1. Coat a large, deep nonstick skillet with nonstick cooking spray, and preheat over medium heat. Add the ground beef, and cook, stirring to crumble, until the meat is no longer pink. Drain off and discard any excess fat.

2. Add all of the remaining ingredients to the skillet, and stir to mix well. Increase the heat to medium-high, and allow the mixture to come to a boil. Then reduce the heat to low, cover, and simmer, stirring occasionally, for about 10 minutes, or until the pasta is tender and most of the liquid has been absorbed. Serve hot.

NUTRITIONAL FACTS (PER 1½-CUP SERVING)
Cal: 311   Carbs: 44 g   Chol: 50 mg   Fat: 4.3 g
Fiber: 6 g   Protein: 24 g   Sodium: 357 mg

Chili Macaroni Skillet

YIELD: 6 SERVINGS

1 pound 95% lean ground beef

1 can (14½ ounces) unsalted tomatoes, crushed

1 can (8 ounces) unsalted tomato sauce

1 can (15 ounces) kidney beans, drained

8 ounces ziti pasta (about 3 cups)

2 cups water

½ cup chopped onion

1 tablespoon chili powder

2 teaspoons instant beef bouillon granules

½ teaspoon dried oregano

½ teaspoon ground cumin

1. Coat a large, deep nonstick skillet with nonstick cooking spray, and preheat over medium heat. Add the ground beef, and cook, stirring to crumble, until the meat is no longer pink. Drain off and discard any excess fat.

2. Add all of the remaining ingredients to the skillet, and stir to mix well. Increase the heat to medium-high, and allow the mixture to come to a boil. Then reduce the heat to low, cover, and simmer, stirring occasionally, for about 12 minutes, or until the ziti is tender and most of the liquid has been absorbed. Serve hot.

NUTRITIONAL FACTS (PER 1½-CUP SERVING)
Cal: 360   Carbs: 51 g   Chol: 46 mg   Fat: 3.9 g
Fiber: 9.5 g   Protein: 29 g   Sodium: 464 mg

Beef and Biscuit Bake

YIELD: 6 SERVINGS

1 pound 95% lean ground beef

1 medium yellow onion, chopped

2¼ cups water, divided

1½ cups frozen (unthawed) whole kernel corn

1½ cups frozen (unthawed) cut green beans

2¼ teaspoons instant beef bouillon granules

½ teaspoon crushed dried thyme or marjoram

¼ teaspoon ground black pepper

¼ cup unbleached flour

BISCUIT TOPPING

1½ cups low-fat biscuit mix

¾ cup plus 2 tablespoons nonfat or
low-fat buttermilk

1. Coat a large oven-proof skillet with nonstick cooking spray, and preheat over medium heat. Add the ground beef, and cook, stirring to crumble, until the meat is no longer pink. Drain off and discard any excess fat.

2. Add the onion to the skillet, and stir to mix. Cook for a minute or 2, or until the onion is crisp-tender.

3. Add 1½ cups of the water and all of the corn, green beans, bouillon granules, thyme or marjoram, and pepper to the meat mixture. Bring to a boil over high heat, reduce the heat to low, and cover. Simmer for about 3 minutes, or until the vegetables are thawed and heated through.

4. Place the remaining ¾ cup of water and all of the flour in a jar with a tight-fitting lid, and shake until smooth. Stir the flour mixture into the meat mixture, and cook, stirring constantly, for about 2 minutes, or until the sauce has thickened. Remove the skillet from the heat, and set aside to keep warm.

5. To make the topping, place the biscuit mix in a medium-sized bowl. Add enough of the buttermilk to form a moderately thick batter, and stir just until the dry ingredients are moistened. Drop heaping tablespoonfuls of batter onto the meat mixture to make 6 biscuits.

6. Bake uncovered at 400°F for about 18 minutes, or until the biscuits are lightly browned and cooked through. Cover with aluminum foil during the last few minutes of baking if the biscuits begin to brown too quickly. Serve hot.

NUTRITIONAL FACTS (PER SERVING)		
Cal: 333 Carbs: 58 g Chol: 42 mg Fat: 4.6 g		
Fiber: 3.2 g Protein: 22 g Sodium: 641 mg		

Skillet Stroganoff

YIELD: 5 SERVINGS

12 ounces 95% lean ground beef
2 cups sliced fresh mushrooms
1/2 cup chopped onion
2 1/4 cups water
1 tablespoon plus 1 1/2 teaspoons tomato paste
2 1/2 teaspoons instant beef bouillon granules
1/4 teaspoon coarsely ground black pepper
6 ounces wide or extra-broad whole wheat ribbon noodles or no-yolk noodles
1 cup nonfat or light sour cream

1. Coat a large, deep nonstick skillet with nonstick cooking spray, and preheat over medium heat. Add the ground beef, and cook, stirring to crumble, until the meat is no longer pink. Drain off and discard any excess fat.

2. Add the mushrooms, onion, water, tomato paste, bouillon granules, and pepper to the skillet, and stir to mix well. Increase the heat to high, and bring the mixture to a boil.

3. Add the noodles to the skillet, and stir gently to mix. Reduce the heat to medium, cover, and simmer, stirring occasionally, for 8 to 10 minutes, or until the noodles are al dente and most of the liquid has been absorbed.

4. Reduce the heat to low, add the sour cream, and stir gently to mix well. Cook for 1 additional minute, or just until the sour cream is heated through. (Add a little more water or broth if the sauce seems too dry.) Serve hot.

NUTRITIONAL FACTS (PER 1 1/4-CUP SERVING)		
Cal: 280 Carbs: 38 g Chol: 36 mg Fat: 3.8 g		
Fiber: 3.6 g Protein: 21 g Sodium: 409 mg		

Mama's Meat Loaf

YIELD: 8 SERVINGS

LOAF

1 1/2 pounds 95% lean ground beef
1 cup finely chopped fresh mushrooms
1/2 cup finely chopped onion
1/2 cup finely chopped green bell pepper
1/2 cup quick-cooking oats
1/4 cup grated nonfat or regular Parmesan cheese
3 egg whites
1 1/2 teaspoons crushed fresh garlic
1 1/2 teaspoons dried Italian seasoning
1/2 teaspoon ground black pepper

TOPPING

1 can (8 ounces) tomato sauce, divided
1 teaspoon sugar
1/2 teaspoon Italian seasoning

1. Place all of the loaf ingredients and 3 tablespoons of the tomato sauce in a large bowl, and mix well. Coat a 9-x-5-inch meat loaf pan with nonstick cooking spray, and press the mixture into the pan to form a loaf.

2. Bake uncovered at 350°F for 35 minutes. Place the remaining tomato sauce, the sugar, and the Italian seasoning in a small bowl, stir to mix, and pour over the meat loaf. Bake for 30 additional minutes, or until the meat is no longer pink inside and a meat thermometer registers 160°F.

3. Remove the loaf from the oven, and let sit for 10 minutes before slicing and serving.

NUTRITIONAL FACTS (PER SERVING)		
Cal: 158 Carbs: 9 g Chol: 48 mg Fat: 4.2 g		
Fiber: 1.4 g Protein: 21 g Sodium: 272 mg		

Spicy Salsa Meat Loaf

YIELD: 8 SERVINGS

LOAF

1½ pounds 95% lean ground beef

¾ cup oat bran or quick-cooking oats

½ cup bottled chunky salsa

½ cup finely chopped onion

¼ cup finely chopped green bell pepper

3 egg whites

¼ teaspoon ground black pepper

2 teaspoons chili powder

TOPPING

½ cup ketchup

¼ cup bottled chunky salsa

1. Place all of the loaf ingredients in a large bowl, and mix well. Coat a 9-x-5-inch meat loaf pan with nonstick cooking spray, and press the mixture into the pan to form a loaf.

2. Bake uncovered at 350°F for 35 minutes. Place all of the topping ingredients in a small bowl, stir to mix, and pour over the meat loaf. Bake for 30 additional minutes, or until the meat is no longer pink inside and a meat thermometer registers 160º.

3. Remove the loaf from the oven, and let sit for 10 minutes before slicing and serving.

NUTRITIONAL FACTS (PER SERVING)
Cal: 158   Carbs: 10 g   Chol: 45 mg   Fat: 4.2 g
Fiber: 1.5 g   Protein: 19 g   Sodium: 322 mg

Pot Roast With Sour Cream Gravy

Top round roast—which is sometimes sold as London broil—is one of the leanest cuts available, and can be easily substituted for brisket and other fatty pot-roast cuts.

YIELD: 8 SERVINGS

2½-pound top round roast or London broil

2 teaspoons crushed fresh garlic, or ½ teaspoon garlic powder

¼ teaspoon coarsely ground black pepper

1 medium yellow onion, thinly sliced

2 bay leaves

¾ cup beef broth

1½ pounds potatoes (about 4 medium), scrubbed and quartered

1¼ pounds carrots (about 6 medium), peeled and cut into 2-inch pieces

GRAVY

Meat drippings

1½ teaspoons instant beef bouillon granules

3 tablespoons unbleached flour

¼ cup water

½ cup nonfat or light sour cream

1. Trim all visible fat from the meat. Rinse the meat with cool water, and pat it dry with paper towels.

Making Moist and Flavorful Low-Fat Meat Loaf

For flavorful, juicy low-fat meat loaf, add lots of finely chopped vegetables—such as onions, mushrooms, green peppers, and grated carrots—to the meat loaf mixture. As the loaf cooks, the chopped vegetables will release their juices into the meat, keeping your meat loaf moist and flavorful. Another great way to trim the fat from your favorite meat loaf is to add some meatless recipe crumbles as a meat extender. You can easily replace eight ounces of ground beef with one cup of recipe crumbles in most meat loaf recipes with no detectable difference. (Read more about these fat-saving products in Chapter 1.) And last but not least, be sure to use a "lean" meat loaf pan for baking your meat loaf. These pans have a perforated inner liner that allows the fat to drain into the bottom of the pan instead of being reabsorbed into the meat.

Spread the garlic or garlic powder over both sides of the meat, and sprinkle with the pepper.

2. Coat a large oven-proof skillet with nonstick cooking spray, and preheat over medium-high heat. Place the meat in the skillet, and brown for 2 to 3 minutes on each side. Remove the skillet from the heat.

3. Spread the onions over the meat. Place the bay leaves in the skillet, and pour the broth into the bottom of the skillet. Cover the skillet tightly with aluminum foil, and bake at 325°F for 1 hour and 15 minutes.

4. Remove the skillet from the oven, and carefully remove the cover. (Steam will escape.) Place the potatoes and carrots around the meat, cover, and return the skillet to the oven for 45 additional minutes, or until the meat and vegetables are tender. Transfer the meat and vegetables to a serving platter, and cover to keep warm.

5. To make the gravy, discard the bay leaves, and pour the meat drippings into a fat separator cup. Then pour the fat-free drippings into a 2-cup measure. (If the meat was well trimmed, there may not be any fat to remove.) If necessary, add water to the defatted drippings to bring the volume up to 1¼ cups.

6. Pour the drippings mixture into a 1-quart saucepan, add the bouillon granules, and bring to a boil over medium heat. Place the flour and water in a jar with a tight-fitting lid, and shake until smooth. Slowly pour the flour mixture into the boiling gravy. Cook and stir with a wire whisk until the gravy is thickened and bubbly.

7. Reduce the heat to low, add the sour cream, and whisk just until heated through. Transfer the gravy to a warmed gravy boat or pitcher, and serve hot with the meat and vegetables.

NUTRITIONAL FACTS (PER SERVING)
Cal: 300   Carbs: 36 g   Chol: 59 mg   Fat: 5.2 g
Fiber: 4.2 g   Protein: 29 g   Sodium: 335 mg

Saucy Stuffed Peppers

YIELD: 6 SERVINGS
6 large green bell peppers

FILLING
1 pound 95% lean ground beef
1 medium onion, chopped
1 tablespoon chili powder
1 teaspoon instant beef bouillon granules
¼ teaspoon ground black pepper
4 cups cooked brown rice

SAUCE
3 cans (8 ounces each) unsalted tomato sauce
2½ teaspoon chili powder
¼ teaspoon salt

1. Coat a large nonstick skillet with nonstick cooking spray, and preheat over medium heat. Add the ground beef, and cook, stirring to crumble, until the meat is no longer pink. Drain off and discard any excess fat.

2. Stir the onion, chili powder, bouillon granules, and pepper into the beef, cover, and continue to cook, stirring frequently, for a few more minutes, or until the onion is tender. (Add a few tablespoons of water or broth if the skillet gets too dry.) Remove the skillet from the heat, and stir in the rice.

3. Cut the tops off the peppers, and remove the seeds and membranes. Divide the filling among the peppers, and replace the pepper tops.

4. To make the sauce, place all of the sauce ingredients in a large bowl, and stir to mix. Place the peppers upright in an 8-x-12-inch casserole dish or Dutch oven, and pour the sauce around the peppers. Cover with aluminum foil and bake at 350°F for 1 hour, or until the peppers are tender. Serve hot.

NUTRITIONAL FACTS (PER SERVING)
Cal: 336   Carbs: 52 g   Chol: 40 mg   Fat: 5.6 g
Fiber: 8 g   Protein: 22 g   Sodium: 306 mg

Shepherd's Pie

YIELD: 6 SERVINGS

1 pound 95% lean ground beef

1$\frac{1}{2}$ cups unsalted tomato sauce

2 teaspoons chili powder

1 teaspoon instant beef bouillon granules

$\frac{1}{2}$ teaspoon dried oregano

1 package (10 ounces) frozen (thawed)
mixed vegetables

TOPPING

1$\frac{1}{2}$ pounds baking potatoes (about 4 medium)

$\frac{1}{2}$ cup nonfat or light sour cream or
plain nonfat yogurt

$\frac{1}{4}$ teaspoon salt

$\frac{1}{8}$ teaspoon ground white pepper

1 cup shredded nonfat or reduced-fat
Cheddar cheese

1. To make the topping, peel the potatoes and cut them into 1-inch pieces. Place in a 2-quart pot, barely cover with water, and bring to a boil over high heat. Reduce the heat to medium, cover, and cook for 10 minutes, or until the potatoes are soft.

2. Drain all but 2 tablespoons of water from the potatoes, reserving the drained water. Add the sour cream or yogurt, salt, and pepper, and mash the potatoes with a potato masher until smooth. If the potatoes are too stiff, add a little of the reserved cooking liquid. Set aside.

3. Coat a large, deep nonstick skillet with nonstick cooking spray, and preheat over medium heat. Add the ground beef, and cook, stirring to crumble, until the meat is no longer pink. Drain off and discard any excess fat.

4. Stir the tomato sauce, chili powder, bouillon granules, and oregano into the beef, and continue to cook and stir just until the mixture is heated through.

5. Coat a 2$\frac{1}{2}$-quart casserole dish with nonstick cooking spray, and spoon the beef mixture into the dish. Arrange the mixed vegetables in a layer over the beef mixture. Then spread the mashed potatoes over the vegetables.

6. Bake uncovered at 350°F for 25 minutes, or until the edges are bubbly. Top with the cheese, and bake for 5 additional minutes, or until the cheese is melted. Remove the dish from the oven, and let sit for 5 minutes before serving.

NUTRITIONAL FACTS (PER 1$\frac{1}{3}$-CUP SERVING)
Cal: 290   Carbs: 36 g   Chol: 54 mg   Fat: 4 g
Fiber: 5 g   Protein: 27 g   Sodium: 489 mg

Savory Swiss Steak

YIELD: 4 SERVINGS

1-pound top round steak

$\frac{1}{3}$ cup unbleached flour

$\frac{1}{4}$ teaspoon salt

$\frac{1}{4}$ teaspoon ground black pepper

Nonstick cooking spray

1 can (14$\frac{1}{2}$ ounces) stewed tomatoes, crushed

1. Trim all visible fat from the meat. Rinse the meat with cool water, and pat it dry with paper towels. Cut the meat into 4 pieces, and use a meat mallet to pound each piece to $\frac{3}{8}$-inch thickness.

2. Place the flour, salt, and pepper in a shallow dish, and stir to mix. Dip the meat in the flour mixture, turning to coat both sides.

3. Coat a large nonstick skillet with nonstick cooking spray, and preheat over medium-high heat. Place the meat in the skillet, and brown for 2 to 3 minutes, or until nicely browned. Spray the top of the beef with the cooking spray, turn, and cook for 2 to 3 additional minutes, or until both sides are browned.

4. Pour the tomatoes over the meat, and reduce the heat to low. Cover and simmer for 45 minutes, or until the meat is very tender. Scrape the bottom of the pan occasionally, adding a little water if the skillet becomes too dry. Serve hot with noodles or brown rice, if desired.

NUTRITIONAL FACTS (PER SERVING)
Cal: 220   Carbs: 15 g   Chol: 70 mg   Fat: 4.4 g
Fiber: 2 g   Protein: 28 g   Sodium: 378 mg

Italian-Style Pot Roast

YIELD: 6 SERVINGS
1³⁄₄-pound top round roast or London broil
2 teaspoons crushed fresh garlic, or 1¹⁄₂ teaspoons garlic powder
¹⁄₄ teaspoon ground black pepper
1 cup chopped onion
1¹⁄₂ cups sliced fresh mushrooms
1 can (1 pound) unsalted tomatoes, crushed
1 can (6 ounces) tomato paste
¹⁄₄ cup water
2 teaspoons dried Italian seasoning
2 teaspoons instant beef bouillon granules

1. Trim all visible fat from the meat. Rinse the meat with cool water, and pat it dry with paper towels. Spread the garlic or garlic powder over both sides of the meat, and sprinkle with the pepper.

2. Coat a large oven-proof skillet with nonstick cooking spray, and preheat over medium-high heat. Place the meat in the skillet, and brown for 2 to 3 minutes on each side. Remove the skillet from the heat.

3. Spread the onions and mushrooms over the meat. Place the tomatoes, tomato paste, water, Italian seasoning, and bouillon granules in a large bowl, and stir to mix. Pour the tomato mixture over the meat and vegetables.

4. Cover the skillet tightly with aluminum foil, and bake at 350°F for 2 hours, or until the meat is tender. Serve hot, accompanying the roast with spaghetti, linguine, or another pasta, if desired.

NUTRITIONAL FACTS (PER SERVING)
Cal: 205   Carbs: 13 g   Chol: 59 mg   Fat: 5 g
Fiber: 3.3 g   Protein: 27 g   Sodium: 361 mg

Herbed Eye of Round Roast

YIELD: 8 SERVINGS
2¹⁄₂-pound beef eye of round roast
1 tablespoon crushed fresh garlic, or ³⁄₄ teaspoon garlic powder
¹⁄₂ teaspoon coarsely ground black pepper
¹⁄₂ cup condensed beef broth, undiluted
¹⁄₄ cup dry red wine or tomato juice
2 bay leaves
1 medium yellow onion, chopped
1 teaspoon dried marjoram
1 teaspoon dried thyme

1. Trim all visible fat from the meat. Rinse the meat with cool water, and pat it dry with paper towels. Spread the garlic or garlic powder over both sides of the meat, and sprinkle with the pepper.

2. Coat a large oven-proof skillet with nonstick cooking spray, and preheat over medium-high heat. Place the meat in the skillet, and brown for several minutes, or until all sides are nicely browned.

3. Remove the skillet from the heat, and pour the broth and the wine or tomato juice into the bottom of the skillet. Add the bay leaves, and sprinkle the onion, marjoram, and thyme over and around the roast. Cover the skillet tightly with aluminum foil, and bake at 325°F for 2 hours, or until the meat is tender.

4. Transfer the roast to a serving platter. Cover the roast loosely with aluminum foil, and let sit for 15 minutes before slicing thinly.

5. Pour the pan juices through a strainer into a fat separator cup. (If the meat was well trimmed, there may not be any fat to remove.) Pour the fat-free drippings into a 1-quart pot, and cook over medium-high heat, stirring occasionally, for about 10 minutes, or until the mixture is reduced to about 1 cup. Transfer the gravy to a warmed gravy boat or pitcher, and serve hot with the roast.

NUTRITIONAL FACTS (PER SERVING)
Cal: 157   Carbs: 4 g   Chol: 59 mg   Fat: 4.9 g
Fiber: 0 g   Protein: 25 g   Sodium: 85 mg

Braised Beef With Hearty Mushroom Sauce

YIELD: 8 SERVINGS

2$\frac{1}{2}$-pound top round roast or London broil

2 teaspoons crushed fresh garlic,
or $\frac{1}{2}$ teaspoon garlic powder

$\frac{1}{2}$ teaspoon coarsely ground black pepper

2 medium yellow onions, chopped

2 medium carrots, peeled and chopped

2 stalks celery, sliced (include the leaves)

$\frac{3}{4}$ teaspoon dried thyme

$\frac{3}{4}$ cup dry red wine

$\frac{1}{2}$ cup water

2$\frac{1}{2}$ teaspoons instant beef bouillon granules

2 bay leaves

GRAVY

Meat drippings

2 cups sliced fresh mushrooms

1. Trim all visible fat from the meat. Rinse the meat with cool water, and pat it dry with paper towels. Spread the garlic or garlic powder over both sides of the meat, and sprinkle with the pepper.

2. Coat a large oven-proof skillet with nonstick cooking spray, and preheat over medium-high heat. Place the meat in the skillet, and brown for 2 to 3 minutes on each side. Remove the skillet from the heat.

3. Arrange the onions, carrots, and celery over and around the meat, and sprinkle the thyme over the top. Place the wine, water, and bouillon granules in a bowl, and stir to mix well. Pour the mixture over and around the meat. Drop 1 bay leaf into the liquid on each side of the roast. Cover the skillet tightly with aluminum foil, and bake at 325°F for 1 hour and 45 minutes to 2 hours, or until the roast is tender.

4. Remove the skillet from the oven and carefully remove the foil. (Steam will escape.) Transfer the meat to a serving platter, and cover to keep warm.

5. To make the gravy, discard the bay leaves, and pour the pan juices into a fat separator cup. (If the meat was well trimmed, there may not be any fat to remove.) Pour 1$\frac{1}{2}$ cups of fat-free drippings into a blender. Transfer the vegetables from the skillet to the blender, and, leaving the lid slightly ajar to allow steam to escape, carefully process the mixture at low speed until smooth. Set aside.

6. Coat a large nonstick skillet with nonstick cooking spray, and preheat over medium-high heat. Add the mushrooms, and stir-fry for about 2 minutes, or just until the mushrooms start to brown and release their liquid. Add the puréed vegetable mixture to the skillet, and reduce the heat to medium. Cook, stirring constantly, for about 2 minutes, or until the mixture begins to boil and is heated through.

7. Cut the meat into $\frac{1}{2}$-inch-thick slices, and arrange the slices slightly overlapping down the center of the platter. Spoon a little of the mushroom sauce over the meat, and serve the remaining sauce separately.

> **NUTRITIONAL FACTS** (PER SERVING)
> Cal: 173   Carbs: 5.3 g   Chol: 59 mg   Fat: 5 g
> Fiber: 1.3 g   Protein: 26 g   Sodium: 282 mg

Tuscan Roast Tenderloin

YIELD: 8 SERVINGS

2 pork tenderloins, 1 pound each

1 tablespoon crushed fresh garlic

1 tablespoon Dijon mustard

1$\frac{1}{2}$ teaspoons dried sage

1$\frac{1}{2}$ teaspoons dried rosemary

$\frac{1}{2}$ teaspoon coarsely ground black pepper

$\frac{1}{4}$ teaspoon salt

SAUCE

$\frac{3}{4}$ cup dry white wine

1$\frac{1}{2}$ cups chicken broth, divided

2 tablespoons plus 2 teaspoons unbleached flour

1 teaspoon Dijon mustard

1 teaspoon balsamic vinegar

1. Trim the tenderloins of any visible fat and membranes. Rinse the meat with cool water, and pat it dry with paper towels.

2. Place the garlic, mustard, sage, rosemary, pepper, and salt in a small bowl, and stir together to form a paste. Spread the paste over the entire surface of the tenderloins.

3. Coat a 9-x-13-inch baking pan with nonstick cooking spray, and place the tenderloins in the pan, spacing them at least 2 inches apart. Bake uncovered at 350°F for about 45 minutes, or until an instant-read thermometer inserted in the center of a tenderloin registers 160°F and the meat is no longer pink inside.

4. Remove the pan from the oven, transfer the tenderloins to a cutting board, and cover loosely with aluminum foil to keep warm.

5. To make the sauce, pour the wine into the roasting pan, and, using a spatula, scrape up the glaze and the browned bits from the bottom of the pan. (Avoid any spots that are charred or blackened.) Pour the mixture into a 1½-quart pot, and cook over medium heat, stirring frequently, for about 5 minutes, or until the mixture is reduced by half.

6. While the wine mixture is reducing, place ¼ cup of the broth and all of the flour in a jar with a tight-fitting lid. Shake until smooth, and set aside.

7. When the wine mixture is reduced by half, add the remaining 1¼ cups of broth to the pot, and bring to a boil over medium heat. Whisk in the flour mixture, and cook, stirring constantly, for about 2 minutes, or until the mixture is thickened and bubbly. Whisk in the mustard and vinegar, and remove the pot from the heat.

8. To serve, slice the tenderloins thinly at an angle, and arrange on a serving platter. Serve hot, accompanied by the sauce.

NUTRITIONAL FACTS (PER SERVING)
Cal: 159   Carbs: 2.3 g   Chol: 67 mg   Fat: 4.2 g
Fiber: 0.1 g   Protein: 24.3 g   Sodium: 275 mg

Sweet and Sour Pork

For variety, substitute skinless chicken breast for the pork.

YIELD: 4 SERVINGS
1-pound pork tenderloin or pork sirloin
1 teaspoon crushed fresh garlic, or ¼ teaspoon garlic powder
¼ teaspoon ground ginger
2 cans (8 ounces each) pineapple chunks in juice, undrained
¼ cup chicken broth
1 medium green bell pepper, cut into thin strips
1 medium yellow onion, cut into thin wedges
1 medium carrot, peeled and diagonally sliced

SAUCE
¼ cup chicken broth
2 tablespoons seasoned rice wine vinegar
2 tablespoons reduced-sodium soy sauce
2 tablespoons light brown sugar
1 tablespoon cornstarch

1. To make the sauce, place all of the sauce ingredients in a small dish, and stir to mix. Set aside.

2. Trim the meat of any visible fat and membranes. Rinse the meat with cool water, and pat it dry with paper towels. Cut the meat into ¾-inch cubes, toss with the garlic and ginger, and set aside.

3. Coat a large nonstick skillet with nonstick cooking spray, and preheat over medium-high heat. Add the pork, and stir-fry for about 4 minutes, or until the pork is nicely browned.

4. Drain the juice from the pineapple, reserving both the juice and the fruit. Add the juice and the chicken broth to the pork, and bring to a boil. Reduce the heat to low, cover, and simmer for about 6 minutes, or until the pork is tender and cooked through.

5. Add the pineapple chunks, green pepper, onion, and carrot to the pork mixture. Cover and cook over medium-low heat for 3 additional minutes, or until the vegetables are crisp-tender.

6. Stir the sauce to mix, and add it to the skillet. Cook, stirring constantly, until the sauce is thickened and bubbly. Serve hot, accompanying the dish with brown rice, if desired.

NUTRITIONAL FACTS (PER 1⅛-CUP SERVING)
Cal: 257   Carbs: 34 g   Chol: 75 mg   Fat: 3.5 g
Fiber: 2.5 g   Protein: 26 g   Sodium: 606 mg

Rosemary Roasted Tenderloin

YIELD: 8 SERVINGS

2 pork tenderloins, 1 pound each

MARINADE

¼ cup frozen (thawed) apple juice concentrate

2 tablespoons Dijon mustard

2 tablespoons fresh rosemary leaves,
or 2½ teaspoons dried

4 cloves garlic, crushed

½ teaspoon coarsely ground black pepper

1. Trim the tenderloins of any visible fat and membranes. Rinse the meat with cool water, and pat it dry with paper towels. Place the tenderloins in a shallow nonmetal dish.

2. Place all of the marinade ingredients in a small bowl, and stir to mix well. Pour the marinade over the meat, turning the tenderloins to coat all sides. Cover and refrigerate for several hours or overnight.

3. When ready to bake, coat a 9-x-13-inch baking pan with nonstick cooking spray, and place the tenderloins in the pan, spacing them at least 2 inches apart. Pour the marinade remaining in the dish over the tenderloins, and bake uncovered at 350°F for about 45 minutes, or until an instant-read thermometer inserted in the center of a tenderloin registers 160°F and the meat is no longer pink inside.

4. Remove the pan from the oven, cover loosely with aluminum foil, and let sit for 5 minutes before slicing thinly at an angle. Serve hot.

NUTRITIONAL FACTS (PER SERVING)
Cal: 144   Carbs: 2 g   Chol: 79 mg   Fat: 4.2 g
Fiber: 0 g   Protein: 34.6 g   Sodium: 76 mg

Jerk Pork Kabobs

YIELD: 6 SERVINGS

1½-pound pork tenderloin or pork sirloin

1 medium red bell pepper, cut into 6 wedges

3 large fresh or frozen (thawed) ears corn
on the cob, cut crosswise into 12 (2-inch) pieces

1 medium green bell pepper, cut into 6 wedges

Nonstick butter-flavored cooking spray

MARINADE

1 medium yellow onion, finely chopped

¼ cup unsweetened pineapple juice

1 tablespoon plus 1 teaspoon brown sugar

1 teaspoon ground allspice

1 teaspoon dried thyme

½ teaspoon coarsely ground black pepper

½ teaspoon salt

¼ teaspoon ground cinnamon

¼ teaspoon ground nutmeg

¼ teaspoon crushed red pepper

1. Place all of the marinade ingredients in a small bowl, and stir to mix well. Set aside.

2. Trim the tenderloin of any visible fat and membranes. Rinse the meat with cool water, and pat it dry with paper towels. Cut the tenderloin into 18 cubes, each about 1½ inches square. Place the meat and the marinade in a shallow nonmetal container, cover, and refrigerate for at least 6 hours or overnight.

3. To assemble the kabobs, thread 1 piece of meat onto a 12-inch skewer. Follow the meat with 1 wedge of red pepper, 1 piece of corn, 1 piece of meat, 1 piece of corn, 1 wedge of green pepper, and finally 1 piece of meat. Repeat to make 6 kabobs. Discard the remaining marinade.

4. Spray the kabobs lightly with the cooking spray, and grill over medium coals or under a broiler for about 10 minutes, turning every 3 minutes, until the meat is no longer pink inside and the vegetables are lightly browned. Serve hot.

NUTRITIONAL FACTS (PER SERVING)
Cal: 223   Carbs: 16 g   Chol: 67 mg   Fat: 4.7 g
Fiber: 3 g   Protein: 26.6 g   Sodium: 140 mg

Pork Tenderloins With Apple-Raisin Stuffing

YIELD: 8 SERVINGS

2 pork tenderloins, 1 pound each

STUFFING

6 slices firm multigrain or oatmeal bread

3/4 cup chopped peeled tart apple (about 1 medium)

1/4 cup dark raisins

1/4 cup finely chopped onion

1/4 cup finely chopped celery (include the leaves)

1/2 teaspoon dried rosemary

1/2 cup chicken broth

BASTING SAUCE

2 tablespoons frozen (thawed) apple juice concentrate

2 teaspoons Dijon mustard

1/2 teaspoon dried rosemary

1. To make the stuffing, place 3 of the bread slices in a blender or food processor, and process into coarse crumbs. There should be 2¼ cups. Cut the remaining bread slices into 1/2-inch cubes. There should be 2½ cups.

2. Place the bread crumbs, bread cubes, apple, raisins, onion, celery, and rosemary in a large bowl, and toss to mix well. Tossing gently, slowly add enough broth to make a moist, but not wet, stuffing that holds together. Set aside.

3. Place all of the basting sauce ingredients in a small bowl, and stir to mix well. Set aside.

4. Trim the tenderloins of any visible fat and membranes. Rinse the meat with cool water, and pat it dry with paper towels.

5. Split each of the tenderloins lengthwise, cutting not quite all the way through, so that each tenderloin can be spread open like a book. Spread half of the stuffing mixture over half of each tenderloin, extending the stuffing all the way to the outer edges of the meat. Fold the facing half of the tenderloin over the stuffing-spread half, and use heavy string to tie the meat together at 2½-inch intervals.

6. Coat a 9-x-13-inch baking pan with nonstick cooking spray, and arrange the tenderloins in the pan, spacing them about 3 inches apart. Bake uncovered at 350°F, occasionally basting with the prepared sauce, for about 50 minutes, or until the meat is no longer pink inside.

7. Remove the pan from the oven, cover loosely with aluminum foil, and let sit for 5 to 10 minutes before slicing 1/2-inch thick. Serve hot.

NUTRITIONAL FACTS (PER SERVING)
Cal: 224   Carbs: 17 g   Chol: 67 mg   Fat: 5 g
Fiber: 2.9 g   Protein: 28.2 g   Sodium: 214 mg

Bueno Black Beans and Rice

YIELD: 5 SERVINGS

8 ounces smoked sausage or kielbasa,
at least 97% lean, thinly sliced (about 1½ cups)

1/2 cup chopped onion

1/2 cup chopped green bell pepper

2¼ cups water or unsalted chicken broth

2 cups quick-cooking brown rice

1 can (15 ounces) black beans, drained

1 bay leaf

1/2 teaspoon dried oregano

1. Coat a large nonstick skillet with nonstick cooking spray, and preheat over medium heat. Add the sausage or kielbasa, onion, and green pepper, and stir to mix. Cover and cook, stirring occasionally, for about 4 minutes, or until the vegetables start to soften.

2. Add all of the remaining ingredients to the skillet, stir to mix well, and bring to a boil. Stir, reduce the heat to low, and cover. Simmer for 8 minutes, or until the rice is tender and the liquid is absorbed.

3. Remove the skillet from the heat, cover, and let stand for 5 minutes. Remove and discard the bay leaf, and serve hot.

NUTRITIONAL FACTS (PER 1¼-CUP SERVING)
Cal: 247   Carbs: 42 g   Chol: 20 mg   Fat: 2.4 g
Fiber: 6.2 g   Protein: 13.4 g   Sodium: 514 mg

Presto Paella

YIELD: 5 SERVINGS

2 cups reduced-sodium chicken broth

1/2 teaspoon loosely packed saffron threads

8 ounces peeled and deveined
raw shrimp or scallops

1 1/4 cups sliced smoked sausage or kielbasa,
at least 97% lean (about 6 ounces)

1/2 cup chopped green bell pepper

1/2 cup chopped onion

1 teaspoon crushed fresh garlic

1/2 teaspoon dried thyme

1/2 teaspoon dried oregano

2 cups quick-cooking brown rice

1/2 cup chopped seeded plum tomatoes
(about 2 medium)

1 cup frozen (thawed) green peas

1. Place the broth and saffron in a blender, and process until the saffron is finely ground and the broth turns bright yellow. Set aside.

2. Rinse the seafood with cool water, and pat it dry with paper towels. Set aside.

3. Coat a large nonstick skillet with nonstick cooking spray, and preheat over medium-high heat. Add the sausage or kielbasa, green pepper, onion, garlic, thyme, and oregano. Stir-fry for about 4 minutes, or just until the sausage is nicely browned and the vegetables begin to soften. Cover the skillet periodically if it begins to dry out. (The steam from the cooking vegetables will moisten the skillet.)

4. Add the rice, tomatoes, seafood, and broth mixture to the skillet. Stir to mix well, and bring the mixture to a boil. Reduce the heat to low, cover, and simmer without stirring for about 7 minutes.

5. Add the peas to the skillet, and stir to mix. Cover and cook for 3 additional minutes, or until the liquid is absorbed and the rice is tender. Remove the skillet from the heat, and let sit covered for 5 minutes before serving.

NUTRITIONAL FACTS (PER 1 1/3-CUP SERVING)
Cal: 274   Carbs: 44 g   Chol: 79 mg   Fat: 2.7 g
Fiber: 4.1 g   Protein: 20 g   Sodium: 575 mg

Jiffy Jambalaya

YIELD: 6 SERVINGS

12 ounces peeled and deveined raw shrimp

1 cup thinly sliced smoked sausage or kielbasa,
at least 97% lean (about 5 ounces)

1/2 cup thinly sliced celery

1/2 cup chopped green bell pepper

1/2 cup chopped onion

1 teaspoon crushed fresh garlic

1/2 teaspoon dried thyme

2 cups quick-cooking brown rice

1 1/3 cups water

1 can (8 ounces) unsalted tomato sauce

1 can (1 pound) red kidney beans, drained

1 1/2 teaspoons Cajun seasoning

1. Rinse the shrimp with cool water, and pat them dry with paper towels. Set aside.

2. Coat a large deep nonstick skillet with nonstick cooking spray, and preheat over medium heat. Add the sausage or kielbasa, celery, green pepper, onion, garlic, and thyme, and stir to mix. Cover and cook, stirring occasionally, for about 4 minutes, or until the vegetables start to soften.

3. Add the shrimp and all of the remaining ingredients to the skillet, and bring the mixture to a boil. Stir, reduce the heat to low, and cover. Simmer for about 8 minutes, or until the rice is tender and the liquid has been absorbed.

4. Remove the skillet from the heat, and let sit covered for 5 minutes before serving.

NUTRITIONAL FACTS (PER 1 1/2-CUP SERVING)
Cal: 319   Carbs: 52 g   Chol: 89 mg   Fat: 2.7 g
Fiber: 9.8 g   Protein: 21 g   Sodium: 433 mg

Cajun Red Beans and Rice

YIELD: 5 SERVINGS

1½ cups sliced smoked sausage or kielbasa, at least 97% lean (about 8 ounces)

⅓ cup chopped onion

⅓ cup chopped green bell pepper

⅓ cup chopped celery

¾ teaspoon dried thyme

1¼ cups water or unsalted chicken broth

1 can (8 ounces) unsalted tomato sauce

1½ cups quick-cooking brown rice

1 can (15 ounces) red kidney beans, drained

1. Coat a large nonstick skillet with nonstick cooking spray, and preheat over medium heat. Add the sausage or kielbasa, onion, green pepper, celery, and thyme, and stir to mix. Cover and cook, stirring occasionally, for about 4 minutes, or until the vegetables begin to soften.

2. While the sausage and vegetables are cooking, place the water or broth and the tomato sauce in a medium-sized bowl, and stir to mix well.

3. Add the rice, beans, and tomato sauce mixture to the skillet, and stir to mix well. Increase the heat to medium-high, and allow the mixture to come to a boil. Reduce the heat to low, cover, and simmer without stirring for 10 minutes, or until the liquid is absorbed and the rice is tender. Remove the skillet from the heat, and let sit for 5 minutes before serving.

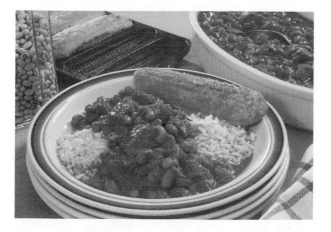

NUTRITIONAL FACTS (PER 1½-CUP SERVING)			
Cal: 365	Carbs: 66 g	Chol: 22 mg	Fat: 3.1 g
Fiber: 12 g	Protein: 20.1 g	Sodium: 485 mg	

Hoppin' John

YIELD: 6 SERVINGS

6 cups water

2 cups dried black-eyed peas, cleaned (page 302)

1½ cups diced ham, at least 97% lean (about 8 ounces)

1 medium yellow onion, chopped

1 teaspoon crushed fresh garlic

1 teaspoon dried sage

1 teaspoon instant ham, chicken, or vegetable bouillon granules

¼ teaspoon ground black pepper

TOPPINGS

¼ cup plus 2 tablespoons finely chopped tomato (optional)

¼ cup plus 2 tablespoons finely chopped scallions (optional)

Tabasco pepper sauce (optional)

1. Place all of the ingredients except for the toppings in a 3-quart pot. Stir to mix, and bring the mixture to a boil over high heat. Lower the heat; cover; and simmer, stirring occasionally, for 1 hour to 1 hour and 15 minutes, or until the beans are soft and the liquid is thick. Add more water if needed. (The liquid should just cover the peas.)

2. Serve hot over brown rice, if desired, garnishing each serving with 1 tablespoon each of tomatoes and scallions. Pass the Tabasco sauce if your family and friends like it hot!

NUTRITIONAL FACTS (PER 1-CUP SERVING)			
Cal: 237	Carbs: 37 g	Chol: 10 mg	Fat: 2.2 g
Fiber: 6.3 g	Protein: 19 g	Sodium: 496 mg	

Shrimp Fried Rice

For variety, substitute diced skinless chicken breast or pork tenderloin for the shrimp.

YIELD: 4 SERVINGS
1 cup diced peeled and deveined raw shrimp (about 6 ounces)
1–2 teaspoons sesame oil
1/2 cup thinly sliced scallions
1/2 cup thinly sliced celery
1 teaspoon dark brown sugar
3 1/2 cups cooked brown rice
3/4 cup frozen (thawed) green peas
3 tablespoons reduced-sodium soy sauce
1/2 cup fat-free egg substitute

1. Rinse the shrimp with cool water, and pat them dry with paper towels.

2. Coat a large nonstick skillet with nonstick cooking spray. Add the sesame oil, and preheat over medium-high heat. Add the shrimp, and stir-fry for about 3 minutes, or until the shrimp turn pink and are thoroughly cooked.

3. Add the scallions, celery, and brown sugar to the skillet, and stir-fry for about 2 minutes, or until the vegetables are crisp-tender. Cover the skillet periodically if it begins to dry out. (The steam released from the cooking vegetables will moisten the skillet.) Add a few teaspoons of water or broth to the skillet only if necessary.

4. Add the rice, peas, and soy sauce to the skillet, and stir-fry for about 1 minute, or just until the mixture is heated through. Add a few teaspoons of water or broth if the skillet becomes too dry.

5. Make a well in the center of the skillet mixture, and respray the center of the skillet lightly. Add the egg substitute. Reduce the heat to medium, and let the egg cook without stirring for a couple of minutes, or just until set. Gently stir the cooked egg into the rice mixture, and serve hot.

NUTRITIONAL FACTS (PER 1 1/2-CUP SERVING)
Cal: 288　Carbs: 48 g　Chol: 60 mg　Fat: 3 g
Fiber: 5.3 g　Protein: 17 g　Sodium: 422 mg

Mediterranean Foil-Baked Fish

YIELD: 4 SERVINGS
4 firm-fleshed fish fillets or steaks (about 5 ounces each), such as orange roughy, grouper, tuna, mahi-mahi, or salmon
2 teaspoons lemon pepper
12 thin slices tomato
12 thin slices onion
1/4 cup sliced black olives
2 tablespoons fresh dill, or 2 teaspoons dried

1. Rinse the fish with cool water, and pat it dry with paper towels.

2. Coat four 12-x-12-inch pieces of heavy-duty aluminum foil with nonstick olive oil cooking spray, and center a fish fillet on the lower half of each piece. Sprinkle 1/2 teaspoon of the lemon pepper over each fillet. Top each fillet with 3 of the tomato slices, 3 of the onion slices, and a tablespoon of olives. Sprinkle a quarter of the dill over the top.

3. Fold the upper half of the foil over the fish to meet the bottom half. Seal the edges together by making a tight 1/2-inch fold; then fold again to double-seal. Allow space for heat circulation and expansion. Use this technique to seal the remaining sides.

4. Arrange the pouches on a baking sheet, and bake at 450°F for about 18 minutes, or until the fish is opaque and the thickest part is easily flaked with a fork. Open each packet by carefully cutting an "X" in the top of the foil (steam will escape), and serve hot.

NUTRITIONAL FACTS (PER SERVING)
Cal: 171　Carbs: 13 g　Chol: 28 mg　Fat: 3.1 g
Fiber: 2.8 g　Protein: 23 g　Sodium: 295 mg

Tempting Tuna Skillet

YIELD: 5 SERVINGS

½ cup plus 2 tablespoons chopped fresh mushrooms
¼ cup plus 2 tablespoons finely chopped onion
¼ teaspoon dried thyme
8 ounces small seashell pasta (about 2¾ cups)
2½ cups reduced-sodium chicken broth
1¼ cups skim or low-fat milk, divided
1 tablespoon plus 1½ teaspoons cornstarch
⅛ teaspoon ground white pepper
3 tablespoons instant nonfat dry milk powder
¾ cup frozen (thawed) green peas
¾ cup shredded or diced nonfat or reduced-fat process Cheddar cheese (about 3 ounces)
1 can (12 ounces) water-packed albacore tuna, drained

1. Spray a large, deep nonstick skillet with nonstick cooking spray, and preheat over medium heat. Add the mushrooms, onion, and thyme, and stir to mix. Cover, and cook, stirring occasionally, for about 3 minutes, or until the vegetables are tender. Add a little water or broth if the skillet becomes too dry.

2. Add the pasta and the broth to the skillet, stir to mix, and increase the heat slightly to bring the mixture to a boil. Reduce the heat to medium-low, cover, and simmer, stirring occasionally, for about 9 minutes, or until the pasta is almost al dente and most of the liquid has been absorbed.

3. While the pasta is cooking, place 2 tablespoons of the milk and all of the cornstarch and pepper in a small bowl. Stir to dissolve the cornstarch, and set aside.

4. Add the remaining 1⅛ cups of milk, the milk powder, and the peas to the skillet, and stir to mix. Increase the heat to medium, and bring the mixture to a boil, stirring frequently. Stir the cornstarch mixture, and add it to the skillet. Cook and stir for a minute or 2, or until the sauce is slightly thickened and bubbly.

5. Reduce the heat to medium-low. Add the cheese to the skillet, and continue to cook, stirring frequently, for a minute or 2, or until the cheese melts.

6. Stir the tuna into the skillet mixture, and cook for another minute, or until the tuna is heated through. Add a little more milk if the mixture seems too dry. Serve hot.

NUTRITIONAL FACTS (PER 1⅓-CUP SERVING)
Cal: 351   Carbs: 44 g   Chol: 31 mg   Fat: 2.6 g
Fiber: 2.7 g   Protein: 35 g   Sodium: 498 mg

Tempting Tuna Casserole

YIELD: 5 SERVINGS

8 ounces small seashell pasta (about 2¾ cups)
1 can (10¾ ounces) low-fat cream of mushroom soup, undiluted
½ cup nonfat or light sour cream
½ cup skim or low-fat milk
¾ cup frozen (thawed) green peas
1 can (9 ounces) water-packed solid white or albacore tuna, drained
½ cup shredded nonfat or reduced-fat Cheddar cheese

1. Cook the pasta al dente according to package directions. Drain well, return to the pot, and set aside.

2. Place the mushroom soup, sour cream, and milk in a medium-sized bowl, and stir to mix well. Add the soup mixture to the pasta, and toss to mix well. Add the peas, and toss gently to mix. Add the tuna, and toss gently to mix.

3. Coat a 2-quart casserole dish with nonstick cooking spray, and spread the mixture evenly in the dish. Cover the dish with aluminum foil.

4. Bake at 375°F for 25 minutes, or until the dish is heated through. Remove the foil, spread the cheese over the top, and bake uncovered for 5 additional minutes, or until the cheese is melted. Serve hot.

NUTRITIONAL FACTS (PER 1¼-CUP SERVING)
Cal: 337   Carbs: 47 g   Chol: 23 mg   Fat: 3.9 g
Fiber: 2.1 g   Protein: 25 g   Sodium: 661 mg

Tuna With Fresh Tomato Sauce

For variety, substitute other fish steaks such as grouper, salmon, or amberjack for the tuna.

YIELD: 4 SERVINGS

4 tuna steaks (about 5 ounces each)

½ teaspoon coarsely ground black pepper

1½ teaspoons crushed fresh garlic

½ cup dry white wine

1 pound fresh plum tomatoes
(about 6 medium), diced

3 tablespoons sliced black olives

1 tablespoon chopped capers

¾ teaspoon dried oregano

¼ teaspoon crushed red pepper

2 anchovy fillets, mashed (optional)

1. Rinse the tuna steaks with cool water, and pat them dry with paper towels. Sprinkle both sides of the steaks with the pepper.

2. Coat a large nonstick skillet with nonstick olive oil cooking spray, and preheat over medium-high heat. Arrange the tuna in the skillet, and cook for 3 to 4 minutes on each side, or until nicely browned. Transfer the tuna to a platter, and cover to keep warm.

3. Reduce the heat under the skillet to medium, and add the garlic. Sauté for about 30 seconds, or just until the garlic begins to turn color. Add the wine, and cook for about 5 minutes, or until the wine is reduced by half.

4. Add the tomatoes, olives, capers, oregano, red pepper, and, if desired, the anchovies to the skillet. Cover and cook, stirring occasionally, for about 5 minutes, or until the tomatoes soften and cook down into a sauce.

5. Return the tuna to the skillet, and reduce the heat to low. Cover and simmer for about 5 minutes, or until the flavors are well blended and the tuna steaks are no longer pink inside. Serve hot with your choice of pasta.

NUTRITIONAL FACTS (PER SERVING)
Cal: 206   Carbs: 6 g   Chol: 63 mg   Fat: 2.4 g
Fiber: 1.5 g   Protein: 34 g   Sodium: 270 mg

Browning Without Fat

Great cooks know that browning enhances many foods by adding a deep color and a rich, full flavor. Unfortunately, the traditional method of browning often requires several tablespoons of oil, butter, or margarine. However, as the recipes in this chapter show, all that extra oil is simply not necessary.

To brown meat, chicken, seafood, or vegetables with virtually no added fat, spray a thin film of nonstick cooking spray over the bottom of a skillet. Then preheat the skillet over medium-high heat, and brown the food as usual. If the food starts to stick, periodically place a lid over the skillet, and the steam released from the cooking food will moisten the skillet. Another option is to add a few teaspoons of water, broth, or wine. If you use both a nonstick skillet and cooking spray, it should not be necessary to add any liquid at all.

When browning foods that have been breaded or floured, brown the bottom of the food as directed above. Then spray the top lightly with cooking spray before turning the food over and browning the second side.

Risotto With Scallops and Spinach

YIELD: 4 SERVINGS

8 ounces raw scallops

1 teaspoon crushed fresh garlic

1¾ cups arborio rice

4⅓ cups unsalted chicken broth

⅛ teaspoon ground black pepper

⅛ teaspoon ground white pepper

Pinch ground nutmeg

½ cup evaporated skim milk

3 tablespoons grated nonfat or regular
Parmesan cheese

1½ cups (packed) chopped fresh spinach

1. Rinse the scallops with cool water, and pat them dry with paper towels.

2. Coat a large nonstick skillet with nonstick butter-flavored cooking spray, and preheat over medium-high heat. Add the garlic and scallops, and stir-fry for about 3 minutes, or until the scallops turn opaque. Remove the scallops from the skillet, and set aside.

3. Place the rice, broth, black pepper, white pepper, and nutmeg in the skillet, and stir to mix. Bring to a boil over medium-high heat. Reduce the heat to low, cover, and simmer without stirring for about 15 minutes, or until most of the liquid has been absorbed.

4. Add the evaporated milk to the skillet, and, if necessary, increase the heat slightly to return the mixture to a simmer. Cook uncovered, stirring frequently, for about 5 minutes, or until the rice is tender but still a little firm to the bite, and most of the liquid has been absorbed. Add a little more broth during cooking if needed, leaving just enough liquid to make the mixture moist and creamy.

5. Return the scallops to the skillet mixture. Add the Parmesan cheese, and stir to mix. If the mixture seems too dry at this point, add a little more evaporated milk or broth. Stir in the spinach, cover, and cook over low heat without stirring for about 2 minutes, or until the spinach is wilted. Serve hot, topping each serving with a rounded teaspoon of additional Parmesan, if desired.

NUTRITIONAL FACTS (PER 1½-CUP SERVING)
Cal: 424   Carbs: 72 g   Chol: 22 mg   Fat: 1.4 g
Fiber: 1.6 g   Protein: 30.8 g   Sodium: 291 mg

Crispy Oven-Fried Fish

YIELD: 4 SERVINGS

1 pound cod, grouper, orange roughy, or other
white fish fillets, cut into 4 equal pieces

¼ cup plus 2 tablespoons fat-free egg substitute

½ cup corn flake crumbs or plain dried bread crumbs

1 teaspoon ground paprika

1–2 teaspoons lemon pepper

Nonstick cooking spray

TANGY TARTAR SAUCE

¼ cup nonfat or reduced-fat mayonnaise

2–3 teaspoons sweet pickle relish

2 teaspoons finely chopped onion

¼ teaspoon dry mustard

1. To make the tartar sauce, place all of the sauce ingredients in a small bowl, and stir to mix well. Cover and chill while you prepare the fish.

2. Rinse the fish with cool water, and pat it dry with paper towels. Set aside.

3. Place the egg substitute in a shallow bowl. Place the corn flake or bread crumbs, paprika, and lemon pepper in another shallow bowl, and stir to mix well. Dip the fish pieces first in the egg substitute and then in the crumb mixture, turning to coat both sides well.

4. Coat a medium-sized baking sheet with nonstick cooking spray, and arrange the fish pieces on the sheet in a single layer. Spray the tops lightly with the cooking spray, and bake at 450°F for about 15 minutes, or until the outside is crisp and golden and the fish flakes easily with a fork. Serve hot, accompanied by the tartar sauce.

NUTRITIONAL FACTS (PER SERVING)
Cal: 159   Carbs: 13 g   Chol: 48 mg   Fat: 0.7 g
Fiber: 0.4 g   Protein: 23 g   Sodium: 357 mg

Risotto With Shrimp and Asparagus

YIELD: 4 SERVINGS
8 ounces cleaned and deveined raw shrimp
1 teaspoon crushed fresh garlic
1½ cups arborio rice
3¼ cups unsalted chicken broth
½ cup dry white wine
⅛ teaspoon ground black pepper
¾ cup 1-inch pieces fresh asparagus, or ¾ cup frozen (thawed) 1-inch pieces asparagus
½ cup evaporated skim milk
3 tablespoons grated nonfat or regular Parmesan cheese

1. Rinse the shrimp with cool water, and pat them dry with paper towels.

2. Coat a large nonstick skillet with nonstick butter-flavored cooking spray, and preheat over medium-high heat. Add the garlic and shrimp, and stir-fry for about 3 minutes, or until the shrimp turn pink. Remove the shrimp from the skillet, and set aside.

3. Place the rice, broth, wine, and pepper in the skillet, and stir to mix. Bring to a boil over medium-high heat. Reduce the heat to low, cover, and simmer without stirring for about 12 minutes, or until about three-fourths of the liquid has been absorbed.

4. Add the asparagus to the skillet, and stir to mix well. Increase the heat to medium-high, and return the mixture to a boil. Reduce the heat to low, cover, and simmer without stirring for about 3 minutes, or until most of the liquid has been absorbed.

5. Add the evaporated milk to the skillet, and, if necessary, increase the heat slightly to return the mixture to a simmer. Cook uncovered, stirring frequently, for about 5 minutes, or until the rice is tender but still a little firm to the bite, and most of the liquid has been absorbed. Add a little more broth during cooking if needed, leaving just enough liquid to make the mixture moist and creamy. Return the shrimp to the skillet, and cook for another minute to heat through.

6. Stir the Parmesan cheese into the risotto. If the mixture seems too dry at this point, add a little more evaporated milk or broth. Serve hot, topping each serving with a rounded teaspoon of additional Parmesan, if desired.

NUTRITIONAL FACTS (PER 1½-CUP SERVING)
Cal: 402   Carbs: 63 g   Chol: 89 mg   Fat: 1.9 g
Fiber: 1.4 g   Protein: 28 g   Sodium: 259 mg

Italian Oven-Fried Scallops

YIELD: 4 SERVINGS
1 pound raw medium-large scallops
¼ cup plus 2 tablespoons fat-free egg substitute
½ cup Italian-style seasoned dried bread crumbs
2 tablespoons Parmesan cheese*
Nonstick olive oil cooking spray
2 tablespoons finely chopped Italian parsley
4 wedges lemon

* In this recipe, use regular Parmesan cheese, not a fat-free product.

1. Rinse the scallops with cool water, and pat them dry with paper towels. Set aside.

2. Place the egg substitute in a shallow dish. Place the bread crumbs and Parmesan cheese in another shallow dish, and stir to mix well. Dip the scallops first in the egg substitute and then in the bread crumb mixture, rolling the scallops in the crumbs to coat all sides evenly. (Note that if the scallops are small, you may need extra crumbs, as there will be more surface area to coat.)

3. Coat a 9-x-13-inch pan with nonstick olive oil cooking spray, and arrange the scallops in a single layer in the pan. Spray the tops lightly with the cooking spray.

4. Bake at 450°F for about 10 minutes, or until the scallops are nicely browned on the outside and opaque on the inside. Remove the pan from the oven and sprinkle with the parsley. Squeeze the lemon over the scallops, and serve hot.

NUTRITIONAL FACTS (PER SERVING)
Cal: 181   Carbs: 13.7 g   Chol: 41 mg   Fat: 2.2 g
Fiber: 0.6 g   Protein: 24 g   Sodium: 481 mg

Savory Stuffed Fish

YIELD: 4 SERVINGS

4 long, thin fish fillets (about 4 ounces each),
such as flounder, sole, or orange roughy

Nonstick butter-flavored cooking spray

Ground paprika

STUFFING

3 slices whole wheat or multigrain bread

1/4 cup finely chopped onion

1/4 cup finely chopped celery

3/4 teaspoon lemon pepper

1/4 teaspoon dried thyme

1/4 cup chicken broth, divided

3/4 cup finely chopped cooked crab meat,
or 1 can (6 ounces) crab meat, drained

1. Rinse the fish with cool water, and pat it dry with paper towels. Set aside.

2. To make the stuffing, tear the bread into pieces, place in a blender or food processor, and process into coarse crumbs. There should be 1 1/2 cups. Adjust the amount if necessary, and set aside.

3. Coat a large nonstick skillet with nonstick cooking spray, and preheat over medium heat. Add the onion, celery, lemon pepper, thyme, and 1 tablespoon of the broth, and stir to mix. Cover and cook, stirring occasionally, for about 3 minutes, or until the vegetables are tender. Add a little more broth if the skillet becomes too dry.

4. Remove the skillet from the heat, and toss the bread crumbs and crab meat into the vegetable mixture. Gently toss in the remaining broth, 1 tablespoon at a time, until the mixture is moist but not wet, and holds together nicely. Add a little more broth or water if needed.

5. Arrange the fish fillets on a flat surface, and spread a quarter of the stuffing over the bottom half of each fillet, gently pressing the stuffing onto the fish so that it holds together. Fold the tops over to enclose the filling, and secure each fillet with a wooden toothpick.

6. Coat a 9-inch nonstick square pan with nonstick butter-flavored cooking spray, and arrange the fillets in the pan. Spray the top of each fillet lightly with the cooking spray, and sprinkle with the paprika. Bake uncovered at 400°F for 20 minutes, or until the fish flakes easily with a fork. Serve hot.

NUTRITIONAL FACTS (PER SERVING)			
Cal: 184	Carbs: 11 g	Chol: 71 mg	Fat: 2.6 g
Fiber: 1.9 g	Protein: 28 g	Sodium: 306 mg	

Grilled Teriyaki Fish

YIELD: 6 SERVINGS

6 firm-fleshed fish steaks (about 5 ounces each),
such as grouper, mahi-mahi, swordfish,
fresh tuna, or amberjack

Nonstick butter-flavored cooking spray

MARINADE

1/2 cup unsweetened pineapple juice

2 tablespoons reduced-sodium soy sauce

2 tablespoons dry sherry

2 tablespoons dark brown sugar

1 scallion, finely minced

1 teaspoon crushed fresh garlic

1 teaspoon minced fresh ginger root,
or 1/3 teaspoon ground ginger

1 teaspoon sesame oil

1. Place all of the marinade ingredients in a small bowl, and stir to mix well. Set aside.

2. Rinse the fish steaks with cool water, and pat them dry with paper towels. Place the steaks in a shallow nonmetal container, and pour the marinade over the steaks, turning to coat all sides. Cover and refrigerate for several hours or overnight.

3. Spray the steaks lightly with the cooking spray, and grill over medium heat, covered, or under a broiler, for about 5 minutes on each side, or until the meat is easily flaked with a fork. Serve hot.

NUTRITIONAL FACTS (PER SERVING)			
Cal: 149	Carbs: 5 g	Chol: 53 mg	Fat: 1.9 g
Fiber: 0 g	Protein: 28 g	Sodium: 146 mg	

Foil-Baked Flounder

*Baking fish in a foil pouch allows the fish to steam
in its own juices, sealing in flavor and nutrients.
In this recipe, vegetables, wine, and herbs—not
fat or salt—provide added flavor and color.*

YIELD: 4 SERVINGS

4 flounder, sole, snapper, or orange roughy fillets
(about 6 ounces each)

2 teaspoons crushed fresh garlic

2 cups snow peas

2 cups thinly sliced carrots (about 2 medium)

1/4 cup chopped scallions

2 tablespoons plus 2 teaspoons minced fresh dill

2 teaspoons butter-flavored sprinkles

1/2 teaspoon ground black pepper

1/4 cup dry white wine

1. Rinse the fish with cool water, and pat it dry with
paper towels.

2. Cut four 8-x-12-inch pieces of heavy-duty aluminum foil, and center a fish fillet on the lower half
of each piece. Spread 1/2 teaspoon of garlic over each
fillet, and top with 1/2 cup of snow peas, 1/2 cup of
carrots, 1 tablespoon of scallions, 2 teaspoons of dill,
1/2 teaspoon of butter sprinkles, 1/8 teaspoon of pepper, and 1 tablespoon of wine.

3. Fold the upper half of the foil over the fish to meet
the bottom half. Seal the edges together by making a
tight 1/2-inch fold; then fold again to double-seal.
Allow space for heat circulation and expansion. Use
this technique to seal the remaining sides.

4. Arrange the pouches on a baking pan or directly
on the oven rack, and bake at 450°F for about 15 minutes, or until the fish is opaque and the thickest part
is easily flaked with a fork. Open each packet by carefully cutting an "X" in the top of the foil (steam will
escape), and serve hot.

NUTRITIONAL FACTS (PER SERVING)
Cal: 223   Carbs: 15 g   Chol: 82 mg   Fat: 2.3 g
Fiber: 3.2 g   Protein: 35 g   Sodium: 176 mg

11. Meatless Main Dishes

No one can dispute the health benefits of meatless eating. People who eat diets rich in veggies and low in fatty meats have a reduced risk of heart disease, high blood pressure, obesity—the list goes on and on. And meatless dishes can be both delicious and satisfying. Pastas, whole grains, beans, cheeses, garden-fresh vegetables, and herbs and spices can be combined to make dishes that are substantial enough for the largest of appetites, and flavorful enough for the fussiest of eaters.

There is one catch, though. Meatless meals made with ingredients like whole milk cheese, full-fat sour cream, and generous amounts of butter, margarine, or oil are no more healthful than meat-based meals. If this is hard to believe, consider this: Just one ounce of full-fat cheese, such as Cheddar, contains more than twice as much fat as a three-ounce serving of top beef round. The solution? Simply replace full-fat milk, cheese, and other dairy products with their low- or no-fat counterparts. By doing this—as well as making a few other simple recipe adjustments— you can enjoy healthy versions of many of your meatless favorites, including creamy macaroni and cheese and eggplant Parmesan. And by adding ultra-lean meat alternatives to your pantry, you can even indulge in a hearty bowl of chili.

As you peruse this chapter, remember that these are just some of the slimmed-down meatless entrées that can be found within the pages of this book. Chapter 2 includes a selection of vegetable omelettes, frittatas, and quiches that are perfect for any meal of the day. Chapter 5 presents a variety of meatless sandwiches, wraps, burritos, and pizzas. And Chapter 9 features an array of delightful vegetarian pasta dishes.

So if you're trying to eliminate meat from your diet—or if you simply want a change from the usual lunch and dinner fare—you've come to the right place. From Black Bean Burritos, to Roasted Ratatouille, to Risotto With Sun-Dried Tomatoes, this chapter will prove to you once and for all that dishes made without meat can be not only healthful and low in fat, but also absolutely delicious.

Swiss Noodle Kugel

YIELD: 6 SERVINGS

6 ounces wide no-yolk noodles

1 package (10 ounces) frozen chopped spinach, thawed and squeezed dry

1 can (4 ounces) sliced mushrooms, drained

1 cup nonfat or low-fat cottage cheese

1 cup shredded nonfat or reduced-fat Swiss cheese

1/4 cup plus 2 tablespoons grated Parmesan cheese, divided*

1 cup fat-free egg substitute

3/4 cup evaporated skim milk

1 pinch ground nutmeg

* In this recipe, use regular Parmesan cheese, not a fat-free product.

1. Cook the noodles al dente according to package directions. Drain well, and return to the pot.

2. Add the spinach, mushrooms, cottage cheese, Swiss cheese, and 3 tablespoons of the Parmesan cheese to the noodles, and toss to mix well.

3. Coat a 2^1/$_2$-quart casserole dish with nonstick cooking spray, and spread the noodle mixture evenly in the dish. Place the egg substitute, evaporated milk, and nutmeg in a small bowl, and stir to mix well. Pour the mixture over the noodles, and sprinkle the remaining 3 tablespoons of Parmesan over the top.

4. Cover the dish with aluminum foil, and bake at 350°F for 50 minutes. Remove the foil, and bake uncovered for 10 additional minutes, or until the top is lightly browned and a sharp knife inserted in the center of the dish comes out clean.

5. Remove the dish from the oven, and let sit for 10 minutes before serving.

NUTRITIONAL FACTS (PER 1¼-CUP SERVING)
Cal: 245   Carbs: 29 g   Chol: 11 mg   Fat: 2.4 g
Fiber: 2 g   Protein: 25 g   Sodium: 475 mg

Low-Fat Egg Foo Yung

For variety, make a nonvegetarian version by adding 1 cup of chopped cooked shrimp or crab meat.

YIELD: 4 SERVINGS

1^1/$_2$ cups fat-free egg substitute

4 cups mung bean sprouts

1 can (8 ounces) water chestnuts, drained and chopped

2 scallions, thinly sliced

1/8 teaspoon ground black pepper

SAUCE

2 teaspoons cornstarch

1 teaspoon dark brown sugar

1 cup unsalted vegetable broth

2 tablespoons reduced-sodium soy sauce or hoisin sauce

1 teaspoon sesame oil

1. To make the sauce, place the cornstarch and brown sugar in a 1-quart saucepan, and stir to mix well. Add the broth, the soy or hoisin sauce, and the sesame oil, and stir until smooth. Place the pan over medium heat, and cook, stirring constantly, until thickened and bubbly. Cover to keep warm, and set aside.

2. Place the egg substitute, sprouts, water chestnuts, scallions, and pepper in a large bowl, and stir to mix well.

3. Coat a griddle or large skillet with nonstick cooking spray, and preheat over medium heat. For each pancake, pour ^{1}/$_2$ cup of the egg mixture onto the griddle, spreading the bean sprouts out evenly to make a 4-inch cake. Cook for 3 minutes, or until the eggs are almost set. Flip the pancake over, and cook for 2 additional minutes, or until the eggs are completely set. As the pancakes are done, transfer them to a serving plate and keep warm in a preheated oven.

4. Serve hot, topping each serving with some of the sauce.

NUTRITIONAL FACTS (PER 2-PANCAKE SERVING)
Cal: 118   Carbs: 15 g   Chol: 0 mg   Fat: 1.5 g
Fiber: 4 g   Protein: 13 g   Sodium: 512 mg

Lentil Crunch Casserole

YIELD: 5 SERVINGS
3/4 cup dried brown lentils, cleaned (page 302)
1 3/4 cups water
1 2/3 cups quick-cooking brown rice
1 2/3 cups vegetable broth
1 cup coarsely chopped fresh mushrooms
2/3 cup chopped onion
2/3 cup thinly sliced celery
1/4 cup chopped toasted walnuts (page 348)
1/2 teaspoon dried thyme
1/4 cup plus 2 tablespoons grated Parmesan cheese, divided*

* In this recipe, use regular Parmesan cheese, not a fat-free product.

1. Place the lentils and water in a 1 1/2-quart pot, and bring to a boil over high heat. Reduce the heat to low, cover, and simmer for 20 to 25 minutes, or until the lentils are tender. Remove the pot from the heat, drain off any excess water, and set aside.

2. Place the rice and broth in a 2 1/2-quart pot, and bring to a boil over high heat. Reduce the heat to low, cover, and simmer for 5 minutes, or until the rice is tender and the liquid has been absorbed. Remove the pot from the heat, and let sit covered for 5 minutes.

3. Add the lentils, mushrooms, onion, celery, walnuts, thyme, and 1/4 cup of the Parmesan to the rice. Toss to mix well.

4. Coat a 2-quart casserole dish with nonstick cooking spray, and spread the rice mixture evenly in the dish. Sprinkle with the remaining 2 tablespoons of Parmesan, cover with aluminum foil, and bake at 350°F for 30 minutes, or until the dish is heated through and the vegetables are crisp-tender. Remove the foil, and bake uncovered for 5 additional minutes, or until the top is lightly browned. Serve hot.

NUTRITIONAL FACTS (PER 1 1/4-CUP SERVING)
Cal: 285 Carbs: 43 g Chol: 5 mg Fat: 7 g
Fiber: 11 g Protein: 15 g Sodium: 373 mg

Spinach and Barley Bake

For variety, substitute brown rice for the barley.

YIELD: 4 SERVINGS
2/3 cup hulled or pearled barley
1 2/3 cups water
1 package (10 ounces) frozen chopped spinach, thawed and squeezed dry
1 cup sliced fresh mushrooms
1 teaspoon crushed fresh garlic
1 1/2 cups nonfat or low-fat cottage cheese
1/4 cup plus 2 tablespoons grated Parmesan cheese, divided*
1/2 cup fat-free egg substitute
1 tablespoon unbleached flour
1/2 teaspoon dried thyme
1/8 teaspoon ground black pepper

* In this recipe, use regular Parmesan cheese, not a fat-free product.

1. Place the barley and water in a 1 1/2-quart pot, and bring to a boil over high heat. Reduce the heat to low, cover, and simmer for about 50 minutes, or until the barley is tender and the liquid has been absorbed.

2. Place the cooked barley and all of the remaining ingredients except for 2 tablespoons of the Parmesan in a large bowl, and stir to mix well. Coat a 1 1/2-quart casserole dish with cooking spray, and spread the mixture evenly in the dish. Sprinkle the remaining Parmesan over the top.

3. Bake uncovered at 375°F for 50 to 60 minutes, or until golden brown and bubbly. Remove the dish from the oven, and let sit for 5 minutes before serving.

NUTRITIONAL FACTS (PER 1 1/4-CUP SERVING)
Cal: 257 Carbs: 34 g Chol: 15 mg Fat: 3.4 g
Fiber: 7 g Protein: 23 g Sodium: 445 mg

Enchilada Pie

YIELD: 6 SERVINGS

1 can (14$\frac{1}{2}$ ounces) Mexican-style stewed tomatoes, crushed

1$\frac{1}{2}$ teaspoons chili powder

10 corn tortillas (6-inch rounds)

1 can (15 ounces) black or pinto beans, rinsed and drained

1$\frac{1}{2}$ cups frozen (thawed) whole kernel corn, or 1 can (15 ounces) whole kernel corn, drained

1 can (4 ounces) chopped green chilies, drained

$\frac{1}{2}$ cup plus 2 tablespoons nonfat or light sour cream

1$\frac{1}{2}$ cups shredded nonfat or reduced-fat Cheddar or Monterey jack cheese

1. Place the tomatoes and chili powder in a small bowl, and stir to mix. Spread $\frac{1}{4}$ cup of the tomato mixture over the bottom of a 10-inch pie pan. Line the bottom of the pan with 4 of the tortillas, overlapping them as needed to make them fit.

2. Spread half of the beans over the tortilla-lined pie pan. Top with half of the corn, half of the chilies, and $\frac{1}{2}$ cup of the tomato mixture. Dot with half of the sour cream, and sprinkle with $\frac{1}{2}$ cup of the cheese. Repeat the layers, this time using only 3 tortillas. Top with the 3 remaining tortillas, and spread the remaining tomatoes over the top.

3. Coat a piece of aluminum foil with nonstick cooking spray, and cover the pan with the foil, coated side down. (This will prevent the tortillas from sticking to the foil.) Bake at 350°F for 35 minutes, or until the dish is heated through. Remove the foil, and sprinkle the remaining $\frac{1}{2}$ cup of cheese over the top. Return the dish to the oven, and bake uncovered for 3 additional minutes, or until the cheese is melted.

4. Remove the dish from the oven, and let sit for 5 minutes before cutting into wedges and serving.

NUTRITIONAL FACTS (PER SERVING)
Cal: 251   Carbs: 42 g   Chol: 3 mg   Fat: 1.5 g
Fiber: 8 g   Protein: 18 g   Sodium: 570 mg

Zucchini-Rice Casserole

YIELD: 6 SERVINGS

2 medium zucchini, halved lengthwise and sliced $\frac{1}{4}$-inch thick (about 2 cups)

1$\frac{1}{2}$ cups sliced fresh mushrooms

$\frac{1}{2}$ cup chopped onion

2 medium plum tomatoes, chopped

1 teaspoon crushed fresh garlic

3 cups cooked brown rice

$\frac{1}{2}$ cup fat-free egg substitute

$\frac{1}{2}$ cup plain nonfat or low-fat yogurt

1 cup shredded nonfat or reduced-fat Swiss or mozzarella cheese

$\frac{1}{8}$ teaspoon ground black pepper

3 tablespoons grated Parmesan cheese*

* In this recipe, use regular Parmesan cheese, not a fat-free product.

1. Coat a large skillet with nonstick cooking spray, and preheat over medium heat. Add the zucchini, mushrooms, onions, tomatoes, and garlic, and cook, stirring constantly, for several minutes, or until the vegetables are tender and most of the liquid has evaporated.

2. Remove the skillet from the heat, and set aside to cool slightly. Stir in first the rice, and then the egg substitute, yogurt, Swiss or mozzarella, and pepper.

3. Coat a 2-quart casserole dish with nonstick cooking spray, and spread the mixture evenly in the dish. Sprinkle the Parmesan over the top, and bake uncovered at 350°F for about 50 minutes, or until browned and bubbly. Remove the dish from the oven, and let sit for 5 minutes before serving.

NUTRITIONAL FACTS (PER 1$\frac{1}{4}$-CUP SERVING)
Cal: 193   Carbs: 29 g   Chol: 6 mg   Fat: 2 g
Fiber: 3 g   Protein: 14 g   Sodium: 278 mg

Mega Macaroni and Cheese

YIELD: 6 SERVINGS

8 ounces ziti pasta (about 3 cups)

2½ cups skim or low-fat milk, divided

3 tablespoons unbleached flour

1½ teaspoons dry mustard

⅛ teaspoon ground black pepper

¼ cup finely chopped onion

1 tablespoon water

8 ounces nonfat or reduced-fat process
Cheddar cheese or reduced-fat Cheddar cheese,
shredded or diced (about 2 cups)

1 jar (2 ounces) chopped pimentos, drained

2 tablespoons seasoned dried bread crumbs

Nonstick butter-flavored cooking spray

1. Cook the pasta al dente according to package directions. Drain well, return to the pot, and cover to keep warm.

2. While the pasta is cooking, place ½ cup of the milk and all of the flour, mustard, and pepper in a jar with a tight-fitting lid. Shake until smooth, and set aside.

3. Place the onion and water in a 2-quart nonstick pot. Cover and cook over medium heat, stirring occasionally, for about 3 minutes, or until the onions are soft.

4. Add the remaining 2 cups of milk to the pot, and bring to a boil over medium heat, stirring constantly. Add the flour mixture, and cook, still stirring, for about 1 minute, or until the mixture begins to boil and thickens slightly. Reduce the heat to medium-low, add the cheese, and stir just until the cheese has melted.

5. Pour the cheese sauce over the pasta. Add the pimentos, and toss to mix well. Coat a 2½-quart casserole dish with nonstick cooking spray, and spread the pasta mixture evenly in the dish. Sprinkle the crumbs over the top, and spray the top with the cooking spray.

6. Bake uncovered at 350°F for about 30 minutes, or until hot and bubbly around the edges. Remove the

dish from the oven, and let sit for 10 minutes before serving.

> **NUTRITIONAL FACTS (PER 1-CUP SERVING)**
> Cal: 255   Carbs: 38 g   Chol: 2 mg   Fat: 1.4 g
> Fiber: 1.5 g   Protein: 20 g   Sodium: 322 mg

Spicy Rice Casserole

YIELD: 6 SERVINGS

¾ cup chopped onion

¾ cup chopped green bell pepper

1 teaspoon crushed fresh garlic

4 cups cooked brown rice

1 can (15 ounces) red kidney beans, pinto beans,
or black beans, drained

1 cup plus 2 tablespoons frozen (thawed)
whole kernel corn

1 can (14½ ounces) Mexican-style stewed tomatoes,
drained and chopped

2 teaspoons chili powder

1 cup shredded nonfat or reduced-fat Cheddar cheese

1. Coat a large nonstick skillet with nonstick cooking spray, and preheat over medium heat. Add the onion, green pepper, and garlic, and stir to mix. Cover the skillet and cook, stirring occasionally, for about 3 minutes, or until the vegetables begin to soften. Add a few teaspoons of water if the skillet seems too dry.

2. Remove the skillet from the heat. Add the rice, beans, corn, tomatoes, and chili powder, and stir to mix well. Add the cheese, and stir to mix well.

3. Coat a 2½-quart casserole dish with nonstick cooking spray, and spread the mixture evenly in the dish. Cover with aluminum foil, and bake at 350°F for 45 minutes, or until the mixture is heated through and the cheese is melted. Remove the dish from the oven, and let sit for 5 minutes before serving.

> **NUTRITIONAL FACTS (PER 1⅓-CUP SERVING)**
> Cal: 318   Carbs: 60 g   Chol: 2 mg   Fat: 1.6 g
> Fiber: 10.7 g   Protein: 16.5 g   Sodium: 348 mg

Black Bean Burritos

YIELD: 4 SERVINGS

1½ cups cooked black beans, or 1 can (15 ounces) black beans, drained

1 teaspoon chili powder

4 flour tortillas (8-inch rounds)

1 cup frozen (thawed) whole kernel corn

½ cup bottled salsa

½ cup shredded nonfat or reduced-fat Cheddar cheese

TOPPINGS

1 cup shredded lettuce

½ cup chopped tomatoes

½ cup nonfat or light sour cream

¼ cup sliced scallions

1. Place the beans and chili powder in a 1-quart pot, and mash lightly with a fork or a potato masher, leaving the beans slightly chunky. Cover and cook over medium heat, stirring occasionally, for about 2 minutes, or until heated through. Set aside.

2. Warm the tortillas according to package directions. Lay a warm tortilla on a flat surface, and spoon a quarter of the beans along the right side of the tortilla, stopping 1½ inches from the bottom. Top the beans with a quarter of the corn.

3. Fold the bottom edge of the tortilla up about 1 inch. (This fold will prevent the filling from falling out.) Then, beginning at the right edge, roll the tortilla up jelly-roll style. Repeat with the remaining ingredients to make 4 burritos.

4. Coat a 9-x-13-inch pan with nonstick cooking spray, and arrange the burritos, seam side down, in a single layer in the pan. Spread the salsa over the tops of the burritos, and sprinkle with the cheese. Cover the pan with aluminum foil.

5. Bake at 350°F for 20 minutes, or until the burritos are heated through and the cheese has melted. Top each burrito with ¼ cup of lettuce, 2 tablespoons of tomatoes, 2 tablespoons of sour cream, and a tablespoon of the scallions, and serve hot.

NUTRITIONAL FACTS (PER BURRITO)

Cal: 286   Carbs: 50 g   Chol: 1 mg   Fat: 2.5 g
Fiber: 8.1 g   Protein: 15 g   Sodium: 467 mg

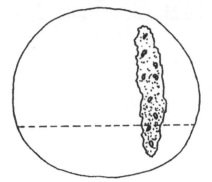

a. Arrange the filling along the right side of the tortilla.

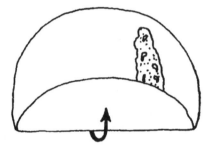

b. Fold the bottom edge of the tortilla up.

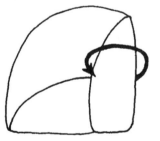

c. Fold the right side over the filling.

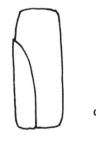

d. Continue folding to form a roll.

MAKING BLACK BEAN BURRITOS

Black Bean Quesadillas

YIELD: 4 SERVINGS

1 can (15 ounces) black beans, drained

2 teaspoons chili powder

1/4 teaspoon ground cumin

1 teaspoon crushed fresh garlic

1 small red bell pepper, cut into thin strips

1 small onion, cut into thin wedges

4 flour tortillas (8-inch rounds)

1 cup shredded nonfat or reduced-fat Cheddar or Monterey Jack cheese

Nonstick olive oil cooking spray

TOPPINGS

1/2 cup nonfat or light sour cream

1/2 cup diced tomato

1/4 cup thinly sliced scallions

4 large pitted black olives, sliced

1. Place the beans, chili powder, and cumin in a medium-sized bowl, and mash with a fork until the mixture has the consistency of refried beans. Set aside.

2. Coat a large nonstick skillet with nonstick cooking spray, and preheat over medium-high heat. Add the garlic, red pepper, and onion, and stir-fry for about 3 minutes, or until the vegetables are crisp-tender. Cover the skillet periodically if it begins to dry out. (The steam from the cooking vegetables will moisten the skillet.) Add a few teaspoons of water only if necessary. Remove the skillet from the heat, and set aside.

3. Arrange the tortillas on a flat surface, and spread a quarter of the bean mixture over the bottom half of each tortilla, extending the filling all the way to the edge. Layer a quarter of the red pepper mixture over the beans on each tortilla. Sprinkle 1/4 cup of cheese over the vegetables. Fold the top half of each tortilla over the bottom half to enclose the filling.

4. Coat a large baking sheet with nonstick cooking spray. Arrange the quesadillas on the sheet, and spray the tops lightly with the cooking spray. Bake uncovered at 400°F for 4 minutes. Turn the quesadillas over, and bake for 5 additional minutes, or until the cheese has melted and the quesadillas are heated through.

5. Transfer the quesadillas to individual serving plates, and top each with 2 tablespoons of the sour cream, 2 tablespoons of the tomatoes, 1 tablespoon of the scallions, and a few olive slices. Serve hot.

NUTRITIONAL FACTS (PER QUESADILLA)
Cal: 332   Carbs: 53 g   Chol: 3 mg   Fat: 3.4 g
Fiber: 9.5 g   Protein: 20 g   Sodium: 595 mg

Spicy Pinto Beans

YIELD: 7 CUPS

2 cups dried pinto beans, cleaned and soaked (page 302)

5 1/2 cups water

1 medium onion, chopped

1 tablespoon chopped or pickled jalapeño peppers

1 teaspoon crushed fresh garlic

1 tablespoon instant ham, chicken, or vegetable bouillon granules

2 teaspoons chili powder

1 1/4 teaspoons ground cumin

2 medium tomatoes, diced

1/3 cup chopped fresh cilantro or scallions (garnish)

1. Place all of the ingredients except for the tomatoes and cilantro in a 3-quart pot, and bring to a boil over high heat. Reduce the heat to low, cover, and simmer, stirring occasionally, for 1 hour and 30 minutes, or until the beans are soft. Periodically check the pot during cooking, and add a little more broth or water if needed.

2. Add the tomatoes to the bean mixture, and cook for 30 additional minutes. Serve hot, topping each serving with some of the cilantro or scallions. If desired, ladle the beans over brown rice.

NUTRITIONAL FACTS (PER 1-CUP SERVING)
Cal: 184   Carbs: 33 g   Chol: 0 mg   Fat: 0.9 g
Fiber: 15 g   Protein: 11 g   Sodium: 289 mg

Bean Basics

If you really want to improve the quality of your diet, think beans. A hearty and satisfying alternative to meat, beans are low in fat, and rich in protein, complex carbohydrates, B vitamins, iron, zinc, copper, and potassium. As for fiber, no other food surpasses beans. Just a half cup of cooked beans provides 4 to 8 grams of fiber—up to four times the amount found in most other plant foods. Beans also help maintain healthy blood sugar and cholesterol levels. As an added bonus, beans keep you feeling full and satisfied long after the meal is over—a definite benefit if you're watching your weight.

Some people avoid eating beans because of "bean bloat." What causes this problem? Complex sugars in beans, called oligosaccharides, sometimes form gas when broken down in the lower intestine. This side effect usually subsides when beans are made a regular part of the diet, and the body becomes more efficient at digesting them. The proper cleaning, soaking, and cooking of dried beans can also help you make beans a delicious and healthful part of your diet.

CLEANING

Because beans are a natural product, packages of dried beans sometimes contain shriveled or discolored beans, as well as small twigs and other items. Before cooking, sort through your beans and discard any discolored or blemished legumes. Rinse the beans well, cover them with water, and discard any that float to the top.

SOAKING

There are two methods used to soak beans in preparation for cooking. If you have time—if you intend to cook your dish the next day, for instance—you may want to use the long method, as this technique is best for reducing the gas-producing oligosaccharides. If dinner is just a cou-ple of hours away, though, the quick method is your best bet. Keep in mind that not all beans must be soaked before cooking. Black-eyed peas, brown and red lentils, and split peas do not require soaking.

The Long Method

After cleaning the beans, place them in a large bowl or pot, and cover them with four times as much water. Soak the beans for at least four hours, and for as long as twelve hours. If soaking them for more than four, place the bowl or pot in the refrigerator. After soaking, discard the water and replace with fresh water before cooking.

The Quick Method

After cleaning the beans, place them in a large pot, and cover them with four times as much water. Bring the pot to a boil over high heat, and continue to boil for two minutes. Remove the pot from the heat, cover, and let stand for one hour. After soaking, discard the water and replace with fresh water before cooking.

COOKING

To cook beans for use in salads, casseroles, and other dishes that contain little or no liquid, clean and soak as described above, discard the soaking water, and replace with two cups of water for each cup of dried beans. When beans are to be cooked in soups or stews that include acidic ingredients—lemon juice, vinegar, or tomatoes, for instance—add these ingredients at the end of the cooking time. Acidic foods can toughen the beans' outer layer, slowing the rate at which the beans cook. You'll know that the beans are done when you can mash them easily with a fork. Keep in mind that old beans may take longer to cook. The use of hard water can also lengthen cooking times. During long cooking times, periodically check the pot, and add more liquid if necessary.

The following table gives approximate cooking times for several different kinds of beans. Need a meal in a hurry? Lentils, split peas, and black-eyed peas require no soaking and cook quickly.

Lentils are the fastest cooking of all legumes; they can be prepared in less than thirty minutes. Split peas cook in less than an hour, and black-eyed peas, in about an hour.

COOKING TIMES FOR DRIED BEANS AND LEGUMES

Bean or Legume	Cooking Time
Black, great northern, kidney, navy, pinto, and white beans, and chickpeas	$1^1/_2$–2 hours
Black-eyed peas*	1–$1^1/_4$ hours
Lentils, brown*	20–30 minutes
Lentils, red*	15–20 minutes
Lima beans, baby	45 minutes–$1^1/_4$ hours
Lima beans, large	1–$1^1/_2$ hours
Split peas*	45 minutes–1 hour

* These beans do not require soaking.

Spicy Lentils and Rice

YIELD: 4 SERVINGS

$1^3/_4$ cups plus 2 tablespoons vegetable or chicken broth, divided

$3/_4$ cup brown lentils, cleaned (page 302)

$1^1/_2$ cups coarsely chopped fresh mushrooms

1 medium yellow onion, chopped

2 teaspoons curry paste

$1^1/_2$ teaspoons crushed fresh garlic

$1/_2$ teaspoon ground cumin

$1/_2$ teaspoon ground ginger

$2^1/_2$ cups cooked brown rice

$3/_4$ cup frozen (thawed) green peas

1. Place $1^1/_2$ cups of the broth and all of the lentils in a $1^1/_2$-quart pot, and bring to a boil over high heat.

Reduce the heat to low, cover, and simmer for about 20 minutes, or until the lentils are tender and the liquid is absorbed. Set aside.

2. Coat a large nonstick skillet with nonstick cooking spray, and preheat over medium heat. Add the mushrooms, onion, curry paste, garlic, cumin, ginger, and 2 tablespoons of the remaining broth. Cover and cook, stirring occasionally, for about 4 minutes, or until the onions and mushrooms are tender.

3. Add the rice, peas, lentils, and remaining $1/_4$ cup of broth to the skillet, and stir to mix. Cook over medium heat, stirring frequently, for about 3 minutes, or until well mixed and heated through. Serve hot.

NUTRITIONAL FACTS (PER 1$1/_3$-CUP SERVING)
Cal: 313   Carbs: 56 g   Chol: 0 mg   Fat: 2.9 g
Fiber: 9.4 g   Protein: 15.6 g   Sodium: 322 mg

Orzo and Vegetable Pie

*This savory pie features a crust made with orzo—
a small pasta that resembles rice.*

YIELD: 6 SERVINGS
2 medium-large zucchini, halved lengthwise and sliced ¼-inch thick (about 2½ cups)
1¼ cups sliced fresh mushrooms
1 cup diced plum tomatoes (about 3 medium)
1 teaspoon crushed fresh garlic
1 teaspoon dried Italian seasoning
⅛ teaspoon ground black pepper
2 tablespoons grated Parmesan cheese*
Nonstick butter-flavored cooking spray
1 cup shredded nonfat or reduced-fat mozzarella cheese

CRUST
8 ounces orzo pasta (about 1 cup)
⅓ cup grated Parmesan cheese*
¼ cup fat-free egg substitute

* In this recipe, use regular Parmesan cheese, not a fat-free product.

1. To make the crust, cook the orzo al dente according to package directions. Drain well, and return to the pot. Add the Parmesan cheese and egg substitute, and stir to mix well.

2. Coat a 9-inch deep dish pie pan with nonstick cooking spray, and place the orzo mixture in the pan. Using the back of a spoon, pat the mixture over the bottom and sides of the pan, forming an even crust. Set aside.

3. Coat a large nonstick skillet with nonstick cooking spray, and preheat over medium heat. Add the zucchini, mushrooms, tomatoes, garlic, Italian seasoning, and pepper, and stir to mix. Cover and cook, stirring occasionally, for about 7 minutes, or until the zucchini is crisp-tender and the tomatoes are soft. Remove the cover, and cook for 3 additional minutes, or until most of the liquid has evaporated.

4. Spread the vegetable mixture evenly over the bottom of the crust, and sprinkle with the Parmesan cheese. Spray the exposed edges of the crust lightly with the cooking spray.

5. Bake uncovered at 400°F for 15 minutes, or until the dish is heated through and the top is lightly browned. Spread the mozzarella evenly over the vegetables, and bake for 5 additional minutes, or until the cheese has melted.

6. Remove the dish from the oven, and let sit for 5 minutes before cutting into wedges and serving.

NUTRITIONAL FACTS (PER SERVING)
Cal: 229   Carbs: 32 g   Chol: 9 mg   Fat: 3.2 g
Fiber: 2.2 g   Protein: 16 g   Sodium: 328 mg

Curried Lentils

YIELD: 5 CUPS
3 cups unsalted chicken broth or water
1 cup dried brown or red lentils, cleaned (page 302)
1 large onion, chopped
2 medium carrots, peeled, halved, and sliced
2 stalks celery, thinly sliced (include the leaves)
1 large Granny Smith apple, peeled and finely chopped
2–3 teaspoons curry paste
1½ teaspoons instant chicken bouillon granules
1 teaspoon crushed fresh garlic

1. Place all of the ingredients in a 2½-quart pot, and bring to a boil over high heat. Reduce the heat to low, cover, and simmer, stirring occasionally, for about 30 minutes, or until the lentils are soft. (If you're using red lentils, cook the mixture for only about 20 minutes.)

2. Serve hot, ladling each serving over brown rice or whole wheat couscous, if desired.

NUTRITIONAL FACTS (PER 1-CUP SERVING)
Cal: 192   Carbs: 32 g   Chol: 0 mg   Fat: 1.8 g
Fiber: 7.2 g   Protein: 12 g   Sodium: 340 mg

Roasted Ratatouille

YIELD: 4 SERVINGS
1⅓ cups brown rice
3⅓ cups water
1 pound fresh plum tomatoes, quartered lengthwise (about 6 medium)
2 cups ¾-inch cubes peeled eggplant (about 1 small)
1 medium-large zucchini, halved lengthwise and sliced ½-inch thick
1 medium green bell pepper, cut into ½-inch-thick strips
1 medium yellow onion, cut into ½-inch-thick wedges
2 teaspoons crushed fresh garlic
1 tablespoon balsamic vinegar
1 tablespoon extra virgin olive oil
¾ teaspoon dried thyme
½ teaspoon salt
⅛ teaspoon ground black pepper
½ cup crumbled nonfat or reduced-fat feta cheese

1. Place the rice and water in a 2½-quart nonstick pot, and bring to a boil over high heat. Stir, reduce the heat to low, and cover. Allow to simmer for 45 to 50 minutes, or until the water is absorbed and the rice is tender. Do not stir during cooking.

2. While the rice is cooking, place the vegetables, garlic, vinegar, olive oil, thyme, salt, and pepper in a large bowl, and toss to mix well.

3. Coat a 9-x-13-inch nonstick roasting pan with nonstick olive oil cooking spray, and spread the vegetable mixture evenly in the pan. Cover the pan with aluminum foil.

4. Bake at 450°F for 15 minutes. Then remove the foil and bake uncovered for 15 additional minutes. Turn the vegetables, and bake for 15 minutes more, or until the tomatoes are soft and the vegetables are nicely browned.

5. Place 1 cup of rice on each of 4 serving plates, and top with 1 cup of the vegetable mixture. Serve hot, topping each serving with 2 tablespoons of the feta cheese.

NUTRITIONAL FACTS (PER SERVING)
Cal: 352   Carbs: 59 g   Chol: 1 mg   Fat: 5.7 g
Fiber: 7 g   Protein: 10.8 g   Sodium: 548 mg

Fiesta Bean Bake

YIELD: 5 SERVINGS
1 teaspoon whole cumin seeds
1 medium zucchini, halved and sliced ¼-inch thick
½ cup chopped onion
¼ cup finely chopped red bell pepper
4 cups cooked brown rice
1 can (15 ounces) pinto or black beans, rinsed and drained
1¼ cups shredded nonfat or reduced-fat Cheddar or Monterey jack cheese, divided

1. Coat a large nonstick skillet with nonstick cooking spray, and preheat over medium-high heat. Add the cumin seeds, and stir-fry for about 1 minute, or until the seeds smell toasted and fragrant. Add the zucchini, onion, and red pepper, and stir-fry for about 2 minutes, or just until the vegetables are crisp-tender.

2. Remove the skillet from the heat, and toss in the rice and beans. Add 1 cup of the cheese to the rice mixture, and toss to mix well.

3. Coat a 2-quart casserole dish with nonstick cooking spray, and spread the rice mixture evenly in the dish. Cover with aluminum foil, and bake at 350°F for about 25 minutes, or until the casserole is heated through. Remove the foil, sprinkle the remaining ¼ cup of cheese over the top, and bake uncovered for 5 additional minutes, or just until the cheese has melted. Serve hot.

NUTRITIONAL FACTS (PER 1⅓-CUP SERVING)
Cal: 299   Carbs: 52 g   Chol: 3 mg   Fat: 1.8 g
Fiber: 8 g   Protein: 18 g   Sodium: 355 mg

Southwestern Black Beans

YIELD: 8 SERVINGS

2½ cups dried black beans,
cleaned and soaked (page 302)

7½ cups water

2 medium yellow onions, chopped

1 large green bell pepper, chopped

2 dried hot red chili pepper pods

2 teaspoons crushed fresh garlic

1 tablespoon instant ham, chicken,
or vegetable bouillon granules

1 tablespoon chili powder

1 teaspoon dried oregano

½ teaspoon ground cumin

¼ teaspoon ground black pepper

3 tablespoons distilled white vinegar

TOPPINGS

¾ cup shredded nonfat or reduced-fat
Cheddar cheese

½ cup nonfat or light sour cream

¼ cup sliced scallions

1. Place all of the ingredients except for the vinegar and toppings in a 4-quart pot, and bring to a boil over high heat. Reduce the heat to low, cover, and simmer, stirring occasionally, for about 2 hours, or until the beans are soft and the liquid is thick. Periodically check the pot during cooking, and add a little more water if needed.

2. Remove the pot from the heat, discard the pepper pods, and stir in the vinegar. Serve hot, topping each serving with a 1½ tablespoons of cheese, 1 tablespoon of sour cream, and 1½ teaspoons of scallions. Serve over brown rice, if desired.

> **NUTRITIONAL FACTS** (PER 1-CUP SERVING)
> Cal: 237   Carbs: 41 g   Chol: 2 mg   Fat: 0.8 g
> Fiber: 16 g   Protein: 16 g   Sodium: 345 mg

Curry in a Hurry

YIELD: 4 SERVINGS

1 can (15 ounces) red kidney beans, rinsed and drained

1¾ cups water

1½ cups quick-cooking brown rice

¾ cup diced carrot

½ cup thinly sliced celery

½ cup chopped onion

2–3 teaspoons curry paste

1 teaspoon instant vegetable or chicken bouillon granules

1. Place all of the ingredients in a large skillet. Stir to mix well, and bring to a boil over high heat. Reduce the heat to low, cover, and simmer for 10 minutes, or until the rice is tender and the liquid has been absorbed.

2. Remove the skillet from the heat, and let sit covered for 5 minutes. Fluff with a fork, and serve hot.

> **NUTRITIONAL FACTS** (PER 1⅓-CUP SERVING)
> Cal: 271   Carbs: 50 g   Chol: 0 mg   Fat: 2.6 g
> Fiber: 11 g   Protein: 11 g   Sodium: 258 mg

Vegetable-Brown Rice Curry

YIELD: 5 SERVINGS

1½ cups small cauliflower florets

1 cup finely chopped peeled tomatoes
(about 1½ medium)

¾ cup chopped onion

½ cup finely chopped carrot

2 tablespoons vegetable or chicken broth

2–3 teaspoons curry paste

2 teaspoons crushed fresh garlic

½ teaspoon ground ginger

¼ teaspoon salt

4 cups cooked brown rice

1 can (15 ounces) red kidney beans, rinsed and
drained, or 1 recipe Crispy Tofu Cubes (page 314)

¾ cup frozen (thawed) green peas

1. Place the cauliflower, tomatoes, onion, carrot, broth, curry paste, garlic, ginger, and salt in a large nonstick skillet. Cover and cook over medium heat, stirring occasionally, for 5 to 7 minutes, or until the vegetables are tender. Add a little more broth if the skillet becomes too dry.

2. Add the rice, beans or tofu, and peas to the skillet. Cook and stir over medium heat until the mixture is heated through, and serve hot.

NUTRITIONAL FACTS (PER 1²/₃-CUP SERVING)
Cal: 318   Carbs: 61 g   Chol: 0 mg   Fat: 3g
Fiber: 12.4 g   Protein: 12 g   Sodium: 382 mg

Jamaican Red Beans

YIELD: 7 CUPS

2 cups dried red kidney beans, cleaned and soaked (page 302)

6 cups water

2 medium onions, chopped

2 stalks celery, thinly sliced (include the leaves)

1 tablespoon instant ham or chicken bouillon granules

2 teaspoons dried thyme

¹/₂ teaspoon ground allspice

¹/₄ teaspoon ground black pepper

2 bay leaves

2–3 dried hot red chili pepper pods

2 tablespoons distilled white vinegar

1. Place all of the ingredients except for the vinegar in a 3-quart pot, and bring to a boil over high heat. Reduce the heat to low, cover, and simmer, stirring occasionally, for 2 hours, or until the beans are soft and the liquid is thick. Add a little more liquid during cooking if needed.

2. Remove the pot from the heat, and discard the bay leaves and pepper pods. Stir in the vinegar, and serve hot, ladling the beans over brown rice, if desired.

NUTRITIONAL FACTS (PER 1-CUP SERVING)
Cal: 193   Carbs: 35 g   Chol: 0 mg   Fat: 0.6 g
Fiber: 12 g   Protein: 12 g   Sodium: 287 mg

Spicy Vegetable Stew

YIELD: 6 SERVINGS

1 can (14¹/₂ ounces) unsalted tomatoes, crushed

1 can (14¹/₂ ounces) vegetable broth

¹/₂ cup tomato paste

1 medium yellow onion, chopped

1 medium green bell pepper, chopped

1 large sweet potato (about 12 ounces), peeled and diced

2¹/₂ cups fresh or frozen (unthawed) cauliflower florets

1 cup fresh or frozen (unthawed) cut green beans

1 can (1 pound) chickpeas, drained

2 teaspoons crushed fresh garlic

1¹/₂ teaspoons ground paprika

¹/₂ teaspoon ground allspice

¹/₄ teaspoon ground cinnamon

¹/₄ cup golden raisins

1. Place all of the ingredients except for the raisins in a 3-quart pot. Stir to mix well, and bring to a boil over high heat. Reduce the heat to low, cover, and simmer for 20 to 25 minutes, or until the vegetables are tender and the flavors are well blended.

2. Add the raisins to the pot, and simmer for 5 additional minutes, or until the raisins are plumped. Serve hot, ladling the stew over whole wheat couscous, bulgur wheat, or brown rice, if desired.

NUTRITIONAL FACTS (PER 1¹/₂-CUP SERVING)
Cal: 188   Carbs: 34 g   Chol: 0 mg   Fat: 2.1 g
Fiber: 7.2 g   Protein: 8 g   Sodium: 448 mg

Savory Stuffed Peppers

YIELD: 4 SERVINGS

4 large green bell peppers

FILLING

1/2 cup plus 1 tablespoon dried brown lentils, cleaned (page 302)

1 cup plus 2 tablespoons unsalted vegetable, chicken, or beef broth

3/4 cup chopped fresh mushrooms

1/4 cup plus 2 tablespoons chopped onion

1/4 cup chopped celery

2 teaspoons crushed fresh garlic

1 teaspoon dried thyme

2 1/2 cups cooked brown rice

1/3 cup grated nonfat or regular Parmesan cheese

1/4 cup chopped roasted soy nuts or walnuts

SAUCE

1/2 teaspoon dried thyme

1/4 teaspoon salt

1 can (1 pound) unsalted tomato sauce

1. To make the filling, place the lentils and broth in a 1-quart pot, and bring to a boil over high heat. Reduce the heat to low, cover, and simmer for 20 minutes, or until the lentils are tender and the broth has been absorbed. Remove the pot from the heat.

2. Coat a large nonstick skillet with nonstick cooking spray, and preheat over medium heat. Add the mushrooms, onion, celery, garlic, and thyme, and stir to mix. Cover and cook, stirring occasionally, for about 3 minutes, or until the mushrooms begin to brown and release their juices. Add a few teaspoons of water or broth if the skillet seems too dry.

3. Remove the skillet from the heat, and stir in first the rice and lentils, and then the Parmesan cheese. Stir in the nuts, and set aside.

4. Cut the tops off the peppers, and remove and discard the seeds and membranes. Divide the filling among the peppers, and replace the pepper tops.

5. To make the sauce, stir the thyme and salt into the tomato sauce. Arrange the peppers upright in an

8-x-8-inch casserole dish, and pour the sauce around the peppers. Cover the pan with aluminum foil, and bake at 350°F for about 1 hour, or until the peppers are tender. Serve hot.

NUTRITIONAL FACTS (PER SERVING)		
Cal: 340 Carbs: 64 g Chol: 6 mg Fat: 3.2 g		
Fiber: 13.6 g Protein: 17.6 g Sodium: 429 mg		

Curried Vegetable Stew

YIELD: 8 CUPS

1 can (19 ounces) chickpeas, drained, or 2 cups cooked chickpeas, divided

1 1/2 cups vegetable or chicken broth, divided

2 cups 1/2-inch cubes white potatoes or butternut squash

2 cups small cauliflower florets

1 cup sliced fresh mushrooms

1 can (14 1/2 ounces) unsalted stewed tomatoes, crushed

2–3 teaspoons curry paste

1 cup frozen (thawed) green peas

1. Place 1/2 cup of the chickpeas and 1/2 cup of the broth in a blender, and process until smooth. Set aside.

2. Place the remaining chickpeas, the remaining broth, and the potatoes or squash, cauliflower, mushrooms, tomatoes with their juice, and curry paste in a 3-quart pot, and bring to a boil over high heat. Reduce the heat to medium-low, cover, and cook, stirring occasionally, for 20 minutes, or until the potatoes or squash and the cauliflower are tender.

3. Add the peas and the chickpea-broth mixture to the pot, and stir to mix. Cover and simmer for 5 to 10 additional minutes, or until the mixture is heated through and the flavors are well blended. Serve hot, ladling the stew over whole wheat couscous, brown rice, or pasta, if desired.

NUTRITIONAL FACTS (PER 1-CUP SERVING)		
Cal: 138 Carbs: 24 g Chol: 0 mg Fat: 2 g		
Fiber: 4.3 g Protein: 7 g Sodium: 304 mg		

Spicy Spaghetti Squash

YIELD: 4 SERVINGS

8-inch spaghetti squash (about 4 pounds)

2 cups chopped tomato (about 2$\frac{1}{2}$ medium)

1$\frac{1}{2}$ cups sliced fresh mushrooms

$\frac{1}{2}$ cup chopped onion

1 teaspoon crushed fresh garlic

1$\frac{1}{2}$ teaspoons dried oregano

$\frac{1}{2}$ teaspoon crushed red pepper

$\frac{1}{4}$ cup grated Parmesan cheese*

1 cup shredded nonfat or reduced-fat
mozzarella cheese

* In this recipe, use regular Parmesan cheese, not a fat-free product.

1. Cut the squash in half lengthwise, and remove the seeds. Coat a large baking sheet with nonstick cooking spray, and place the squash halves cut side down on the sheet. Bake at 375°F for 40 minutes, or until the squash is easily pierced with a sharp knife.

2. Remove the squash from the oven, and let it sit until cool enough to handle. Scoop out the pulp, and transfer it to a large bowl. Use a fork to separate the pulp into strands, and set aside.

3. Place the tomato, mushrooms, onion, garlic, and spices in a large skillet. Place over medium heat, cover, and cook, stirring occasionally, for 6 to 8 minutes, or until the vegetables are tender.

4. Spoon the tomato mixture over the squash, and toss gently to mix well. Add the Parmesan cheese, and toss gently to mix.

5. Coat a 2-quart casserole dish with nonstick cooking spray, and spread the mixture evenly in the dish. Bake uncovered at 350°F for 30 minutes, or until heated through. Top with the mozzarella, and bake for 5 additional minutes, or until the cheese has melted. Serve hot.

NUTRITIONAL FACTS (PER SERVING)

Cal: 179   Carbs: 25 g   Chol: 8 mg   Fat: 3 g
Fiber: 5.2 g   Protein: 15 g   Sodium: 415 mg

Mushroom Risotto Milanese

YIELD: 5 SERVINGS

1 teaspoon crushed fresh garlic

2 cups sliced fresh mushrooms

2 cups arborio rice

5 cups unsalted beef, chicken,
or vegetable broth

$\frac{1}{8}$ teaspoon ground black pepper

$\frac{1}{4}$ teaspoon loosely packed
saffron threads (optional)

$\frac{1}{2}$ cup plus 2 tablespoons evaporated skim milk

$\frac{1}{4}$ cup grated nonfat or regular Parmesan cheese

1. Coat a 3-quart pot with nonstick butter-flavored cooking spray, and preheat over medium-high heat. Add the garlic and mushrooms, and sauté for about 3 minutes, or just until the mushrooms begin to brown and start to release their juices. (Add a little white wine or broth if the pot becomes too dry.)

2. Stir the rice, broth, pepper, and, if desired, the saffron into the mushrooms, and bring to a boil. Reduce the heat to low, cover, and simmer without stirring for about 15 minutes, or until most of the liquid has been absorbed.

3. Add the evaporated milk to the pot, and, if necessary, increase the heat slightly to return the mixture to a simmer. Cook uncovered, stirring frequently, for about 5 minutes, or until the rice is tender but still a little firm to the bite, and most of the liquid has been absorbed. Add a little more broth during cooking if needed, leaving just enough liquid to make the mixture moist and creamy.

4. Stir the Parmesan into the risotto. If the mixture seems too dry at this point, add a little more evaporated milk or broth. Serve hot, topping each serving with a rounded teaspoon of additional Parmesan, if desired.

NUTRITIONAL FACTS (PER 1⅓-CUP SERVING)

Cal: 340   Carbs: 67 g   Chol: 2 mg   Fat: 0.6 g
Fiber: 1.3 g   Protein: 15.7 g   Sodium: 189 mg

Risotto With Sun-Dried Tomatoes

YIELD: 5 SERVINGS

1/4 cup plus 1 tablespoon chopped sun-dried tomatoes (not packed in oil)
1/4 cup plus 1 tablespoon boiling water
1 teaspoon crushed fresh garlic
1/3 cup finely chopped shallot or onion
2 cups arborio rice
4 1/2 cups unsalted chicken or vegetable broth
1/2 cup dry white wine
1/8 teaspoon ground black pepper
1 pinch ground white pepper
1/2 cup plus 2 tablespoons evaporated skim milk
1/4 cup grated nonfat or regular Parmesan cheese
2 tablespoons finely chopped Italian parsley

1. Place the sun-dried tomatoes in a small bowl, and pour the boiling water over the tomatoes. Let sit for about 10 minutes, or until the tomatoes have plumped.

2. Coat a 3-quart pot with nonstick butter-flavored cooking spray, and preheat over medium heat. Add the garlic and the shallot or onion, and sauté for about 1 minute, or until the garlic begins to turn color and the shallot or onion starts to soften. (Add a little white wine or chicken broth if the pot becomes too dry.)

3. Stir the rice, broth, wine, black pepper, and white pepper into the garlic mixture, and bring to a boil over medium-high heat. Reduce the heat to low, cover, and simmer without stirring for about 15 minutes, or until the most of the liquid has been absorbed.

4. Add the evaporated milk to the pot, and, if necessary, increase the heat slightly to return the mixture to a simmer. Cook uncovered, stirring frequently, for about 5 minutes, or until the rice is tender but still a little firm to the bite, and most of the liquid has been absorbed. Add a little more broth during cooking if needed, leaving just enough liquid to make the mixture moist and creamy.

5. Drain any excess liquid from the sun-dried toma-

toes, and add them to the risotto. Stir in the Parmesan and parsley. If the mixture seems too dry at this point, add a little more evaporated milk or broth. Serve hot, topping each serving with a rounded teaspoon of additional Parmesan, if desired.

NUTRITIONAL FACTS (PER 1⅓-CUP SERVING)			
Cal: 377	Carbs: 69 g	Chol: 3 mg	Fat: 1 g
Fiber: 1.5 g	Protein: 18.1 g	Sodium: 260 mg	

Eggplant Parmesan

YIELD: 6 SERVINGS

2 large eggplants (1 pound each)
1/2 cup fat-free egg substitute
1/2 cup Italian-style seasoned dried bread crumbs
1/4 cup plus 2 tablespoons grated nonfat or regular Parmesan cheese, divided
2 tablespoons unbleached flour
Nonstick olive oil cooking spray
1 recipe Chunky Garden Marinara Sauce (page 235), 1 recipe Arrabbiata Sauce (page 233), or 3 1/2 cups bottled marinara sauce
1 cup shredded nonfat or reduced-fat mozzarella cheese

1. Trim the ends off the eggplants, but do not peel. Cut each eggplant crosswise into 9 rounds, each 1/2-inch thick. Set aside.

2. Place the egg substitute in a shallow bowl. Place the bread crumbs, 1/4 cup of the Parmesan, and the flour in another shallow bowl, and stir to mix well. Dip the eggplant slices first in the egg substitute, and then in the crumb mixture, turning to coat both sides.

3. Coat a large baking sheet with nonstick olive oil cooking spray, and arrange the eggplant slices in a single layer on the sheet. Spray the tops of the slices lightly with the cooking spray, and bake at 400°F for 15 to 20 minutes, or until the slices are golden brown and tender.

4. While the eggplant is baking, place the sauce in a medium-sized pot, and cook over medium heat, stirring frequently, until heated through. Remove the sauce from the heat, and cover to keep warm.

5. Spoon a thin layer of sauce over the bottom of a 9-x-13-inch baking pan. Arrange the baked eggplant slices in the pan, slightly overlapping them to fit in a single layer. Pour the remaining sauce over the eggplant. Then sprinkle with the remaining Parmesan and the mozzarella.

6. Bake uncovered at 400°F for about 5 minutes, or until the cheese is melted. Serve hot with your choice of pasta.

NUTRITIONAL FACTS (PER SERVING)
Cal: 190   Carbs: 31 g   Chol: 6 mg   Fat: 1.1 g
Fiber: 6.6 g   Protein: 15.4 g   Sodium: 570 mg

Eggplant Pastitsio

YIELD: 6 SERVINGS

MACARONI MIXTURE

6 ounces elbow macaroni (about 1 1/3 cups)

1/3 cup grated nonfat or regular Parmesan cheese

3 tablespoons fat-free egg substitute

FILLING

2 cups diced peeled eggplant
(about 1 medium-small)

1/2 cup chopped onion

1 can (8 ounces) tomato sauce

2 tablespoons tomato paste

2 tablespoons vegetable broth or water

1 1/2 teaspoons crushed fresh garlic

1 teaspoon dried oregano

1/4 teaspoon ground cinnamon or allspice

1/4 teaspoon ground black pepper

SAUCE

1 cup skim or low-fat milk

1/2 cup evaporated skim milk

1/3 cup grated nonfat Parmesan cheese,
or 1/4 cup regular Parmesan cheese
mixed with 1 tablespoon cornstarch

1/2 cup plus 2 tablespoons fat-free egg substitute

1. To make the filling, place all of the filling ingredients in a 2-quart pot. Stir to mix, and bring to a boil over high heat. Reduce the heat to low, cover, and simmer for about 30 minutes, or until the eggplant is soft and the mixture is thick. Remove the pot from the heat, and set aside.

2. While the filling is simmering, cook the macaroni al dente according to package directions. Drain well, and return to the pot. Add the Parmesan cheese and egg substitute, stir to mix well, and set aside.

3. To make the sauce, place the milk and evaporated milk in a 1-quart pot. Place the pot over medium heat, and cook, stirring constantly, until the mixture begins to boil. Add the Parmesan, and continue to cook and stir for another minute, or until the mixture thickens slightly. Reduce the heat to low.

4. Place the egg substitute in a small bowl. Stir 1/2 cup of the hot milk mixture into the egg substitute. Return the mixture to the pot, and cook, still stirring, for another minute or 2, or until the mixture thickens slightly. *Do not allow the mixture to come to a boil.* Remove the pot from the heat, and set aside.

5. To assemble the dish, coat an 8-inch square casserole dish with nonstick cooking spray. Spread half of the macaroni mixture evenly over the bottom of the dish. Top with all of the filling, followed by the remaining macaroni mixture. Spoon the sauce evenly over the macaroni.

6. Bake uncovered at 350°F for about 30 minutes, or until the sauce layer is set and a sharp knife inserted in the center of the sauce layer comes out clean.

7. Remove the dish from the oven, and let sit for 5 minutes before cutting into squares and serving.

NUTRITIONAL FACTS (PER SERVING)
Cal: 219   Carbs: 36 g   Chol: 7 mg   Fat: 1.1 g
Fiber: 4.5 g   Protein: 16 g   Sodium: 417 mg

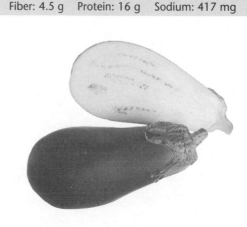

Vegetarian Fried Rice

YIELD: 5 SERVINGS

2 teaspoons vegetable oil (optional)
1½ teaspoons crushed fresh garlic
1½ cups sliced fresh mushrooms
1 cup thinly sliced celery
½ cup plus 2 tablespoon sliced scallions
1¼ cups frozen (thawed) green peas
1 recipe Crispy Tofu Cubes (page 314)
4 cups cooked brown rice
¼ cup reduced-sodium soy sauce

1. Coat a large nonstick skillet with nonstick cooking spray or with the vegetable oil, and preheat over medium-high heat. Add the garlic, mushrooms, celery, and scallions, and stir-fry for about 3 minutes, or until the vegetables are crisp-tender. Cover the skillet periodically if it begins to dry out. (The steam from the cooking vegetables will moisten the skillet.) Add a few teaspoons of broth or water to the skillet only if necessary.

2. Add the peas and tofu to the skillet mixture, and toss to mix well. Add the rice and soy sauce, and cook, tossing gently, for another minute or 2, or until the mixture is thoroughly heated and the flavors are well blended. Add a little broth or water if the mixture seems too dry. Serve hot.

NUTRITIONAL FACTS (PER 1½-CUP SERVING)
Cal: 281   Carbs: 47 g   Chol: 0 mg   Fat: 4.6 g
Fiber: 5.4 g   Protein: 15 g   Sodium: 473 mg

Two-Bean Chili

YIELD: 8 CUPS

1 cup texturized vegetable protein (TVP)
⅞ cup vegetable or beef broth
1 large onion, chopped
1 large green bell pepper, chopped
1 can (14½ ounces) tomatoes, crushed
1 can (1 pound) unsalted tomato sauce
1 can (1 pound) red kidney beans, drained
1 can (1 pound) pinto beans, drained
2–3 tablespoons chili powder
1 teaspoon dried oregano
½ teaspoon ground cumin
1 cup shredded nonfat or reduced-fat Cheddar cheese (optional)

1. Place the TVP and broth in a 3-quart pot, and bring to a boil over high heat. Remove the pot from the heat, and let sit for 5 minutes, or until the liquid has been absorbed.

2. Add all of the remaining ingredients except for the cheese to the TVP mixture, and stir to mix well. Place over high heat, and bring to a boil. Reduce the heat to low, cover, and simmer for 25 to 30 minutes, or until the vegetables are tender.

3. Serve hot, topping each serving with some of the cheese, if desired.

NUTRITIONAL FACTS (PER 1-CUP SERVING)
Cal: 156   Carbs: 24 g   Chol: 0 mg   Fat: 0.8 g
Fiber: 11 g   Protein: 13 g   Sodium: 433 mg

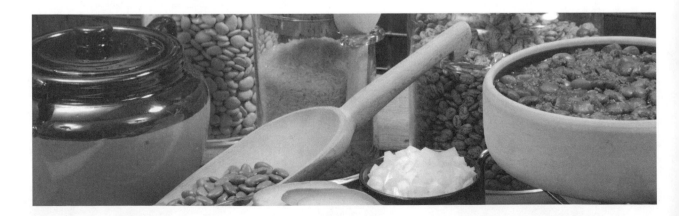

Tofu Chop Suey

YIELD: 5 SERVINGS

1 pound reduced-fat or regular firm or extra-firm tofu,
frozen, thawed, and squeezed dry (below)

Nonstick cooking spray

2 teaspoons crushed fresh garlic

1 medium yellow onion,
cut into thin wedges

1 cup diagonally sliced carrots

1 cup diagonally sliced celery

1 small green bell pepper, cut into thin strips

1½ cups sliced fresh mushrooms

2 cups fresh mung bean sprouts

SAUCE

1 cup vegetable or chicken broth

¼ cup reduced-sodium soy sauce

3 tablespoons dry sherry

2 tablespoons dark brown sugar

2–3 teaspoons dark (roasted) sesame oil

1 teaspoon ground ginger

1 tablespoon plus 1 teaspoon cornstarch

1. Cut the tofu into ½-inch cubes, and arrange the cubes in a shallow nonmetal container.

2. To make the sauce, place all of the sauce ingredients except for the cornstarch in a small bowl, and stir to mix well. Pour ¼ cup of the sauce mixture over the tofu, tossing to mix, and set aside for 10 minutes. (The tofu will soak up the sauce.) Add the cornstarch to the remaining sauce, stir to dissolve the cornstarch, and set aside.

3. Coat a large baking sheet with nonstick cooking spray. Arrange the tofu cubes in a single layer over the baking sheet, and spray the tops lightly with the cooking spray.

4. Bake at 375°F for 10 minutes. Turn the cubes, and bake for 10 additional minutes, or until nicely browned and crisp. Set aside.

5. Coat a large deep nonstick skillet or nonstick wok with nonstick cooking spray, and preheat over medium-high heat. Add the garlic, onion, carrots, celery,

green pepper, and mushrooms, and stir-fry for about 4 minutes, or until crisp-tender. Cover the skillet or wok periodically if it begins to dry out. (The steam from the cooking vegetables will moisten the skillet.) Add a few teaspoons of water or broth only if necessary.

6. Add the bean sprouts to the skillet or wok, and stir-fry for another minute or 2, or just until the sprouts start to wilt.

7. Stir the sauce, and add it to the skillet. Stir-fry the mixture for another minute or 2, or until the sauce thickens. Add the tofu cubes, and toss to mix well. Serve hot over brown rice, if desired.

NUTRITIONAL FACTS (PER 1⅔-CUP SERVING)
Cal: 162   Carbs: 17 g   Chol: 0 mg   Fat: 5.5 g
Fiber: 3 g   Protein: 11.6 g   Sodium: 532 mg

Adding Texture to Tofu

Not crazy about tofu? Try freezing it. Freezing causes tofu to take on a meaty, chewy texture that is perfect for stir-fries, stews, and chilies, and is also wonderful when grilled or baked. Freezing also improves tofu's ability to soak up flavorful marinades and sauces.

To freeze tofu, place the unopened container in the freezer for at least twenty-four hours, and for as long as several months. Keep in mind that when frozen, tofu takes on a yellowish color, but that this color will disappear when the product is thawed.

To thaw frozen tofu, place it in the refrigerator for approximately twenty-four hours, or thaw at room temperature by immersing it in cool water. When it is thawed, press the tofu between your palms to squeeze out any excess liquid. The tofu is now ready to marinate or cook. Freeze only nonsilken firm and extra-firm tofu. Soft and silken tofus are not suitable for freezing.

Teriyaki Tofu

YIELD: 5 SERVINGS

1 pound reduced-fat or regular firm or extra-firm tofu, frozen, thawed, and squeezed dry (page 313)

Nonstick cooking spray

MARINADE

1 cup unsweetened pineapple juice

3 tablespoons reduced-sodium soy sauce

1 tablespoon plus 1 teaspoon dark brown sugar

2 teaspoons crushed fresh garlic

1 teaspoon ground ginger, or 1 tablespoon freshly grated ginger root

1 tablespoon plus 1 teaspoon peanut butter, or 2 teaspoons dark (roasted) sesame oil (optional)

1. To make the marinade, place all of the marinade ingredients in a blender, and process for about 30 seconds, or until well mixed.

2. Cut the block of tofu crosswise into 10 slices. Place the tofu slices in a shallow nonmetal container, and pour the marinade over the tofu, lifting the tofu slices to allow the marinade to flow beneath them. Cover and refrigerate for at least 2 hours.

3. When ready to cook the tofu, coat a large baking sheet with nonstick cooking spray. Remove the tofu from the marinade, reserving the marinade, and arrange the tofu in a single layer on the sheet. Spray the tops lightly with the cooking spray.

4. Bake at 375°F for 15 minutes. Turn the slices, and cook for 10 to 15 additional minutes, or until nicely browned on both sides. (The longer the slices bake, the firmer and crisper they will become.)

5. A few minutes before the tofu is done, place the remaining marinade in a nonstick 1-quart pot, and bring to a boil over medium heat. Cook uncovered, stirring frequently, for several minutes, or until the marinade is reduced by almost half.

6. Arrange the baked tofu on a serving platter. Pour the marinade over the slices, and serve hot.

NUTRITIONAL FACTS (PER SERVING)
Cal: 144   Carbs: 16 g   Chol: 0 mg   Fat: 4 g
Fiber: 0 g   Protein: 11.2 g   Sodium: 393 mg

Crispy Tofu Cubes

Tofu prepared this way has a pleasant crispy-chewy texture. Use Crispy Tofu Cubes instead of meat in stir-fries, stews, and casseroles.

YIELD: 5 SERVINGS

1 pound reduced-fat or regular firm or extra-firm tofu

Nonstick cooking spray

MARINADE

3/4 cup vegetable, chicken, or beef broth

2 tablespoons reduced-sodium soy sauce

1 teaspoon ground ginger, or 1 tablespoon freshly grated ginger root

1 teaspoon crushed fresh garlic

1 teaspoon dark (roasted) sesame oil (optional)

1. Cut the tofu into 1/2-inch cubes, and arrange the cubes in a single layer in a shallow nonmetal container.

2. To make the marinade, place all of the marinade ingredients in a small bowl, and stir to mix well. Pour the marinade over the tofu cubes, and set aside at room temperature for 30 minutes, or cover and refrigerate for several hours or overnight.

3. Coat a large nonstick baking sheet with nonstick cooking spray. Remove the tofu cubes from the marinade, and discard the marinade. Arrange the tofu cubes in a single layer over the baking sheet, and spray the tops with the cooking spray.

4. Bake at 375°F for 10 minutes. Turn the cubes and bake for 20 additional minutes, or until golden brown and crisp on the outside and chewy on the inside. (The longer the cubes bake, the crisper and chewier they will become.) If you are using frozen thawed tofu for this recipe, bake for only about 20 minutes, turning after 10 minutes, as the frozen tofu is more porous and will cook faster.

5. Remove the tofu cubes from the oven. They are now ready to add to stir-fries, stews, casseroles, and other dishes.

NUTRITIONAL FACTS (PER SERVING)
Cal: 73   Carbs: 2.5 g   Chol: 0 mg   Fat: 4 g
Fiber: 0 g   Protein: 8.3 g   Sodium: 156 mg

12. *Deceptively Decadent Desserts*

Dessert is one of the simplest yet greatest pleasures of life. But, as everyone knows, most desserts are loaded with fat, sugar, and calories, leaving little place for them in a healthy diet. Take your typical chocolate fudge cake, for instance. With two cups of granulated sugar, four cups of powdered sugar, almost a half pound of chocolate, a stick of butter, and a cup of oil, even a moderate portion contains over 500 calories and nearly 30 grams of fat! Other desserts like cheesecake, chocolate mousse, buttery pastry, and streusel-topped pies are generally no better.

Does this mean you must give up dessert to live a healthy low-fat lifestyle? Definitely not. After all, what good is healthier living if you are deprived of the foods you love? As you will see, with just a little thought, you can have your dessert and eat it, too. The goodies in this chapter combine wholesome ingredients with creative cooking techniques to bring you the best of both worlds—great taste *and* good nutrition.

Each and every one of the following recipes is designed to keep fat and calories to a minimum, to use only moderate amounts of sugar, and to provide a respectable amount of nutrients. For instance, many of the fruit desserts in this chapter provide a full serving of fruit. Delightfully sweet toppings for crisps, cobblers, and fruit pies include nutrient-rich ingredients like whole grain flours, oats, wheat germ, and nuts. Rich and creamy custards, puddings, cheesecake, and frozen desserts feature nonfat and low-fat dairy products that add calcium and protein—but not unwanted fat—to your diet. And cakes are made super-moist and tender with ingredients like puréed fruits, juices, nonfat sour cream, and nonfat buttermilk—not unhealthy amounts of shortening or oil.

So get ready to enjoy sweet satisfaction without an excess of calories, fat, or sugar. From Classic Berry-Topped Cheesecake to Sour Cream Apple Pie, you will find a galaxy of deceptively decadent desserts that are right for any occasion. Skip dessert? There's no need—not once you know the secrets of healthy cooking.

Cappuccino Cheesecake

YIELD: 12 SERVINGS

CRUST

6 large (2½-x-5-inch) reduced-fat
chocolate graham crackers

2 tablespoons sugar

1 tablespoon tub-style nonfat margarine,
or 1 tablespoon plus 1½ teaspoons
reduced-fat margarine or light butter

¼ cup honey crunch wheat germ or
finely chopped toasted almonds (page 348)

FILLING

2 blocks (8 ounces each) nonfat cream cheese,
softened to room temperature

2 teaspoons vanilla extract

2 tablespoons coffee liqueur

¾ teaspoon instant coffee granules

2 tablespoons plus 2 teaspoons cornstarch

1 tablespoon cocoa powder

¼ teaspoon ground cinnamon

1 can (14 ounces) fat-free or low-fat sweetened
condensed milk

½ cup plus 2 tablespoons fat-free egg substitute

1 cup vanilla yogurt cheese (page 12)

TOPPING

3 cups fresh raspberries or sliced fresh strawberries

¼ cup plus 2 tablespoons chocolate syrup

1. To make the crust, break the graham crackers into pieces, place in the bowl of a food processor, and process into fine crumbs. Measure the crumbs. There should be ¾ cup. (Adjust the amount if needed.)

2. Return the crumbs to the food processor, add the sugar, and process for a few seconds to mix well. Add the margarine or butter, and process for about 20 seconds, or until moist and crumbly. Add the wheat germ or almonds, and process for a few seconds to mix well.

3. Coat a 9-inch springform pan with nonstick cooking spray, and use the back of a spoon to press the mixture against the bottom and sides of the pan, forming an even crust. (Periodically dip the spoon in sugar, if necessary, to prevent sticking.) Then use your fingers to finish pressing the crust firmly against the bottom and sides of the pan.

4. Bake at 350°F for about 8 minutes, or until the edges feel firm and dry. Set aside to cool to room temperature before filling.

5. To make the filling, place the cream cheese and vanilla extract in a large bowl, and beat with an electric mixer until smooth.

6. Place the liqueur and coffee granules in a small bowl, and stir to dissolve the coffee granules. Add the liqueur mixture to the cream cheese mixture, and beat to mix well.

7. Sprinkle the cornstarch over the cheese mixture, and beat to mix well. Sprinkle the cocoa and cinnamon over the cheese mixture, and beat to mix well. Add the sweetened condensed milk, and beat to mix well. Add the egg substitute, and beat to mix well. Finally, add the yogurt cheese, and beat to mix well.

8. Spread the cheesecake batter evenly over the crust, and bake at 325°F for about 1 hour, or until the center is firm to the touch. (If you use a dark pan instead of a shiny one, reduce the oven temperature to 300°F.) Turn the oven off, and allow the cake to cool in the oven with the door ajar for 1 hour. Remove the cake from the oven, cover, and chill for at least 8 hours, or until firm.

9. When ready to serve, run a sharp, thin-bladed knife between the cheesecake and the collar of the pan. Remove the collar, and cut the cheesecake into wedges. Top each serving with ¼ cup of the berries. Then drizzle 1½ teaspoons of the chocolate syrup over the top, and serve.

NUTRITIONAL FACTS (PER SERVING)		
Cal: 246	Carbs: 45 g	Chol: 6 mg Fat: 1.4 g
Fiber: 1.8 g	Protein: 13 g	Sodium: 281 mg

Classic Berry-Topped Cheesecake

YIELD: 12 SERVINGS

CRUST

6 large (2½-x-5-inch) reduced-fat graham crackers

2 tablespoons sugar

1 tablespoon tub-style nonfat margarine,
or 1 tablespoon plus 1½ teaspoons
reduced-fat margarine or light butter

¼ cup honey crunch wheat germ or finely toasted
almonds or walnuts (page 348)

FILLING

2 blocks (8 ounces each) nonfat cream cheese,
softened to room temperature

2 teaspoons vanilla extract

2 tablespoons plus 1 teaspoon cornstarch

1 teaspoon dried grated lemon rind,
or 1 tablespoon fresh

1 can (14 ounces) fat-free or low-fat sweetened
condensed milk

½ cup plus 2 tablespoons fat-free egg substitute

1 cup vanilla yogurt cheese (page 12)

TOPPING

2 cups fresh strawberry halves or
fresh whole raspberries

¼ cup plus 2 tablespoons seedless strawberry
or raspberry jam

1. To make the crust, break the graham crackers into pieces, place in the bowl of a food processor, and process into fine crumbs. Measure the crumbs. There should be ¾ cup. (Adjust the amount if needed.)

2. Return the crumbs to the food processor, add the sugar, and process for a few seconds to mix well. Add the margarine or butter, and process for about 20 seconds, or until moist and crumbly. Add the wheat germ or nuts, and process for a few seconds to mix well.

3. Coat a 9-inch springform pan with nonstick cooking spray, and use the back of a spoon to press the crumb mixture against the bottom and sides of the pan, forming an even crust. (Periodically dip the spoon in sugar, if necessary, to prevent sticking.) Then use your fingers to finish pressing the crust firmly against the bottom and sides of the pan.

4. Bake at 350°F for about 8 minutes, or until the edges feel firm and dry. Set aside to cool to room temperature before filling.

5. To make the filling, place the cream cheese and vanilla extract in a large bowl, and beat with an electric mixer until smooth. Sprinkle the cornstarch and lemon rind over the cheese mixture, and beat until smooth. Add the sweetened condensed milk, and beat until smooth. Add the egg substitute, and beat until smooth. Finally, add the yogurt cheese, and beat until smooth.

6. Spread the cheesecake batter evenly over the crust, and bake at 325°F for about 1 hour, or until the center is firm to the touch. (If you use a dark pan instead of a shiny one, reduce the oven temperature to 300°F.) Turn the oven off, and allow the cake to cool in the oven with the door ajar for 1 hour. Remove the cake from the oven, cover, and chill for at least 6 hours, or until firm.

7. Arrange the berries in concentric circles over the top of the cheesecake. Place the jam in a small pot, and place over medium heat. Cook, stirring constantly, for about 1 minute, or until the jam is runny. Drizzle the jam over the berries, and chill for at least 2 additional hours.

8. When ready to serve, run a sharp, thin-bladed knife between the cheesecake and the collar of the pan. Remove the collar, cut the cheesecake into wedges, and serve.

NUTRITIONAL FACTS (PER SERVING)
Cal: 231   Carbs: 42 g   Chol: 6 mg   Fat: 1 g
Fiber: 0.8 g   Protein: 13 g   Sodium: 314 mg

Lite and Luscious Lemon Cheesecake

YIELD: 10 SERVINGS

CRUST

6 large (2½-x-5-inch) reduced-fat graham crackers

2 tablespoons sugar

1 tablespoon tub-style nonfat margarine, or 1 tablespoon plus 1½ teaspoons reduced-fat margarine or light butter

¼ cup honey crunch wheat germ or finely chopped toasted almonds or walnuts (page 348)

FILLING

2 blocks (8 ounces each) nonfat cream cheese, softened to room temperature

1½ teaspoons vanilla extract

3 tablespoons cornstarch

1 can (14 ounces) fat-free or low-fat sweetened condensed milk

½ cup plus 2 tablespoons fat-free egg substitute

⅓ cup lemon juice

1½ teaspoons freshly grated lemon rind, or ½ teaspoon dried

TOPPING

1 package (10 ounces) frozen (thawed) sweetened raspberries or strawberries

1. To make the crust, break the graham crackers into pieces, place in the bowl of a food processor, and process into fine crumbs. Measure the crumbs. There should be ¾ cup. (Adjust the amount if needed.)

2. Return the crumbs to the food processor, add the sugar, and process for a few seconds to mix well. Add the margarine or butter, and process for about 20 seconds, or until moist and crumbly. Add the wheat germ or nuts, and process for a few seconds to mix well.

3. Coat a 9-inch springform pan with nonstick cooking spray, and use the back of a spoon to press the crumb mixture against the bottom and sides of the pan, forming an even crust. (Periodically dip the spoon in sugar, if necessary, to prevent sticking.) Then use your fingers to finish pressing the crust firmly against the bottom and sides of the pan.

4. Bake at 350°F for about 8 minutes, or until the edges feel firm and dry. Set aside to cool to room temperature before filling.

5. To make the filling, place the cream cheese and vanilla extract in a large bowl, and beat with an electric mixer until smooth. Sprinkle the cornstarch over the cheese mixture, and beat until smooth. Add the sweetened condensed milk, and beat to mix well. Add the egg substitute, and beat to mix well. Finally, add the lemon juice and lemon rind, and beat to mix well.

6. Spread the cheesecake batter evenly over the crust, and bake at 325°F for about 50 minutes, or until the center is firm to the touch. (If you use a dark pan instead of a shiny one, reduce the oven temperature to 300°F.) Turn the oven off, and allow the cake to cool in the oven with the door ajar for 1 hour. Remove the cake from the oven, cover, and chill for at least 8 hours, or until firm.

7. When ready to serve, run a sharp, thin-bladed knife between the cheesecake and the collar of the pan. Remove the collar, and cut the cheesecake into wedges. Top each serving with some of the berries, and serve.

NUTRITIONAL FACTS (PER SERVING)

Cal: 253   Carbs: 48 g   Chol: 6 mg   Fat: 1 g
Fiber: 1.7 g   Protein: 13.1 g   Sodium: 357 mg

VARIATION

To make Coconut Key Lime Cheesecake, substitute shredded sweetened coconut for the wheat germ or nuts in the crust, and substitute key lime juice and rind for the lemon juice and rind in the filling.

NUTRITIONAL FACTS (PER SERVING)

Cal: 254   Carbs: 48 g   Chol: 6 mg   Fat: 1.4 g
Fiber: 1.6 g   Protein: 13 g   Sodium: 363 mg

No-Bake Cherry Cheesecake

YIELD: 8 SERVINGS

1 prebaked Lite Graham Cracker Pie Crust (page 330) made with plain or chocolate graham crackers

FILLING

2 blocks (8 ounces each) nonfat cream cheese or soft curd farmer cheese, softened to room temperature

1/2 cup sugar

1 teaspoon vanilla extract

1 tablespoon plus 1 teaspoon lemon juice

1 teaspoon unflavored gelatin

TOPPING

1 can (20 ounces) light (reduced-sugar) cherry pie filling

1. To make the filling, place the cream cheese or farmer cheese, sugar, and vanilla extract in the bowl of a food processor, and process until smooth. Set aside.

2. If using a microwave oven, place the lemon juice in a small microwave-safe bowl, and microwave uncovered at high power for about 30 seconds, or until the juice comes to a boil. If using a stovetop, place the juice in a small pot, and place over medium heat for about 30 seconds, or until it comes to a boil. Remove the pot from the heat. Sprinkle the gelatin over the lemon juice and stir for about 1 minute, or until the gelatin is completely dissolved.

3. Add the gelatin mixture to the cheese mixture, and process until well mixed. Spread the cheese filling evenly over the crust, cover, and chill for at least 3 hours, or until set.

4. Spread the cherry pie filling over the top of the cheesecake, extending it all the way to the edges of the cake. Chill for at least 1 additional hour before cutting into wedges and serving.

NUTRITIONAL FACTS (PER SERVING)

Cal: 263   Carbs: 49 g   Chol: 4 mg   Fat: 3.5 g
Fiber: 1.2 g   Protein: 10 g   Sodium: 430 mg

Creamy Cheesecakes Without the Fat

There's something about cheesecake that can turn even the most humdrum meal into a special event. But with up to 500 calories and 40 grams of fat per slice, a piece of this popular confection can easily blow your fat budget for the entire day! Even worse, most of this fat is the saturated, artery-clogging type. But don't fear. Creamy, delicious, ultra-light cheesecakes can now be made using nonfat cream cheese.

To defat your favorite cheesecake recipe, substitute a block-style nonfat cream cheese like Philadelphia Free for the full-fat cream cheese on a one-for-one basis. Since the nonfat cheese contains more water than the full-fat product, you will need to add 1 to 1 1/2 tablespoons of flour or 1 1/2 to 2 1/2 teaspoons of cornstarch to the batter for each 8-ounce block of nonfat cream cheese used. This should produce a firm, nicely-textured cake that is rich and creamy, yet remarkably low in fat and calories.

Slashing Fat in Half

Looking for a simple way to slash the fat in cakes and other baked goods? Try replacing the butter, margarine, or other solid shortening in cakes, muffins, quick breads, cookies, and other treats with half as much oil. For instance, if a recipe calls for 1/2 cup of butter, use 1/4 cup of oil instead. Bake as usual, checking the product for doneness a few minutes before the end of the usual baking time. This technique makes it possible to produce moist and tender cakes, breads, and biscuits; crisp cookies; and tender pie crusts—all with about half the original fat.

Banana Fudge Cake

YIELD: 18 SERVINGS

1½ cups sugar

1¼ cups unbleached flour

¾ cup oat flour

½ cup Dutch processed cocoa powder

1½ teaspoons baking soda

½ teaspoon salt

1½ cups mashed very ripe banana (about 3 large)

½ cup coffee, cooled to room temperature

¼ cup walnut or vegetable oil

2 egg whites, lightly beaten

1½ teaspoons vanilla extract

GLAZE

1½ cups powdered sugar

4½ teaspoons Dutch processed cocoa powder

2 tablespoons skim milk

1 teaspoon vanilla extract

¼ cup plus 2 tablespoons chopped walnuts (optional)

1. Place the sugar, flours, cocoa, baking soda, and salt in a large bowl, and stir to mix well. Add the banana, coffee, oil, egg whites, and vanilla extract, and stir to mix well.

2. Coat a 9-x-13-inch pan with nonstick cooking spray, and spread the batter evenly in the pan. Bake at 325°F for 35 to 40 minutes, or just until the top springs back when lightly touched, and a wooden toothpick inserted in the center of the cake comes out clean or coated with a few fudgy crumbs. Allow the cake to cool to room temperature.

3. To make the glaze, place all of the glaze ingredients in a small bowl, and stir to mix well, adding a little more milk if needed to bring the mixture to a thick, frostinglike consistency. If using a microwave oven, place the glaze in a microwave-safe bowl, and heat uncovered at high power for 60 seconds, or until runny. If using a conventional stovetop, place the glaze in a small saucepan, and, stirring constantly, cook over medium heat for 60 seconds, or until runny. Drizzle the glaze over the cake, and allow to harden before cutting into squares and serving.

> **NUTRITIONAL FACTS (PER SERVING)**
> Cal: 198   Carbs: 41 g   Chol: 0 mg   Fat: 3.7 g
> Fiber: 2 g   Protein: 2.6 g   Sodium: 178 mg

Classic Carrot Cake

YIELD: 18 SERVINGS

2 cups unbleached flour

1½ cups sugar

1 teaspoon baking soda

1 teaspoon baking powder

1½ teaspoons ground cinnamon

¼ teaspoon salt

½ cup plus 1 tablespoon fat-free egg substitute

½ cup orange or apple juice

⅓ cup vegetable oil

1 teaspoon vanilla extract

3 cups (not packed) grated carrots (about 6 medium)

½ cup golden or dark raisins

½ cup chopped toasted pecans or walnuts
(page 348) (optional)

FROSTING

1½ blocks (8 ounces each) nonfat or reduced-fat
cream cheese, softened to room temperature

¼ cup plus 2 tablespoons sugar

½ teaspoon vanilla extract

2 tablespoons instant vanilla pudding mix*

1½ cups nonfat or light whipped topping

* Omit the pudding mix if you are using reduced-fat cream cheese rather than a nonfat brand.

1. Place the flour, sugar, baking soda, baking powder, cinnamon, and salt in a large bowl, and stir to mix well. Stir in the egg substitute, fruit juice, vegetable oil, and vanilla extract. Fold in the carrots, raisins, and, if desired, the nuts.

2. Coat a 9-x-13-inch pan with nonstick cooking spray, and spread the mixture evenly in the pan. Bake at 300°F for about 40 minutes, or just until the top springs back when lightly touched and a wooden toothpick inserted in the center of the cake comes out clean. Allow the cake to cool to room temperature.

3. To make the frosting, place the cream cheese, sugar, and vanilla extract in a medium-sized bowl, and beat with an electric mixer until smooth. Add the pudding mix, and beat until smooth. (If you are using reduced-fat cream cheese rather than a nonfat brand, omit the pudding mix, and, if needed, beat in a teaspoon or 2 of milk to soften the mixture.) Gently fold in the whipped topping.

4. Immediately spread the frosting over the cooled cake, and refrigerate for at least 2 hours before cutting into squares and serving.

NUTRITIONAL FACTS (PER SERVING)
Cal: 220   Carbs: 40 g   Chol: 1 mg   Fat: 4.2 g
Fiber: 1 g   Protein: 5.3 g   Sodium: 266 mg

VARIATION

To make Pineapple Carrot Cake, drain and discard 2 tablespoons of juice from an 8-ounce can of crushed pineapple. Substitute the remaining juice and the pineapple for the orange or apple juice in the batter.

NUTRITIONAL FACTS (PER SERVING)
Cal: 220   Carbs: 40 g   Chol: 1 mg   Fat: 4.2 g
Fiber: 1.1 g   Protein: 5.3 g   Sodium: 266 mg

Cassata Alla Siciliana (Sicilian Cake)

YIELD: 10 SERVINGS

1 fat-free vanilla loaf cake or low-fat pound cake
(15 ounces, or about 4-x-7 inches)

¼ cup plus 2 tablespoons orange juice
or amaretto liqueur

FILLING

15 ounces nonfat or low-fat ricotta cheese

¼ cup sugar

1 teaspoon vanilla extract

¼ cup finely chopped dried cherries or apricots

¼ cup finely chopped semi-sweet chocolate chips

GLAZE

¾ cup powdered sugar

2 tablespoons Dutch processed cocoa powder

2 tablespoons skim or low-fat milk

1. Using a bread knife, cut the cake horizontally to create 4 layers. Arrange the 3 bottom layers on a flat surface, and sprinkle each layer with 2 tablespoons of the orange juice or liqueur. Set aside.

2. To make the filling, place the ricotta, sugar, and vanilla extract in a food processor, and process until smooth. Transfer the mixture to a bowl, and stir in the cherries or apricots and the chocolate chips.

3. To assemble the cake, place the bottom cake layer on a serving plate, and spread with a third of the filling. Repeat with the next 2 layers and the remaining filling. Top with the last layer, and cover the cake with plastic wrap or aluminum foil. Chill for 8 hours or overnight, or until the filling is firm.

4. To make the glaze, place the sugar and cocoa in a small bowl, and stir to mix well. Stir in enough of the milk to make a thick glaze. If using a microwave oven, place the glaze in a microwave-safe bowl, and heat uncovered at high power for 30 seconds, or until hot and runny. If using a conventional stovetop, place the glaze in a small saucepan, and, stirring constantly, cook over medium heat for 30 seconds, or until hot and runny.

5. Spread the glaze over the top of the chilled cake, allowing some of the mixture to drip down the sides. Allow the glaze to cool for 5 minutes before slicing and serving, or return the cake to the refrigerator and chill until ready to serve.

NUTRITIONAL FACTS (PER SERVING)
Cal: 223   Carbs: 44 g   Chol: 3 mg   Fat: 1.3 g
Fiber: 0.8 g   Protein: 8.8 g   Sodium: 169 mg

Lemon Cream Cake

YIELD: 16 SERVINGS

1 box (1 pound, 2.25 ounces) reduced-fat or regular lemon or yellow cake mix

1 package (4-serving size) instant lemon pudding mix

1 cup nonfat or light sour cream

3/4 cup fat-free egg substitute

1/2 cup water

3 tablespoons lemon juice

GLAZE

1/2 cup powdered sugar

1 teaspoon lemon juice

2 teaspoons nonfat or light sour cream

1. Place the cake mix and pudding mix in a large bowl, and stir to mix well. Add the sour cream, egg substitute, water, and lemon juice, and beat with an electric mixer for about 2 minutes, or until well mixed.

2. Coat a 12-cup bundt pan with nonstick cooking spray, and spread the batter evenly in the pan. Bake at 350°F for about 40 minutes, or just until the top springs back when lightly touched and a wooden toothpick inserted in the center of the cake comes out clean. Be careful not to overbake.

3. Allow the cake to cool in the pan for 45 minutes. Then invert onto a serving platter and cool to room temperature.

4. To make the glaze, place all of the glaze ingredients in a small bowl, and stir to mix well. If using a microwave oven, place the glaze in a microwave-safe bowl, and heat uncovered at high power for 25 seconds, or until hot and runny. If using a conventional stovetop, place the glaze in a small saucepan, and, stirring constantly, cook over medium heat for about 25 seconds, or until hot and runny.

5. Drizzle the hot glaze over the cake. Allow the cake to sit for at least 15 minutes before slicing and serving.

NUTRITIONAL FACTS (PER SERVING)
Cal: 186   Carbs: 39 g   Chol: 0 mg   Fat: 1.5 g
Fiber: 0.4 g   Protein: 2.7 g   Sodium: 323 mg

Royal Raspberry Cake

For variety, substitute chocolate or lemon cake and pudding mix for the white cake mix and the white chocolate pudding mix. Use chocolate or lemon yogurt in the frosting.

YIELD: 16 SERVINGS

1 box (1 pound, 2.25 ounces) reduced-fat or regular white cake mix

1 package (4-serving size) instant white chocolate pudding mix

1 1/4 cups water

1/2 cup nonfat or light sour cream

3 egg whites

FILLING

1 package (10 ounces) frozen (thawed) sweetened raspberries

1 1/2 teaspoons cornstarch

2 tablespoons raspberry or amaretto liqueur

FROSTING

2 1/4 cups nonfat or light whipped topping

3/4 cup nonfat or low-fat raspberry or white chocolate yogurt

3 tablespoons sliced toasted almonds (page 348) (optional)

1. Place the cake mix and pudding mix in a large bowl, and stir to mix well. Add the water, sour cream, and egg whites, and beat with an electric mixer for 2 minutes, or until well mixed.

2. Coat three 9-inch round cake pans with nonstick cooking spray, and divide the batter among the pans, spreading it evenly. Bake at 325°F for about 25 minutes, or just until the tops spring back when lightly touched and a wooden toothpick inserted in the center of the cakes comes out clean. Be careful not to overbake. Allow the cakes to cool to room temperature in the pans.

3. To make the filling, transfer 1 tablespoon of the juice from the raspberries to a small bowl. Stir in the cornstarch, and set aside.

4. Place the berries and the remaining juice in a 1-quart pot, and place the pot over medium heat. Cook, stirring frequently, until the mixture comes to a boil and the berries begin to break down. Stir in the cornstarch mixture, and cook for another minute or 2, or until thickened and bubbly. Stir in the liqueur, remove from the heat, and allow to cool to room temperature.

5. To assemble the cake, place one layer, with the top side down, on a serving plate. Spread half of the raspberry filling over the cake layer. Place a second layer over the first, top side down, and spread with the remaining raspberry filling. Place the third layer on the cake, top side up.

6. To make the frosting, place the whipped topping in a medium-sized bowl, and gently fold in the yogurt. Spread the frosting over the top and sides of the cake, swirling the frosting with a knife. Sprinkle the almonds over the top of the cake, if desired. Cover and refrigerate for at least 2 hours before serving.

NUTRITIONAL FACTS (PER SERVING)
Cal: 214   Carbs: 45 g   Chol: 0 mg   Fat: 1.9 g
Fiber: 1.2 g   Protein: 3.3 g   Sodium: 337 mg

Sour Cream-Coconut Bundt Cake

YIELD: 16 SERVINGS

1 box (1 pound, 2.25 ounces) reduced-fat or regular yellow, white, or chocolate cake mix

1 package (4-serving size) instant coconut pudding mix*

1 cup nonfat or light sour cream

3/4 cup fat-free egg substitute

3/4 cup water

GLAZE

1/2 cup powdered sugar

1 tablespoon nonfat or light sour cream

1/2 teaspoon coconut-flavored extract

2 tablespoons shredded sweetened coconut

* If you cannot find coconut pudding mix, substitute 1 package of instant vanilla pudding mix plus 3/4 teaspoon of coconut-flavored extract and 2 tablespoons of finely shredded coconut.

1. Place the cake mix and pudding mix in a large bowl, and stir to mix well. Add the sour cream, egg substitute, and water, and beat with an electric mixer for about 2 minutes, or until well mixed.

2. Coat a 12-cup bundt pan with nonstick cooking spray, and spread the batter evenly in the pan. Bake at 350°F for about 40 minutes, or just until the top springs back when lightly touched and a wooden toothpick inserted in the center of the cake comes out clean. Be careful not to overbake.

3. Allow the cake to cool in the pan for 45 minutes. Then invert onto a serving platter and cool to room temperature.

4. To make the glaze, place the powdered sugar, sour cream, and coconut extract in a small bowl, and stir to mix well. If using a microwave oven, place the glaze in a microwave-safe bowl, and heat uncovered at high power for 30 seconds, or until hot and runny. If using a conventional stovetop, place the glaze in a small saucepan, and, stirring constantly, cook over medium heat for about 30 seconds, or until hot and runny.

5. Drizzle the hot glaze over the cake, and sprinkle the glaze with the coconut. Allow the cake to sit for at least 15 minutes before slicing and serving.

NUTRITIONAL FACTS (PER SERVING)
Cal: 188   Carbs: 38.4 g   Chol: 0 mg   Fat: 2 g
Fiber: 0.5 g   Protein: 3 g   Sodium: 281 mg

Macaroon Swirl Cake

YIELD: 18 SERVINGS

1 stick (1/2 cup) reduced-fat margarine or light butter

1 2/3 cups sugar

2 egg whites

1 1/2 teaspoons vanilla extract

2 cups unbleached flour

3/4 cup oat bran

2 teaspoons baking powder

3/4 teaspoon baking soda

1 1/2 cups nonfat or low-fat buttermilk

1/4 cup sweetened flaked coconut

3/4 teaspoon coconut extract

1/4 cup plus 2 tablespoons Dutch processed cocoa powder

GLAZE

1/2 cup powdered sugar

2 teaspoons skim or low-fat milk

1/2 teaspoon coconut extract

1 tablespoon sweetened flaked coconut

1. Place the margarine or butter and the sugar in the bowl of an electric mixer, and beat until smooth. Beat in the egg whites and vanilla extract until smooth, and set aside.

2. Place the flour, oat bran, baking powder, and baking soda in a medium-sized bowl, and stir to mix well. Add the flour mixture and the buttermilk to the margarine mixture, and beat just until well mixed.

3. Remove 1 cup of the batter, and place it in a small bowl. Stir in the flaked coconut and coconut extract, and set aside.

4. Add the cocoa to the large bowl of batter, and beat just until well mixed.

5. Coat a 12-cup bundt pan with nonstick cooking spray. Pour two-thirds of the cocoa batter into the pan, spreading the batter evenly. Top with the coconut batter, followed by the remaining cocoa batter.

6. Bake at 350°F for 40 minutes, or just until a wooden toothpick inserted in the center of the cake comes out clean. Allow the cake to cool in the pan for 40 minutes. Then invert onto a serving plate, and cool to room temperature.

7. To make the glaze, place the powdered sugar, milk, and coconut extract in a small bowl, and stir until smooth. If using a microwave oven, place the glaze in a microwave safe-bowl, and heat uncovered at high power for 30 seconds, or until hot and runny. If using a conventional stovetop, place the glaze in a small saucepan, and, stirring constantly, cook over medium heat for 30 seconds, or until hot and runny.

8. Drizzle the glaze over the cake, and sprinkle the coconut over the top of the glaze. Allow the glaze to harden for at least 15 minutes before slicing and serving.

NUTRITIONAL FACTS (PER SERVING)
Cal: 183   Carbs: 36 g   Chol: 0 mg   Fat: 3.6 g
Fiber: 1.5 g   Protein: 3.5 g   Sodium: 170 mg

Using Coconut in Low-Fat Recipes

Loaded with saturated fat, coconut oil has long been strictly off limits in heart-healthy diets. Does this mean that the meat of the coconut is also taboo? Not necessarily. While coconut does contain coconut oil—one cup of shredded sweetened coconut contains about 33 grams of fat, or about 7 teaspoons of oil—small amounts of coconut may be added to recipes, especially if the recipe contains little or no other added fat.

Instead of totally eliminating this flavorful ingredient from your favorite recipes, try to decrease the amount used. For example, rather than thickly covering a cake's frosting with coconut, sprinkle the coconut sparingly over the top or just around the edges of the cake. This will enhance the flavor and appearance of the cake without adding too much fat. A little coconut-flavored extract added to batters, frostings, and fillings will also reduce the amount of coconut needed.

Piña Colada Cake

YIELD: 16 SERVINGS
1 box (1 pound, 2.25 ounces) reduced-fat or regular yellow cake mix
1 package (4-serving size) instant coconut pudding mix*
1 can (8 ounces) crushed pineapple, undrained
1 cup nonfat or light sour cream
3/4 cup fat-free egg substitute
1/4 cup water

SYRUP

1/2 cup fat-free or low-fat sweetened condensed milk
1/4 cup light rum
1/2 teaspoon coconut-flavored extract

FROSTING

2 cups nonfat or light whipped topping
1 container (8 ounces) piña colada or coconut-flavored nonfat yogurt (7/8 cup)
1/4 cup shredded sweetened coconut

* If you cannot find coconut pudding mix, substitute 1 package of instant vanilla pudding mix plus 3/4 teaspoon of coconut-flavored extract and 2 tablespoons of finely shredded coconut.

1. Place the cake mix and pudding mix in a large bowl, and stir to mix well. Add the pineapple with its liquid and the sour cream, egg substitute, and water, and beat with an electric mixer for about 2 minutes, or until well mixed.

2. Coat a 9-x-13-inch pan with nonstick cooking spray, and spread the batter evenly in the pan. Bake at 350°F for about 33 minutes, or just until the top springs back when lightly touched and a wooden toothpick inserted in the center of the cake comes out clean. Be careful not to overbake.

3. Allow the cake to cool in the pan for 20 minutes. Using a small knife, poke holes in the cake at 1/2-inch intervals.

4. To make the syrup, place all of the syrup ingredients in a small bowl, and stir to mix well. Slowly pour the syrup over the cake, allowing it to be absorbed into the cake. Allow the cake to cool to room temperature.

5. To make the frosting, place the whipped topping in a medium-sized bowl, and gently fold in the yogurt. Spread the mixture over the cake, swirling the frosting with a knife. Sprinkle the coconut over the top. Cover and refrigerate for at least 3 hours before cutting into squares and serving.

NUTRITIONAL FACTS (PER SERVING)
Cal: 240   Carbs: 48 g   Chol: 0 mg   Fat: 2.6 g
Fiber: 0.6 g   Protein: 4.6 g   Sodium: 305 mg

Citrus Pound Cake

For variety, add 2 tablespoons of poppy seeds to the batter.

YIELD: 16 SERVINGS
1 box (1 pound, 2.25 ounces) reduced-fat or regular lemon or yellow cake mix
1 box (4-serving size) instant lemon pudding mix
1 can (11 ounces) mandarin orange sections, undrained
3/4 cup fat-free egg substitute
3 tablespoons powdered sugar (optional)

1. Place the cake mix and pudding mix in a large bowl, and stir to mix well. Add the mandarin oranges with their liquid and the egg substitute, and beat with an electric mixer for about 2 minutes, or until the ingredients are well mixed and the oranges are pulverized.

2. Coat a 12-cup bundt pan with nonstick cooking spray, and spread the batter evenly in the pan. Bake at 350°F for about 40 minutes, or just until the top springs back when lightly touched and a wooden toothpick inserted in the center of the cake comes out clean. Be careful not to overbake.

3. Allow the cake to cool in the pan for 45 minutes. Then invert onto a serving platter and cool to room temperature. If desired, sift the powdered sugar over the top just before slicing and serving.

NUTRITIONAL FACTS (PER SERVING)
Cal: 168   Carbs: 36 g   Chol: 0 mg   Fat: 1.5 g
Fiber: 0.4 g   Protein: 2 g   Sodium: 306 mg

Minty Mocha-Fudge Cake

YIELD: 18 SERVINGS

1 1/2 cups sugar

1 1/2 cups unbleached flour

1 cup oat flour

1/2 cup Dutch processed cocoa powder

1 1/2 teaspoons baking soda

1/2 teaspoon salt

1 2/3 cups coffee, cooled to room temperature

1/2 cup chocolate syrup

1/4 cup vegetable oil

1 tablespoon distilled white vinegar

2 teaspoons vanilla extract

GLAZE

1 1/2 cups powdered sugar

1 tablespoon Dutch processed cocoa powder

2 tablespoons skim or low-fat milk

1/2 teaspoon vanilla extract

3 drops peppermint extract

1. Place the sugar, flours, cocoa, baking soda, and salt in a large bowl, and stir to mix well. Set aside.

2. Place the coffee, chocolate syrup, vegetable oil, vinegar, and vanilla extract in a medium-sized bowl, and stir to mix well. Add the coffee mixture to the flour mixture, and stir with a wire whisk until well mixed. (The batter will be thin.)

3. Coat a 9-x-13-inch pan with nonstick cooking spray, and pour the batter into the pan. Bake at 350°F for 40 minutes, or just until the top springs back when lightly touched, and a wooden toothpick inserted in the center of the cake comes out clean or coated with a few fudgy crumbs. Allow to cool to room temperature.

4. To make the glaze, place all of the glaze ingredients in a small bowl, and stir to mix well, adding a little more milk if needed to bring the mixture to a thick, frostinglike consistency. If using a microwave oven, place the glaze in a microwave-safe bowl, and heat uncovered at high power for 60 seconds, or until runny. If using a conventional stovetop, place the glaze in a small saucepan, and, stirring constantly, cook over medium heat for 60 seconds, or until runny. Drizzle the glaze over the cake, and allow the glaze to harden for at least 15 minutes before slicing and serving.

NUTRITIONAL FACTS (PER SERVING)
Cal: 190   Carbs: 38 g   Chol: 0 mg   Fat: 3.6 g
Fiber: 1.7 g   Protein: 2.4 g   Sodium: 172 mg

VARIATION

To make Almond Mocha Fudge Cake, substitute 1/2 teaspoon of almond extract for the peppermint extract in the glaze, and add 1/4 cup plus 2 tablespoons of chopped toasted almonds when mixing the glaze.

NUTRITIONAL FACTS (PER SERVING)
Cal: 208   Carbs: 39 g   Chol: 0 mg   Fat: 5.1 g
Fiber: 2.1 g   Protein: 3.1 g   Sodium: 172 mg

Old-Fashioned Strawberry Shortcake

For variety, substitute diced peaches for the strawberries, and amaretto for the raspberry or orange liqueur. Or substitute fresh raspberries or blueberries for part of the strawberries.

YIELD: 6 SERVINGS

BISCUITS

1 cup unbleached flour

1/3 cup sugar

1/4 cup oat bran

2 teaspoons baking powder

2–3 tablespoons chilled reduced-fat margarine or light butter, cut into pieces

1/2 cup plus 1 tablespoon nonfat or low-fat buttermilk

BERRY MIXTURE

4 cups sliced strawberries

1/3 cup sugar

2 tablespoons Chambord (raspberry) liqueur or orange liqueur (optional)

TOPPING

1 cup nonfat or light whipped topping

1/3 cup nonfat or low-fat vanilla yogurt

1. To make the berry mixture, place 1 cup of the strawberries in a medium-sized bowl. Add the sugar, and mash with a fork. Add the remaining berries and, if desired, the liqueur, and stir to mix well. Cover and chill for 2 to 5 hours to allow the juices to develop.

2. To make the topping, place the whipped topping in a small bowl, and gently fold in the yogurt. Cover and chill until ready to serve.

3. To make the biscuits, place the flour, sugar, oat bran, and baking powder in a medium-sized bowl, and stir to mix well. Using a pastry cutter or 2 knives, cut in the margarine or butter just until the mixture resembles coarse crumbs. Add the buttermilk, and stir just until moistened. Add a little more buttermilk if needed to make a moderately thick batter.

4. Coat a medium-sized baking sheet with nonstick cooking spray, and drop heaping tablespoons of the batter onto the sheet to make 6 biscuits. Bake at 400°F for about 15 minutes, or until the biscuits are lightly browned. Be careful not to overbake. Remove the biscuits from the oven, and let sit for 5 minutes.

5. To assemble the desserts, use a serrated knife to split each biscuit open, and place each biscuit bottom on an individual dessert plate. Top the biscuit half with 1/4 cup of the berry mixture, the top half of the biscuit, and 2 more tablespoons of the berry mixture. Crown with a dollop of the topping. Repeat with the remaining ingredients to make 6 desserts, and serve immediately.

NUTRITIONAL FACTS (PER SERVING)
Cal: 252   Carbs: 53 g   Chol: 2 mg   Fat: 3 g
Fiber: 3.6 g   Protein: 4.9 g   Sodium: 227 mg

Applesauce Spice Cake

YIELD: 18 SERVINGS

1 stick (1/2 cup) reduced-fat margarine
or light butter, softened to room temperature

1 1/2 cups light brown sugar

1/4 cup plus 2 tablespoons fat-free egg substitute

2 teaspoons vanilla extract
1 1/4 cups unbleached flour
1 1/4 cups oat flour
2 teaspoons baking powder
1 teaspoon baking soda
1 teaspoon ground cinnamon
1/2 teaspoon ground nutmeg
1 cup unsweetened applesauce
1/2 cup apple butter
1/2 cup dark raisins or chopped dates
1/2 cup chopped toasted walnuts or pecans (page 348) (optional)

GLAZE
1 1/2 cups powdered sugar
1/4 cup apple butter

1. Place the margarine or butter in a large bowl. Using an electric mixer, beat in the brown sugar 1/2 cup at a time. Add the egg substitute and vanilla extract, and beat to mix well. Set aside.

2. Place the flours, baking powder, baking soda, cinnamon, and nutmeg in a medium-sized bowl, and stir to mix well. Add the flour mixture, the applesauce, and the apple butter to the margarine mixture, and stir with a wooden spoon just until well mixed. Stir in the raisins or dates and, if desired, the nuts.

3. Coat a 9-x-13-inch pan with nonstick cooking spray, and spread the batter evenly in the pan. Bake at 325°F for about 35 minutes, or just until the top springs back when lightly touched and a wooden toothpick inserted in the center of the cake comes out clean. Be careful not to overbake. Remove the cake from the oven, and set aside.

4. To make the glaze, place the powdered sugar and apple butter in a medium-sized bowl, and stir to mix well. Spread the glaze over the hot cake. Allow the cake to cool to room temperature before serving.

NUTRITIONAL FACTS (PER SERVING)
Cal: 225   Carbs: 48 g   Chol: 0 mg   Fat: 2.9 g
Fiber: 1.6 g   Protein: 2.5 g   Sodium: 172 mg

Applesauce Gingerbread

YIELD: 18 SERVINGS

1½ cups unbleached flour

1 cup whole wheat pastry flour

¾ cup sugar

2 teaspoons baking soda

2½ teaspoons ground ginger

1 teaspoon ground cinnamon

1 teaspoon ground allspice

¼ teaspoon salt

1½ cups unsweetened applesauce

1 cup molasses

¼ cup vegetable oil

2 egg whites, lightly beaten

1. Place the flours, sugar, baking soda, spices, and salt in a large bowl, and stir to mix well. Add all of the remaining ingredients, and stir with a wire whisk to mix well. Set the batter aside for 10 minutes.

2. Coat a 9-x-13-inch pan with nonstick cooking spray. Whisk the batter for 15 seconds, and spread it evenly in the pan. Bake at 325°F for about 40 minutes, or just until the top springs back when lightly touched and a wooden toothpick inserted in the center of the cake comes out clean.

3. Allow the cake to cool for at least 30 minutes. Cut into squares and serve warm or at room temperature with a light whipped topping, if desired.

NUTRITIONAL FACTS (PER SERVING)
Cal: 174   Carbs: 34 g   Chol: 0 mg   Fat: 3.1 g
Fiber: 1.3 g   Protein: 2.3 g   Sodium: 185 mg

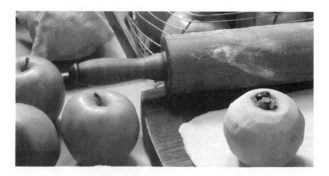

Lite and Luscious Key Lime Pie

YIELD: 8 SERVINGS

1 prebaked Lite Graham Cracker Pie Crust (page 330) made with plain graham crackers

FILLING

¼ cup fat-free egg substitute

1⅛ teaspoons unflavored gelatin

½ cup key lime juice, divided

1 can (14 ounces) fat-free or low-fat sweetened condensed milk

TOPPING

1 cup nonfat or light whipped topping (optional)

2 tablespoons shredded sweetened coconut (optional)

1. To make the filling, place the egg substitute in a blender, and sprinkle the gelatin over the egg. Set aside for 2 minutes to allow the gelatin to soften.

2. Place ¼ cup of the lime juice in a small bowl. If using a microwave oven, microwave uncovered on high for about 1 minute, or until the juice comes to a boil. If using a conventional stovetop, place the juice in a small pot, and cook over medium heat for about 1 minute, or until it comes to a boil.

3. Add the boiling lime juice to the blender, place the lid on, and blend for about 1 minute, or until the ingredients are well mixed and the gelatin is completely dissolved. Add the remaining ¼ cup of lime juice, and blend for about 30 seconds, or until well mixed. Add the condensed milk, and blend for about 1 minute, or until well mixed. Immediately pour the filling into the crust.

4. Cover and chill for at least 6 hours, or until set, before cutting into wedges and serving. Top each serving with 2 tablespoons of whipped topping and a sprinkling of coconut, if desired.

NUTRITIONAL FACTS (PER SERVING)
Cal: 253   Carbs: 50 g   Chol: 2 mg   Fat: 3.1 g
Fiber: 0.4 g   Protein: 6.7 g   Sodium: 218 mg

Pleasing Pie Crusts

Meringue Tart Shells

These light-as-air shells have always been fat-free, and make an elegant base for fresh fruits, puddings, and a variety of other fillings.

YIELD: 8 SHELLS
3 egg whites, brought to room temperature
1/4 teaspoon cream of tartar
Pinch salt
3/4 cup sugar
3/4 teaspoon vanilla extract

1. Place the egg whites, cream of tartar, and salt in a medium-sized bowl, and beat with an electric mixer until soft peaks form when the beaters are raised.

2. Gradually add the sugar, a tablespoon at a time, while beating continuously, until all of the sugar has been incorporated, the mixture is glossy, and stiff peaks form when the beaters are raised. (The total beating time will be about 7 minutes.) Beat in the vanilla extract.

3. Place a sheet of waxed paper over the bottom of a large baking sheet, and drop the meringue onto the sheet in 8 mounds, spacing the mounds about 4 inches apart. Using the back of a spoon, spread each mound into a 3 1/2-inch circle, creating a center that is about 1/2 inch thick and building up the sides to about 1 1/4 inches in height.

4. Bake at 250°F for 1 hour, or until the shells are creamy white and firm to the touch. Turn the oven off, and allow the shells to cool in the oven for 1 hour with the door closed. Fill as desired. (Note that the shells may be prepared the day before you plan to use them, and stored in an airtight container until ready to fill.)

NUTRITIONAL FACTS (PER SHELL)
Cal: 79   Carbs: 18.8 g   Chol: 0 mg   Fat: 0 g
Fiber: 0 g   Protein: 1.3 g   Sodium: 34 mg

VARIATION

To make Almond Meringue Tart Shells, reduce the vanilla extract to 1/2 teaspoon, and add 1/2 teaspoon of almond extract along with the vanilla. Gently fold 1/4 cup of finely ground toasted almonds into the finished meringue. Then shape and bake as directed in the recipe.

NUTRITIONAL FACTS (PER SHELL)
Cal: 102   Carbs: 19.6 g   Chol: 0 mg   Fat: 2.1 g
Fiber: 0 g   Protein: 2.1 g   Sodium: 34 mg

Flaky Oat Pie Crust

This pie crust has less than half the fat of a traditional crust, with a tender flaky texture. Fill it with precooked fillings or with fillings that require baking.

YIELD: ONE 9-INCH PIE CRUST
1/2 cup plus 2 tablespoons quick-cooking oats
1/2 cup plus 1 tablespoon unbleached flour
1/8 teaspoon salt
2–3 tablespoons vegetable oil (try walnut oil for extra flavor)
2 tablespoons skim or low-fat milk

1. Place the oats, flour, and salt in a medium-sized bowl, and stir to mix. Add the oil and milk, and stir just until the mixture is moist and crumbly, and holds together when pinched.

2. Coat a 9-inch deep dish pie pan with nonstick cooking spray. Pinch off pieces of dough and press them in a thin layer against the sides of the pan. Then fill in the bottom with the remaining dough.

3. For a prebaked crust, prick the crust with a fork at 1-inch intervals, and bake at 400°F for about 12 minutes, or until lightly browned. Allow the crust to cool to room temperature before filling. When a prebaked crust is not desired, simply fill and bake the crust as directed in the recipe.

NUTRITIONAL FACTS (PER ⅛ CRUST)
Cal: 83   Carbs: 10 g   Chol: 0 mg   Fat: 3.7 g
Fiber: 0.8 g   Protein: 2 g   Sodium: 38 mg

Lite Graham Cracker Pie Crust

Fill this crust only with precooked or no-cook fillings, such as puddings.

YIELD: ONE 9-INCH PIE CRUST

10 large (2½-x-5-inch) reduced-fat
plain or chocolate graham crackers

3 tablespoons sugar

3 tablespoons reduced-fat margarine
or light butter, cut into pieces (do not melt)

1. Break the crackers into pieces, place in the bowl of a food processor, and process into fine crumbs. Measure the crumbs. There should be 1¼ cups. (Adjust the amount if necessary.)

2. Return the crumbs to the food processor, add the sugar, and process for a few seconds to mix well. Add the margarine or butter, and process for about 20 seconds, or until the mixture is moist and crumbly, and holds together when pinched. If the mixture seems too dry, mix in more margarine, ½ teaspoon at a time, until the proper consistency is reached.

3. Coat a 9-inch pie pan with cooking spray, and use the back of a spoon to press the mixture against the bottom and sides of the pan, forming an even crust. (Periodically dip the spoon in sugar, if necessary, to prevent sticking.) Then use your fingers to finish pressing the crust firmly against the bottom and sides of the pan.

4. Bake at 350°F for 9 minutes, or until the edges feel firm and dry. Cool to room temperature before filling.

NUTRITIONAL FACTS (PER ⅛ CRUST)
Cal: 106   Carbs: 19 g   Chol: 0 mg   Fat: 3 g
Fiber: 0.3 g   Protein: 1.3 g   Sodium: 152 mg

Strawberry Angel Tarts

YIELD: 8 TARTS

8 Meringue Tart Shells, plain or almond
(page 329)

2 cups nonfat or light whipped topping

3 cups sliced fresh strawberries

½ cup seedless strawberry jam

1. Place one tart shell on each of 8 serving plates. Fill the center of each tart shell with ¼ cup of the whipped topping; then place ¼ cup plus 2 tablespoons of the strawberries over the topping, allowing a few of the berry slices to tumble down the sides.

2. Place the jam in a small pot. Cook over medium heat, stirring constantly, for about 1 minute, or until runny. Drizzle 1 tablespoon of the jam over the fruit, and serve immediately.

NUTRITIONAL FACTS (PER TART)
Cal: 176   Carbs: 42 g   Chol: 0 mg   Fat: 0.8 g
Fiber: 1.2 g   Protein: 1.8 g   Sodium: 52 mg

VARIATION
To make Raspberry Angel Tarts, substitute fresh raspberries for the strawberries, and chocolate syrup or seedless raspberry jam for the strawberry jam. (Do not heat the chocolate syrup; just drizzle it over the berries straight from the bottle.)

NUTRITIONAL FACTS (PER TART)
Cal: 172   Carbs: 41 g   Chol: 0 mg   Fat: 1 g
Fiber: 2.2 g   Protein: 2.1 g   Sodium: 62 mg

Mocha Meringue Tarts

YIELD: 8 SERVINGS

8 Meringue Tart Shells, plain or almond (page 329)

1 quart nonfat or low-fat mocha
or cappuccino ice cream

2 cups fresh raspberries

$\frac{1}{2}$ cup chocolate syrup

1. Place each tart on an individual serving dish, and place a $\frac{1}{2}$-cup scoop of ice cream in the center of each tart.

2. Scatter $\frac{1}{4}$ cup of berries over and around the ice cream in each tart, and drizzle 1 tablespoon of the chocolate syrup over the top. Serve immediately.

NUTRITIONAL FACTS (PER SERVING)
Cal: 224   Carbs: 51 g   Chol: 2 mg   Fat: 0.5 g
Fiber: 1.6 g   Protein: 4.9 g   Sodium: 107 mg

Sour Cream Apple Pie

YIELD: 8 SERVINGS

1 unbaked Flaky Oat Pie Crust (page 329)

FILLING

1 cup nonfat or light sour cream

$\frac{1}{2}$ cup sugar

$\frac{1}{4}$ cup fat-free egg substitute

2 tablespoons unbleached flour

1 teaspoon vanilla extract

4 cups sliced peeled golden Delicious or
Rome apples (about 6 medium)

$\frac{1}{4}$ cup golden raisins (optional)

TOPPING

$\frac{1}{4}$ cup honey crunch wheat germ
or chopped walnuts

3 tablespoons whole wheat pastry flour

3 tablespoons light brown sugar

$\frac{1}{2}$ teaspoon ground cinnamon

1 tablespoon frozen (thawed)
apple juice concentrate

1. To make the filling, place the sour cream, sugar, egg substitute, flour, and vanilla extract in a large bowl, and stir to mix well. Add the apples and, if desired, the raisins, and toss to mix well.

2. Spread the mixture evenly in the pie shell. Spray a square of aluminum foil with nonstick cooking spray, and cover the pie loosely with the foil, placing it sprayed side down. Bake at 400°F for 25 minutes, or until the filling begins to set around the edges.

3. While the pie is baking, make the topping by placing the wheat germ or walnuts, flour, brown sugar, and cinnamon in a small bowl, and stirring to mix well. Add the juice concentrate, and stir until the mixture is moist and crumbly.

4. Remove the pie from the oven, remove and discard the foil, and sprinkle the pie with the topping. Reduce the oven temperature to 375°F, and bake uncovered for 25 to 30 additional minutes, or until the topping is nicely browned and the filling just starts to bubble around the edges.

5. Allow the pie to cool for at least 1 hour before cutting into wedges and serving. Serve warm or at room temperature, refrigerating any leftovers.

NUTRITIONAL FACTS (PER SERVING)
Cal: 234   Carbs: 45 g   Chol: 0 mg   Fat: 4.2 g
Fiber: 2.7 g   Protein: 5.2 g   Sodium: 65 mg

Frozen Mocha Pie

For variety, substitute raspberry ripple or chocolate ice cream for the cappuccino ice cream.

YIELD: 8 SERVINGS

$\frac{1}{4}$ cup chocolate syrup

2 tablespoons coffee or amaretto liqueur

2 cups nonfat or light whipped topping

4 ounces ladyfingers (about 16 whole cookies)

4 cups nonfat or low-fat cappuccino ice cream,
slightly softened

1 teaspoon cocoa powder (garnish)

1. To make the syrup, place the chocolate syrup and liqueur in a small bowl, and stir to mix well. Set aside.

2. To make the topping, place the whipped topping in a medium-sized bowl, and gently fold in 1 tablespoon of the chocolate syrup mixture. Set aside.

3. To assemble the pie, first split each of the ladyfingers in half lengthwise. (Most ladyfingers come presplit.) Line the bottom and sides of a 9-inch deep dish pie pan with about two-thirds of the ladyfinger halves, arranging them split side-up. Drizzle half of the chocolate syrup mixture over the ladyfingers that line the bottom of the pan.

4. Spread the ice cream over the ladyfingers. Then top with the remaining ladyfingers, this time arranging them split side-down.

5. Drizzle the remaining chocolate syrup mixture over the ladyfingers layer. Then spread the whipped topping mixture over the syrup, swirling the topping.

6. Cover the pie loosely with aluminum foil, and freeze for several hours or overnight. When ready to serve, sprinkle the cocoa over the top of the pie. Cut the pie into wedges, place the wedges on individual serving plates, and allow to sit at room temperature for 5 minutes before serving.

> **NUTRITIONAL FACTS (PER SERVING)**
> Cal: 202   Carbs: 42 g   Chol: 27 mg   Fat: 1.4 g
> Fiber: 0.4 g   Protein: 4.4 g   Sodium: 176 mg

Very Strawberry Pie

YIELD: 8 SERVINGS

1 prebaked Lite Graham Cracker Pie Crust (page 330) made with plain graham crackers

FILLING

5 cups halved strawberries

GLAZE

1/2 cup sugar

3 tablespoons cornstarch

1 cup cran-strawberry juice or another strawberry juice blend

1/2 teaspoon unflavored gelatin

1. To make the glaze, place the sugar and cornstarch in a 1-quart pot, and stir to mix well. Add the juice, and stir until the cornstarch is dissolved. Bring the mixture to a boil over medium heat, stirring constantly with a whisk. Reduce the heat to low, and cook and stir for 1 minute, or until the mixture is thickened and bubbly.

2. Remove the glaze from the heat, and sprinkle the gelatin over the top. Whisk for about 1 minute, or until the gelatin is completely dissolved. Set aside to cool to room temperature.

3. Place the berries in a large bowl. Stir the glaze, and pour it over the berries, tossing gently to coat.

4. Spread the strawberry mixture over the prepared crust, and chill for several hours, or until the glaze is set. Serve cold.

> **NUTRITIONAL FACTS (PER SERVING)**
> Cal: 211   Carbs: 45 g   Chol: 0 mg   Fat: 3.4 g
> Fiber: 2.5 g   Protein: 1.8 g   Sodium: 154 mg

> **TIME-SAVING TIP**
> To save time and effort, substitute 1 1/3 cups of ready-made strawberry glaze for the homemade glaze.

Praline Pumpkin Pie

YIELD: 8 SERVINGS

1 unbaked Flaky Oat Pie Crust (page 329)

FILLING

1 1/2 cups mashed cooked or canned pumpkin

3/4 cup light brown sugar

2 1/2 teaspoons pumpkin pie spice*

1 1/2 teaspoons vanilla extract

1 cup plus 2 tablespoons evaporated skim milk

1/2 cup fat-free egg substitute

TOPPING

3 tablespoons light brown sugar

3 tablespoons honey crunch wheat germ or finely chopped toasted pecans (page 348)

* If you don't have any pumpkin pie spice on hand, you can use 1 1/2 teaspoons of ground cinnamon, 1/2 teaspoon of ground nutmeg, and 1/2 teaspoon of ground ginger.

1. To make the topping, place the brown sugar and the wheat germ or pecans in a small bowl, and stir to mix well. Set aside.

2. To make the filling, place the pumpkin, brown sugar, pie spice, and vanilla extract in a large bowl, and whisk to mix well. Add the milk and egg substitute, and whisk again to mix.

3. Pour the filling into the crust, and bake uncovered at 400°F for 15 minutes. Reduce the oven temperature to 350ºF, and bake for an additional 20 minutes. Sprinkle the topping over the pie, and bake for about 25 additional minutes, or until a sharp knife inserted in the center of the pie comes out clean.

4. Allow the pie to cool to room temperature before cutting into wedges and serving. Or refrigerate and serve chilled.

NUTRITIONAL FACTS (PER SERVING)

Cal: 229   Carbs: 43 g   Chol: 1 mg   Fat: 4.1 g
Fiber: 2.4 g   Protein: 6.2 g   Sodium: 99 mg

Apricot-Apple Turnovers

YIELD: 20 PASTRIES

CRUSTS

10 sheets (about 12 x 18 inches) phyllo pastry (about 8 ounces)

Nonstick butter-flavored cooking spray

2 tablespoons powdered sugar (optional)

FILLING

3 cups chopped peeled golden Delicious or Rome apples (about 4 medium)

½ cup apricot preserves

2 tablespoons water, divided

1 tablespoon cornstarch

GLAZE

1 tablespoon plus 1 teaspoon fat-free egg substitute

1 tablespoon plus 1 teaspoon sugar

1. To make the filling, place the apples, apricot preserves, and 1 tablespoon of the water in a 2-quart pot. Stir to mix well, cover, and cook over medium-low heat, stirring occasionally, for about 5 minutes, or until the apples are tender.

2. Place the cornstarch and remaining tablespoon of water in a small bowl, and stir to dissolve the cornstarch. Add the cornstarch mixture to the simmering apple mixture, and cook, stirring constantly, for about 1 minute, or until the mixture is thick and bubbly. Remove the pot from the heat, and set aside to cool to room temperature.

3. To make the glaze, place the egg substitute and sugar in a small bowl. Stir to mix well, and set aside.

4. Spread the phyllo dough out on a clean, dry surface, with the short end facing you. Cut the phyllo lengthwise into 4 long strips, each measuring about 3 x 18 inches. Cover the dough with plastic wrap to prevent it from drying out as you work. (Remove strips as you need them, being sure to re-cover the remaining dough.)

5. Remove 2 strips of phyllo dough and stack 1 on top of the other. Spray the top strip lightly with the cooking spray. Spread 1 level tablespoon of the filling over the bottom right-hand corner of the double phyllo strip. Fold the filled corner up and over to the left, so that the corner meets the left side of the strip. Continue folding in this manner until you form a triangle of dough. Repeat with the remaining filling and dough to make 20 pastries. (At this point, the turnovers may be frozen for future use. See the Time-Saving Tip below.)

6. Coat a large baking sheet with nonstick cooking spray, and arrange the pastries seam side down on the sheet. Brush the top of each pastry with some of the glaze.

7. Bake at 375°F for 12 to 15 minutes, or until golden brown. Allow to cool for at least 15 minutes before serving warm. Sift the powdered sugar over the turnovers just before serving, if desired.

NUTRITIONAL FACTS (PER PASTRY)

Cal: 59   Carbs: 12.3 g   Chol: 0 mg   Fat: 0.8 g
Fiber: 0.4 g   Protein: 0.8 g   Sodium: 50 mg

TIME-SAVING TIP
To save time the day you bake Apricot-Apple Turnovers, prepare the pastries ahead of time to the point of baking, and arrange them in single layers in airtight containers, separating the layers with sheets of waxed paper. Then place the pastries in the freezer until needed. When ready to bake, arrange the frozen pastries on a coated sheet and allow them to sit at room temperature for 45 minutes before baking.

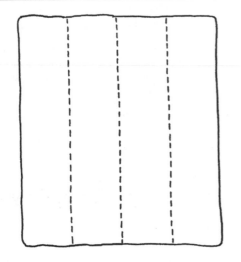

a. Cut the dough into 4 strips.

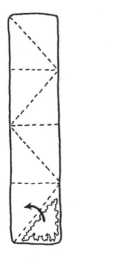
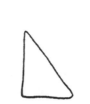

b. Fold the filled corner up and over.

c. Continue folding to form a triangle.

MAKING APRICOT-APPLE TURNOVERS

Apple-Raisin Crisp

For variety, substitute dates, dried pitted cherries, dried cranberries, or chopped dried apricots for the raisins.

YIELD: 8 SERVINGS

4³⁄₄ cups sliced peeled apples
(about 6¹⁄₂ medium)

¹⁄₃ cup dark raisins

¹⁄₃ cup light brown sugar

1¹⁄₂ teaspoons cornstarch

2 tablespoons water

TOPPING

¹⁄₄ cup plus 2 tablespoons quick-cooking oats

¹⁄₄ cup plus 2 tablespoons whole wheat pastry flour

¹⁄₃ cup light brown sugar

¹⁄₂ teaspoon ground cinnamon

2 tablespoons frozen (thawed) apple juice concentrate or maple syrup

¹⁄₃ cup honey crunch wheat germ, chopped toasted pecans (page 348), or chopped walnuts

1. To make the filling, place the apples and raisins in a large bowl, and toss to mix well. Set aside.

2. Place the brown sugar and cornstarch in a small bowl, and stir to mix well. Sprinkle the mixture over the fruit, and toss to mix well. (If the fruit is tart, you may need to add another couple of tablespoons of sugar.) Add the water, and toss to mix well. Coat a 9-inch deep dish pie pan with nonstick cooking spray, and spread the fruit mixture evenly in the pan. Set aside.

3. To make the topping, place the oats, flour, brown sugar, and cinnamon in a small bowl, and stir to mix well. Add the juice concentrate or maple syrup, and stir until the mixture is moist and crumbly. (If the mixture seems too dry, add more juice concentrate or maple syrup, ¹⁄₄ teaspoon at a time, until the proper consistency is reached.) Stir in the wheat germ or nuts. Sprinkle the topping over the filling.

4. Bake uncovered at 375°F for 35 to 40 minutes, or until the filling is bubbly and the topping is golden brown. Cover loosely with aluminum foil during the last few minutes of baking if the topping starts to brown too quickly. Allow to cool at room temperature for at least 15 minutes, and serve warm or at room temperature.

NUTRITIONAL FACTS (PER SERVING)
Cal: 160   Carbs: 37 g   Chol: 0 mg   Fat: 1 g
Fiber: 2.8 g   Protein: 2.7 g   Sodium: 7 mg

Summer Fruit Crisp

YIELD: 8 SERVINGS

4 cups sliced peeled peaches or nectarines (about 6 medium)
1 cup fresh or frozen (unthawed) blueberries, raspberries, or pitted sweet cherries
1/3 cup sugar
1 tablespoon cornstarch

TOPPING

1/4 cup plus 2 tablespoons quick-cooking oats
1/4 cup plus 2 tablespoons whole wheat pastry flour
1/4 cup plus 2 tablespoons light brown sugar
1/2 teaspoon ground cinnamon
2 tablespoons chilled tub-style nonfat margarine, or 3 tablespoons reduced-fat margarine or light butter, softened to room temperature
1/3 cup honey crunch wheat germ or chopped toasted pecans (page 348)

1. To make the filling, place the peaches or nectarines and the blueberries, raspberries, or cherries in a large bowl, and toss to mix well. Set aside.

2. Place the sugar and cornstarch in a small bowl, and stir to mix well. Sprinkle the mixture over the fruit, and toss to mix well. (If the fruit is tart, you may need to add another couple of tablespoons of sugar.) Coat a 9-inch deep dish pie pan with nonstick cooking spray, and spread the fruit mixture evenly in the pan. Set aside.

3. To make the topping, place the oats, flour, brown sugar, and cinnamon in a small bowl, and stir to mix well. Add the margarine or butter, and stir until the mixture is moist and crumbly. (If the mixture seems too dry, add more margarine or butter, 1/2 teaspoon at a time, until the proper consistency is reached.) Stir in the wheat germ or pecans. Sprinkle the topping over the filling.

4. Bake uncovered at 375°F for 35 to 40 minutes, or until the filling is bubbly and the topping is golden brown. Cover loosely with aluminum foil during the last few minutes of baking if the topping starts to brown too quickly. Allow to cool at room temperature for at least 15 minutes, and serve warm or at room temperature.

NUTRITIONAL FACTS (PER SERVING)
Cal: 163   Carbs: 37 g   Chol: 0 mg   Fat: 1 g
Fiber: 3.4 g   Protein: 3.2 g   Sodium: 27 mg

Phyllo Apple Dumplings

YIELD: 6 SERVINGS

3 tablespoons sugar
1/4 teaspoon ground cinnamon
6 medium golden Delicious or Rome apples
3 tablespoons dark raisins, dried cranberries, or chopped dried apricots
3 tablespoons toasted chopped almonds, pecans, or walnuts (page 348)
5 tablespoons honey, divided
6 sheets (about 12 x 18 inches) phyllo pastry (about 5 ounces)
Nonstick butter-flavored cooking spray

1. Place the sugar and cinnamon in a small bowl, and stir to mix well. Set aside.

2. Starting at the stem end, core the apples without cutting through the opposite end. Then peel the apples, and set aside.

3. Place the dried fruit and nuts in a small bowl, and toss to mix well. Stuff 1 tablespoon of the mixture into the cavity of each apple, and drizzle 1 teaspoon of honey over the fruit-and-nut mixture. Set aside.

4. Spread the phyllo dough out on a clean, dry surface, with the short end facing you. Cover the dough with plastic wrap to prevent it from drying out as you work. (Remove the sheets as you need them, being sure to re-cover the remaining dough.)

5. Remove 1 sheet of the phyllo dough, and lay it on a clean dry surface. Spray the sheet lightly with the cooking spray, and sprinkle with 1 teaspoon of the cinnamon mixture. Fold the bottom up to form a double layer of phyllo measuring approximately 12 x 9 inches.

6. Stand an apple upright in the center of the folded phyllo sheet. Bring 1 corner of the sheet up and over the top of the apple and down the other side. Repeat with the other 3 corners to completely cover the apple. Use your hands to press the phyllo dough over the apple to make it conform to the shape of the apple. Repeat this procedure with the remaining ingredients to make 6 phyllo-wrapped apples.

7. Coat a large baking sheet with nonstick cooking spray, and stand the wrapped apples upright on the sheet. Spray the tops and sides of the apples lightly with the cooking spray, and sprinkle with the remaining sugar mixture. (Note that you can prepare the recipe up to this point, cover the apples with plastic wrap, and refrigerate for up to 6 hours before baking, if desired.)

8. Bake uncovered at 350°F for 35 minutes, or until the phyllo is nicely browned and the apples are tender when pierced with a sharp knife. Cover the apples loosely with aluminum foil during the last 10 minutes of baking if they begin to brown too quickly.

9. Remove the apples from the oven, and allow to cool for 10 minutes. To serve, cut each apple in half lengthwise and drizzle with $1^1/_2$ teaspoons of the remaining honey. As an alternative, try topping the apples with a scoop of low-fat vanilla ice cream. Serve warm.

NUTRITIONAL FACTS (PER SERVING)
Cal: 224   Carbs: 47 g   Chol: 1 mg   Fat: 3.9 g
Fiber: 2.7 g   Protein: 2.5 g   Sodium: 94 mg

Cranberry-Pear Crumble

YIELD: 8 SERVINGS

$4^1/_2$ cups diced peeled pears (about 5 medium)

$^1/_2$ cup coarsely chopped fresh or frozen (unthawed) cranberries

$^1/_3$ cup light brown sugar

2 teaspoons cornstarch

TOPPING

$^1/_4$ cup plus 2 tablespoons quick-cooking oats

$^1/_4$ cup plus 2 tablespoons whole wheat pastry flour

$^1/_3$ cup light brown sugar

$^1/_2$ teaspoon ground cinnamon

2 tablespoons frozen (thawed) orange juice concentrate

$^1/_3$ cup honey crunch wheat germ or chopped toasted pecans (page 348)

1. To make the filling, place the pears and cranberries in a large bowl, and toss to mix well. Set aside.

2. Place the brown sugar and cornstarch in a small bowl, and stir to mix well. Sprinkle the mixture over the fruit, and toss to mix. (If the fruit is tart, you may need to add another couple of tablespoons of sugar.) Coat a 9-inch deep dish pie pan with nonstick cooking spray, and spread the fruit mixture evenly in the pan. Set aside.

3. To make the topping, place the oats, flour, brown sugar, and cinnamon in a small bowl, and stir to mix well. Add the juice concentrate, and stir until the mixture is moist and crumbly. (If the mixture seems too dry, add more juice concentrate, $^1/_4$ teaspoon at a time, until the proper consistency is reached.) Stir in the wheat germ or pecans. Sprinkle the topping over the filling.

4. Bake uncovered at 375°F for 35 to 40 minutes, or until the filling is bubbly and the topping is golden brown. Cover loosely with aluminum foil during the last few minutes of baking if the topping starts to brown too quickly. Allow to cool at room temperature for at least 15 minutes before serving warm.

NUTRITIONAL FACTS (PER SERVING)
Cal: 163   Carbs: 38 g   Chol: 0 mg   Fat: 1.1 g
Fiber: 3.8 g   Protein: 2.9 g   Sodium: 5 mg

California Crumble

YIELD: 6 SERVINGS

1 can (1 pound) sliced peaches in juice, drained

1 can (1 pound) apricot halves in juice, drained

3 tablespoons light brown sugar

1/4 cup plus 1 tablespoon dark raisins, chopped dates, dried pitted cherries, or chopped pitted prunes

TOPPING

1/4 cup plus 2 tablespoons quick-cooking oats

1/4 cup plus 2 tablespoons whole wheat pastry flour

1/3 cup light brown sugar

1/2 teaspoon ground cinnamon

2 tablespoons chilled tub-style nonfat margarine, or 3 tablespoons reduced-fat margarine or light butter, softened to room temperature

1/3 cup honey crunch wheat germ or chopped toasted almonds or walnuts (page 348)

1. To make the filling, cut the peaches and apricots into bite-sized pieces, and place them in a large bowl. Add the brown sugar, and toss to mix well. Add the raisins, dates, cherries, or prunes, and toss to mix well.

2. Coat a 9-inch deep dish pie pan with nonstick cooking spray, and spread the fruit mixture evenly in the pan. Set aside.

3. To make the topping, place the oats, flour, brown sugar, and cinnamon in a small bowl, and stir to mix well. Add the margarine or butter, and stir until the mixture is moist and crumbly. (If the mixture seems too dry, add more margarine or butter, 1/2 teaspoon at a time, until the proper consistency is reached.) Stir in the wheat germ or nuts. Sprinkle the topping over the filling.

4. Bake uncovered at 375°F for 30 to 35 minutes, or until the filling is bubbly and the topping is golden brown. Cover loosely with aluminum foil during the last few minutes of baking if the topping starts to brown too quickly. Allow to cool at room temperature for at least 15 minutes, and serve warm or at room temperature.

NUTRITIONAL FACTS (PER SERVING)		
Cal: 186 Carbs: 40 g Chol: 0 mg Fat: 1.3 g		
Fiber: 3.4 g Protein: 4.2 g Sodium: 38 mg		

Biscuit-Topped Blueberry Cobbler

For variety, substitute blackberries or pitted sweet cherries for the blueberries.

YIELD: 8 SERVINGS

5 cups fresh or frozen (partially thawed) blueberries

1/4 cup plus 2 tablespoons sugar

1 tablespoon plus 1/2 teaspoon cornstarch

1 tablespoon plus 1 teaspoon frozen (thawed) orange juice concentrate

BISCUIT TOPPING

3/4 cup plus 2 tablespoons unbleached flour

1/4 cup oat bran or quick-cooking oats

1/3 cup plus 1 1/2 teaspoons sugar, divided

1 3/4 teaspoons baking powder

1/2 cup plus 2 tablespoons nonfat or low-fat buttermilk

Pinch ground cinnamon

1. To make the filling, place the blueberries in a large bowl. Set aside.

2. Place the sugar and cornstarch in a small bowl, and stir to mix well. Sprinkle the mixture over the fruit, and toss to mix well. (If the fruit is tart, you may need to add another couple of tablespoons of sugar.) Add the juice concentrate, and toss to mix well.

3. Coat a 2-quart casserole dish with nonstick cooking spray, and spread the fruit mixture evenly in the dish. Cover the dish with aluminum foil, and bake at 375°F for 30 to 40 minutes, or until hot and bubbly.

4. To make the biscuit topping, place the flour, oat bran or oats, 1/3 cup of the sugar, and the baking powder in a medium-sized bowl, and stir to mix well. Add just enough of the buttermilk to make a moderately thick batter, stirring just until the dry ingredients are moistened.

5. Drop heaping tablespoonfuls of the batter onto the hot fruit filling to make 8 biscuits. Combine the remaining 1½ teaspoons of sugar and the cinnamon in a small bowl, and stir to mix well. Sprinkle the mixture over the biscuit topping.

6. Bake uncovered at 375°F for 18 to 20 minutes, or until the biscuits are lightly browned. Allow to cool at room temperature for at least 10 minutes before serving warm.

NUTRITIONAL FACTS (PER SERVING)
Cal: 190   Carbs: 46 g   Chol: 0 mg   Fat: 0.7 g
Fiber: 3.2 g   Protein: 3.1 g   Sodium: 120 mg

Cherry-Vanilla Cobbler

YIELD: 8 SERVINGS
5 cups fresh or frozen (partially thawed) pitted sweet cherries
⅓ cup sugar
1 tablespoon plus 1 teaspoon cornstarch
¼ cup white grape juice

BISCUIT TOPPING
¾ cup unbleached flour
⅓ cup oat bran or quick-cooking oats
¼ cup sugar
1½ teaspoons baking powder
¾ cup plus 1 tablespoon nonfat or low-fat vanilla yogurt

1. To make the filling, place the cherries in a large bowl. Set aside.

2. Place the sugar and cornstarch in a small bowl, and stir to mix well. Sprinkle the mixture over the fruit, and toss to mix well. (If the fruit is tart, you may need to add another couple of tablespoons of sugar.) Add the juice, and toss to mix well.

3. Coat a 2-quart casserole dish with nonstick cooking spray, and spread the fruit mixture evenly in the dish. Cover the dish with aluminum foil, and bake at 375°F for 30 to 40 minutes, or until hot and bubbly.

4. To make the biscuit topping, place the flour, oat bran or oats, sugar, and baking powder in a medium-

sized bowl, and stir to mix well. Add just enough of the yogurt to make a moderately thick batter, stirring just until the dry ingredients are moistened. Drop heaping tablespoonfuls of the batter onto the hot fruit filling to make 8 biscuits.

5. Bake uncovered at 375°F for 18 to 20 minutes, or until the biscuits are lightly browned. Allow to cool at room temperature for at least 10 minutes before serving warm.

NUTRITIONAL FACTS (PER SERVING)
Cal: 198   Carbs: 46 g   Chol: 1 mg   Fat: 0.9 g
Fiber: 3.3 g   Protein: 3.8 g   Sodium: 108 mg

Spiced Peach Cobbler

For variety, substitute pears for the peaches.

YIELD: 8 SERVINGS
1 tablespoon plus 1½ teaspoons cornstarch
½ cup plus 2 tablespoons peach nectar or white grape juice, divided
¼ cup plus 2 tablespoons sugar
½ teaspoon ground cinnamon
¼ teaspoon ground nutmeg
5½ cups sliced peeled peaches (about 7 medium)
¼ cup dark raisins

BISCUIT TOPPING
¾ cup plus 2 tablespoons unbleached flour
¼ cup oat bran or quick-cooking oats
¼ cup plus 1½ teaspoons sugar, divided
1¾ teaspoons baking powder
½ cup nonfat or low-fat vanilla yogurt
3 tablespoons reduced-fat margarine or light butter, melted

1. To make the filling, place the cornstarch and 2 tablespoons of the nectar or juice in a small bowl, and stir to dissolve the cornstarch. Set aside.

2. Place the sugar and spices in a 3-quart pot, and stir to mix well. Add the remaining ½ cup of nectar or juice, and stir to mix well. Add the peaches, and bring to a boil over medium-high heat, stirring frequently. Reduce the heat to medium-low, cover, and simmer, stirring occasionally, for about 5 minutes, or just until the peaches are tender. Stir in the raisins.

3. Stir the cornstarch mixture, and slowly pour it into the boiling peach mixture, stirring constantly. Cook and stir for another minute, or until the mixture has thickened. Remove the pot from the heat, cover, and set aside.

4. To make the biscuit topping, place the flour, oat bran or oats, 1/4 cup of the sugar, and the baking powder in a medium-sized bowl, and stir to mix well. Place the yogurt and the margarine or butter in a small bowl, and stir to mix well. Add the yogurt mixture to the flour mixture, and stir just until the dry ingredients are moistened.

5. Coat a 2-quart baking dish with nonstick cooking spray, and spread the hot peach mixture evenly in the dish. Drop heaping tablespoonfuls of the batter onto the fruit filling to make 8 biscuits. Sprinkle the remaining 1 1/2 teaspoons of sugar over the biscuit topping.

6. Bake uncovered at 375°F for about 20 minutes, or until the biscuits are lightly browned. Allow to cool at room temperature for at least 10 minutes before serving warm.

NUTRITIONAL FACTS (PER SERVING)
Cal: 227   Carbs: 51 g   Chol: 1 mg   Fat: 2.4 g
Fiber: 3.4 g   Protein: 3.6 g   Sodium: 145 mg

Glazed Mocha Brownies

YIELD: 12 BROWNIES

1 tablespoon hot tap water

1 teaspoon instant coffee granules

2/3 cup oat flour

1/4 cup Dutch processed cocoa powder

2 tablespoons instant nonfat dry milk powder

1 pinch baking soda

1/8 teaspoon salt

3/4 cup light brown sugar

1/4 cup plus 2 tablespoons fat-free egg substitute

1/4 cup chocolate syrup

1 1/2 teaspoons vanilla extract

1/3 cup toasted chopped pecans or almonds (page 348) (optional)

GLAZE

1/2 cup powdered sugar

1/2 teaspoon vanilla extract

1/4 teaspoon instant coffee granules

2 teaspoons skim or low-fat milk

1. To make the batter, place the hot water and coffee granules in a small bowl, and stir to mix well. Set aside.

2. Place the flour, cocoa powder, milk powder, baking soda, and salt in a medium-sized bowl, and stir to mix well. Add the brown sugar, and stir to mix well. Use the back of a wooden spoon to press out any lumps in the brown sugar. Add the egg substitute, chocolate syrup, vanilla extract, and coffee mixture, and stir to mix well. Set the batter aside for 15 minutes.

3. If desired, stir the nuts into the batter. Coat the bottom only of an 8-x-8-inch pan with nonstick cooking spray, and spread the mixture in the pan. Bake at 325°F for about 22 minutes, or just until the edges are firm and the center is almost set. Be careful not to overbake. Allow to cool to room temperature.

4. To make the glaze, place the powdered sugar in a small bowl. Place the vanilla extract in another small bowl, add the coffee granules, and stir to dissolve the granules. Add the vanilla mixture and the milk to the sugar, and stir to mix well, adding a little more milk if the glaze seems too thick. Microwave on high power for about 30 seconds, or until hot and runny.

5. Drizzle the hot glaze back and forth over the cooled brownies. Allow the brownies to sit for at least 15 minutes before cutting into squares and serving. For easier cutting, rinse the knife off periodically.

NUTRITIONAL FACTS (PER BROWNIE)
Cal: 115   Carbs: 25 g   Chol: 0 mg   Fat: 0.6 g
Fiber: 1.3 g   Protein: 2.2 g   Sodium: 56 mg

Cream Cheese Marble Brownies

YIELD: 24 BROWNIES

1 package (about 1 pound, 5 ounces)
low-fat fudge brownie mix

1 block (8 ounces) nonfat cream cheese,
softened to room temperature

1/3 cup sugar

1 tablespoon unbleached flour

3 tablespoons fat-free egg substitute

1 teaspoon vanilla extract

1. Prepare the brownie mix as directed on the package. Coat the bottom only of a 9-x-13-inch pan with nonstick cooking spray, and spread the mixture evenly in the pan. Set aside.

2. Place the cream cheese and sugar in a medium-sized bowl, and beat with an electric mixer until smooth. Add the flour, and beat to mix well. Add the egg substitute and vanilla extract, and beat to mix well.

3. Pour the cheese mixture over the brownie batter in an "S" pattern. Then draw a knife through the batter to create a marbled effect.

4. Bake at 325°F for 30 to 33 minutes, or just until the edges are firm and the center is almost set. Be careful not to overbake.

5. Allow the brownies to cool to room temperature before cutting into squares and serving. For easier cutting, rinse the knife off periodically.

NUTRITIONAL FACTS (PER BROWNIE)
Cal: 119   Carbs: 23 g   Chol: 0 mg   Fat: 1.5 g
Fiber: 0.7 g   Protein: 3.1 g   Sodium: 132 mg

Toasted Coconut Meringues

YIELD: 24 COOKIES

2/3 cup shredded sweetened coconut

2 large egg whites, warmed to room temperature

1/8 teaspoon cream of tartar

1/8 teaspoon salt

1/4 cup plus 2 tablespoons sugar

1/2 teaspoon coconut-flavored extract

1/2 teaspoon vanilla extract

1. Spread the coconut in a thin layer on a small baking sheet, and bake at 350°F, stirring occasionally, for about 5 minutes, or until the coconut turns light golden brown. Remove from the oven and set aside to cool to room temperature.

2. Place the egg whites in the bowl of an electric mixer, and beat on high speed until foamy. Add the cream of tartar and salt, and continue beating until soft peaks form. Still beating, slowly add the sugar, 1 tablespoon at a time. Beat the mixture just until stiff peaks form when the beaters are raised. Beat in the extracts.

3. Remove the beaters from the meringue mixture, and fold in the coconut.

4. Line a large baking sheet with aluminum foil. (Do not grease the sheet or coat it with cooking spray.) Drop heaping teaspoonfuls of the mixture onto the baking sheet, spacing them 1 inch apart.

5. Bake at 250°F for 45 minutes, or until firm to the touch. Turn the oven off, and allow the meringues to cool in the oven for 2 hours with the door closed. Remove the pans from the oven, and peel the meringues from the foil. Serve immediately, or transfer to an airtight container.

NUTRITIONAL FACTS (PER COOKIE)
Cal: 26   Carbs: 4.3 g   Chol: 0 mg   Fat: 0.8 g
Fiber: 0.1 g   Protein: 0.4 g   Sodium: 22 mg

VARIATIONS

To make Toasted Almond Meringues, substitute almond-flavored extract for the coconut extract, and substitute 1/2 cup sliced toasted almonds for the coconut.

NUTRITIONAL FACTS (PER COOKIE)
Cal: 27   Carbs: 3.6 g   Chol: 0 mg   Fat: 1.2 g
Fiber: 0.3 g   Protein: 0.7 g   Sodium: 17 mg

To make Toasted Pecan Meringues, omit the coconut-flavored extract and increase the vanilla extract to 1 teaspoon. Substitute 1/2 cup of chopped toasted pecans for the coconut.

NUTRITIONAL FACTS (PER COOKIE)
Cal: 30   Carbs: 3.6 g   Chol: 0 mg   Fat: 1.7 g
Fiber: 0.2 g   Protein: 0.5 g   Sodium: 17 mg

To make Chocolate Chip Meringues, omit the coconut-flavored extract and increase the vanilla extract to 1 teaspoon. Substitute $1/2$ cup of semi-sweet, milk chocolate, mint chocolate, or white chocolate chips for the coconut.

NUTRITIONAL FACTS (PER COOKIE)
Cal: 30   Carbs: 5.3 g   Chol: 0 mg   Fat: 1 g
Fiber: 0.2 g   Protein: 0.4 g   Sodium: 17 mg

Citrus Sugar Cookies

YIELD: 36 COOKIES

$1/4$ cup plus 1 tablespoon reduced-fat margarine or light butter, softened to room temperature

$1/2$ cup plus 2 tablespoons sugar

3 tablespoons frozen (thawed) orange juice concentrate

1 teaspoon vanilla extract

1 cup plus 2 tablespoons unbleached flour

$3/4$ cup oat bran

$1/4$ cup instant nonfat dry milk powder

$3/4$ teaspoon baking soda

1 teaspoon dried grated lemon rind, or 1 tablespoon fresh

COATING

1 tablespoon plus $1 1/2$ teaspoons sugar

1. Place the margarine or butter, sugar, juice concentrate, and vanilla extract in a large bowl, and beat with an electric mixer until smooth. Set aside.

2. Place the flour, oat bran, milk powder, baking soda, and lemon rind in a medium-sized bowl, and stir to mix well. Add the flour mixture to the margarine mixture, and beat to mix well. (Add 1 to 2 teaspoons of additional orange juice concentrate if the mixture seems too dry.)

3. Place the sugar coating in a small shallow dish, and set aside.

4. Coat a baking sheet with nonstick cooking spray. Using your hands, shape the dough into 1-inch balls.

(If the dough is too sticky to handle, place it in the freezer for a few minutes.) Roll the balls in the sugar coating; then arrange on the baking sheet, spacing them $1 1/2$ inches apart. Using the bottom of a glass, flatten each ball to $1/4$-inch thickness.

5. Bake at 300°F for about 14 minutes. To check for doneness, lift a cookie from the sheet with a spatula. The bottom should be lightly browned. Cool the cookies on the pan for 2 minutes. Then transfer the cookies to wire racks, and cool completely. Serve immediately, or transfer to an airtight container.

NUTRITIONAL FACTS (PER COOKIE)
Cal: 45   Carbs: 8.8 g   Chol: 0 mg   Fat: 0.9 g
Fiber: 0.4 g   Protein: 0.9 g   Sodium: 39 mg

Molasses Spice Cookies

YIELD: 40 COOKIES

$1/4$ cup plus 2 tablespoons reduced-fat margarine or light butter, softened to room temperature

$2/3$ cup light brown sugar

$1/4$ cup molasses

1 tablespoon unsweetened applesauce

1 teaspoon vanilla extract

2 cups whole wheat pastry flour

2 tablespoons instant nonfat dry milk powder

$3/4$ teaspoon baking soda

$1 1/4$ teaspoons ground ginger

$1 1/4$ teaspoons ground cinnamon

COATING

2 tablespoons sugar

1. Place the margarine or butter, brown sugar, molasses, applesauce, and vanilla extract in a large bowl, and beat with an electric mixer until smooth. Set aside.

2. Place the flour, milk powder, baking soda, ginger, and cinnamon in a medium-sized bowl, and stir to mix well. Add the flour mixture to the margarine mixture, and beat to mix well. (Add a couple of teaspoons of additional applesauce if the mixture seems too dry.)

3. Place the sugar coating in a small shallow dish, and set aside.

4. Coat a baking sheet with nonstick cooking spray. Using your hands, shape the dough into 1-inch balls. (If the dough is too sticky to handle, place it in the freezer for a few minutes.) Roll the balls in the sugar coating; then arrange on the baking sheet, spacing them 1 1/2 inches apart. Using the bottom of a glass, flatten each ball to 1/4-inch thickness.

5. Bake at 300°F for about 14 minutes. To check for doneness, lift a cookie from the sheet with a spatula. The bottom should be lightly browned. Cool the cookies on the pan for 2 minutes. Then transfer the cookies to wire racks, and cool completely. Serve immediately, or transfer to an airtight container.

> **NUTRITIONAL FACTS (PER COOKIE)**
> Cal: 47　Carbs: 8.9 g　Chol: 0 mg　Fat: 0.9 g
> Fiber: 0.8 g　Protein: 0.9 g　Sodium: 38 mg

Maple Oatmeal Cookies

YIELD: 40 COOKIES

1 cup whole wheat pastry flour
1 cup quick-cooking oats
2/3 cup sugar
1 teaspoon baking soda
1/2 teaspoon ground cinnamon
1/4 teaspoon ground nutmeg
1/4 cup maple syrup
1/4 cup water
2 tablespoons vegetable oil
1 teaspoon vanilla extract
1/2 cup dark raisins
1/2 cup chopped toasted walnuts or pecans (page 348)

1. Place the flour, oats, sugar, baking soda, cinnamon, and nutmeg in a large bowl, and stir to mix well. Add the maple syrup, water, oil, and vanilla extract, and stir to mix well. Finally, add the raisins and nuts, and stir to mix well.

2. Coat a baking sheet with nonstick cooking spray. Drop rounded teaspoonfuls of dough onto the sheet, placing them 1 1/2 inches apart. Slightly flatten each cookie with the tip of a spoon.

3. Bake at 300°F for about 15 minutes, or until lightly browned. Cool the cookies on the pan for 2 minutes. Then transfer the cookies to wire racks, and cool completely. Serve immediately, or transfer to an airtight container.

> **NUTRITIONAL FACTS (PER COOKIE)**
> Cal: 57　Carbs: 9 g　Chol: 0 mg　Fat: 1.8 g
> Fiber: 0.8 g　Protein: 0.9 g　Sodium: 26 mg

Triple Chocolate Biscotti

YIELD: 28 BISCOTTI

1 2/3 cups whole wheat pastry flour
3/4 cup sugar
1/3 cup Dutch processed cocoa powder
2 teaspoons baking powder
1/4 teaspoon baking soda
1/4 cup plus 1 tablespoon fat-free egg substitute
1/4 cup chocolate syrup
2 teaspoons vanilla extract
1/2 cup semi-sweet, milk chocolate, or white chocolate chips
1/2 cup chopped toasted pecans, hazelnuts, walnuts, or almonds (page 348) (optional)

1. Place the flour, sugar, cocoa, baking powder, and baking soda in a large bowl, and stir to mix well. Set aside.

2. Place the egg substitute, chocolate syrup, and vanilla extract in a small bowl, and stir to mix well. Add the egg mixture, chocolate chips, and, if desired, the nuts to the flour mixture, and stir just until the dry ingredients are moistened and the dough holds together. Add a little more egg substitute if the mixture seems too dry.

3. Spray your hands with nonstick cooking spray, and divide the dough into 2 pieces. Shape each piece into a 9-x-2 1/2-inch log. Coat a large baking sheet with the cooking spray, and place the logs on the sheet, spacing them 4 inches apart to allow for spreading. Bake at 325°F for 25 to 30 minutes, or until lightly browned and firm to the touch.

4. Using a spatula, carefully transfer the logs to a wire rack, and allow to cool at room temperature for 10 minutes. Then place the logs on a cutting board, and use a serrated knife to slice them diagonally into $1/2$-inch-thick slices.

5. Arrange the slices in a single layer on an ungreased baking sheet, cut side down. Bake for 6 minutes at 325°F. Turn the slices and bake for 6 additional minutes, or until dry and crisp.

6. Transfer the biscotti to wire racks, and cool completely. Serve immediately, or transfer to an airtight container.

NUTRITIONAL FACTS (PER BISCOTTI)
Cal: 74   Carbs: 15.8 g   Chol: 0 mg   Fat: 1.5 g
Fiber: 1.4 g   Protein: 2 g   Sodium: 54 mg

Maple-Date Drops

YIELD: 42 COOKIES
1 cup plus 2 tablespoons whole wheat pastry flour
$3/4$ cup sugar
1 teaspoon baking soda
$1/2$ teaspoon ground cinnamon
$1/3$ cup maple syrup
$1/4$ cup orange or apple juice
1 teaspoon vanilla extract
2 cups raisin bran cereal
$1/2$ cup chopped dates, dark raisins, or chopped dried apricots
$2/3$ cup chopped toasted pecans or walnuts (page 348)

1. Place the flour, sugar, baking soda, and cinnamon in a large bowl, and stir to mix well. Add the maple syrup, juice, and vanilla extract, and stir to mix well. Finally, add the cereal, dried fruit, and nuts, and stir to mix well.

2. Coat a baking sheet with nonstick cooking spray. Drop rounded teaspoonfuls of dough onto the sheet, placing them $1 1/2$ inches apart. Slightly flatten each cookie with the tip of a spoon. (Note that the dough will be slightly crumbly, so that you may have to press it together slightly to make it hold its shape.)

3. Bake at 325°F for about 14 minutes, or until lightly browned. Cool the cookies on the pan for 2 minutes. Then transfer the cookies to wire racks, and cool completely. Serve immediately, or transfer to an airtight container.

NUTRITIONAL FACTS (PER COOKIE)
Cal: 58   Carbs: 11 g   Chol: 0 mg   Fat: 1.4 g
Fiber: 1.1 g   Protein: 0.9 g   Sodium: 47 mg

Chocolate Flavor With a Fraction of the Fat

For rich chocolate flavor with minimum fat, substitute cocoa powder for high-fat baking chocolate. Simply use 3 tablespoons of cocoa powder plus 1 tablespoon of water or another liquid to replace each ounce of baking chocolate in cakes, brownies, puddings, and other goodies. You'll save 111 calories and 13.5 grams of fat for each ounce of baking chocolate you replace!

For the deepest, darkest, richest chocolate desserts, use Dutch processed cocoa. Dutching, a process that neutralizes the natural acidity in cocoa, results in a darker, sweeter, more mellow-flavored cocoa. Look for a brand name like Hershey's Dutch Processed European Style cocoa. Like regular cocoa, this product has only half a gram of fat per tablespoon—although some brands do contain more fat. Dutched cocoa can be substituted for regular cocoa in any recipe, and since it has a smoother, sweeter flavor, you may find that you can reduce the sugar in your recipe by up to 25 percent.

Maple Snickerdoodles

YIELD: 40 COOKIES

1/4 cup plus 2 tablespoons reduced-fat margarine
or light butter, softened to room temperature

3/4 cup sugar

3 tablespoons maple syrup

1 tablespoon lemon juice

1 1/2 teaspoons vanilla extract

1 1/4 cups unbleached flour

3/4 cup plus 2 tablespoons oat bran

1/4 cup instant nonfat dry milk powder

3/4 teaspoon baking soda

COATING

1 tablespoon plus 1 1/2 teaspoons sugar

1 1/2 teaspoons ground cinnamon

1. Place the margarine or butter, sugar, maple syrup, lemon juice, and vanilla extract in a large bowl, and beat with an electric mixer until smooth. Set aside.

2. Place the flour, oat bran, milk powder, and baking soda in a medium-sized bowl, and stir to mix well. Add the flour mixture to the margarine mixture, and beat to mix well.

3. To make the coating, place the sugar and cinnamon in a small shallow dish, and stir to mix well. Set aside.

4. Coat a baking sheet with nonstick cooking spray. Using your hands, shape the dough into 1-inch balls. (If the dough is too sticky to handle, place it in the freezer for a few minutes.) Roll the balls in the sugar coating; then arrange on the baking sheet, spacing them 1 1/2 inches apart. Using the bottom of a glass, flatten each ball to 1/4-inch thickness.

5. Bake at 300°F for about 14 minutes. To check for doneness, lift a cookie from the sheet with a spatula. The bottom should be lightly browned. Cool the cookies on the pan for 2 minutes. Then transfer the cookies to wire racks, and cool completely. Serve immediately, or transfer to an airtight container.

NUTRITIONAL FACTS (PER COOKIE)
Cal: 48   Carbs: 9.4 g   Chol: 0 mg   Fat: 0.9 g
Fiber: 0.4 g   Protein: 0.9 g   Sodium: 37 mg

Fat-Free Marshmallow Treats

YIELD: 18 BARS

1 tablespoon nonfat margarine, or 1 tablespoon
plus 1 1/2 teaspoons reduced-fat margarine

6 cups miniature marshmallows

6 cups crisp rice cereal, regular
or cocoa-flavored

1. Coat a 4-quart pot with nonstick butter-flavored cooking spray. Add the margarine and marshmallows, cover, and cook over low heat without stirring for 3 minutes. Then remove the lid and continue to cook, stirring constantly, for 2 to 3 additional minutes, or until the mixture is melted and smooth.

2. Remove the pot from the heat, and stir in the cereal. Coat a 9-x-13-inch pan with nonstick cooking spray, and use the back of a wooden spoon to pat the mixture firmly into the pan. (Coat the spoon with cooking spray to help prevent sticking.)

3. Allow the mixture to cool to room temperature before cutting into squares. Serve immediately, or store in an airtight container in single layers separated by sheets of waxed paper.

NUTRITIONAL FACTS (PER BAR)
Cal: 86   Carbs: 20.7 g   Chol: 0 mg   Fat: 0.1 g
Fiber: 0.1 g   Protein: 0.8 g   Sodium: 81 mg

VARIATION

To make Peanut Butter Marshmallow Treats, add 1/4 cup plus 2 tablespoons of reduced-fat or regular peanut butter to the pot along with the margarine and marshmallows.

NUTRITIONAL FACTS (PER BAR)
Cal: 116   Carbs: 23 g   Chol: 0 mg   Fat: 1.9 g
Fiber: 0.5 g   Protein: 2.2 g   Sodium: 106 mg

Peach Bavarian

For variety, substitute canned apricots or canned dark sweet cherries and apricot or cherry gelatin for the canned peaches and peach gelatin.

YIELD: 6 SERVINGS
1 can (1 pound) sliced peaches in juice or light syrup, undrained
1 package (4-serving size) regular or sugar-free peach gelatin
1 cup nonfat or low-fat peach yogurt
2 cups nonfat or light whipped topping

1. Drain the peaches, reserving the juice. Dice the peaches and set aside.

2. Place $3/4$ cup of the reserved peach juice in a small pot. (If there is not enough juice, add water to bring the volume to $3/4$ cup.) Bring the mixture to a boil over high heat.

3. Pour the boiling juice into a large bowl. Sprinkle the gelatin over the top, and stir for about 3 minutes, or until the gelatin is completely dissolved. Set the mixture aside for about 20 minutes, or until it reaches room temperature.

4. When the gelatin mixture has cooled to room temperature, whisk in the yogurt. Chill for 15 minutes. Stir the mixture; it should be the consistency of pudding. If it is too thin, return it to the refrigerator for a few minutes.

5. When the gelatin mixture has reached the proper consistency, stir it with a wire whisk until smooth. Gently fold in first the diced peaches, and then the whipped topping.

6. Divide the mixture among six 8-ounce wine glasses, cover, and chill for at least 3 hours, or until set, before serving.

NUTRITIONAL FACTS (PER $3/4$-CUP SERVING)
Cal: 161   Carbs: 36.7 g   Chol: 0 mg   Fat: 0.9 g
Fiber: 1.3 g   Protein: 3.3 g   Sodium: 77 mg

Black Forest Pudding

For variety, substitute vanilla loaf cake or low-fat pound cake and vanilla pudding mix for the chocolate cake and pudding mix.

YIELD: 9 SERVINGS
2 cups skim or low-fat milk
1 package (4-serving size) cook-and-serve or instant chocolate or white chocolate pudding mix, regular or sugar-free
8 slices ($1/2$-inch each) fat-free chocolate loaf cake
2 tablespoons amaretto or hazelnut liqueur
1 can (20 ounces) light (reduced-sugar) cherry pie filling

TOPPING
$1 1/2$ cups nonfat or light whipped topping
$3/4$ cup regular or sugar-free nonfat or low-fat vanilla yogurt
3 tablespoons sliced toasted almonds (page 348) (optional)

1. Use the milk to prepare the pudding according to package directions. Cover the mixture and chill for at least 2 hours for cook-and-serve pudding or 30 minutes for instant pudding, or until chilled and thickened.

2. Arrange 4 of the cake slices in a single layer over the bottom of a 2-quart glass bowl, and drizzle 1 tablespoon of liqueur over the cake. Spread half of the pudding over the cake, and follow with a layer of half of the pie filling. Repeat the cake, liqueur, pudding, and pie filling layers.

3. To make the topping, place the whipped topping in a medium-sized bowl, and gently fold in the yogurt. Spread the mixture over the top of the pie filling.

4. Cover the dish, and chill for at least 3 hours. If desired, sprinkle the almonds over the top just before serving.

NUTRITIONAL FACTS (PER $3/4$-CUP SERVING)
Cal: 222   Carbs: 48 g   Chol: 1 mg   Fat: 1 g
Fiber: 0.8 g   Protein: 4.8 g   Sodium: 224 mg

Polenta Pudding

YIELD: 8 SERVINGS
¼ cup plus 2 tablespoons yellow cornmeal
2½ cups skim or low-fat milk
1 cup evaporated skim milk
¼ cup plus 2 tablespoons honey
1 cup fat-free egg substitute
⅓ cup golden raisins or chopped dried apricots
2 teaspoons vanilla extract
Ground nutmeg (garnish)

1. Place the cornmeal in a 2½-quart pot, and slowly stir in the milk and the evaporated milk. Cook over medium heat, stirring constantly, for 10 to 12 minutes, or until the mixture comes to a boil. Reduce the heat to low and continue cooking for 2 additional minutes, or until slightly thickened. Slowly stir in the honey.

2. Place the egg substitute in a small bowl, and stir in 1 cup of the hot cornmeal mixture. Slowly stir the egg mixture into the pudding, and continue cooking and stirring for 2 minutes, or until slightly thickened. Remove the pot from the heat, and stir in the raisins or apricots and the vanilla extract.

3. Coat a 2-quart round casserole dish with nonstick cooking spray. Pour the pudding mixture into the dish, and sprinkle with the nutmeg. Place the dish in a pan filled with 1 inch of hot water.

4. Bake uncovered at 350°F for 1 hour, or until set. When done, a sharp knife inserted midway between the center of the pudding and the rim of the dish will come out clean.

5. Allow the pudding to cool at room temperature for at least 30 minutes. Serve warm, or refrigerate for several hours and serve chilled. Refrigerate any leftovers.

NUTRITIONAL FACTS (PER ⅔-CUP SERVING)
Cal: 156　Carbs: 30 g　Chol: 2 mg　Fat: 0.5 g
Fiber: 0.8 g　Protein: 9 g　Sodium: 150 mg

Cherry Risotto Pudding

YIELD: 6 SERVINGS
3 cups skim or low-fat milk
½ cup plus 1 tablespoon arborio rice
¼ cup plus 1 tablespoon dried cherries
¼ cup plus 2 tablespoons evaporated skim milk
¼ cup plus 2 tablespoons fat-free egg substitute
¼ cup plus 2 tablespoons sugar
1 teaspoon vanilla extract

1. Place the milk and rice in a heavy 2-quart pot, and place over medium heat. Cook, stirring frequently, until the mixture comes to a boil. Reduce the heat to low, cover, and simmer, stirring occasionally, for about 25 minutes, or until most of the milk has been absorbed and the rice is tender.

2. Add the dried cherries to the rice mixture, cover, and cook for about 2 minutes, or until the cherries start to soften.

3. Place the evaporated milk, egg substitute, sugar, and vanilla extract in a small bowl, and stir to mix well. Slowly stir the evaporated milk mixture into the rice mixture. Cook and stir for 3 to 5 minutes, or until the mixture is thick and creamy.

4. Remove the pot from the heat, and allow to cool for 10 minutes. Stir the pudding, and spoon into dessert dishes. Serve warm.

NUTRITIONAL FACTS (PER ¾-CUP SERVING)
Cal: 199　Carbs: 40 g　Chol: 3 mg　Fat: 0.5 g
Fiber: 0.6 g　Protein: 8.5 g　Sodium: 107 mg

VARIATION

To make Apple-Raisin Risotto, cook the rice and milk as directed in step 1, adding 1 cup of chopped peeled Granny Smith or Rome apples after the mixture has cooked for 15 minutes. Substitute ¼ cup of dark or golden raisins for the cherries, and top each serving with a sprinkling of cinnamon or nutmeg.

NUTRITIONAL FACTS (PER ¾-CUP SERVING)
Cal: 187　Carbs: 39 g　Chol: 3 mg　Fat: 0.4 g
Fiber: 0.7 g　Protein: 8 g　Sodium: 107 mg

Rum-Raisin Bread Pudding

¼ cup dark raisins

2 tablespoons light rum

4 cups ½-inch cubes firm multigrain or oatmeal bread (about 5 ounces)

1 can (12 ounces) evaporated skim milk

½ cup skim or low-fat milk

¼ cup plus 2 tablespoons fat-free egg substitute

¼ cup plus 2 tablespoons light brown sugar

1 teaspoon vanilla extract

1 tablespoon sugar

1. Place the raisins and rum in a small bowl, and stir to mix well. Set aside for at least 15 minutes.

2. Place the bread cubes in a large bowl and set aside.

3. Place the evaporated milk, milk, egg substitute, brown sugar, and vanilla extract in a large bowl, and whisk until smooth. Pour the milk mixture over the bread cubes, and set aside for 10 minutes.

4. Stir the raisin mixture into the bread mixture. Coat a 1½-quart casserole dish with nonstick cooking spray, and pour the mixture into the dish. Sprinkle the sugar over the pudding.

5. Bake uncovered at 350°F for about 1 hour, or until a sharp knife inserted in the center of the dish comes out clean. Allow to cool at room temperature for 45 minutes before serving. Serve warm or at room temperature, refrigerating any leftovers.

NUTRITIONAL FACTS (PER ¾-CUP SERVING)
Cal: 184   Carbs: 33 g   Chol: 2 mg   Fat: 0.4 g
Fiber: 1.1 g   Protein: 8.4 g   Sodium: 227 mg

Sour Cream and Apple Bread Pudding

For variety, substitute diced peaches for the apples.

5 cups ½-inch cubes firm multigrain or French bread (about 6 ounces)

1¾ cups skim or low-fat milk

½ cup nonfat or light sour cream

½ cup plus 2 tablespoons fat-free egg substitute

¼ cup plus 2 tablespoons sugar

1½ teaspoons vanilla extract

¾ cup diced peeled apples (about 1 medium)

¼ cup golden or dark raisins

TOPPING

1 tablespoon plus 1½ teaspoons sugar

⅛ teaspoon ground cinnamon

1. Place the bread cubes in a large bowl and set aside.

2. Place the milk, sour cream, egg substitute, sugar, and vanilla extract in a large bowl, and whisk until smooth. Pour the milk mixture over the bread cubes, and set aside for 10 minutes.

3. Stir the apples and raisins into the bread mixture. Coat a 2-quart casserole dish with nonstick cooking spray, and pour the mixture into the dish.

4. To make the topping, place the sugar and cinnamon in a small bowl, and stir to mix well. Sprinkle the topping over the pudding.

5. Bake uncovered at 350°F for about 1 hour, or until a sharp knife inserted in the center of the dish comes out clean. Allow to cool at room temperature for 45 minutes before serving. Serve warm or at room temperature, refrigerating any leftovers.

NUTRITIONAL FACTS (PER ¾-CUP SERVING)
Cal: 161   Carbs: 32 g   Chol: 1 mg   Fat: 0.9 g
Fiber: 1.8 g   Protein: 6.7 g   Sodium: 180 mg

Delightful Peach Trifle

YIELD: 9 SERVINGS

PUDDING MIXTURE

2 cups skim or low-fat milk

1 package (4-serving size) cook-and-serve
or instant vanilla pudding mix,
regular or sugar-free

PEACH MIXTURE

2 cups diced peeled fresh peaches

1 tablespoon sugar

2 tablespoons amaretto liqueur

CAKE MIXTURE

8 slices (1/2-inch each) fat-free vanilla loaf cake
or low-fat pound cake

2 tablespoons plus 2 teaspoons raspberry jam

TOPPING

1 1/2 cups nonfat or light whipped topping

3/4 cup regular or sugar-free nonfat
or low-fat vanilla yogurt

3 tablespoons sliced toasted almonds
(optional)

1. Use the milk to prepare the pudding according to package directions. Cover the mixture and chill for at least 2 hours for cook-and-serve pudding or 30 minutes for instant pudding, or until chilled and thickened.

2. To make the peach mixture, place the peaches, sugar, and liqueur in a medium-sized bowl, and stir to mix well. Set the mixture aside for 15 minutes to allow the juices to develop.

3. To make the cake mixture, arrange the cake slices on a flat surface, and spread each slice with 1 teaspoon of the jam.

4. To assemble the trifle, arrange half of the cake slices, jam side up, in a single layer over the bottom of a 2-quart glass bowl. Spread half of the peach mixture over the cake slices, and cover the peaches with half of the pudding. Repeat the cake, peach, and pudding layers.

5. To make the topping, place the whipped topping in a medium-sized bowl, and gently fold in the yogurt. Swirl the mixture over the top of the trifle, cover, and chill for at least 3 hours. If desired, sprinkle the almonds over the top just before serving.

NUTRITIONAL FACTS (PER 3/4-CUP SERVING)
Cal: 205   Carbs: 45 g   Chol: 2 mg   Fat: 0.8 g
Fiber: 1 g   Protein: 4.3 g   Sodium: 206 mg

Nutty Nutrition

It's true—nuts are loaded with fat. In fact, one cup of nuts contains close to 800 calories and 70 grams of fat. Does this mean that you should never eat nuts again? Definitely not. Everyone needs some fat to maintain good health, and nuts provide the essential fats we need in their most wholesome and natural form.

Concerned about heart disease? You will be happy to know that nuts are naturally cholesterol-free and that their fat is mostly unsaturated, so they do not raise blood cholesterol levels. In fact, a number of studies have shown that eating an

ounce of nuts (3 to 4 tablespoons) at least five times per week may reduce your risk of heart disease by about 35 percent.

If you look at the nutritional profile of nuts, it's easy to see how these tasty morsels might protect against heart disease, as well as many other health problems. Nuts are rich in a variety of nutrients that many people do not eat in sufficient amounts. For instance, nuts provide important minerals like magnesium, copper, zinc, and manganese, and are a good source of vitamin E. Nuts are also one of the best dietary sources of boron, which can

Razzleberry Trifle

YIELD: 10 SERVINGS

2 tablespoons Chambord or amaretto liqueur

PUDDING MIXTURE

3 cups skim or low-fat milk

1 package (6-serving size) cook-and-serve
or instant vanilla pudding mix,
regular or sugar-free

BERRY MIXTURE

2$\frac{1}{2}$ cups sliced fresh strawberries

1 cup fresh or frozen (thawed) raspberries

2 tablespoons sugar

CAKE MIXTURE

10 slices ($\frac{1}{2}$-inch each) fat-free vanilla loaf cake
or low-fat pound cake

$\frac{1}{4}$ cup low-sugar raspberry jam

TOPPING

1$\frac{1}{2}$ cups nonfat or light whipped topping

$\frac{3}{4}$ cup nonfat or low-fat vanilla yogurt

3 tablespoons sliced toasted almonds
(optional)

1. Use the milk to prepare the pudding according to package directions. Cover the mixture and chill for at least 2 hours for cook-and-serve pudding or 30 minutes for instant pudding, or until chilled and thickened.

2. To make the berry mixture, place the strawberries, raspberries, and sugar in a medium-sized bowl, and stir to mix well. Set the mixture aside for 20 minutes to allow the juices to develop.

3. To make the cake mixture, arrange the cake slices on a flat surface, and spread each slice with some of the jam.

4. To assemble the trifle, drizzle the liqueur down the sides and over the bottom of a 3-quart trifle bowl or other decorative glass bowl. Arrange half of the cake slices, jam side up, over the bottom of the bowl. Top first with half of the berries, and then with half of the pudding. Repeat the layers.

5. To make the topping, place the whipped topping in a medium-sized bowl, and gently fold in the yogurt. Swirl the mixture over the top of the trifle, cover, and chill for at least 2 hours. If desired, sprinkle the almonds over the top just before serving.

NUTRITIONAL FACTS (PER 1-CUP SERVING)
Cal: 215   Carbs: 46 g   Chol: 1 mg   Fat: 1 g
Fiber: 2 g   Protein: 5 g   Sodium: 288 mg

---

help prevent osteoporosis. And Brazil nuts are the richest known source of selenium, a powerful antioxidant. In addition, nuts supply a variety of phytochemicals—beneficial compounds found only in plant foods that protect against cancer, heart disease, and many other health problems.

Because of their nutritional value, their crunch, and their great taste, nuts are included in many of the recipes in this book, from salads and main dishes to breads, muffins, and desserts. And as you can see from the nutritional analysis of the recipes, when included in low-fat recipes like the ones in this book, nuts will not blow your fat or calorie budgets.

To bring out the flavor of both nuts and seeds, try toasting them. Toasting intensifies the flavors of nuts and seeds so much that you can halve the amount used. Simply arrange the nuts or seeds in a single layer on a baking sheet, and bake at 350°F for 8 to 10 minutes (5 to 6 minutes for chopped nuts) or until lightly browned with a toasted, nutty smell. Watch the nuts closely during the last couple of minutes of baking, as they tend to brown quickly. To save time, toast a large batch and store the extras in an airtight container in the refrigerator. That way, you'll always have a supply ready for all your cooking adventures.

Tiramisu

A creamy custard replaces the traditional high-fat mascarpone cheese and egg filling in this luscious Italian dessert. To save time, substitute 3 cups of made-from-mix vanilla or white chocolate pudding for the homemade custard.

YIELD: 6 SERVINGS

18 ladyfingers (about 4½ ounces)

2 teaspoons Dutch processed cocoa powder

¾ cup nonfat or light whipped topping (optional)

CUSTARD

3 cups skim or low-fat milk, divided

½ cup instant nonfat dry milk powder

3 tablespoons cornstarch

¼ cup plus 2 tablespoons sugar

½ teaspoon dried grated orange rind

Pinch ground nutmeg

¼ cup plus 2 tablespoons fat-free egg substitute

1½ teaspoons vanilla extract

COFFEE MIXTURE

¼ cup plus 2 tablespoons espresso or strong black coffee, cooled to room temperature

¼ cup orange liqueur

2 tablespoons Dutch processed cocoa powder

1. To make the custard, place ½ cup of the milk and all of the milk powder and cornstarch in a small jar with a tight-fitting lid. Shake the mixture until smooth, and set aside.

2. Place the remaining 2½ cups of milk in a 2-quart pot. Add the sugar, orange rind, and nutmeg, and cook over medium heat, stirring constantly, until the mixture just begins to boil. Add the cornstarch mixture, and cook, still stirring, for about 2 minutes, or until the mixture returns to a boil and thickens slightly. Reduce the heat to low.

3. Place the egg substitute in a small bowl. Remove ½ cup of the hot milk mixture from the pot, and stir it into the egg substitute. Return the mixture to the pot, and cook, stirring constantly, for 2 to 3 minutes, or until the mixture thickens slightly.

4. Remove the pot from the heat, and stir in the vanilla extract. Then, stirring every 10 minutes, allow the custard to cool for about 30 minutes. Transfer the custard to a covered container, and refrigerate for at least 2 hours, or until well chilled.

5. To make the coffee mixture, place the coffee, liqueur, and cocoa in a small bowl, and stir until smooth. Set aside.

6. To assemble the desserts, coarsely crumble 1½ ladyfingers into the bottom of each of six 10-ounce balloon wine glasses. Top the ladyfingers with 2½ teaspoons of the coffee mixture, and ¼ cup of the custard. Repeat the layers. Then sift a little cocoa over the top of each dessert.

7. Serve immediately, or cover and refrigerate until ready to serve. If desired, top each serving with 2 tablespoons of the whipped topping just before serving.

NUTRITIONAL FACTS (PER SERVING)
Cal: 241   Carbs: 43 g   Chol: 40 mg   Fat: 1.6 g
Fiber: 1.2 g   Protein: 10 g   Sodium: 151 mg

Spiced Pumpkin Flan

YIELD: 6 SERVINGS

½ cup sugar

1 can (12 ounces) evaporated skim milk

½ cup mashed cooked or canned pumpkin

½ cup plus 1 tablespoon fat-free egg substitute

¼ cup orange juice

½ cup light brown sugar

2 teaspoons vanilla extract

1 teaspoon pumpkin pie spice

1. To make the caramel sauce, place the ½ cup of sugar in a heavy 1-quart saucepan. Cook over medium-high heat without stirring for about 1 minute, shaking the saucepan occasionally, until the sugar begins to liquefy around the edges. Reduce the heat to medium, and cook, stirring constantly, for another minute or 2, or until the sugar has completely liquefied and has turned a golden caramel color. Be careful not to cook the sugar too long, as it will continue to cook and darken after you remove it from the heat.

2. Immediately pour about 1 tablespoon of the caramel mixture into the bottom of each of six 6-ounce custard cups. (Be aware that the caramel mixture will be very hot!) Swirl each cup to coat the bottom and about ¹⁄₂ inch up the sides with the caramel mixture. Set the cups aside for 10 minutes to allow the caramel mixture to harden.

3. To make the custard, place all of the remaining ingredients in a blender, and process until smooth. Pour the custard mixture into the caramel-lined cups.

4. Place the custards in a 9-x-13-inch baking pan, and add hot tap water to the pan until it reaches halfway up the sides of the custard cups. Bake at 350°F for about 45 minutes, or until a sharp knife inserted slightly off center in the custards comes out clean.

5. Remove the custards from the pan, and allow to cool to room temperature. Cover with plastic wrap, and chill for at least 24 hours before serving. (During this time, the hardened caramel sauce will become liquid.)

6. To serve, carefully run a sharp knife around the edge of the custards, taking care not to cut into the pudding itself. Invert the cups onto individual serving plates, allowing the sauce to flow over and around the custards. Serve immediately.

NUTRITIONAL FACTS (PER SERVING)
Cal: 177   Carbs: 38 g   Chol: 2 mg   Fat: 0.2 g
Fiber: 0.6 g   Protein: 6.8 g   Sodium: 109 mg

Crème Caramel

YIELD: 4 SERVINGS
²⁄₃ cup sugar, divided
¹⁄₄ cup plus 2 tablespoons fat-free egg substitute
1¹⁄₂ teaspoons vanilla extract
1 can (12 ounces) evaporated skim milk

1. To make the caramel sauce, place ¹⁄₃ cup of the sugar in a heavy 1-quart saucepan. Cook over medium-high heat without stirring for about 1 minute, shaking the saucepan occasionally, until the sugar begins to liquefy around the edges. Reduce the heat to medium, and cook, stirring constantly, for another minute or 2, or until the sugar has completely liquefied and has turned a golden caramel color. Be careful not to cook the sugar too long, as it will continue to cook and darken after you remove it from the heat.

2. Immediately pour about 1 tablespoon of the caramel mixture into the bottom of each of four 6-ounce custard cups. (Be aware that the caramel mixture will be very hot!) Swirl each cup to coat the bottom and about ¹⁄₂-inch up the sides with the caramel mixture. Set the cups aside for 10 minutes to allow the caramel mixture to harden.

3. To make the custard, place the egg substitute, the remaining ¹⁄₃ cup of sugar, and the vanilla extract in a small bowl, and stir to dissolve the sugar. Set aside.

4. Place the evaporated milk in a 1-quart pot, and cook over medium heat, stirring frequently, just until the milk begins to boil. Remove the pot from the heat, and slowly whisk in the egg substitute mixture. Pour the custard into the caramel-lined cups.

5. Place the custards in a 9-x-9-inch baking pan, and add hot tap water to the pan until it reaches halfway up the sides of the custard cups. Bake at 325°F for about 50 minutes, or until a sharp knife inserted slightly off center in the custards comes out clean.

6. Remove the custards from the pan, and allow to cool to room temperature. Cover with plastic wrap, and chill for at least 24 hours before serving. (During this time, the hardened caramel sauce will become liquid.)

7. To serve, carefully run a sharp knife around the edge of the custards, taking care not to cut into the pudding itself. Invert the cups onto individual serving plates, allowing the sauce to flow over and around the custards. Serve immediately.

NUTRITIONAL FACTS (PER SERVING)
Cal: 205   Carbs: 43 g   Chol: 3 mg   Fat: 0.2 g
Fiber: 0 g   Protein: 8.7 g   Sodium: 135 mg

Strawberries n'Cream

For variety, substitute raspberry gelatin and frozen raspberries for the strawberry gelatin and frozen strawberries.

YIELD: 6 SERVINGS

1 package (10 ounces) frozen (thawed) sweetened sliced strawberries, undrained

1/2 cup boiling water

1 package (4-serving size) regular or sugar-free strawberry gelatin

1/2 cup plus 2 tablespoons nonfat or light sour cream

2 cups nonfat or light whipped topping

1. Drain the strawberries, reserving the juice. Set both the strawberries and the juice aside.

2. Pour the boiling water into a blender, and sprinkle the gelatin over the top. Cover with the lid, and carefully blend at low speed for about 30 seconds, or until the gelatin is completely dissolved. Allow the mixture to sit in the blender for about 20 minutes, or until it reaches room temperature.

3. When the gelatin mixture has cooled to room temperature, add the sour cream and the reserved juice from the strawberries, and blend for about 30 seconds, or until well mixed. Pour the mixture into a large bowl, and chill for 15 minutes. Stir the mixture; it should be the consistency of pudding. If it is too thin, return it to the refrigerator for a few minutes.

4. When the gelatin mixture has reached the proper consistency, stir it with a wire whisk until smooth. Gently fold in first the strawberries, and then the whipped topping.

5. Divide the mixture among six 8-ounce wine glasses, cover, and chill for at least 3 hours, or until set, before serving.

NUTRITIONAL FACTS (PER 3/4-CUP SERVING)
Cal: 162   Carbs: 36 g   Chol: 0 mg   Fat: 0.9 g
Fiber: 0.9 g   Protein: 2.5 g   Sodium: 67 mg

Presto Peach Ice Cream

YIELD: 4 SERVINGS

1/2 cup nonfat or light sour cream

1/3 cup sugar

1 teaspoon vanilla extract

1 bag (1 pound) frozen (unthawed) sliced peaches

1. Place the sour cream, sugar, and vanilla extract in a small bowl, and stir to mix well. Set aside.

2. Dice the frozen peaches into 3/4-inch chunks. Place the peaches in the bowl of a food processor, and process for a couple of minutes, or until finely ground.

3. Add the sour cream mixture to the food processor, and process for a couple of minutes, or until the mixture is light, creamy, and smooth. Serve immediately. Freeze leftovers in a covered container, and let sit at room temperature for about 10 minutes, or until slightly softened, before serving.

NUTRITIONAL FACTS (PER 3/4-CUP SERVING)
Cal: 143   Carbs: 34 g   Chol: 0 mg   Fat: 0.1 g
Fiber: 2 g   Protein: 2.6 g   Sodium: 22 mg

Sicilian Ice Cream Sundaes

YIELD: 6 SERVINGS

2 cups fresh or frozen (thawed) raspberries

2 tablespoons sugar

2 tablespoons Chambord, amaretto, or Frangelico liqueur

12 ladyfingers

1 quart nonfat or low-fat vanilla ice cream

3 tablespoons chocolate syrup

1. Place the raspberries, sugar, and liqueur in a medium-sized bowl, and mash them together. Set aside.

2. Crumble 1 ladyfinger into the bottom of each of six 10-ounce balloon wine glasses. Spoon 1 1/2 tablespoons of the raspberry mixture over the ladyfinger in each glass, and top with 1/3 cup of the ice cream. Repeat the ladyfinger, raspberry, and ice cream layers.

3. Drizzle 1$\frac{1}{2}$ teaspoons of chocolate syrup over the top of each sundae, and serve immediately.

NUTRITIONAL FACTS (PER SERVING)
Cal: 244   Carbs: 51 g   Chol: 25 mg   Fat: 0.9 g
Fiber: 2 g   Protein: 7 g   Sodium: 35 mg

Orange Burst Granita

Granita—an icy Italian confection—is always fat-free. As an added virtue, this version uses no refined sugar and is bursting with fresh orange flavor.

YIELD: 4 SERVINGS
3 cups freshly squeezed orange juice
$\frac{1}{4}$ cup plus 2 tablespoons frozen (thawed) orange juice concentrate

1. Pour the orange juice and juice concentrate into an 8-inch square pan, and stir to mix well.

2. Place the pan in the freezer, and freeze for 25 minutes, or until ice crystals begin to form around the sides of the pan. Using a spoon, stir the frozen crystals from around the edges and bottom of the pan back into the liquid portion. Repeat the scraping process every 20 minutes for about 2 hours, or until the mixture is icy and granular.

3. Spoon the granita into four 10-ounce balloon wine glasses, and serve immediately.

NUTRITIONAL FACTS (PER $\frac{7}{8}$-CUP SERVING)
Cal: 126   Carbs: 29.5 g   Chol: 0 mg   Fat: 0.3 g
Fiber: 0.6 g   Protein: 2 g   Sodium: 3 mg

TIME-SAVING TIP
To make Orange Burst Granita with less fuss, pour the juice mixture into 2 ice cube trays, and freeze for at least 3 hours, or until frozen solid. (Remove the cubes from the trays and transfer them to freezer bags if you want to partially prepare the granita several days ahead of time.) Just before serving, place the ice cubes in the bowl of a food processor, and process for several minutes, pulsing and scraping the mixture down the sides of the bowl until small crystals are formed. Spoon the granita into serving dishes, and serve immediately.

Simple Peach Sorbet

For variety, substitute canned apricots for the peaches.

YIELD: 6 SERVINGS
2 cans (15 ounces each) sliced peaches in juice, undrained
$\frac{1}{2}$ cup plus 2 tablespoons frozen (thawed) white grape juice concentrate

1. Place the peaches with their juice and the juice concentrate in a blender, and blend until smooth.

2. If using an ice cream maker, pour the mixture into a 1$\frac{1}{2}$-quart ice cream maker, and proceed as directed by the manufacturer. If you do not own an ice cream maker, follow steps 3 through 5.

3. To make the sorbet in your freezer, pour the mixture into an 8-inch square pan. Cover the pan with aluminum foil, and place in the freezer for at least 8 hours, or until the mixture is frozen solid. (You can prepare the mixture a few days ahead of time, if you prefer.) Remove the frozen mixture from the freezer, and allow it to sit at room temperature for about 10 minutes, or until thawed enough to break into chunks.

4. Break the mixture into chunks, and place in the bowl of a food processor or electric mixer. Process or beat for several minutes, or until the mixture is light, creamy, and smooth. (Note that, depending on the capacity of your food processor, you may have to process the mixture in 2 batches.)

5. Return the mixture to the pan, cover, and return to the freezer. Freeze for at least 4 hours, or until firm.

6. Scoop the sorbet into individual serving dishes. (If it seems too solid, let it sit for 5 to 10 minutes at room temperature before scooping.) Serve immediately.

NUTRITIONAL FACTS (PER $\frac{3}{4}$-CUP SERVING)
Cal: 150   Carbs: 37 g   Chol: 0 mg   Fat: 0 g
Fiber: 2.4 g   Protein: 1.1 g   Sodium: 6 mg

Burst-of-Berries Sorbet

YIELD: 6 SERVINGS

5 cups sliced fresh strawberries, or 1½ pounds frozen (slightly thawed) unsweetened strawberries

½ cup plus 2 tablespoons sugar

½ cup cranberry juice cocktail

¼ cup Chambord liqueur

1. Place the strawberries, sugar, and cranberry juice cocktail in a 2½-quart pot, and stir to mix well. Cover and cook over medium heat, stirring occasionally, for about 5 minutes, or until the strawberries are soft and the liquid is syrupy. Allow the mixture to cool to room temperature.

2. Place the cooled strawberry mixture in a blender or food processor. Add the liqueur, and process until smooth.

3. If using an ice cream maker, pour the mixture into a 1½-quart ice cream maker, and proceed as directed by the manufacturer. If you do not own an ice cream maker, follow steps 4 through 6.

4. To make the sorbet in your freezer, pour the mixture into an 8-inch square pan. Cover the pan with aluminum foil, and place in the freezer for at least 8 hours, or until the mixture is frozen solid. (You can prepare the mixture a few days ahead of time, if you prefer.) Remove the frozen mixture from the freezer, and allow it to sit at room temperature for about 10 minutes, or until thawed enough to break into chunks.

5. Break the mixture into chunks, and place in the bowl of a food processor or electric mixer. Process or beat for several minutes, or until the mixture is light, creamy, and smooth. (Note that, depending on the capacity of your food processor, you may have to process the mixture in 2 batches.)

6. Return the mixture to the pan, cover, and return to the freezer. Freeze for at least 4 hours, or until firm.

7. Scoop the sorbet into individual serving dishes. (If it seems too solid, let it sit for 5 to 10 minutes at room temperature before scooping.) Serve immediately.

NUTRITIONAL FACTS (PER ¾-CUP SERVING)			
Cal: 169	Carbs: 38 g	Chol: 0 mg	Fat: 0.6 g
Fiber: 3.2 g	Protein: 0.9 g	Sodium: 3 mg	

Strawberry Angel Parfaits

YIELD: 5 SERVINGS

10 ounces frozen (thawed) sliced sweetened strawberries

5 slices (½-inch each) angel food cake

3⅓ cups nonfat or low-fat vanilla ice cream

1. Place 1 tablespoon of the strawberries in the bottom of each of five 10-ounce balloon wine glasses.

2. Crumble a half-slice of cake over the berries in each glass. Top the cake with ⅓ cup of ice cream, and then spoon 2 tablespoons of strawberries over the ice cream.

3. Repeat the cake, ice cream, and strawberry layers, and serve immediately.

NUTRITIONAL FACTS (PER SERVING)			
Cal: 248	Carbs: 56.4 g	Chol: 2 mg	Fat: 0.3 g
Fiber: 1.5 g	Protein: 7.3 g	Sodium: 214 mg	

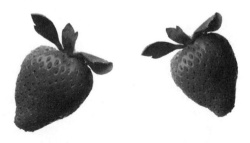

Banana Pudding Parfaits

For variety, substitute chocolate pudding and chocolate wafers for the vanilla pudding and vanilla wafers.

YIELD: 4 SERVINGS
2 cups skim or low-fat milk
1 package (4-serving size) cook-and-serve or instant vanilla pudding mix, regular or sugar-free
1¼ cups sliced bananas (about 1¼ large)
16 reduced-fat vanilla wafers
½ cup nonfat or light whipped topping (optional)

1. Use the milk to prepare the pudding according to package directions. Cover the mixture and chill for at least 2 hours for cook-and-serve pudding or 30 minutes for instant pudding, or until chilled and thickened.

2. To assemble the parfaits, spoon 1 tablespoon of pudding into the bottom of each of four 8-ounce wine or parfait glasses. Top the pudding with 2½ tablespoons of sliced bananas, 2 crumbled vanilla wafers, and a scant ¼ cup of pudding. Repeat the banana, wafer, and pudding layers.

3. Serve immediately, topping each serving with a rounded tablespoon of whipped topping, if desired. Or cover each glass with plastic wrap and chill for up to 2 hours before serving.

NUTRITIONAL FACTS (PER 1-CUP SERVING)
Cal: 237 Carbs: 51 g Chol: 2 mg Fat: 2.1 g
Fiber: 1.1 g Protein: 5.6 g Sodium: 229 mg

Metric Conversion Tables

Common Liquid Conversions

Measurement	=	Milliliters
1/4 teaspoon	=	1.25 milliliters
1/2 teaspoon	=	2.50 milliliters
3/4 teaspoon	=	3.75 milliliters
1 teaspoon	=	5.00 milliliters
1 1/4 teaspoons	=	6.25 milliliters
1 1/2 teaspoons	=	7.50 milliliters
1 3/4 teaspoons	=	8.75 milliliters
2 teaspoons	=	10.0 milliliters
1 tablespoon	=	15.0 milliliters
2 tablespoons	=	30.0 milliliters

Measurement	=	Liters
1/4 cup	=	0.06 liters
1/2 cup	=	0.12 liters
3/4 cup	=	0.18 liters
1 cup	=	0.24 liters
1 1/4 cups	=	0.30 liters
1 1/2 cups	=	0.36 liters
2 cups	=	0.48 liters
2 1/2 cups	=	0.60 liters
3 cups	=	0.72 liters
3 1/2 cups	=	0.84 liters
4 cups	=	0.96 liters
4 1/2 cups	=	1.08 liters
5 cups	=	1.20 liters
5 1/2 cups	=	1.32 liters

Converting Fahrenheit to Celsius

Fahrenheit	=	Celsius
200–205	=	95
220–225	=	105
245–250	=	120
275	=	135
300–305	=	150
325–330	=	165
345–350	=	175
370–375	=	190
400–405	=	205
425–430	=	220
445–450	=	230
470–475	=	245
500	=	260

Conversion Formulas

LIQUID When You Know	Multiply By	To Determine
teaspoons	5.0	milliliters
tablespoons	15.0	milliliters
fluid ounces	30.0	milliliters
cups	0.24	liters
pints	0.47	liters
quarts	0.95	liters

WEIGHT When You Know	Multiply By	To Determine
ounces	28.0	grams
pounds	0.45	kilograms

Index